BASIC SCIENCE FOR THE MRCS

A revision guide for surgical trainees

BASIC SCIENCE FOR THE MRCS

A revision guide for surgical trainees

FOURTH EDITION

Michael S. Delbridge MBChB (Hons) MD FRCS (Vascular)

Consultant Vascular and Endovascular Surgeon
Norfolk and Norwich University Hospital, Norwich, UK

Wissam Al-Jundi MBBS MSc MEd MBA FRCS (Vascular)

Consultant Vascular and Endovascular Surgeon
Norfolk and Norwich University Hospital, Norwich, UK
Honorary Senior Lecturer, University of East Anglia, Norwich, UK

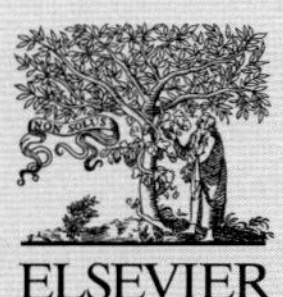

ELSEVIER

First edition 2006
Second edition 2012
Third edition 2018

Notices

Practitioners and researchers must always rely on their own experience and knowledge in evaluating and using any information, methods, compounds or experiments described herein. Because of rapid advances in the medical sciences, in particular, independent verification of diagnoses and drug dosages should be made. To the fullest extent of the law, no responsibility is assumed by Elsevier, authors, editors or contributors for any injury and/or damage to persons or property as a matter of products liability, negligence or otherwise, or from any use or operation of any methods, products, instructions, or ideas contained in the material herein.

ISBN: 978-0-7020-8540-6

Content Strategist: Alexandra Mortimer
Content Project Manager: Taranpreet Kaur
Design: Renee Duenow
Marketing Manager: Deborah Watkins

Printed in India

Last digit is the print number: 9 8 7 6 5 4 3 2

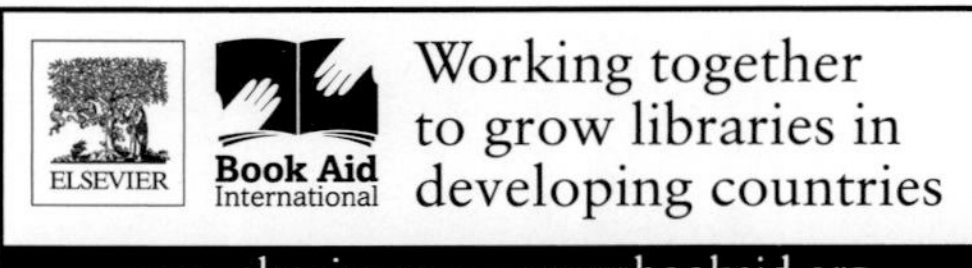

CONTENTS

PREFACE

The authors are grateful to the publishers, Elsevier, for the invitation to produce a fourth edition of *Basic Science for the MRCS*.

The book is a concise revision guide to the core basic sciences which comprise the essential knowledge for those entering surgical training. It is a basic requirement that every surgical trainee has a thorough understanding of the basic principles of anatomy, physiology and pathology irrespective of which speciality within surgery they intend to pursue as a career. It is equally important that they understand the clinical application of the basic sciences. This revision guide has been written with this in mind, using a bullet-point style which we hope will make it easier for the reader to revise the essential facts.

Much has changed both in the undergraduate curriculum and in the post-graduate examination system since the first edition was published 16 years ago. In this fourth edition, the chapters have been updated where appropriate and sections expanded to cover topics which are particularly relevant to examinations. As most examinations are Objective Structured Clinical Examinations (OSCEs), each chapter has OSCE scenario questions at the end with sample answers provided in an appendix at the back of the book. More than 20 new OSCE scenarios have been added to this edition. In addition, to accompany this edition there is an online question bank within the Student Consult eBook comprising over 200 Single Best Answer questions (SBAs) based on each chapter in the book. The reader can access the section from the Table of Contents in the eBook.

No book of this length could hope to be comprehensive and we have therefore concentrated on the topics that tend to be recurring examination themes. As with previous editions, this book has been written primarily as a means of rapid revision for the surgical trainee. However, it should also prove useful for those in higher surgical training, as well as for the surgically inclined, well-motivated medical student. We hope that this fourth edition will provide a simple and straightforward approach to the basic science that underpins surgical training.

Michael S. Delbridge
Wissam Al-Jundi

ACKNOWLEDGEMENTS

We are extremely grateful to the publishers, Elsevier, and in particular to Alexandra Mortimer, Content Strategist, for her support and help with this project. We are also grateful to the following colleagues at the Sheffield Teaching Hospitals NHS Foundation Trust who provided help, advice and criticism: Dr Paul Zadik, Consultant Microbiologist; Dr TC Darton, NIHR Academic Clinical Research Fellow, Infectious Diseases and Medical Microbiology; Mr BM Shrestha, Consultant General and Transplant Surgeon. We would also like to thank our consultant radiologist colleagues, who provided images: Dr Matthew Bull, Dr Peter Brown, Dr James Hampton, Dr Robert Cooper and Dr Rebecca Denoronha. Mr Raftery would like to thank his secretary, Mrs Denise Smith, for the long hours and hard work she has put in typing and re-typing the manuscript, and Anne Raftery for collating and organizing the whole manuscript into its final format. The task could not have been completed without them.

The figures in this book come from a variety of sources, and many are reproduced from other publications, with permission, as follows:

Fig. 3.9 from the University of Michigan Medical School, with kind permission of Thomas R. Gest, PhD

Figs 13.10A, 13.10B and 13.11 from Crossman & Neary (2000) *Neuroanatomy: An Illustrated Colour Text*, 2nd edn. Churchill Livingstone, Edinburgh

Figs 3.11 and 4.14, and Tables 6.1 and 6.3 from Easterbrook (1999) *Basic Medical Sciences for MRCP Part 1*, 2nd edn. Churchill Livingstone, Edinburgh

Fig. 9.1 from Hoffman & Cranefield (1960) *Electrophysiology of the Heart*. McGraw-Hill, New York (now public domain)

Figs 4.20, 4.24, 5.25, 6.5 and 6.6 from Jacob (2002) *Atlas of Human Anatomy*. Churchill Livingstone, Edinburgh

Figs 8.1, 8.12B, 8.12C, 10.3, 10.4, 10.5, 10.6, 10.7, 11.1, 11.3, 13.1, 13.5 and 13.6 from McGeown (2002) *Physiology*, 2nd edn. Churchill Livingstone, Edinburgh

Figs 8.3 and 8.4 from Pocock & Richards (2004) *Human Physiology: The Basis of Medicine*, 2nd edn. Oxford University Press, Oxford

Figs 1.1, 1.2, 1.3, 1.4, 1.5, 1.6, 1.7, 1.8, 1.9, 1.11, 1.13, 1.14, 2.1, 2.2, 2.3, 2.4, 2.7, 2.8, 2.9, 2.10, 2.12, 2.13, 2.14, 2.17, 2.18, 2.19, 2.20, 2.21, 2.22, 2.23, 2.24, 2.25, 2.27, 2.28, 2.29, 2.30, 2.31, 2.32, 5.1, 5.2, 5.7, 5.8, 5.16, 5.17, 6.1, 6.2, 6.3, 6.4, 6.7, 6.8, 6.9, 6.10, 6.11, 6.12, 6.13, 6.15, 8.2, 8.6, 8.10, 8.12A, 9.2, 9.4, 9.6, 11.4, 12.1, 12.4, 13.8, 19.2, 20.1, 20.2, 20.3, 21.1, 22.1, 22.2 and 22.3 from Raftery (ed) (2000) *Applied Basic Science for Basic Surgical Training*. Churchill Livingstone, Edinburgh

Fig. 17.2 and A.3 (Q&A) from Pretorius & Solomon (2011) *Radiology Secrets Plus*, 3rd edn. Elsevier, Philadelphia

Figs 5.35, 6.14, 22.2 & A.5 (Q&A), 22.3 & A.6 (Q&A) and 22.5 & A.7 (Q&A) from Raftery, Delbridge & Wagstaff (2011) *Pocketbook of Surgery*, 4th edn. Churchill Livingstone, Edinburgh

Figs 1.10, 3.1, 3.2, 3.3, 3.4, 3.8, 3.12, 4.1, 4.2, 4.3, 4.4, 4.6, 4.7, 4.8, 4.9, 4.11, 4.12, 4.13, 4.15, 4.16, 5.3, 5.4, 5.5, 5.9, 5.10, 5.11, 5.13, 5.14, 5.21, 5.22, 5.24, 5.26, 5.27, 5.28, 5.29, 5.30, 5.31 and 6.16 from Rogers (1992) *Textbook of Anatomy*. Churchill Livingstone, Edinburgh

Fig. 13.4 from Stevens & Lowe (2000) *Pathology*, 2nd edn. Mosby, Edinburgh

Figs 15.1 and 15.2, and Boxes 15.1 and 15.2 from Underwood (ed) (2004) *General and Systematic Pathology*, 4th edn. Churchill Livingstone, Edinburgh

SECTION I

Anatomy

1

The Thorax

DEVELOPMENT

Heart and Great Vessels

Heart (Fig. 1.1)

- Paired endothelial tubes fuse to become the primitive heart tube.
- Primitive heart tube develops in the pericardial cavity and divides into five regions:
  - sinus venosus
  - atrium
  - ventricle
  - bulbus cordis
  - truncus arteriosus.
- Heart tube elongates in pericardial cavity becoming U-shaped and then S-shaped.
- Sinus venosus becomes incorporated into the atrium.
- Bulbus cordis becomes incorporated into the ventricle.
- Boundary tissue between the primitive single atrial cavity and single ventricle grows out as dorsal and ventral endocardial cushions.
- The endocardial cushions meet in the midline, dividing the common atrioventricular (AV) orifice into a right (tricuspid) and left (mitral) orifice.
- An interventricular septum develops from the apex up towards the endocardial cushions.
- In the atrium a partition, the septum primum, grows down to fuse with the endocardial cushions. Before fusion is complete, a hole appears in the upper part of the septum primum that is called the foramen secundum.
- A second incomplete membrane, the septum secundum, then develops to the right of the septum primum but is never complete. It has a free lower edge that extends low enough for it to overlap the foramen secundum in the septum primum and eventually close it.
- The two overlapping defects in the septa form the valvelike foramen ovale.
- The septum secundum acts as a valvelike structure, allowing blood to go straight from the right to the left side of the heart in the fetus.
- At birth, where there is an increased blood flow through the lungs and a rise in left atrial pressure, the septum primum is pushed across to close the foramen ovale.
- The septum primum and septum secundum usually fuse, obliterating the foramen ovale and leaving a small residual dimple (the fossa ovalis).

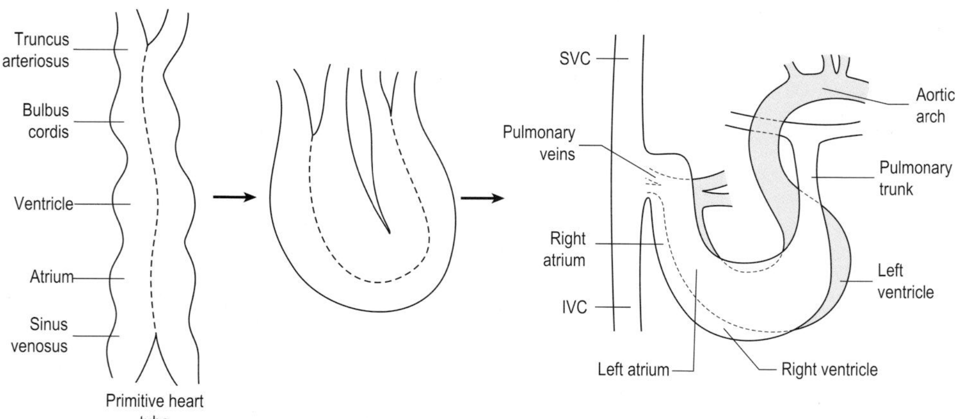

Fig. 1.1 The development of the heart. IVC, Inferior vena cava; SVC, superior vena cava.

- The sinus venosus joins the atria, becoming the two venae cavae on the right and the four pulmonary veins on the left.

Great Vessels (Fig. 1.2)

- Truncus arteriosus gives off six pairs of arches.
- These curve round the pharynx to join the dorsal aortae, which fuse distally into the descending aorta.
- First and second arches disappear completely.
- Third arch remains as carotid artery.
- Fourth arch becomes subclavian artery on the right and aortic arch on the left (giving off the left subclavian artery).
- Fifth arch disappears.
- Sixth arch (ventral part) becomes right and left pulmonary arteries with a connection to dorsal aorta disappearing on the right, but continuing as the ductus arteriosus on the left connecting with the aortic arch.
- The above developmental anatomy explains the different positions of the recurrent laryngeal nerves on each side. On the right, the fifth and sixth arches disappear to leave the nerve hooked round the fourth, i.e. subclavian artery. On the left it remains hooked round the sixth arch (ligamentum arteriosum in the adult).

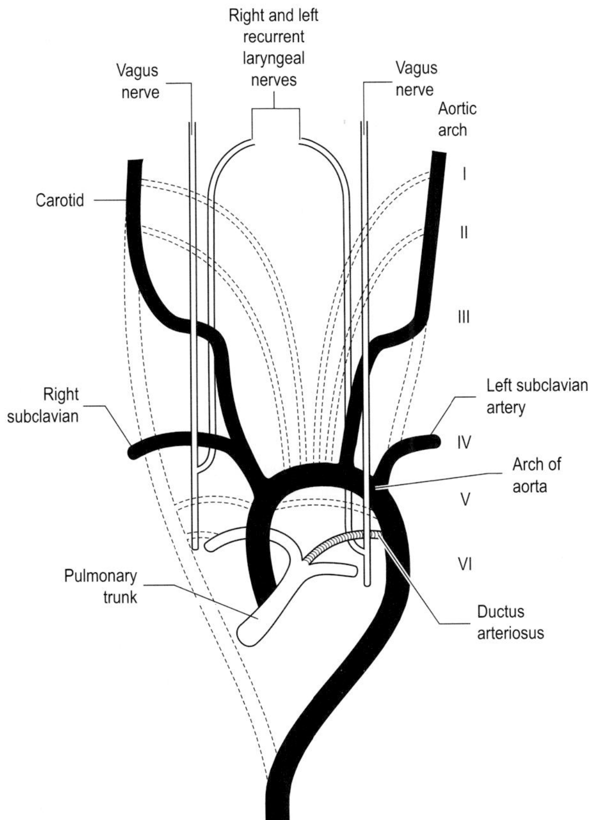

Fig. 1.2 The development of the aortic arches.

Fetal Circulation (Fig. 1.3)

- Oxygenated blood travels from the placenta along the umbilical vein.
- Most blood bypasses the liver in the ductus venosus, joining the inferior vena cava (IVC) and then travelling to the right atrium.
- Most of the blood passes through the foramen ovale into the left atrium so that oxygenated blood can enter the aorta.
- The remainder goes through the right ventricle with returning systemic venous blood into the pulmonary trunk.
- In the fetus the unexpanded lungs present high resistance to flow so that blood in the pulmonary trunk tends to pass down the low-resistance ductus arteriosus into the aorta.
- Blood returns to the placenta via the umbilical arteries (branches of the internal iliac arteries).
- At birth, when the baby breathes, the left atrial pressure rises, pushing the septum primum against the septum secundum and closing the foramen ovale.
- Blood flow through the pulmonary artery increases and becomes poorly oxygenated as it now receives systemic venous blood.
- Pulmonary vascular resistance is abruptly lowered as lungs inflate and the ductus arteriosus is obliterated over the next few hours to days.
- Ligation of the umbilical cord causes thrombosis of the umbilical artery, vein and ductus venosus.

Congenital Anomalies

Malposition

- Dextrocardia: mirror image of normal anatomy.
- Situs inversus: inversion of all viscera.

Left-to-Right Shunt

Atrial septal defect (ASD)

- Fusion between the septum primum and septum secundum usually takes place about 3 months after birth.
- May be incomplete in 10% of the population.
- If the septum secundum is too short to cover the foramen secundum in the septum primum and ASD persists after the primum and septum secundum are pressed together at birth, this results in an ostium secundum defect, which allows shunting of blood from the left to the right atrium.
- ASD may also result if the septum primum fails to fuse with the endocardial cushions.

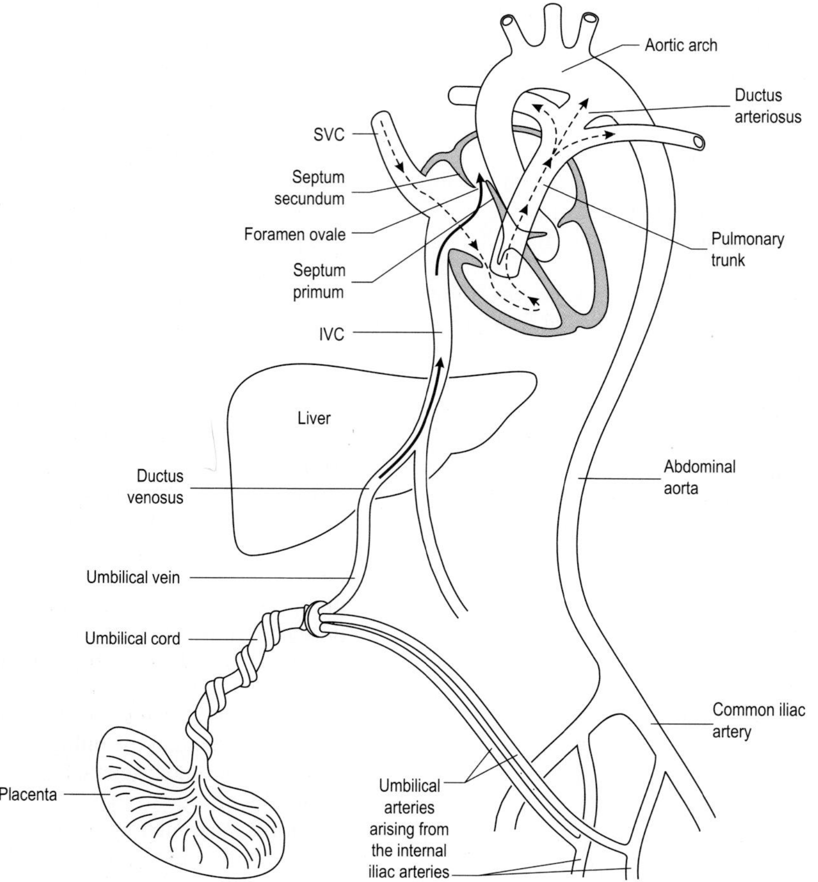

Fig. 1.3 The fetal circulation. IVC, Inferior vena cava; SVC, superior vena cava.

- This is an ostium primum defect lying immediately above the AV boundary and may be associated with a ventricular septal defect (VSD).

Ventricular septal defect

- This is the most common abnormality.
- Small defects occurring in the muscular part of the septum may close.
- Larger ones occurring in the membranous part of the septum just below the aortic valves may require repair.

Patent ductus arteriosus (PDA)

- The ductus may fail to close after birth.
- This should be surgically corrected because it causes increased load on the left ventricle and pulmonary hypertension.
- In open surgery to close a patent ductus, care must be taken to avoid the left recurrent laryngeal nerve.

Eisenmenger's syndrome

- Pulmonary hypertension may cause reversed flow (right-to-left shunting).
- This is due to an increased pulmonary flow resulting from either ASD, VSD or PDA.
- When cyanosis occurs as a result of this mechanism it is known as Eisenmenger's syndrome.

Right-to-Left Shunt (Cyanotic)

Fallot's tetralogy

- Fallot's tetralogy consists of:
  - VSD
  - stenosed pulmonary outflow track
  - a wide aorta which overrides the right and left ventricles
  - right ventricular hypertrophy.

- Because there is a right-to-left shunt across the VSD there is usually cyanosis at an early stage.
- The degree of cyanosis depends mainly on the severity of the pulmonary outflow obstruction.

Other congenital anomalies

Coarctation of the aorta

- Caused by abnormality of obliterative process, which normally occludes ductus arteriosus.
- Hypertension in upper part of body with weak, delayed femoral pulses.
- Extensive collaterals develop to try and bring blood from upper to lower part of body.
- Enlarged intercostal arteries cause notching of the inferior borders of the rib seen on chest X-ray.

Abnormalities of valves

- Any valve may be imperfectly formed.
- May cause stenosis or complete occlusion.
- Pulmonary and aortic valves are more frequently affected than mitral and tricuspid.

The Diaphragm (Fig. 1.4)

The diaphragm develops from the fusion of four parts:

1. septum transversum (the fibrous central tendon)
2. the mesentery of the foregut (the area adjacent to the vertebral column becomes the crura and median part)
3. ingrowth from the body wall
4. the pleuroperitoneal membrane (a small dorsal part). These close the primitive communications between pleura and peritoneal cavities.

Clinical Points

Different types of congenital diaphragmatic hernias occur, depending on which section has failed to close.

- Posterolateral hernia through the foramen of Bochdalek (the pleuroperitoneal membrane)—more common on the left.
- A hernia through a deficiency of the whole central tendon.
- A hernia through the foramen of Morgagni anteriorly between xiphoid and costal origins.
- A hernia through a congenitally large oesophageal hiatus.

THORACIC CAGE

The thoracic cage is formed by:

- vertebral column behind
- ribs and intercostal spaces on either side
- sternum and costal cartilages in front.

Ribs

- There are 12 pairs.
- Ribs 1–7 connect via their costal cartilages with the sternum. These are 'true' ribs articulating directly with the sternum.
- Ribs 8–10 articulate with their costal cartilages, each with the rib above. These are 'false' ribs as they do not articulate directly with the sternum.
- Ribs 11 and 12 are free anteriorly. These are 'floating ribs' as they have no anterior articulation.
- A typical rib comprises:
  - a head with two articular facets for articulation with the corresponding vertebra and the vertebra above

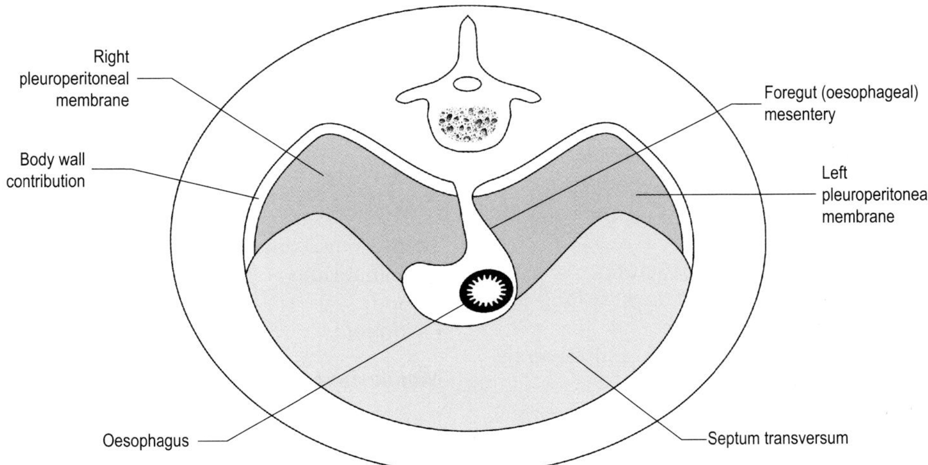

Fig. 1.4 The development of the diaphragm.

- a neck giving attachment to the costotransverse ligament
- a tubercle with a smooth facet for articulation with the transverse process of the corresponding vertebra
- a shaft flattened from side to side possessing an angle which marks the lateral limit of attachment of erector spinae. The shaft possesses a groove on its lower surface, the subcostal groove, in which the vessels and nerves lie.

Atypical ribs

First rib

- Shortest, flattest and most curved.
- Flattened from above downwards.
- Bears a prominent tubercle on the inner border of its upper surface for insertion of scalenus anterior.
- In front of the scalene tubercle the subclavian vein crosses the rib.
- Behind the scalene tubercle is the subclavian groove where the subclavian artery and lowest trunk of the brachial plexus are related to the rib.
- The neck of the first rib is crossed by (medial to lateral): sympathetic trunk; superior intercostal artery; and T1 to the brachial plexus.
- First digitation of serratus anterior attaches to outer edge.
- Suprapleural membrane (Sibson's fascia) is attached to inner border.

Second rib

- Less curved than first.
- Twice as long.

Tenth rib

- Only one articular facet on head.

Eleventh and twelfth ribs

- Short.
- No tubercles.
- Only single facet on head.
- Eleventh rib has shallow subcostal groove.
- Twelfth rib has no subcostal groove and no angle.

Clinical Points

Rib Fractures

- May damage underlying or related structures.
- Fracture of any rib may lead to trauma to lung and development of pneumothorax.
- Fracture of left lower ribs (ninth, tenth and eleventh) may traumatize the spleen.
- Fracture of right lower ribs may traumatize the right lobe of the liver.
- Rib fractures may also traumatize related intercostal vessels leading to haemothorax.

Coarctation of the Aorta

- Collateral vessels develop between vessels above and below the block.
- The superior intercostal artery, derived from the costocervical trunk of the subclavian artery, supplies blood to the intercostal arteries of the aorta, bypassing the narrowed aorta.
- As a consequence, the intercostal vessels dilate and become more tortuous because of increased flow eroding the lower border of the ribs, giving rise to notching which can be seen on X-ray.

Cervical Ribs

- Incidence of 1:200.
- May be bilateral in 1:500.
- Rib may be complete, articulating with the transverse process of the seventh cervical vertebra behind and the first rib in front.
- Occasionally a cervical rib may have a free distal extremity or may be only represented by a fibrous band.
- Cervical ribs may cause vascular or neurological symptoms.
- Vascular consequences include poststenotic dilatation of the subclavian artery, causing local turbulence, thrombosis and possibility of distal emboli.
- Subclavian aneurysm may also arise.
- Pressure on vein may result in subclavian vein thrombosis.
- Pressure on the lower trunk of the brachial plexus may result in paraesthesia of dermatomal distribution of C8/T1 together with wasting of small muscles of hands (myotome T1).

Costal Cartilages

- Upper seven connect ribs to sternum.
- 8, 9 and 10 connect ribs to cartilage immediately above.
- Composed of hyaline cartilage and add resilience to thoracic cage, protecting it from more frequent fractures.
- Calcify with age; irregular areas of calcification seen on chest X-ray.

Sternum

The sternum consists of three parts:

- manubrium
- body
- xiphoid.

Manubrium

- Approximately triangular in shape.
- Articulates with medial end of clavicle.
- First costal cartilage and upper part of second articulate with manubrium.

- Articulates with body of sternum at manubriosternal joint (angle of Louis).

Relations

- Anterior boundary of superior mediastinum.
- Lowest part is related to arch of aorta.
- Upper part is related to left brachiocephalic vein; left brachiocephalic artery; left common carotid artery; left subclavian artery.
- Laterally it is related to the lungs and pleura.

Body

- Composed of four pieces (sternebrae).
- Lateral margins are notched to receive most of the second and third to seventh costal cartilages.

Relations

- On the right side of the median plane, the body is related to the right pleura and the thin anterior border of the right lung, which intervenes between it and the pericardium.
- On the left side of the median plane, the upper two pieces are related to the pleura and left lung; the lower two pieces are related directly to the pericardium.

Xiphoid

- Small and cartilaginous well into adult life.
- May become prominent if patient loses weight.

Clinical Points

- Sternal puncture is used to obtain bone marrow from the body of the sternum; one should be aware of the posterior relations!
- The sternum is split for access to the heart and occasionally a retrosternal goitre, thymus or ectopic parathyroid tissue.
- The xiphoid may become more prominent when a patient loses weight (naturally or due to disease). The patient may present in clinic because they have noticed a lump, which was previously covered in fat.

Intercostal Spaces (Fig. 1.5)

- A typical intercostal space contains three muscles comparable to those of the abdominal wall.
- External intercostal muscle: passes downwards and forwards from the rib above to the rib below; deficient in front where it is replaced by the anterior intercostal membrane.
- Internal intercostal muscle: passes downwards and backwards; deficient behind where it is replaced by the posterior intercostal membrane.
- Innermost intercostal muscle: may cover more than one intercostal space.

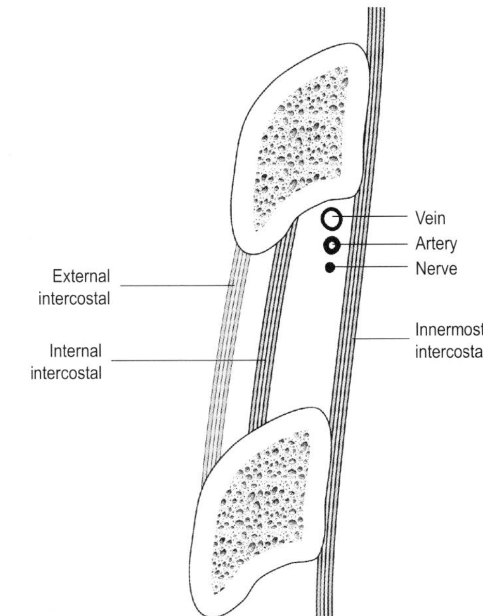

Fig. 1.5 An intercostal space. A needle passed into the chest immediately above a rib will avoid the neurovascular bundle.

- The neurovascular bundle lies between the internal and the innermost intercostal.
- The neurovascular bundle consists of (from above down): the vein, artery and nerve; the vein lying directly in the groove on the undersurface of the corresponding rib.

Clinical Points

- Insertion of a chest drain should be close to the upper border of the rib below the intercostal space to avoid the neurovascular bundle.
- Irritation of the intercostal nerves (anterior primary rami of the thoracic nerves) may give rise to pain referred to the front of the chest wall or abdomen in the region of the termination of the nerves.

TRACHEA (Fig. 1.6)

- Extends from lower border of cricoid cartilage (level of the sixth cervical vertebra) to termination into two main bronchi (level of fifth thoracic vertebra)—11 cm long.
- Composed of fibroelastic tissue and is prevented from collapsing by a series of U-shaped cartilaginous rings,

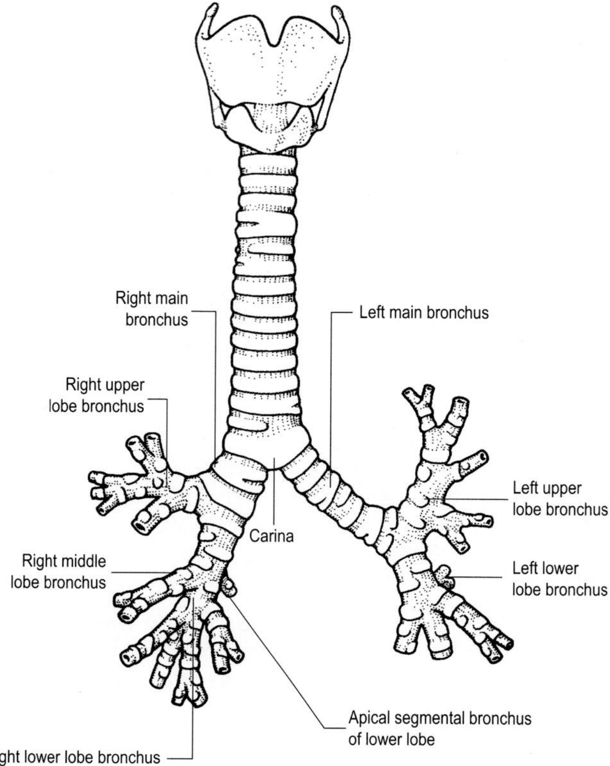

Fig. 1.6 The trachea and bronchi.

open posteriorly, the ends being connected by smooth muscle (trachealis).
- Lined by columnar ciliated epithelium containing numerous goblet cells.

Relations

In the Neck

- Anteriorly: isthmus of thyroid gland over second to fourth tracheal rings, inferior thyroid veins, sternohyoid, sternothyroid.
- Laterally: lobes of thyroid gland, carotid sheath.
- Posteriorly: oesophagus, recurrent laryngeal nerves in the groove between the trachea and oesophagus.

In the Thorax

- Anteriorly: brachiocephalic artery and left common carotid artery, left brachiocephalic vein, thymus.
- Posteriorly: oesophagus, recurrent laryngeal nerves.
- Right side: vagus nerve, azygos vein, pleura.
- Left side: aortic arch, left common carotid artery, left subclavian vein, left recurrent laryngeal nerve, pleura.

BRONCHI (Fig. 1.6)

The trachea terminates at the level of the sternal angle, dividing into right and left bronchi.

Right main bronchus:
- wider, shorter and more vertical than left
- approximately 2.5 cm long
- passes downwards and laterally behind ascending aorta and superior vena cava (SVC) to enter hilum of lung
- azygos vein arches over it from behind to enter SVC
- pulmonary artery lies first below and then anterior to it
- gives off upper lobe bronchus before entering lung
- divides into bronchi to middle and inferior lobes within the lung.

Left main bronchus:
- approximately 5 cm long
- passes downwards and laterally below arch of aorta, in front of oesophagus and descending aorta

- gives off no branches until it enters hilum of lung, where it divides into bronchi to upper and lower lobes
- pulmonary artery lies at first anterior to, and then above, the bronchus.

Clinical Points

- The trachea may be displaced or compressed by pathological enlargement of adjacent structures, e.g. thyroid, arch of aorta.
- The trachea may be displaced if the mediastinum is pushed across, e.g. by tension pneumothorax displacing it to the opposite side.
- Calcification of tracheal rings may occur in the elderly and be visible on X-ray.
- Because the right main bronchus is wider and more vertical, foreign bodies are more likely to be aspirated into this bronchus.
- Distortion and widening of the carina (angle between the main bronchi), seen at bronchoscopy, usually indicates enlargement of the tracheobronchial lymph nodes at the bifurcation by carcinoma.

Anatomy of Tracheostomy

- Either a vertical or cosmetic transverse skin incision may be employed.
- A vertical incision is made downwards from the cricoid cartilage passing between the anterior jugular veins.
- A transverse cosmetic skin crease incision may be used placed halfway between the cricoid cartilage and suprasternal notch.
- The incision goes through the skin and superficial fascia (in the transverse incision, platysma will be located in the lateral part of the incision).
- The pretracheal fascia is split longitudinally.
- Bleeding may be encountered from the anterior relations at this point, namely anastomosis between anterior jugular veins across the midline, inferior thyroid veins, thyroidea ima artery (when present).
- In the young child, the brachiocephalic artery, the left brachiocephalic vein and the thymus may be apparent in the lower part of the wound.
- After splitting the pretracheal fascia and retracting the strap muscles, the isthmus of the thyroid will be encountered and may be either retracted upwards or divided between clamps to expose the cartilages of the trachea.
- An opening is then made in the trachea to admit the tracheostomy tube.

THE LUNGS

- Conical in shape.
- Conform to shape of pleural cavities.
- Each has a blunt apex extending above the sternal end of the first rib.
- Each has a concave base related to the diaphragm.
- Each has a convex parietal surface related to the ribs.
- Each has a concave mediastinal surface related to the pericardium.
- Each has a thin anterior border overlapping the pericardium and deficient on the left at the cardiac notch.
- Each has a hilum where the bronchi and vessels pass to and from the root.
- Each has a rounded posterior border that occupies the groove by the side of the vertebrae.

Right Lung

- Slightly larger than the left.
- Divided into three lobes—upper, middle and lower—by the oblique and horizontal fissures.

Left Lung

- Has only an oblique fissure and therefore only two lobes.
- The anterior border has a notch produced by the heart (cardiac notch).
- The equivalent of the middle lobe of the right lung in the left lung is the lingula, which lies between the cardiac notch and oblique fissure.

Roots of the Lungs

- Comprise the principal bronchus, the pulmonary artery, the two pulmonary veins, the bronchial arteries and veins, pulmonary plexuses of nerves, lymph vessels, bronchopulmonary lymph nodes.
- Chief structures composing the root of each lung are arranged in a similar manner from before backwards on both sides, i.e. the upper of the two pulmonary veins in front; pulmonary artery in the middle; bronchus behind.
- Arrangement differs from above downwards on the two sides:
  - right side from above downwards: upper lobe bronchus, pulmonary artery, right principal bronchus, lower pulmonary vein
  - left side: pulmonary artery, bronchus, lower pulmonary vein.
- Visceral and parietal pleura meet as a sleeve surrounding the structures passing to and from the lung. This sleeve hangs down inferiorly at the pulmonary ligament. It allows for expansion of the pulmonary veins with increased blood flow.

BRONCHOPULMONARY SEGMENTS (Fig. 1.7)

- Each lobar bronchus divides to supply the bronchopulmonary segments of the lung.

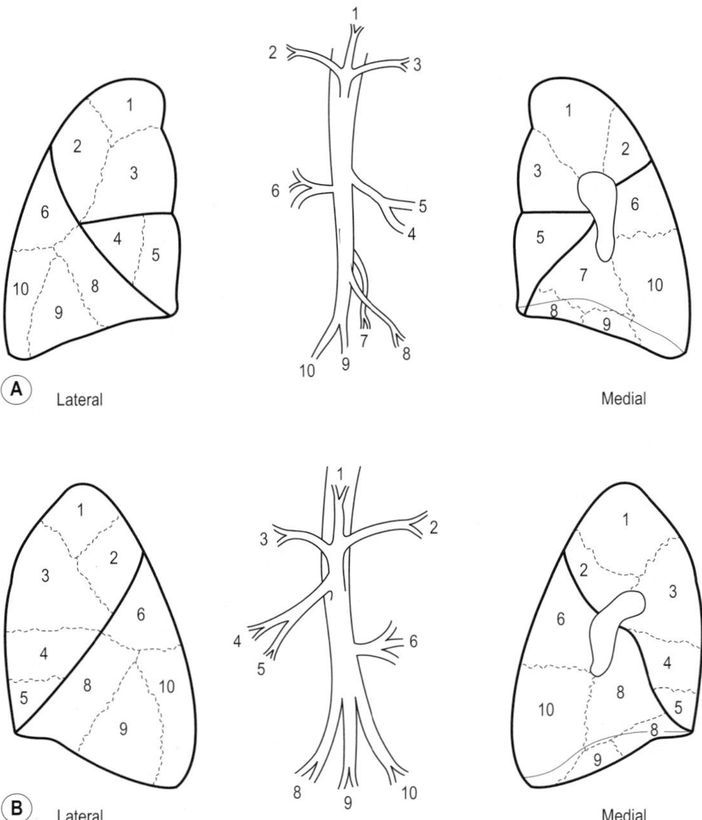

Fig. 1.7 Bronchi and bronchopulmonary segments for the lungs. Divisions of the main bronchi in the centre, with corresponding pulmonary segments on the surfaces. (A) Right lung upper lobe: 1 = apical, 2 = posterior, 3 = anterior; middle lobe, 4 = lateral, 5 = medial; lower lobe, 6 = apical, 7 = medial basal (cardiac), 8 = anterior basal, 9 = lateral basal, 10 = posterior basal. (B) Left lung upper lobe: 1, 2 = apicoposterior, 3 = anterior; lingula (middle lobe), 4 = superior, 5 = inferior; lower lobe, 6 = apical, 8 = anterior basal, 9 = lateral basal, 10 = posterior basal.

- There are 10 bronchopulmonary segments for each lung.
- Each is supplied by a segmental bronchus, artery and vein.
- There is no communication with adjacent segments.
- It is possible to remove an individual segment without interfering with the function of adjacent segments.
- There is little bleeding or alveolar air leak from the raw lung surface if excision takes place accurately along the boundaries (marked by intersegmental veins).
- Each segment is wedge-shaped with the apex at the hilum and the base at the lung surface.
- Each segment takes its name from that of the supplying segmental bronchus.

Blood Supply

- Pulmonary trunk arises from the right ventricle.
- Directed upwards in front of the ascending aorta.
- Passes upwards and backwards on the left of the ascending aorta to reach concavity of the aortic arch.
- Divides in front of the left main bronchus into right and left branches.

Right Pulmonary Artery

- Passes in front of oesophagus to the root of the right lung behind the ascending aorta and SVC.
- At the root of the lung it lies in front of and between the right main bronchus and its upper lobe branch.
- Divides into three branches, one for each lobe.

Left Pulmonary Artery

- Connected at its origin with the arch of the aorta via the ligamentum arteriosum.
- Runs in front of the left main bronchus and descending aorta.
- Left recurrent laryngeal nerve loops below the aortic arch in contact with the ligamentum arteriosum.

Bronchial Arteries

- Supply the air passages.
- Branches of the descending aorta.

PLEURA

- Each pleural cavity is composed of a thin serous membrane invaginated by the lung.
- The visceral pleura is intimately related to the lung surface and is continuous with the parietal layer over the root of the lung.
- The parietal layer is applied to the inner aspect of the chest wall, diaphragm and mediastinum.
- Below the root of the lung the pleura forms a loose fold known as the pulmonary ligament, which allows for distension of the pulmonary vein.
- The lungs conform to the shape of the pleural cavities but do not occupy the full cavity as this would not allow expansion as in full inspiration.
- The two pleural cavities are totally separate from one another.

Surface Anatomy of Pleura and Lungs

Pleura

- Cervical pleura extends above the sternal end of the first rib.
- It follows a curved line drawn from the sternoclavicular joint to the junction of the inner third and the outer two-thirds of the clavicle, the apex arising 2.5 cm above the clavicle.
- Line of pleural reflection passes behind the sternoclavicular joint on each side to meet in the midline at the angle of Louis (second costal cartilage level).
- The right pleural edge passes vertically down to the level of the sixth costal cartilage and crosses:
  - eighth rib in midclavicular line
  - tenth rib in midaxillary line
  - twelfth rib at the lateral border of erector spinae.
- Left pleural edge arches laterally at the fourth costal cartilage and descends lateral to the border of the sternum whence it follows a path similar to the right.
- Medial end of the fourth and fifth left intercostal spaces are therefore not covered by pleura.
- The pleura descends below the twelfth rib at its medial extremity.

Lungs

- Apex of the lung follows the line of cervical pleura.
- Anterior border of the right lung corresponds to the right mediastinal pleura.
- Anterior border of the left lung has a distinct notch (cardiac notch), which passes behind the fifth and sixth costal cartilages.
- The lower border of the lung (midway between inspiration and expiration) crosses:
  - sixth rib in the midclavicular line
  - eighth rib in the midaxillary line
  - tenth rib at the lateral border of erector spinae.
- The oblique fissure is represented by the medial border of the scapula with the arm fully elevated (abducted) or by a line drawn from 2.5 cm lateral to the fifth thoracic vertebrae to the sixth costal cartilage, about 4 cm from the midline.
- The horizontal fissure of the right lung passes horizontally and medially from the oblique fissure at the level of the fourth costal cartilage.

Clinical Points

- The pleura rises above the clavicle into the neck. It may be injured by a stab wound, the surgeon's knife or insertion of a subclavian or internal jugular line.
- A needle passing through the left fourth and fifth intercostal spaces immediately lateral to the sternal edge will enter the pericardium without traversing the pleura.
- The pleura descends below the medial extremity of the twelfth rib and therefore may be inadvertently opened in the loin approach to the kidney or adrenal gland.

Nerve Supply of Pleura

- Receives nerve supply from structures to which it is attached.
- Visceral pleura obtains an autonomic supply from the branches of the vagus nerve supplying the lung and is sensitive only to stretching.
- Parietal pleura receives somatic innervation from the intercostal nerves.
- Diaphragmatic pleura is supplied by the phrenic nerve.
- Parietal pleura and diaphragmatic pleura are therefore sensitive to pain.

Clinical Points

- Pain from the parietal pleura of the chest wall may be referred via the intercostal nerves to the abdomen, e.g. right lower lobar pneumonia may irritate the parietal pleura and refer pain to the right lower abdomen, mimicking acute appendicitis; irritation of the diaphragmatic pleura may refer pain to the tip of the shoulder [irritating the phrenic nerve (C3, 4, 5) and referring pain to the dermatomal distribution of C4 at the shoulder tip].

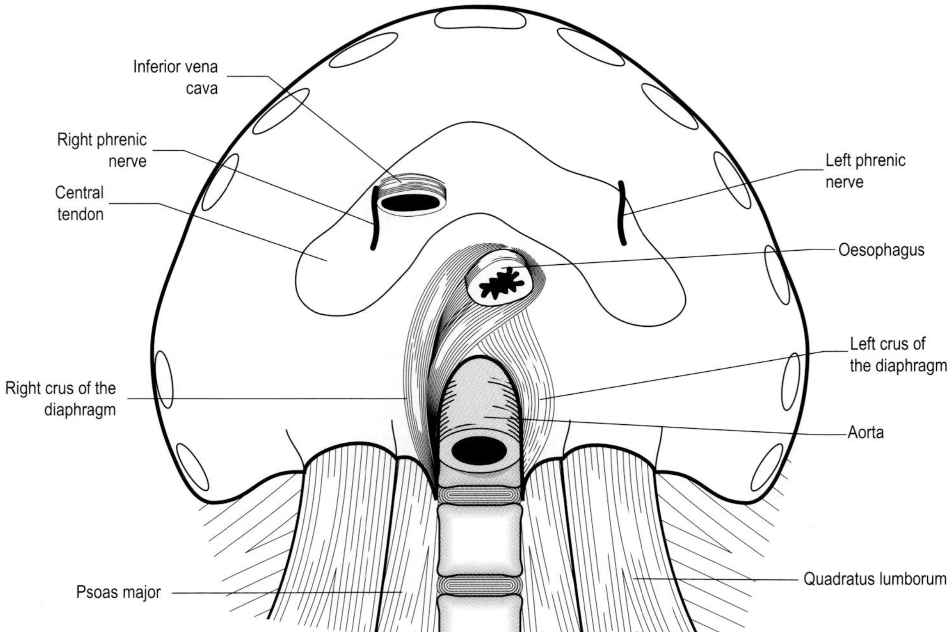

Fig. 1.8 The inferior aspect of the diaphragm.

THE DIAPHRAGM (Fig. 1.8)

- Dome-shaped septum separating the thorax from the abdomen.
- Composed of a peripheral muscular part and a central tendon.
- Muscular part arises from crura, arcuate ligaments, ribs and sternum.
- Right crus arises from the front of the bodies of the first three lumbar vertebrae and the intervening intervertebral discs.
- Left crus arises from the first and second lumbar vertebrae and the intervening disc.
- The lateral arcuate ligament is a condensation of the fascia over quadratus lumborum.
- The medial arcuate ligament is a condensation of the fascia of psoas major.
- The medial borders of the medial arcuate ligament join anteriorly over the aorta as the median arcuate ligament.
- The costal part is attached to the inner aspect of the lower six ribs.
- The sternal portion arises as two small slips from the back of the xiphoid process.
- The central tendon is trefoil in shape and receives insertion of muscular fibres. Above, it fuses with the pericardium.
- There are three main openings in the diaphragm:
  - aortic (strictly speaking the aortic 'opening' is not in the diaphragm, but lies behind it): lies at the level of T12; it transmits the abdominal aorta, the thoracic duct and often the azygos vein
  - oesophageal: lies in the right crus of the diaphragm at the level of T10. Transmits oesophagus, vagus nerves and branches of the left gastric artery and vein
  - IVC opening: lies at T8 level in the central tendon of the diaphragm. Transmits IVC and right phrenic nerve.
- Greater and lesser splanchnic nerves pierce the crura.
- Sympathetic chain passes behind the medial arcuate ligament lying on psoas major.

Nerve Supply

- Phrenic nerve (C3, 4, 5): the phrenic nerve is the sole motor nerve supply to the diaphragm. The sensory innervation of the central tendon of the diaphragm is via the phrenic nerve but the periphery of the diaphragm is supplied by the lower six intercostal nerves.
- Irritation of the diaphragm (e.g. in peritonitis or pleurisy) results in referred pain to the cutaneous area of supply, i.e. the shoulder tip via C4 dermatome.
- Damage to the nerve (e.g. in the neck) leads to paralysis of the diaphragm. Clinical examination reveals dullness to percussion at the base on the affected side and absent

breath sounds. This is due to the diaphragm being elevated as seen on chest X-ray. Paradoxical movement of the diaphragm occurs on respiration.

ANATOMY OF RESPIRATION

- Thoracic breathing: movements of rib cage.
- Abdominal breathing: contraction of diaphragm.

Thoracic Breathing

- 'Pump handle' action of ribs. Anterior ends of ribs are raised and, as these are below the posterior end, this increases the anteroposterior diameter of the thorax.
- 'Bucket handle' action of ribs. Ribs 4–7 are raised. As the centre of these ribs is normally below the anterior and posterior ends, the transverse diameter of the chest is increased when they move upwards.

Abdominal Breathing

- Muscular fibres of the diaphragm contract and the central tendon descends, increasing the vertical diameter of the thorax.
- As the central tendon descends it is arrested by the liver.
- The central tendon is now fixed and acts as the origin for muscle fibres, which now elevate the lower six ribs.
- Combination of thoracic and abdominal breathing increases all diameters of the thorax.
- The negative intrapleural pressure is increased and the lung expands.

Inspiration

- Quiet inspiration is a combination of thoracic and abdominal respiration.
- Forced inspiration (e.g. asthma) brings into action the accessory muscles of respiration, i.e. sternocleidomastoid, scalenes, pectoralis major, pectoralis minor, serratus anterior.

Expiration

- Elastic recoil of lung tissue and chest wall.
- Forced expiration (e.g. coughing and trumpet playing) requires use of muscles, i.e. rectus abdominis, external and internal obliques, transversus abdominis, latissimus dorsi.

THE HEART (Fig. 1.9)

- Roughly conical in shape, lying obliquely in the middle mediastinum.
- Attached at its base to the great vessels, otherwise lies free in pericardial sac.
- Base directed upwards, backwards, to the right.
- Apex directed downwards, forwards, to the left.
- Consists of four chambers: right and left atria, right and left ventricles.

Viewed from the front it has three surfaces and three borders.

Three surfaces:

- anterior: right atrium, right ventricle and narrow strip of left ventricle, auricle of left atrium

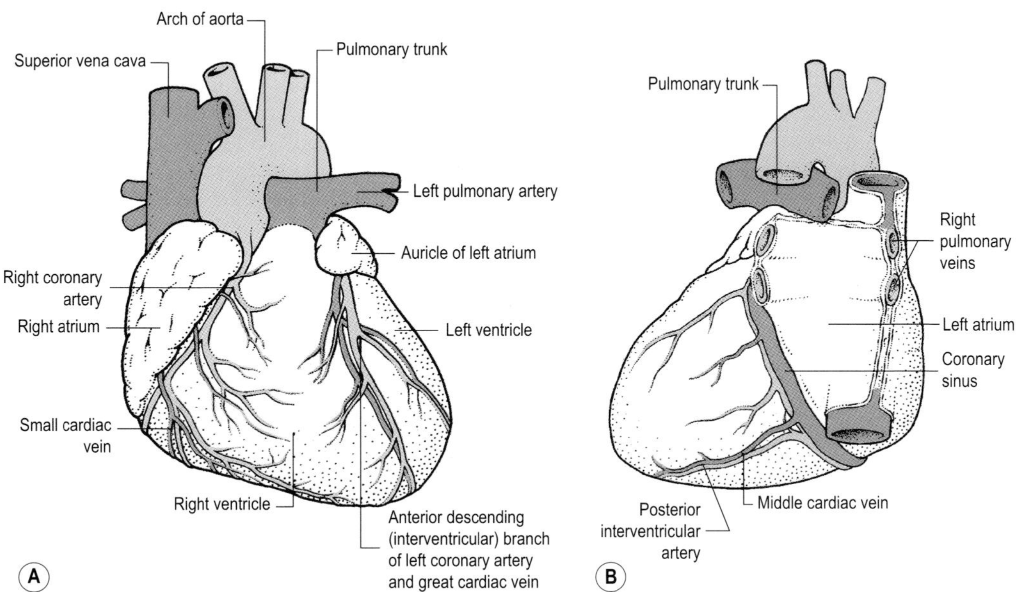

Fig. 1.9 The heart and great vessels in (A) anterior and (B) posterior view.

- posterior (base): left ventricle, left atrium with four pulmonary veins entering it
- inferior (diaphragmatic surface): right atrium with IVC entering it and lower part of ventricles.

Three borders:

- right: right atrium with IVC and SVC
- inferior: right ventricle and apex of left ventricle
- left: left ventricle, auricle of left atrium.

Chambers of Heart

Right Atrium

- Receives blood from IVC, SVC, coronary sinus, anterior cardiac vein.
- Crista terminalis runs between cavae–muscular ridge, separating smooth-walled posterior part of atrium (derived from sinus venosus) from rougher area (due to pectinate muscles) derived from true atrium.
- The fossa ovalis (the site of the fetal foramen ovale) is an oval depression on the interatrial septum.

Right Ventricle

- Thicker-walled than atrium.
- Communicates with atrium via tricuspid valve.
- Connects with pulmonary artery via pulmonary valve.
- Tricuspid valve has three cusps: septal, anterior, posterior.
- Atrial surface of valve is smooth but ventricular surfaces have fibrous cords, the chordae tendineae, which attach them to papillary muscles on the ventricular wall. They prevent eversion of the cusps in the atrium during ventricular contraction.
- Moderator band is a muscle bundle crossing from the interventricular septum to the anterior wall of the heart.
- Moderator band may prevent overdistension of ventricle. Conducts right branch of the AV bundle to anterior wall of ventricle.
- Infundibulum is the outflow tract of the ventricle. Directed upwards and to the right towards the pulmonary trunk.
- Pulmonary orifices guarded by the pulmonary valve consisting of three semilunar cusps.

Left Atrium

- Smaller than the right.
- Consists of principal cavity and auricle.
- Auricle extends forwards and to the right, overlapping the commencement of the pulmonary trunk.
- Four pulmonary veins open into the cavity (two from each lung: superior and inferior).
- Shallow depression on septal surface corresponds to fossa ovalis of right atrium.
- Largely smooth-walled, except for ridges in the auricle owing to underlying pectinate muscles.

Left Ventricle

- Longer and more conical than right with thicker wall (three times thicker).
- Communicates with atrium via mitral valve.
- Connects with aorta via aortic valve.
- Mitral valve has two cusps: anterior (larger) and posterior.
- Chordae tendineae run from the ventricular surfaces of cusps to papillary muscles.
- Aortic valve is stronger than pulmonary valve. Has three cusps—anterior, right and left posterior—each having a central nodule in its free edge and a sinus or dilatation in the aortic wall alongside each cusp.
- The mouths of the right and left coronary arteries are seen opening into the anterior and left posterior aortic sinuses, respectively.

Fibrous Skeleton of the Heart

- The AV orifice is bound together by a figure-of-eight conjoined fibrous ring.
- Acts as a fibrous skeleton for attachment of valves and muscles of atria and ventricles.
- Helps to maintain shape and position of heart.

Conducting System

- Sinoatrial (SA) node situated in right atrial wall at upper end of crista terminalis (SA node = pacemaker of heart).
- From SA node, cardiac impulse spreads to reach AV node.
- AV node lies in interatrial septum immediately above opening of coronary sinus.
- Cardiac impulse is conducted to ventricles via AV bundle (of His).
- AV bundle passes through fibrous skeleton of heart to membranous part of interventricular septum, where it divides into right and left branch.
- Left AV bundle is larger and both run under endocardium to activate all parts of the ventricular muscle.
- Papillary muscles contract first and then wall and septum in a rapid sequence from apex towards outflow tract, both ventricles contracting together.
- AV bundle is normally the only pathway through which impulse can reach ventricles.

Blood Supply of Heart (see Fig. 1.9)

Right Coronary Artery

- Arises from anterior aortic sinus.
- Passes to the right of the pulmonary trunk between it and the auricle.
- Runs along the AV groove around the inferior border of the heart and anastomoses with the left coronary artery at the posterior interventricular groove.

- Branches include:
  - marginal branch along the lower border of the heart
  - posterior interventricular (posterior descending) branch, which runs forward in the inferior interventricular groove to anastomose near the apex with the corresponding branch of the left coronary artery.

Left Coronary Artery

- Arises from the left posterior aortic sinus.
- Larger than the right coronary artery.
- Main stem varies in length (4–10 mm).
- Passes behind and then to the left of the pulmonary trunk.
- Reaches the left part of the AV groove.
- Initially lies under cover of the left auricle where it divides into two equally sized branches.
- Branches:
  - anterior interventricular (left anterior descending): runs down to the apex in the anterior interventricular groove supplying the wall of the ventricles, to anastomose with the posterior interventricular artery
  - circumflex: continues round the left side of the heart in the AV groove to anastomose with the terminal branches of the right coronary artery.
- Occlusion of the left coronary artery will lead to rapid demise.

Variations

- Left coronary and circumflex arteries may be larger and longer than usual and give off the posterior intraventricular artery before anastomosing with the right coronary artery, which is smaller than usual (known as 'left dominance'; occurs in 10% of population).
- Right and left coronary arteries may have equal contribution to posterior interventricular artery (known as codominance; occurs in 10% of population).
- Left main stem may divide into three branches. The third lies between the anterior interventricular and circumflex arteries and may be large, supplying the lateral wall of the left ventricle.
- In just under 60% of the population the SA node is supplied by the right coronary artery, while in just under 40% it is supplied by the circumflex artery. In 3% it has a dual supply.
- The AV node is supplied by the right coronary artery in 90% and the circumflex in 10%.

Venous Drainage (see Fig. 1.9)

- Venae cordis minimae: tiny veins draining directly into the chambers of the heart.
- Anterior cardiac veins: small, open directly into the right atrium.
- Coronary sinus:
  - main venous drainage
  - lies in posterior AV groove
  - opens into the right atrium just to the left of the mouth of the IVC.
- Tributaries of coronary sinus:
  - great cardiac vein: ascends in anterior interventricular groove next to anterior interventricular artery
  - middle cardiac vein: drains posterior and inferior surfaces of heart and lies next to the posterior interventricular artery
  - small cardiac vein: accompanies marginal artery and drains into termination of coronary sinus.

Nerve Supply of Heart

- Sympathetic (cardioaccelerator).
- Vagus (cardioinhibitor).

Clinical Point

- Cardiac pain is experienced not only in the chest but is referred down the inner side of the left arm and up to the neck and jaw. Cardiac pain is referred to areas of the body surface which send sensory impulses to the same level of the spinal cord that receives cardiac sensation. The sensory fibres from the heart travel through the cardiac plexus, sympathetic chain and up to the dorsal root ganglia of T1–4. Excitation of spinothalamic tract cells in the upper thoracic segments contribute to the anginal pain experienced in the chest and inner aspect of the arm via dermatomes T1–4. Cardiac vagal afferent fibres synapse in the nucleus of the tractus solitarius of the medulla and then descend to excite upper cervical spinothalamic tract cells. This innervation contributes to the angina pain experienced in the area of the neck and jaw.

PERICARDIUM

Fibrous

Heart and roots of the great vessels are contained within the conical fibrous pericardium.

- Apex: fuses with adventitia of great vessels about 5 cm from the heart.
- Base: fuses with central tendon of the diaphragm.

Relations

- Anterior sternum: third to sixth costal cartilages, thymus, anterior edges of lungs and pleura.
- Posterior: oesophagus, descending aorta, T5–8 vertebrae.
- Lateral: roots of lung, phrenic nerves, mediastinal pleura.

Serous

- The fibrous pericardium is lined by a parietal layer of serous pericardium.
- The parietal layer is reflected to cover the heart and roots of great vessels to become continuous with visceral layer of serous pericardium.

Oblique and Transverse Sinuses (Fig. 1.10)

At the pericardial reflections, veins are surrounded by one sleeve of pericardium and arteries by another.

Transverse Sinus

- Lies between the aorta and pulmonary trunk in front, and the SVC and left atrium behind.

Oblique Sinus

- Bounded by the pulmonary veins.
- Forms a recess between pericardium and left atrium.

Clinical Points

- Fibrous pericardium can stretch gradually if there is gradual enlargement of the heart.
- Sudden increase in pericardial contents as in sudden bleeds: stretching does not occur and cardiac function is embarrassed (cardiac tamponade).

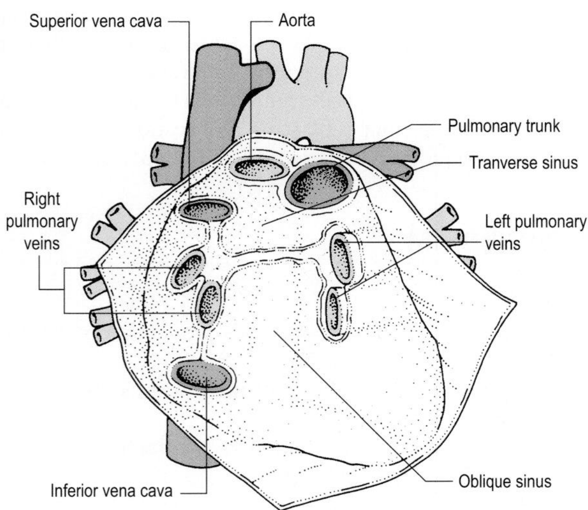

Fig. 1.10 The posterior surface of the pericardial cavity after removal of the heart. The reflection of the pericardium around the great vessels is shown. (From Rogers AW. Textbook of Anatomy. Churchill Livingstone, Edinburgh, 1992, with permission.)

Surface Anatomy of Heart

- Superior: line from second left costal cartilage 1.2 cm from sternal edge to third right costal cartilage, 1.2 cm from sternal edge.
- Inferior: line from the sixth right costal cartilage 1.2 cm from sternal edge to fifth left intercostal space, 9 cm from midline (i.e. position of apex beat).
- Left border: curved line joining second left costal cartilage 1.2 cm from sternal edge to fifth left intercostal space, 9 cm from midline.
- Right border: curved line joining third right costal cartilage 1.2 cm from sternal edge to sixth right costal cartilage, 1.2 cm from sternal edge.

MEDIASTINUM (Fig. 1.11)

The space between the two pleural cavities is called the mediastinum. It is divided into:

- superior mediastinum
- anterior mediastinum
- middle mediastinum
- posterior mediastinum.

Superior Mediastinum

Boundaries are:

- anterior: manubrium sterni
- posterior: first four thoracic vertebrae
- above: continues up to root of neck
- below: continues with inferior mediastinum at level of horizontal line drawn through angle of Louis.

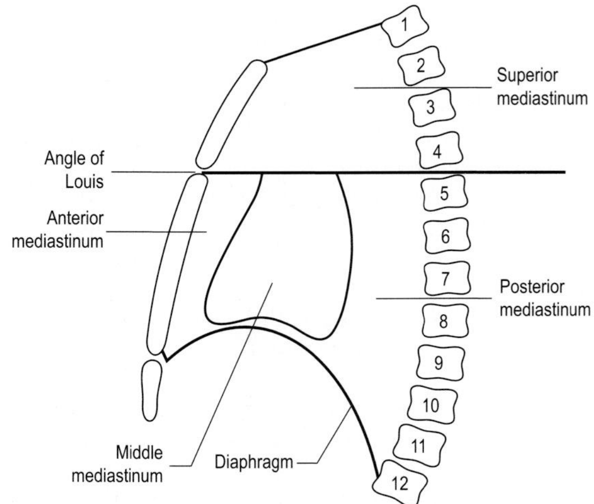

Fig. 1.11 The divisions of the mediastinum.

Contents:
- lower end of trachea
- oesophagus
- thoracic duct
- aortic arch
- innominate artery
- part of carotid and subclavian arteries
- innominate veins
- upper part of SVC
- phrenic and vagus nerves
- left recurrent laryngeal nerves
- cardiac nerves
- lymph nodes
- remnants of thymus gland.

Anterior Mediastinum

Boundaries are:
- anterior: sternum
- posterior: pericardium.

Contents:
- part of the thymus gland in children
- anterior mediastinal lymph nodes.

Middle Mediastinum

Boundaries are:
- anterior: anterior mediastinum
- posterior: posterior mediastinum.

Contents:
- heart
- great vessels
- phrenic nerves
- pericardiophrenic vessels.

Posterior Mediastinum

Boundaries are:
- anterior: pericardium, roots of lungs, diaphragm below
- posterior: vertebral column from lower border of fourth to twelfth vertebrae
- above: horizontal plane drawn through the angle of Louis
- below: diaphragm.

Contents:
- descending thoracic aorta
- oesophagus
- vagus and splanchnic nerves
- azygos vein
- hemiazygos vein
- thoracic duct
- mediastinal lymph nodes.

Fig. 1.12 shows some of the structures in the anterior, middle and posterior mediastinum.

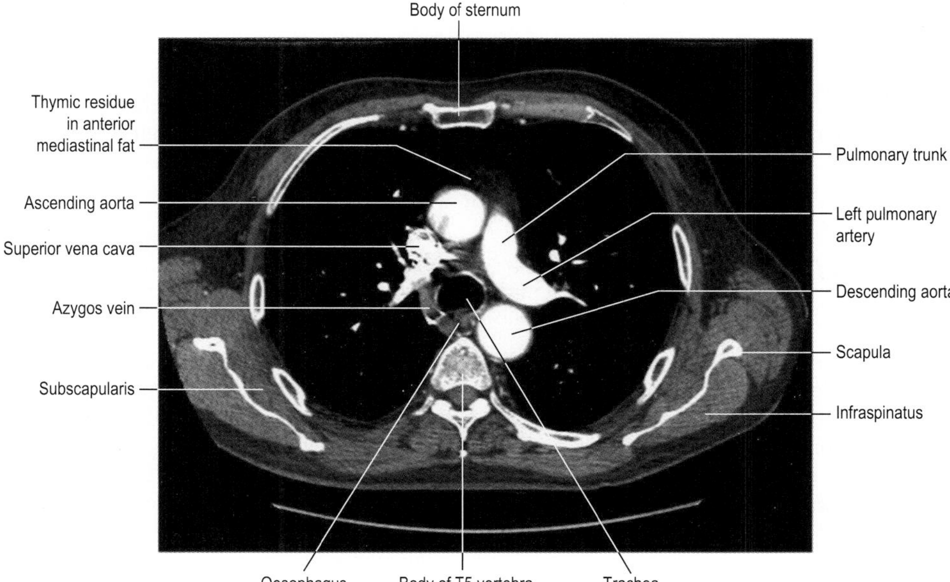

Fig. 1.12 Contrast CT at the level of the fifth thoracic vertebra showing some of the structures in the anterior, middle and posterior mediastinum.

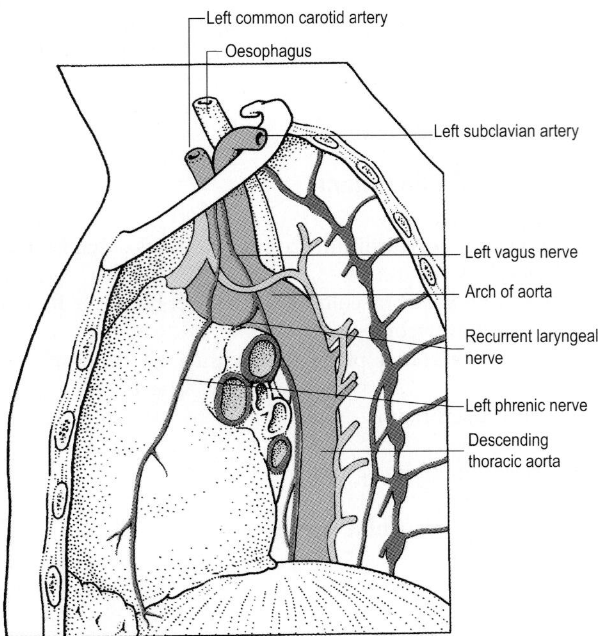

Fig. 1.13 The mediastinum seen from the left side.

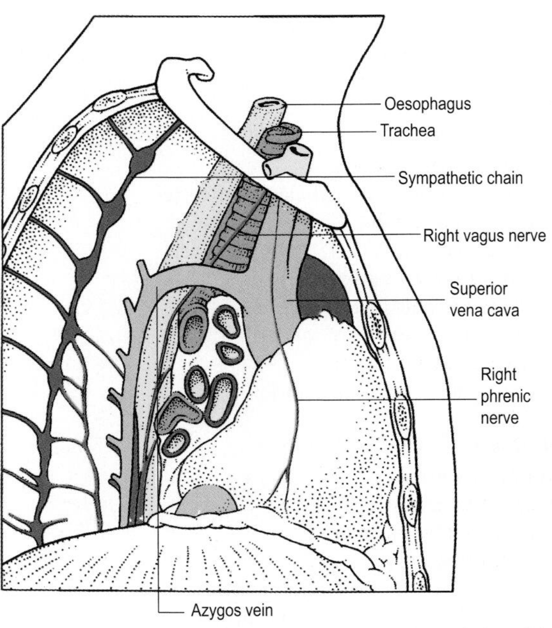

Fig. 1.14 The mediastinum seen from the right side.

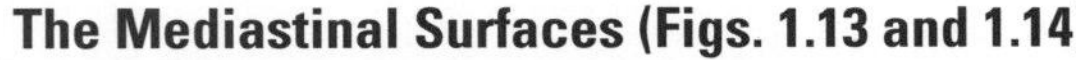

The Mediastinal Surfaces (Figs. 1.13 and 1.14)

Because of the arrangements of structures in the mediastinum, it appears differently when viewed from left and right sides.

The Angle of Louis

The angle of Louis (manubriosternal junction) is an important anatomical landmark. It corresponds to the plane of T4, which is an important landmark. The following occur at T4:

- commencement and termination of aortic arch
- bifurcation of trachea
- junction of superior and inferior mediastinum
- second costosternal joint
- confluence of azygos vein with superior vena cava
- thoracic duct runs from right to left
- ligamentum arteriosum lies on this plane.

OSCE SCENARIOS

OSCE Scenario 1.1

A 19-year-old male is admitted with a right-sided spontaneous pneumothorax. He has a past history of a treated coarctation of the aorta. He requires a chest drain.

1. Describe the anatomy of a typical intercostal space.
2. Why is this knowledge important in your technique of insertion of an intercostal drain?
3. What is the 'triangle of safety' when inserting a chest drain?
4. Explain the anatomical basis for notching of the lower border of a rib seen on a chest X-ray of a patient with coarctation of the aorta.

OSCE Scenario 1.2

A 35-year-old male sustains a crushing upper abdominal injury in a road traffic accident. On admission to A&E he has a tachycardia of 120 and a systolic blood pressure of 90 mmHg. He is complaining of abdominal and bilateral shoulder tip pain. Urgent CT scan reveals liver and splenic trauma as well as a ruptured left hemidiaphragm.

1. Describe the three origins of the muscular part of the diaphragm.
2. At what vertebral levels do the oesophagus and the IVC pass through the diaphragm?
3. What is the nerve supply of the diaphragm?

4. Explain why in some cases irritation of the diaphragm may result in referred pain to the shoulder while in others it may result in referred pain to the abdomen.

OSCE Scenario 1.3

A 60-year-old female undergoes a right open nephrectomy via a loin approach through the bed of the twelfth rib. A postoperative chest X-ray shows a small right pneumothorax.

1. Describe the surface anatomy of the pleura.
2. Why has this patient developed a right pneumothorax?
3. At which other site, other than surgery on the thorax, may surgery or trauma result in a pneumothorax?

OSCE Scenario 1.4

A 22-year-old male is brought to A&E with a penetrating injury in the left third intercostal space, anterior to the mid-axillary line. His blood pressure is 80/40, pulse rate 140 beats/min and has muffled hear sounds and distended neck veins. A diagnosis of cardiac tamponade is established.

1. Describe the surface anatomy of the heart.
2. Why does cardiac tamponade result in drop in the blood pressure and clinical shock?
3. Describe how you would treat a cardiac tamponade.

OSCE Scenario 1.5

An 18-month-old girl developed sudden-onset bouts of cough and wheezes. A bowl of peanuts was found nearby while she was playing unwitnessed. She was rushed to A&E and found to be conscious but distressed, tachypnoeic and wheezy. A chest X-ray revealed a collapsed lung.

1. In which main bronchus a foreign body is more likely to be dislodged and why?
2. In relation to the surface anatomy, where does the trachea commence and terminate?
3. Describe briefly how you would treat the patient.

Answers in Appendix pages 431–433

Please check your eBook at https://studentconsult.inkling.com/ for more self-assessment questions. See inside cover for registration details.

2

The Abdomen, Pelvis and Perineum

DEVELOPMENT

Development of the Gut

The gut develops from a primitive endodermal tube. It is divided into three parts:

- foregut: extends to the entry of the bile duct into the duodenum (supplied by the coeliac axis)
- midgut: extends to distal transverse colon (supplied by superior mesenteric artery)
- hindgut: extends to ectodermal part of anal canal (supplied by inferior mesenteric artery).

Foregut

- Starts to divide into the oesophagus and the laryngotracheal tube during the 4th week.
- If it fails to do so correctly, there may be pure oesophageal atresia (8% of cases), or atresia associated with tracheo-oesophageal fistula (the commonest, 80% of cases), the fistula being between the lower end of the trachea and the distal oesophagus (Fig. 2.1).
- Distal to the oesophagus, the foregut dilates to form the stomach.
- Rotates so that the right wall of the stomach now becomes its posterior surface, forming the lesser sac behind.
- Vagus nerves rotate with the stomach so that the right vagus nerve becomes posterior and the left anterior.
- As the stomach rotates to the left, so the duodenum swings to the right, its mesentery fusing with the peritoneum of the posterior abdominal wall, leaving all but the first inch retroperitoneal.

Midgut (Fig. 2.2)

- Enlarges rapidly in early fetal life, becoming too big for the developing abdominal cavity, and herniates into the umbilical cord.
- The apex of the herniated bowel is continuous with the vitellointestinal duct into the yolk sac.
- While the midgut is within the cord it rotates 90° counterclockwise around the axis of the superior mesenteric artery, bringing the third and fourth parts of the duodenum across to the left of the midline behind the superior mesenteric artery; this part of the duodenum is now fixed retroperitoneally.
- The midgut returns to the abdomen at the 10th week and during this time it continues to rotate counterclockwise through a further 180°, bringing the ascending colon to the right side of the abdomen with the caecum lying immediately below the liver.
- The caecum descends into its definitive position in the right iliac fossa, pulling the colon with it.
- The mesenteries of the ascending and descending colon blend with the posterior abdominal wall, except for the sigmoid colon, which retains a mesentery.

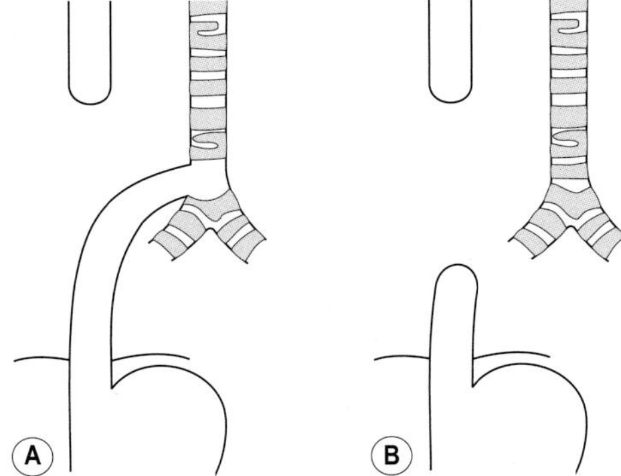

Fig. 2.1 Types of oesophageal atresia. (A) Oesophageal atresia with distal tracheo-oesophageal fistula—most common type, with an incidence of 80%. (B) Isolated oesophageal atresia—second commonest, with an incidence of about 8%.

Clinical Points

- In early fetal life, growth obliterates the lumen of the developing gut. It then recanalizes. If recanalization is incomplete, areas of atresia or stenosis may result.
- The communication between the primitive midgut and yolk sac may persist as a Meckel's diverticulum. This

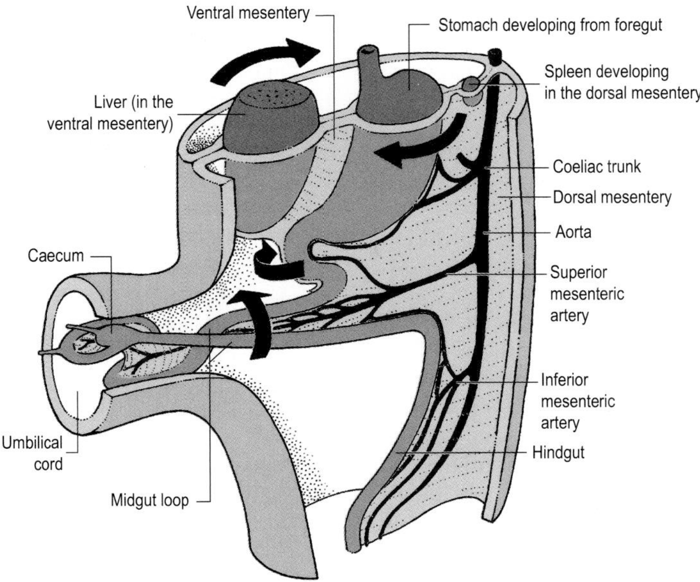

Fig. 2.2 The developing gut and mesentery seen from the left. The midgut is in the umbilical cord. The arrows show the direction of rotation for the foregut and midgut.

may occasionally be attached to the back of the umbilicus by a fibrous cord, a remnant of the vitellointestinal duct (this may act as a fixed point for small bowel volvulus).
- Rarely, the Meckel's diverticulum may open onto the skin at the umbilicus.
- Malrotation occurs when the sequence described above fails to occur or is incomplete. The duodenojejunal (DJ) flexure may not become fixed retroperitoneally and hangs freely from the foregut, lying to the right of the abdomen. The caecum may also be free and may obstruct the second part of the duodenum because of peritoneal bands (of Ladd) passing across it. The base of the mesentery is then very narrow as it is not fixed at either end, and the whole of the midgut may twist around its own blood supply, i.e. volvulus neonatorum.
- Persistence of midgut herniation at the umbilicus may occur after birth, i.e. exomphalos.

Anal Canal

- Rectum, anus and genitourinary tracts develop at the end of the 9th week by separation of these structures within the cloaca (Fig. 2.3).
- Urorectal septum divides the cloaca into bladder anteriorly and rectum (hindgut) posteriorly.
- Anal canal develops from the end of the hindgut (endoderm) and an invagination of ectoderm, the proctodeum.
- At its caudal end, the urorectal septum reaches the cloacal membrane and divides it into anal and urogenital membranes.
- The anal membrane separates the hindgut from the proctodeum (anal pit).

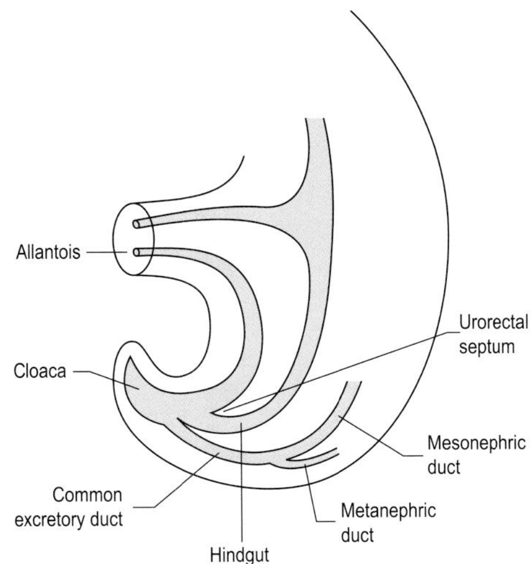

Fig. 2.3 The connections between cloaca (rudimentary bladder) and allantois. The urachus is the embryonic remnant of this connection.

- Eventually the anal membrane breaks down and continuity is established between the anal pit and the hindgut.
- Failure of the anal membrane to rupture or anal pit to develop results in imperforate anus.

The Kidneys and Ureter (Fig. 2.4)

- Pronephros develops at the 3rd week; it is transient and never functions.
- Mesonephros develops at the 4th week; this also degenerates but its duct persists in the male to form the epididymis and vas deferens.
- Metanephros develops at the 5th week in the pelvis. Metanephric duct arises as a diverticulum from the lower end of the mesonephric duct.
- Metanephric duct (ureteric bud) invaginates the metanephros, undergoing repeated branching to develop into the ureter, pelvis, calyces and collecting tubules.
- Collecting tubules fuse with the proximal part of the tubular system and glomeruli which are developing from the metanephros.
- The mesonephric duct loses its connection with the renal tract.
- The kidney develops in the pelvis, eventually migrating upwards, its blood supply moving cranially with it, initially being from the iliac arteries and eventually from the aorta.

Development Anomalies

- Failure of fusion of the derivatives of the ureteric bud with the derivatives of the metanephros may give rise to autosomal recessive form of polycystic kidney.

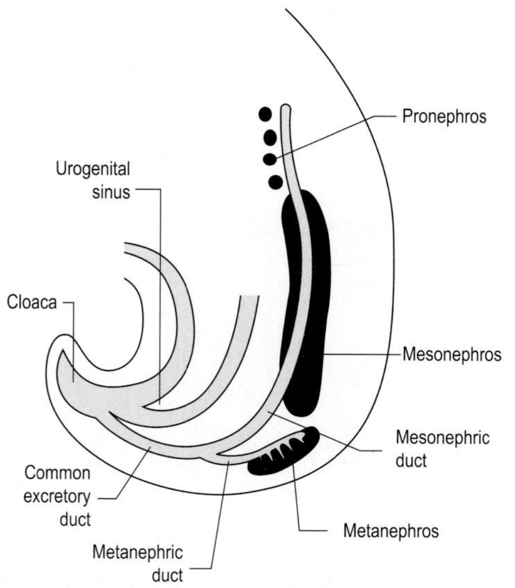

Fig. 2.4 Development of the pronephros, mesonephros, metanephros and their ducts.

- The kidney may fail to migrate cranially, resulting in pelvic kidney.
- One or more of the distal arteries may persist, giving rise to aberrant renal arteries (occasionally one may persist from the common iliac artery).
- The two metanephric masses may fuse in the midline, resulting in a horseshoe kidney.
- The ureteric bud may branch early, giving rise to double ureter. Rarely, the extra ureter may open ectopically into the vagina or urethra, resulting in urinary incontinence.
- The metanephros may fail to develop on one side, resulting in congenital absence of the kidney.

Bladder and Urethra

Bladder

- Urinary bladder is formed partly from the cloaca and partly from the ends of the mesonephric ducts.
- The anterior part of the cloaca is divided into three parts:
  - cephalic: vesicourethral
  - middle: pelvic portion
  - caudal: phallic portion.
- The latter two constitute the urogenital sinus.
- The ureter and mesonephric duct come to open separately into the vesicourethral portion.
- The mesonephric duct participates in the formation of the trigone and dorsal wall of the prostatic urethra.
- The remainder of the vesicourethral portion forms the body of the bladder and part of the prostatic urethra.
- The apex of the bladder is prolonged to the umbilicus as the urachus (where the primitive bladder joins the allantois).

Urethra

- In the female, the whole of the urethra is derived from the vesicourethral portion of the cloaca.
- In the male, the prostatic part of the urethra cranial to the prostatic utricle is derived from the vesicourethral part of the cloaca and the incorporated caudal ends of the mesonephric duct.
- The remainder of the prostatic urethra and the membranous urethra are derived from the urogenital sinus.
- The succeeding portion as far as the glans is formed by fusion of the genital (urethral) folds enclosing the phallic portion of the urogenital sinus (Fig. 2.5).
- The terminal part of the urethra develops within the glans, which in turn develops from the genital tubercle.

Clinical Points

- Failure of fusion of the genital folds results in persistence of the urethral groove. This is known as hypospadias and occurs in varying degrees, e.g. complete

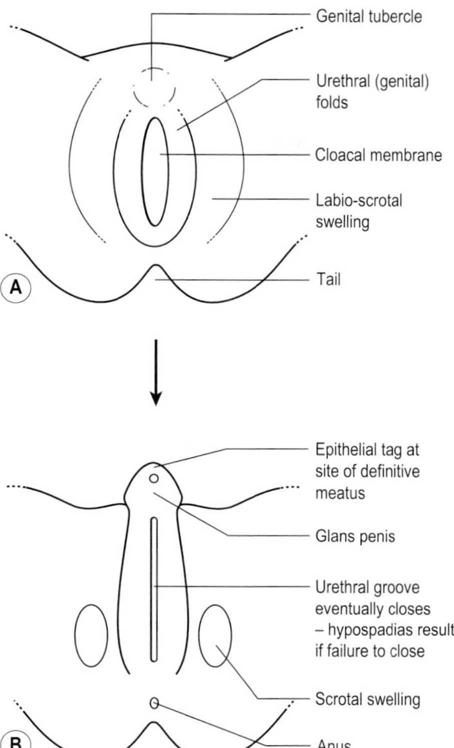

Fig. 2.5 Development of the penis and urethra. (A) Undifferentiated stage of development of external genitalia. (B) Fusion of the urethral folds and penis development. The glans develops from the genital tubercle.

groove, open or just a narrow urethral orifice on the undersurface of the penile shaft.

- Epispadias occurs where the dorsal wall of the urethra is partially or completely absent and is caused by failure of infraumbilical mesodermal development. In extreme cases this results in ectopia vesicae where the trigone of the bladder and ureteric orifices are exposed on the abdominal wall and is associated with cleft pelvis, e.g. no symphysis pubis.

Testis

- Develops as a mesodermal ridge on the posterior abdominal wall medial to the mesonephros (urogenital ridges).
- Links with mesonephric duct, which forms the epididymis, vas deferens and ejaculatory ducts.
- Undergoes descent from the posterior abdominal wall to the scrotum.
- In the 3rd intrauterine month it lies in the pelvis.
- In the 7th intrauterine month it passes down the inguinal canal.
- Reaches the scrotum by the end of the 8th month.
- Guided into scrotum by the gubernaculum, a mesenchymatous column which extends from the lower pole of the developing testis to the scrotal fascia.
- 'Slides' down into the scrotum behind a prolongation of peritoneum, i.e. the processus vaginalis.
- The processus vaginalis obliterates at birth, leaving its distal portion to cover the testis as the tunica vaginalis.

Clinical Points

- Testis develops on posterior abdominal wall and its blood supply, lymphatic drainage and nerve supply remain associated with the posterior abdominal wall.
- The testis may descend into an ectopic position and may be found at the root of the penis, in the perineum or in the upper thigh.
- The testis may fail to descend and may be found anywhere along its course, either intra-abdominally, within the inguinal canal or at the external ring.
- Processus vaginalis may fail to obliterate or may become partially obliterated, resulting in a variety of hydroceles (Fig. 2.6).

ANTERIOR ABDOMINAL WALL

Superficial Fascia of Abdominal Wall

- Only superficial fascia on abdominal wall.
- Two layers in lower abdomen:
  - superficial fatty layer (Camper's fascia)
  - deep fibrous layer (Scarpa's fascia).
- Superficial fascia extends onto penis and scrotum.
- Scarpa's fascia is attached to the deep fascia of thigh 2.5 cm below the inguinal ligament.
- Extends into perineum as Colles' fascia.
- Colles' fascia is attached to the perineal body, perineal membrane and laterally to the rami of the pubis and ischium.

Clinical Points

- In rupture of the bulbous urethra, urine tracks into the scrotum, perineum and penis and into abdominal wall deep to Scarpa's fascia. It does not track into the thigh because of the attachment of Scarpa's fascia to the deep fascia of the thigh.
- An ectopic testis in the groin cannot descend any lower into the thigh because of the attachment of Scarpa's fascia to the deep fascia of the thigh.

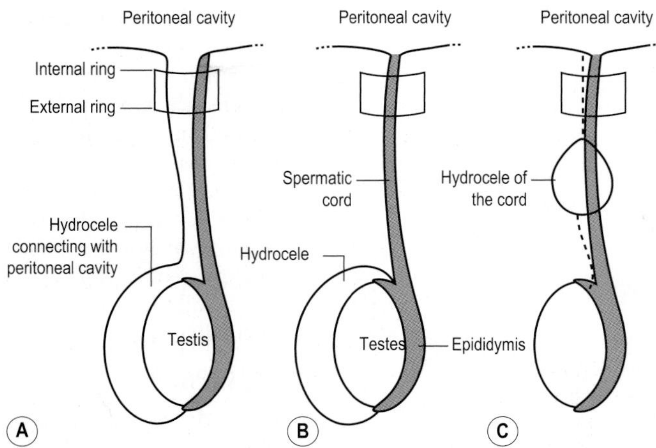

Fig. 2.6 Types of hydrocele. (A) Congenital. (B) Vaginal. (C) Hydrocele of the cord (a similar lesion exists in the female—a hydrocele of the canal of Nuck).

Abdominal Wall Muscles (Fig. 2.7)

- Abdominal wall consists of three sheets of muscle.
- Fleshy laterally and aponeurotic in front and behind.
- As aponeuroses pass forward they ensheath the rectus abdominis muscle.

Rectus Abdominis

- Origin: fifth, sixth, seventh costal cartilages.
- Insertion: pubic crest.
- Three tendinous intersections:
  - level of xiphoid
  - level of umbilicus
  - halfway between the two.
- Tendinous intersections adhere to the anterior sheath but not the posterior sheath.

External Oblique

- Origin: outer surface of lower eight ribs.
- Insertion: linea alba, pubic crest, pubic tubercle, anterior half of iliac crest.
- Between anterior superior and iliac spine and pubic tubercle, its recurved lower border forms the inguinal ligament.
- Fibres run downwards and medially.

Internal Oblique

- Origin: lumbar fascia, anterior two-thirds of iliac crest and lateral two-thirds of inguinal ligament.
- Insertion: linea alba and pubic crest via conjoint tendon.
- Fibres run upwards and medially at right angles to external oblique.

Transversus Abdominis

- Origin: deep surface of lower sixth costal cartilages (interdigitating with diaphragm), lumbar fascia, anterior two-thirds of iliac crest, lateral third of inguinal ligament.
- Insertion: linea alba and pubic crest via the conjoint tendon.

Nerve Supply of Abdominal Muscles

- Rectus and external oblique supplied by lower sixth thoracic nerves.
- Internal oblique and transversus supplied by lower sixth thoracic nerves and iliohypogastric and ilioinguinal nerves.

Rectus Sheath (See Fig. 2.7)

- The lower border of the posterior aponeurotic part of the sheath is marked by a crescentic line, the arcuate line of Douglas (halfway between umbilicus and pubic symphysis).
- At this point the inferior epigastric vessels enter the sheath.
- The rectus sheath fuses in the midline to form the linea alba, which runs from the xiphisternum to the pubic symphysis.

Clinical Points

- A Spigelian hernia emerges at the lateral part of the rectus sheath at the level of the arcuate line of Douglas.
- The epigastric vessels (superior and inferior) are applied to the posterior surface of the rectus muscle. Rupture of

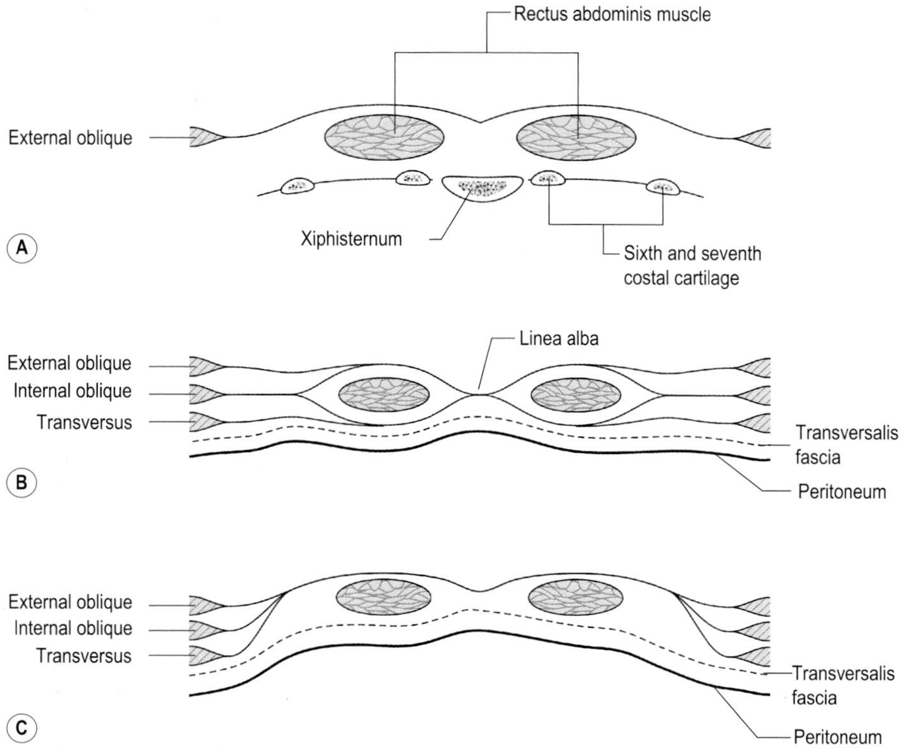

Fig. 2.7 The formation of the rectus sheath. (A) Above the costal margin. (B) Above the arcuate line. (C) Below the arcuate line.

these with violent contraction of the rectus muscle leads to a rectus sheath haematoma.

THE ANATOMY OF ABDOMINAL INCISIONS

Midline

- Through linea alba skirting the umbilicus.
- Excellent for routine and rapid access.
- Linea alba virtually bloodless.
- Structures encountered:
  - skin
  - subcutaneous fat
  - superficial fascia (two layers in lower abdomen)
  - linea alba
  - extraperitoneal fat
  - peritoneum.

Subcostal (Kocher's)

- Right side (cholecystectomy), left side (elective splenectomy), both sides connected (kidneys: anterior approach).
- Incision 2.5 cm below and parallel to costal margin extending laterally to lateral border of rectus or further.
- Structures encountered:
  - skin
  - subcutaneous fat
  - superficial fascia
  - anterior rectus sheath
  - rectus abdominis
  - posterior rectus sheath
  - extraperitoneal fat
  - peritoneum.
- Ninth intercostal nerve is present in lateral part of wound. Damage to it may result in weakness and atrophy of upper rectus with predisposition to incisional hernia.

Gridiron Incision (Muscle-Splitting)

- Used for appendicectomy.
- Centred on McBurney's point (two-thirds of the way along a line drawn from the umbilicus to the anterior superior iliac spine).

- Structures encountered:
  - skin
  - Camper's fascia
  - Scarpa's fascia at lower end of incision
  - external oblique aponeurosis
  - internal oblique muscle
  - transversus muscle
  - extraperitoneal fat
  - peritoneum.

Paramedian Incision

- Use is declining.
- Two and a half centimetres lateral to and parallel to midline.
- Structures encountered:
  - above the arcuate line (of Douglas):
    - skin
    - superficial fascia
    - anterior rectus sheath and tendinous intersections (segmental vessels enter here and bleeding will be encountered)
    - rectus muscle (which is retracted laterally)
    - posterior rectus sheath
    - extraperitoneal fat
    - peritoneum
  - below arcuate line posterior rectus sheath consists of transversalis fascia alone.

Pararectus Incision (Battle Incision)

- Used occasionally for appendicectomy; more often for open insertion of peritoneal dialysis catheters (Tenckhoff catheter for continuous ambulatory peritoneal dialysis).
- Incision at lateral border of rectus below umbilical level.
- Structures encountered:
  - skin
  - Camper's fascia
  - Scarpa's fascia
  - anterior rectus sheath
  - rectus muscle (retracted medially)
  - posterior rectus sheath
  - extraperitoneal fat
  - peritoneum.
- Extending the incision may damage nerves entering sheath to supply rectus, with consequent weakening of muscle.

INGUINAL CANAL

- Oblique passage in lower abdominal wall.
- Passes from deep to superficial inguinal rings.
- About 4 cm long.
- Transmits the spermatic cord and ilioinguinal nerve in the male and the round ligament of the uterus and ilioinguinal nerve in the female.

Relations

- Anteriorly:
  - skin
  - Camper's fascia
  - Scarpa's fascia
  - external oblique aponeurosis
  - internal oblique in lateral third of canal.
- Posteriorly:
  - medially: conjoint tendon
  - laterally: transversalis fascia.
- Above:
  - lower arching fibres of internal oblique and transversus.
- Below:
  - lower recurved edge of external oblique, i.e. inguinal ligament.

Deep Inguinal Ring

- Defect in transversalis fascia.
- Lies 1 cm above midpoint of inguinal ligament.
- Immediately lateral to inferior epigastric vessels.

Superficial Inguinal Ring

- V-shaped defect in inguinal ligament.
- Lies above and medial to pubic tubercle.

Spermatic Cord

This contains:

- Three layers of fascia:
  - external spermatic fascia from the external oblique aponeurosis
  - cremasteric fascia and cremaster from the internal oblique aponeurosis
  - internal spermatic fascia from the transversalis fascia.
- Three arteries:
  - testicular artery
  - cremasteric artery
  - the artery to the vas.
- Three nerves:
  - genital branch of the genitofemoral to cremaster
  - sympathetic nerves
  - ilioinguinal nerve (actually lies on the cord and not within it).
- Three other structures:
  - vas deferens
  - pampiniform plexus of veins
  - lymphatics.

FEMORAL CANAL

- Medial compartment of the femoral sheath.
- Femoral sheath is prolongation of transversalis fascia anteriorly and iliacus fascia posteriorly prolonged over the femoral artery, vein and canal (but *not* the nerve).
- Upper opening of femoral canal is the femoral ring, which will just admit the tip of the little finger.
- Boundaries of the femoral ring are:
  - anterior: inguinal ligament (of Poupart)
  - posteriorly: pectineal ligament (of Astley Cooper)
  - laterally: femoral vein
  - medially: lacunar ligament (of Gimbernat); occasionally an abnormal obturator artery runs in close relationship to the lacunar ligament and is in danger during surgery for femoral hernia.
- Contents of femoral canal:
  - fat
  - lymphatics
  - lymph node (Cloquet's node).
- Functions:
  - dead space for expansion of femoral vein
  - pathway for lymphatics of lower limb to external iliac nodes.

Surgical Anatomy of Hernias

- An indirect inguinal hernia passes through the deep inguinal ring along the inguinal canal and into the scrotum (if large).
- An indirect hernia is covered by the layers of the cord.
- A direct hernia bulges through the posterior wall of the canal medial to the inferior epigastric artery through Hesselbach's triangle.
- Boundaries of Hesselbach's triangle are:
  - laterally: inferior epigastric artery
  - inferiorly: inguinal ligament
  - medially: lateral border of rectus abdominis.
- Distinction between direct and indirect inguinal hernia at operation depends on relationship of sac to the inferior epigastric vessels: direct hernia is medial, indirect lies lateral to the artery.
- Clinical distinction between inguinal and femoral hernias depends on the relationship to the pubic tubercle: inguinal hernias lie above and medially, femoral hernias lie below and laterally.
- Clinical distinction between direct and indirect hernias can be made by reducing the hernia and applying pressure over the deep inguinal ring (1 cm above the midpoint of the inguinal ligament). Pressure over the deep ring should control an indirect hernia when the patient coughs. If a bulge appears medial to the point of finger pressure, then it is a direct hernia.
- The femoral ring is narrow and the lacunar ligament forms a 'sharp' medial border. Therefore, irreducibility and strangulation are more common in a femoral hernia (also, femoral hernias are more likely to be of the Richter type).
- In the female, the pelvis is wider and the canal therefore larger. Femoral hernias are consequently more common in the female.

PERITONEAL CAVITY

- The peritoneum is the serous membrane of the peritoneal cavity.
- Consists of a parietal layer and a visceral layer.
- Visceral layer covers contained organs.
- Parietal layer lines abdominal and pelvic wall.
- Lined by mesothelium (simple squamous epithelium).
- Divided into two cavities: a main cavity, i.e. the greater sac, and a smaller cavity, the lesser sac (omental bursa).

Greater Sac of Peritoneum

- Below the umbilicus the peritoneum contains three folds:
  - median umbilical fold (owing to obliterated urachus)
  - medial umbilical fold (obliterated umbilical artery)
  - lateral umbilical fold (inferior epigastric artery).
- Peritoneum of pelvis is continuous with that of abdominal cavity.
- It completely encloses sigmoid colon, forming sigmoid mesocolon.
- Applied to front and sides of upper third of the rectum.
- Applied to the front of the middle third of the rectum.
- In male, reflected onto base and upper part of bladder.
- In female, reflected onto upper part of posterior vaginal wall and over posterior, upper and anterior surface of uterus onto bladder.
- Between uterus and rectum is rectouterine pouch (of Douglas).
- Peritoneum passes off lateral margins of uterus to pelvic wall, forming broad ligaments with fallopian tubes in upper border.
- Falciform ligament passes upwards from umbilicus and slightly to right of midline to liver (containing the ligamentum teres in its free edge).
- Passes into groove between quadrate lobe and left lobe of liver.
- Traced superiorly, the two layers of the falciform ligament separate: the right limb joins the upper layer of the coronary ligament, the left forms the anterior layer of the left triangular ligament.
- Above the umbilicus the peritoneum sweeps upwards and over the diaphragm to be reflected onto the liver and the right side of the abdominal oesophagus.

- Peritoneal reflexions of the liver are described further in the section on the liver.
- After enclosing the liver the peritoneum descends from the porta hepatis as a double layer, i.e. the lesser omentum.
- This then separates to enclose the stomach, reforming again on the greater curvature, and then loops downwards again, turning upwards and attaching to the length of the transverse colon, forming the greater omentum (Fig. 2.8).
- The lower leaf of the greater omentum continues upwards, enclosing the transverse colon as the transverse mesocolon.
- At the base of the transverse mesocolon the double layer divides again.
- The upper leaf passes over the abdominal wall and upwards to reflect onto the liver.
- The lower leaf passes downwards to cover the pelvic viscera and join with the peritoneum of the anterior abdominal wall.
- The peritoneum of the posterior abdominal wall is interrupted as it is reflected along the small bowel from the DJ flexure to the ileocaecal junction, forming the mesentery of the small intestine.
- The lines of peritoneal reflexion are shown in Fig. 2.9.

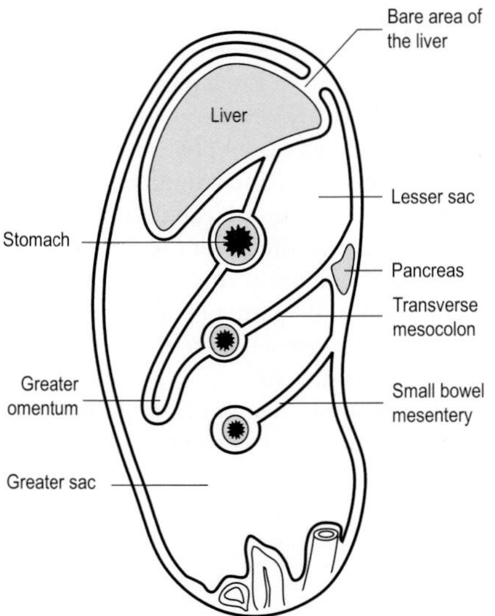

Fig. 2.8 A longitudinal section of the peritoneal cavity, showing the lesser and greater sacs and peritoneal reflexions.

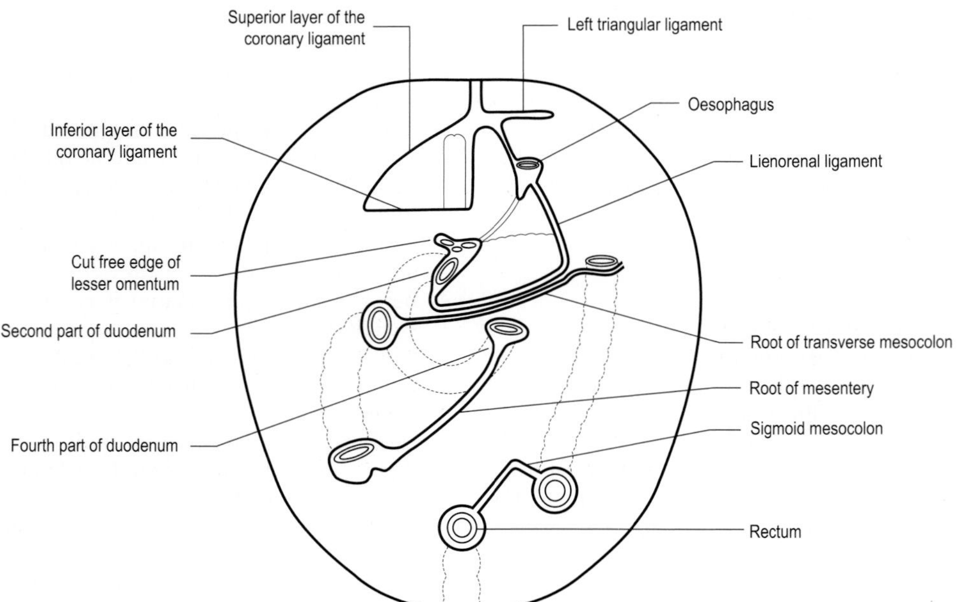

Fig. 2.9 The posterior abdominal wall. The lines of reflexion of the peritoneum are shown. The liver, stomach, spleen and intestines have been removed.

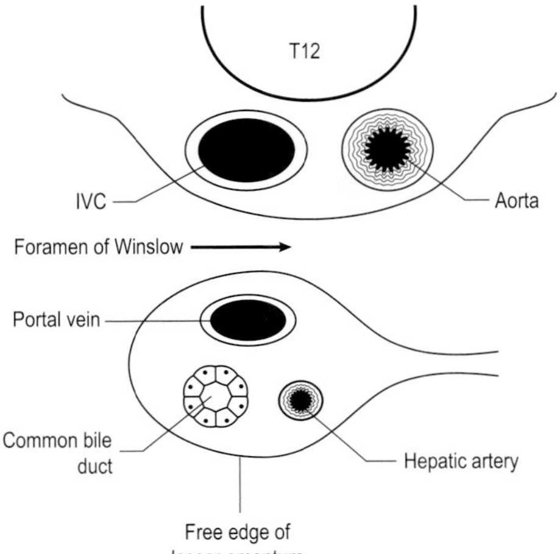

Fig. 2.10 A transverse section through the foramen of Winslow (epiploic foramen). IVC, Inferior vena cava.

Lesser Sac (Omental Bursa)

Relations

- Anteriorly: lesser omentum and stomach.
- Superiorly: superior recess whose anterior border is the caudate lobe of the liver.
- Inferiorly: projects downwards to transverse mesocolon.
- To the left: spleen, gastrosplenic and lienorenal ligaments.
- To the right: opens into the greater sac via the epiploic foramen.

Epiploic Foramen (Foramen of Winslow; Fig. 2.10)

- Anteriorly: free edge of lesser omentum containing bile duct to the right, hepatic artery to the left and portal vein behind.
- Posteriorly: inferior vena cava (IVC).
- Inferiorly: first part of duodenum.
- Superiorly: caudate process of the liver.

Clinical Points

- The hepatic artery can be compressed between finger and thumb in the free edge of the lesser omentum (Pringle's manoeuvre). This is useful if the cystic artery is torn during cholecystectomy or if there is gross haemorrhage following liver trauma.

SUBPHRENIC SPACES

- Potential spaces below liver in relation to diaphragm, which may be site of collections or abscesses (subphrenic abscesses).
- Two spaces are directly subphrenic, the other two spaces are subhepatic.
- Right and left subphrenic spaces lie between the diaphragm and liver and are separated by the falciform ligament.
- Right subhepatic space (renal well of Rutherford Morrison) is bounded by:
  - above: liver with attached gall bladder
  - behind: posterior abdominal wall and kidney
  - below: duodenum.
- The left subhepatic space is the lesser sac.

Clinical Points

- Subphrenic abscesses may result from perforated peptic ulcers, perforated appendicitis, perforated diverticulitis.
- On the right side, infected fluid tracks along the right paracolic gutter into the right subhepatic space when the patient is recumbent.
- The left subhepatic space (lesser sac) may distend with fluid with perforated posterior gastric ulcer or acute pancreatitis (pseudocyst of the pancreas).
- Most subphrenic abscesses are drained percutaneously nowadays under ultrasound or computerized tomography (CT) control.
- If surgery is required, posterior abscesses can be accessed by an incision below or through the bed of the 12th rib; anterior abscesses can be accessed by an incision below and parallel to the costal margin.

POSTERIOR ABDOMINAL WALL

The posterior abdominal wall is made up of bony and muscular structures. The bones are:

- bodies of the lumbar vertebrae
- the sacrum
- the wings of the ilium.

The muscles are:

- the posterior part of the diaphragm
- psoas major
- quadratus lumborum
- iliacus.

Important structures on the posterior abdominal wall include:

- abdominal aorta
- IVC
- kidneys
- suprarenal glands
- lumbar sympathetic chain.

The diaphragm has been described in the section on the thorax, and the kidneys and suprarenal glands are dealt with elsewhere in this chapter.

Psoas Major

Psoas major is a massive fusiform muscle extending from the lumbar region of the vertebral column across the pelvic brim and under the inguinal ligament to the thigh.

- Origin: transverse processes of all lumbar vertebrae and the sides of the bodies and intervening discs from T12 to L5 vertebrae.
- Insertion: into the tip of the lesser trochanter of the femur.
- Nerve supply: L2, L3.
- Action: flexion and medial rotation of extended thigh.
- Important relations of psoas include:
  - psoas sheath enclosing muscle and extending beneath inguinal ligament
  - lumbar nerves forming lumbar plexus in substance of muscle
  - important structures lie on it, such as ureter, gonadal vessels, IVC
  - tendon lies in front of hip joint with bursa intervening and lies directly behind femoral artery
  - a retrocaecal or retrocolic appendix lying anteriorly.

Quadratus Lumborum

- Origin: iliolumbar ligament and adjacent portion of iliac crest.
- Insertion: medial half of lower border of 12th rib and by four small tendons into the transverse processes of the upper four lumbar vertebrae.
- Anterior relations of quadratus lumborum include:
  - colon
  - kidney
  - subcostal, iliohypogastric, ilioinguinal nerve lie in front of the fascia covering it.

Iliacus

- Origin: greater part of iliac fossa extending onto sacrum.
- Insertion: lateral aspect of tendon of psoas major onto lesser trochanter of femur.
- Nerve supply: branch of femoral nerve (L2, L3).

Clinical Points

- Femoral artery lies on psoas tendon and can be palpated and compressed against it at this point.
- Psoas sheath is attached around origin of psoas major. Pus from tuberculous infection of the lumbar vertebra may track down the sheath and present as a swelling below the inguinal ligament (psoas abscess).
- An inflamed retrocaecal or retrocolic appendix lies in contact with psoas—the resulting spasm in the muscle leads to persistent flexion of the hip and pain on attempted extension (psoas test).

ABDOMINAL AORTA (Fig. 2.11)

- Extends from 12th thoracic vertebra to left side of front of body at fourth lumbar vertebra where it divides into the common iliac arteries.
- Enters abdomen between crura of diaphragm lying throughout its course against the vertebral bodies.

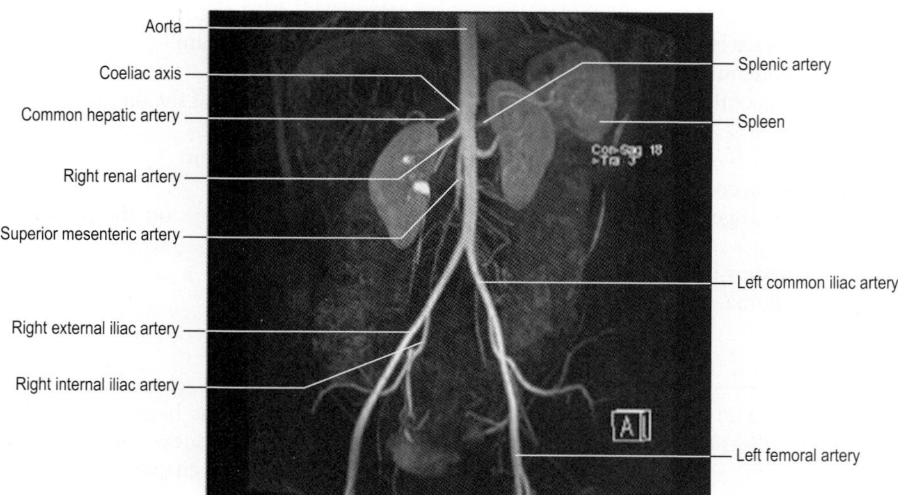

Fig. 2.11 Magnetic resonance angiogram showing the main branches of the abdominal aorta.

- Relations:
  - anterior from above down: lesser omentum, stomach, coeliac plexus, pancreas, splenic vein, left renal vein, third part of duodenum, root of mesentery, coils of small intestine, aortic plexus, peritoneum
  - posterior: bodies of upper four lumbar vertebra, left lumbar veins, cisterna chyli
  - right side: IVC, thoracic duct, azygos vein, right sympathetic trunk
  - left side: left sympathetic trunk.

  The branches of the aorta are:
- Anterior unpaired branches passing to the viscera:
  - coeliac axis: giving off the hepatic artery, splenic artery, left gastric artery
  - superior mesenteric artery
  - inferior mesenteric artery.
- Lateral paired branches:
  - suprarenal artery
  - renal artery
  - gonadal artery.
- Paired branches to the parietes:
  - inferior phrenic arteries
  - four lumbar arteries.
- Terminal branches:
  - common iliac arteries
  - median sacral artery.

Common Iliac Artery

- Arises at bifurcation of aorta at level of body of fourth lumbar vertebra.
- Bifurcates at level of sacroiliac joint into internal and external iliac artery.
- Anterior relations:
  - peritoneum
  - small intestine
  - ureters
  - sympathetic nerves.
- Differences between right and left common iliac arteries:
  - right common iliac artery is the longer, the aorta being on the left side of the spine
  - on the right side lie the IVC and right psoas
  - right common iliac vein is at first behind but to the right at upper part
  - left common iliac vein crosses behind right common iliac artery
  - left common iliac artery is crossed anteriorly by inferior mesenteric artery
  - left common iliac vein is below and medial to left common iliac artery.

External Iliac Artery

- Runs along brim of pelvis on medial side of psoas major.
- Passes below the inguinal ligament to form the femoral artery.
- Gives off inferior epigastric artery immediately before passing below the inguinal ligament.

Internal Iliac Artery

- Passes backwards and downwards into the pelvis between ureter anteriorly and internal iliac vein posteriorly.
- At upper border of greater sciatic notch divides into anterior and posterior branch.
- Branches supply:
  - pelvic organs
  - perineum
  - buttock
  - anal canal.

Inferior Vena Cava

- Formed by junction of two common iliac veins behind the right common iliac artery at the level of the fifth lumbar vertebra.
- Lies to the right of the aorta as it ascends.
- Separated from aorta by right crus of diaphragm when aorta passes behind the diaphragm.
- IVC passes through diaphragm at level T8, traverses the pericardium and drains into the right atrium.
- Anterior relations include:
  - mesentery
  - third part of duodenum
  - pancreas
  - first part of duodenum
  - portal vein
  - posterior surface of liver
  - diaphragm
  - from above down the following arteries: hepatic, right testicular, right colic, right common iliac.
- Posterior relations include:
  - vertebral column
  - right crus of diaphragm and psoas major
  - right sympathetic trunk
  - right renal artery
  - right lumbar arteries
  - right suprarenal arteries
  - right inferior phrenic artery
  - right suprarenal gland
  - to the left: the aorta.

  The IVC receives the following tributaries:
- lumbar branches
- right gonadal vein
- right renal vein
- left renal vein
- right suprarenal vein
- phrenic vein
- hepatic vein.

Lumbar Sympathetic Chain

- Commences deep to the medial arcuate ligament of the diaphragm as a continuation of the thoracic sympathetic chain.
- Lies against the bodies of the lumbar vertebrae overlapped on the right side by the IVC and on the left side by the aorta.
- The lumbar arteries lie deep to the chain but the lumbar veins may cross superficial to it.
- Below the chain passes deep to the iliac vessels to continue as the sacral trunk in front of the sacrum.
- Inferiorly the right and left chain converge and unite in front of the coccyx to end in the ganglion impar.
- Branches from the sympathetic chain pass as follows:
  - to the plexuses around the abdominal aorta
  - to the hypogastric plexus (presacral nerves) to supply the pelvic viscera via plexuses of nerves distributed along the internal iliac artery and its branches.

Clinical Points

- Resection of abdominal aortic aneurysm and extensive pelvic dissection may remove aortic and hypogastric plexuses and hence compromise ejaculation.
- Lumbar sympathectomy may be carried out for plantar hyperhidrosis or vasospastic conditions of the lower limb. Usually the second, third and fourth ganglia are excised with the intermediate chain.

PELVIC FLOOR AND WALL

The muscles of the pelvic floor and wall comprise:

- Pelvis:
  - levator ani
  - coccygeus.
- Pelvic wall:
  - piriformis (on the front of the sacrum)
  - obturator internus (on the lateral wall of the true pelvis).

Piriformis and obturator internus act on the femur and are described with the muscles of the lower limb.

Levator Ani

The levator ani muscles arise from the side wall of the pelvis and are thin sheets of muscle which meet in the midline and close the greater part of the outlet of the pelvis (posterior part of the pelvic diaphragm) (Fig. 2.12).

Origin

- Back of body of pubis.
- Spine of ischium.
- Between these from the fascia covering obturator internus along a thickening between the above two points.

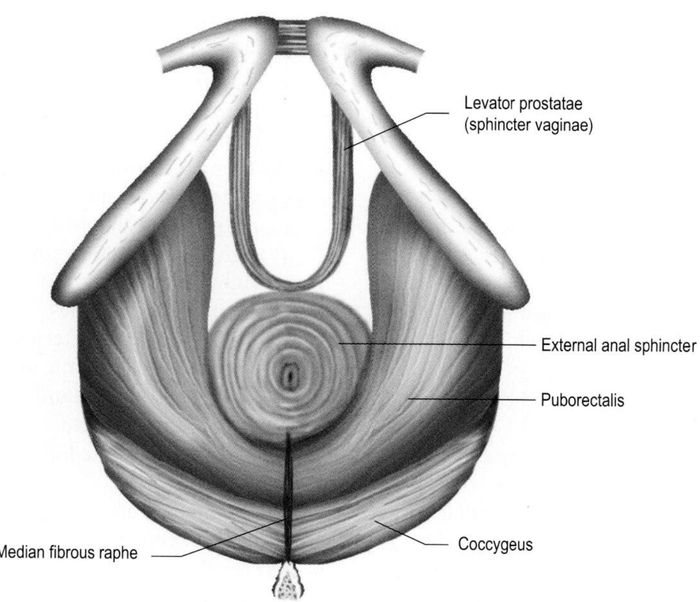

Fig. 2.12 Levator ani viewed from below.

Insertion

- Forms a sling around the prostate (levator prostatae) or vagina (sphincter vaginae) inserting into the perineal body.
- Forms a sling around the rectum and anus inserting into and reinforcing the deep part of the anal sphincter at the anorectal ring (puborectalis).
- Into the sides of the coccyx and to a median fibrous raphe stretching between the apex of the coccyx and the anorectal junction.

Nerve supply

- Perineal branch of S4 on pelvic surface, and branch of the inferior rectal and perineal division of the pudendal nerve on the perineal surface.

Actions

- Acts as principal support of pelvic floor.
- Supports pelvic viscera and resists downwards pressure of abdominal muscles.
- Has a sphincter action on the rectum and vagina.
- Assists in increasing intra-abdominal pressure during defecation, micturition and parturition.

Coccygeus

- Small triangular muscle behind and in the same plane as levator ani.

Origin

- Spine of ischium.

Insertion

- Side of coccyx and lowest part of sacrum.
- Muscle has same attachments as sacrospinous ligament.

Nerve supply

- Perineal branch of S4.

Action

- Holds the coccyx in its natural forwards position.
- Pelvic fascia.
- Parietal pelvic fascia is a strong membrane covering the muscles of pelvic wall and is attached to bones at margins of muscles.
- Visceral pelvic fascia is loose and cellular over movable structures, e.g. levator ani, bladder, rectum.
- It is strong and membranous over fixed or nondistensible structures, e.g. prostate.

PERINEUM

The perineum comprises:

- The anterior (urogenital) perineum.
- The posterior (anal) perineum.

Urogenital Triangle (The Anterior Perineum)

- Triangle formed by the ischiopubic inferior rami and a line joining the ischial tuberosities which passes just in front of the anus (Fig. 2.13).

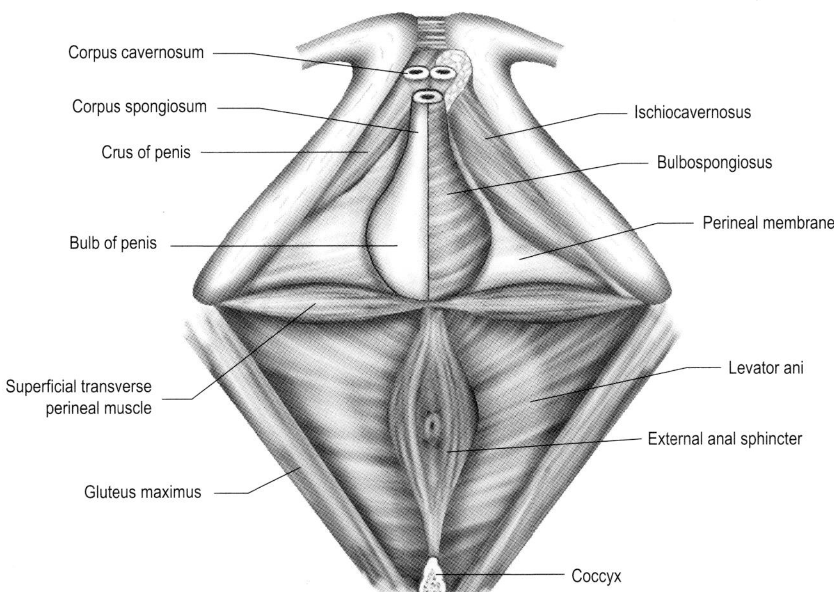

Fig. 2.13 The male perineum viewed from below. On the right side the muscles have been removed to display the crus and bulb of the penis.

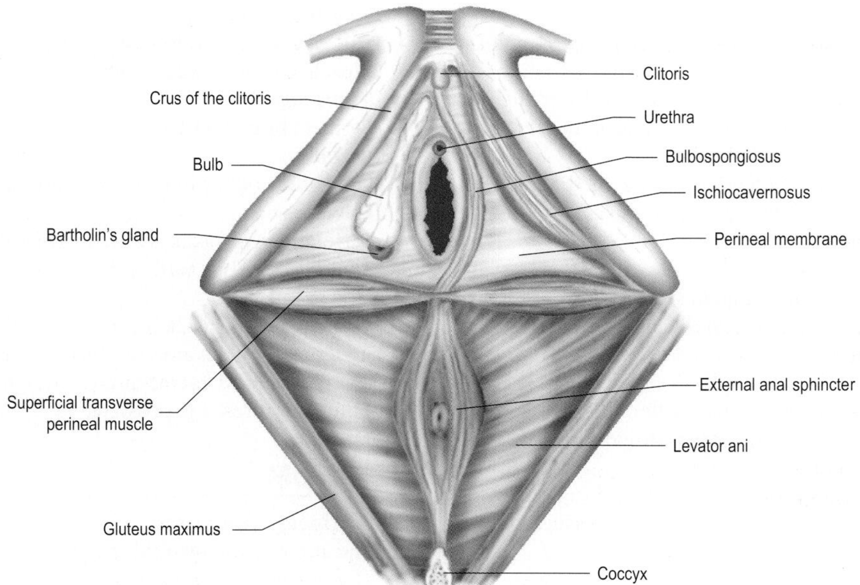

Fig. 2.14 The female perineum. On the right side the muscles have been removed to display the bulb of the vestibule and Bartholin's glands.

- The perineal membrane (the inferior fascia of the urogenital diaphragm) is a strong fascial sheath attached to the sides of this triangle.
- The perineal membrane is pierced by:
  - urethra in the male
  - urethra and vagina in the female.
- Deep to the perineal membrane is the external urethral sphincter composed of striated muscle fibres which surrounds the membranous urethra.
- The deep perineal pouch encloses the external urethral sphincter.
- Below the external urethral sphincter is the perineal membrane, while above is an indefinite layer of fascia, i.e. the superior fascia of the urogenital diaphragm.
- In the male, the deep perineal pouch contains the bulbourethral glands (of Cowper) whose ducts pierce the perineal membrane to open into the bulbous urethra.
- The pouch also contains the deep transverse perineal muscles.
- Superficial to the perineal membrane is the superficial perineal pouch.

Superficial Perineal Pouch

In the male, this contains:

- The bulb of the penis, which is attached to the undersurface of the perineal membrane; bulbospongiosus muscle covers the corpus spongiosum.
- The crura of the penis, which are attached at the angle between the insertion of the perineal membrane and ischiopubic rami; each crus is surrounded by an ischiocavernous muscle.
- Superficial transverse perineal muscle running transversely from the perineal body to the ischial ramus.
- The same muscles are present in the female but are less well developed (Fig. 2.14).

Perineal Body

- Fibromuscular nodule lying in the midline between anterior and posterior perineum.
- Attached to it are:
  - anal sphincter
  - levator ani
  - bulbospongiosus
  - transverse perineal muscles.
- Important site of insertion of levator ani; tearing of perineal body during childbirth will considerably weaken the pelvic floor.

The Posterior (Anal) Perineum

- Triangular area lying between the ischial tuberosities on each side and the coccyx.
- It contains the following:
  - anus and its sphincters
  - levator ani
  - ischiorectal fossa.

Ischiorectal Fossa

This is a space between the anal canal and side wall of the pelvis.

- Its boundaries are:
  - medially: fascia over levator ani and the external anal sphincter
  - laterally: fascia over obturator internus
  - anteriorly: extends forwards as a prolongation deep to the urogenital diaphragm
  - posteriorly: limited by the sacrotuberous ligaments and the origin of gluteus maximus from this ligament.
- Floor is formed from skin and subcutaneous fat.
- Contains mainly fat and is crossed by the inferior rectal vessels and nerves from lateral to medial side.
- The internal pudendal vessel and pudendal nerve lie on the lateral wall of the fossa in the pudendal canal (of Alcock), a tunnel of fascia which is continuous with the fascia overlying obturator internus.

Clinical Points

- Infection of the ischiorectal space may occur from boils or abscesses on the perianal skin, from lesions within the rectum and anal canal, from pelvic collections bursting through levator ani.
- The fossae communicate with one another behind the anus, allowing infection to pass readily from one fossa to another.
- The pudendal nerves can be blocked in Alcock's canal on either side, giving regional anaesthesia in forceps delivery.

Penis

The penis is divided into:

- root
- body
- glans.

Root

- The root is attached at:
  - perineal membrane
  - the pubic rami by two strong processes, the crura
  - the symphysis pubis by the suspensory ligament.

Glans

- Forms the extremity of the penis.
- At its summit is the opening of the urethra—the external meatus.
- Passing from the lower margin of the glans is a fold of mucous membrane continuous with the prepuce called the frenulum.
- At the base of the glans is a projecting edge or corona, behind which is a constriction.
- The skin of the penis is attached to the neck of the glans and doubles up on itself forming the prepuce or foreskin.

Body

- Part of the penis between the root and glans. The body comprises:
  - corpora cavernosa
  - corpus spongiosum.

Corpora cavernosa

- Placed dorsally.
- Connected together in anterior three-quarters with septum of penis intervening.
- Separated behind to form the two crura, which are attached along the medial margins of the ischial and pubic rami.
- Anteriorly, the corpora cavernosa fit into the base of the glans.
- There is a groove on the upper surface for the dorsal vein of the penis and another groove on the lower surface for the corpus spongiosum.
- Corpora cavernosa are attached to the pubic symphysis by the suspensory ligament.

Corpus spongiosum

- Commences at the perineal membrane by an enlargement, i.e. the bulb.
- Runs forward in the groove on the undersurface of the corpora cavernosa, expanding over their extremities to form the glans.
- The bulb lies below the perineal membrane and is surrounded by the bulbospongiosus muscle.
- The urethra pierces the bulb on its upper surface and runs forwards in the middle of the corpus spongiosum.

URETHRA

Male Urethra

The male urethra is 20 cm long and is divided into:

- prostatic urethra
- membranous urethra
- spongy urethra.

Prostatic Urethra

- Passes through the prostate gland from base to apex.
- Three centimetres long.
- Bears the urethral crest on the posterior wall, on each side of which is the shallow depression, the prostatic sinus, into which 15–20 prostatic ducts empty.
- In the centre of the urethral crest is a prominence (verumontanum), into which opens the prostatic utricle.
- The ejaculatory ducts formed by the union of the duct of the seminal vesicle and the terminal part of the vas deferens open on either side of the prostatic utricle.

Membranous Urethra

- Two centimetres in length.
- Contained between perineal membrane and pelvic fascia.
- Surrounded by and pierces the external sphincter urethrae.

Spongy Urethra

- Fifteen centimetres long.
- Traverses corpus spongiosum of penis.
- Passes upwards and forwards to lie below pubic symphysis and then in flaccid state, bends downwards and forwards.
- The ducts of the bulbourethral glands open on its floor.
- The urethral canal enlarges just behind the external meatus, i.e. the fossa navicularis.
- The lumen of this part of the urethra is transverse except at its meatus (narrowest part) where it is vertical, hence the spiral stream of urine.

Clinical Point

- Where the urethra passes beneath the pubis, it may be ruptured by a fall astride an object which crushes it against the edges of the symphysis (straddle injury).

Female Urethra

- Four centimetres long.
- Traverses the sphincter urethrae and lies immediately in front of the vagina.
- Its external meatus opens 2.5 cm behind the clitoris and between the labia minora.

The Vulva

The vulva is the term applied to the female external genitalia.

- The mons pubis is the eminence in front of the pubis covered in hair.
- The labia majora:
  - two prominent folds extending from the mons to the perineum
  - externally covered with hair and skin, internally with mucous membrane
  - they are the equivalent of the male scrotum.
- The labia minora:
  - lie between the labia majora as lips of soft skin which meet posteriorly in a sharp fold at the fourchette
  - surround the clitoris, the upper fold forming the prepuce of the clitoris, the lower ones attached to the glans, being the frenulum of the clitoris.
- Vestibule:
  - area enclosed by the labia minora
  - contains the urethral orifice, which lies immediately behind the clitoris
  - contains the vaginal orifice.
- Vaginal orifice:
  - guarded in the virgin by a thin mucosal fold—the hymen
  - hymen is perforated to allow menstruation
  - following childbirth, the only remnants of the hymen are a few tags named the carunculae myrtiformes.
- Clitoris:
  - corresponds somewhat in structure to the penis
  - contains two corpora cavernosa attached to the pubic rami
  - free extremity or glans is formed by the corpus spongiosum.
- The greater vestibular glands (Bartholin's glands):
  - analogous to bulbourethral glands in male
  - pea-sized mucus-secreting glands lying deep to the posterior part of the labia majora
  - ducts open on the labia minora external to the hymen
  - impalpable when healthy but obvious and palpable when inflamed or distended
  - each gland is overlapped by the bulb of the vestibule, a mass of erectile tissue equivalent to bulbospongiosus of the male
  - this erectile tissue passes forward under cover of bulbospongiosus around the sides of the vagina to the root of the clitoris.

SCROTUM

- Contains the testicles suspended by the spermatic cord.
- The skin shows a median raphe.
- A fibrous septum divides the scrotum into two cavities.
- The left cavity is longer than the right, the left testicle hanging lower.
- Skin is thin, pigmented, rugose and contains numerous sebaceous glands.
- The subcutaneous tissue is devoid of fat but contains the dartos muscle.

Clinical Points

- Scrotal subcutaneous tissue is continuous with the fascia of the abdominal wall and perineum; extravasation of urine or blood deep to this plane gravitates into the scrotum, hence frequent bruising of scrotum following hernia repair.
- Tissues of scrotum are extremely lax and because of its dependent position it fills with oedema fluid in cardiac or renal failure.

TESTIS AND EPIDIDYMIS

- Each testis is ovoid, measuring 4 cm from upper to lower pole, 3 cm anteroposteriorly and 2.5 cm from medial to lateral surface.

- Left testis lies at a lower level than the right within the scrotum.
- Covered by a fibrous white capsule, the tunica albuginea.
- Covering this is a double serous membrane into which the testis became invaginated in fetal life, i.e. the tunica vaginalis testis.
- Septae pass from the tunica albuginea dividing the testis into lobules, each lobule containing one to three tightly coiled tubules, i.e. the seminiferous tubules, in which sperm is produced.
- Testes lie outside the body because spermatogenesis requires a temperature below that of the body. Failure of the testes to descend properly leads to a malfunction in spermatogenesis and relative infertility.
- At the hilum of the testis, the seminiferous tubules drain into an irregular series of ducts called the rete testis from which afferent tubules arise, transporting the sperm into the head of the epididymis.
- Epididymis lies along posterior border of testis to its lateral side.
- Epididymis divided into head, body and tail inferiorly.
- Medially, there is a distinct groove, the sinus epididymis, between it and the testis.
- The epididymis is covered by the tunica vaginalis except at its posterior margin which is free.
- Sperm passes from the epididymis through the vasa, which join with the seminal vesicles prior to forming the common ejaculatory ducts.
- Testis and epididymis each may bear, at their upper extremities, a small stalked body named, respectively, the appendix testis and the appendix epididymis (hydatid of Morgagni).

Blood Supply

- Testicular artery arising from the aorta at the level of the renal vessels.
- Testicular artery anastomoses with artery to vas (which supplies the vas deferens and epididymis), which arises from the inferior vesical branch of the internal iliac artery.
- Anastomosis between these two arteries means that ligation of the testicular artery is not necessarily followed by testicular atrophy.
- Venous drainage is via the pampiniform plexus of veins, which usually becomes a single vessel, the testicular vein, at the deep inguinal ring.
- Right testicular vein drains into the IVC; the left into the left renal vein.

Lymphatic Drainage

- Accompany testicular veins to drain into para-aortic nodes.

Coverings of the Testis

In the surgical approach to the testis via the scrotum the following structures are encountered:

- scrotal skin
- dartos muscle
- external spermatic fascia
- cremaster muscle in cremasteric fascia
- internal spermatic fascia
- parietal layer of tunica vaginalis
- once the parietal layer of the tunica vaginalis has been incised, the visceral layer of the tunica vaginalis is seen covering the white tunica albuginea.

Clinical Points

- The testis arises at the level of L2/3 on the posterior abdominal wall. In its development it takes its vascular supply, lymphatic supply and nerve supply from this region; hence lymphatic drainage is to the para-aortic nodes, and pain from the kidney may radiate down to the scrotum and, conversely, testicular pain may radiate to the loin.
- A rapidly developing varicocele may be a presenting sign of tumour of the left kidney; tumour invades the left renal vein and blocks the drainage of the left testicular vein into the left renal vein.
- Congenital anomalies of descent of the testis are explained under embryology at the beginning of this chapter.

Vas Deferens (Ductus Deferens)

- Commences at the inferior pole of the testis as the continuation of the epididymis.
- Approximately 45 cm long.
- Thick muscular tube, which transports sperm from the epididymis to the ejaculatory ducts within the prostate gland.
- Passes through the scrotum and inguinal canal, and comes to lie on the lateral wall of the pelvis.
- At this point, lies immediately below the peritoneum of the lateral wall of the pelvis.
- Then runs towards tip of ischial spine.
- Turns medially to base of bladder.
- Vas ends by uniting with the ducts of the seminal vesicles to become the common ejaculatory duct.
- This occurs at the most superior and posterior aspect of the prostate gland.
- The common ejaculatory duct traverses the prostate to open into the prostatic urethra at the verumontanum on either side of the utricle.

ABDOMINAL VISCERA

The relationships of abdominal viscera to one another in the upper abdomen are shown in Figs. 2.15 and 2.16.

Oesophagus

Although only a small part of this is contained within the abdominal cavity, it will be dealt with here in its entirety. The oesophagus extends from the lower border of the cricoid cartilage to the cardiac orifice of the stomach. It is about 25 cm long. It has three parts:

- cervical
- thoracic
- abdominal.

Cervical

- Passes downwards and slightly to left.

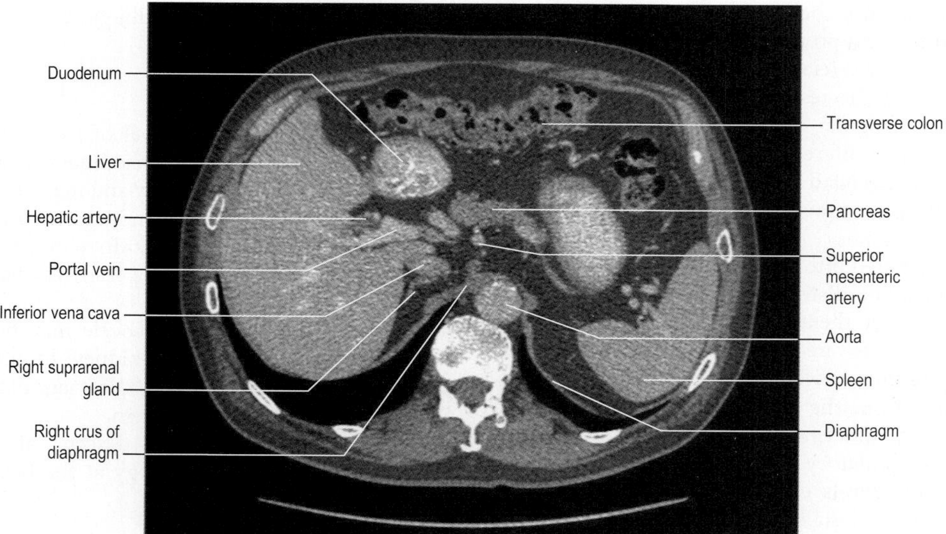

Fig. 2.15 CT scan passing through the body of the 11th thoracic vertebra.

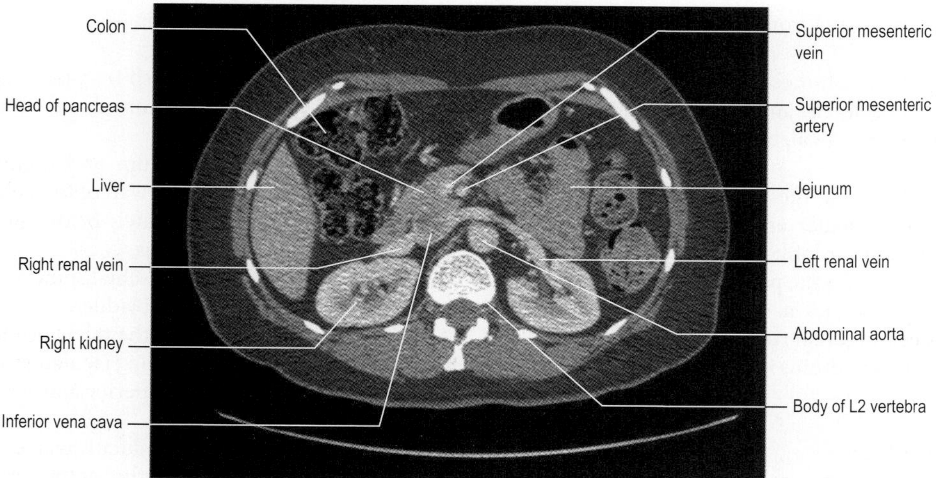

Fig. 2.16 CT scan passing through the body of the second lumbar vertebra.

- Anterior relations:
  - trachea
  - thyroid gland.
- Posterior relations:
  - lower cervical vertebrae
  - prevertebral fascia.
- To the left:
  - left common carotid artery
  - left inferior thyroid artery
  - left subclavian artery
  - thoracic duct.
- To the right:
  - right common carotid artery
  - recurrent laryngeal nerves lie on either side in the groove between trachea and oesophagus.

Thoracic

- Oesophagus passes downwards through the superior and posterior mediastinum.
- Initially passes to the right to reach the midline opposite T5.
- Then passes downwards, forwards and to the left to reach to the oesophageal hiatus in the diaphragm at T10.
- The two vagus nerves form a plexus on the surface of the oesophagus in the posterior mediastinum, the left being anterior and the right posterior.
- Anterior relations:
  - left common carotid artery
  - trachea
  - left main bronchus, which constricts it
  - pericardium separating it from left atrium and the diaphragm.
- Posterior relations:
  - thoracic vertebrae
  - thoracic duct
  - hemiazygos vein
  - the descending aorta below.
- To the left side:
  - left subclavian artery
  - aortic arch
  - left vagus nerve and its recurrent laryngeal branch
  - thoracic duct
  - left pleura.
- To the right side:
  - right pleura
  - azygos vein.

Abdominal

- Passes through oesophageal opening in the right crus of the diaphragm at level T10.
- Lies in a groove on the posterior surface of the left lobe of the liver with the left crus of the diaphragm behind.
- Covered anteriorly and to left with peritoneum.
- Anterior vagus nerve is closely applied to the surface behind its peritoneal covering.
- Posterior vagus nerve is at a little distance from the posterior surface of the oesophagus.

Blood Supply

- In the neck: from the inferior thyroid arteries.
- In the thorax: from branches of the aorta.
- In the abdomen: from the left gastric and inferior phrenic arteries.
- Venous drainage:
  - cervical part to inferior thyroid veins
  - thoracic part to azygos veins
  - abdominal part to azygos vein (systemic) and partly to the left gastric veins (portal).

Nerve Supply

- Upper third: parasympathetics via recurrent laryngeal nerve and sympathetic nerves from the middle cervical ganglion via the inferior thyroid artery.
- Below the root of the lung, the vagi and sympathetic nerves contribute to the oesophageal plexus.

Microscopic Structure

The oesophagus consists of:

- Mucous membrane lined by stratified squamous epithelium (occasionally there is gastric mucosa in the lower part of the oesophagus).
- Submucosa containing mucous glands.
- Muscular layer consisting of inner circular and outer longitudinal muscle.
- In the upper third, muscle is striated, producing rapid contraction and swallowing.
- In the lower two-thirds, it is composed of smooth muscle exhibiting peristalsis.
- Outer layer of loose areolar tissue.

Clinical Points

- There are three narrow points in the oesophagus at which foreign bodies may impact:
  - commencement of the oesophagus (17 cm from the upper incisor teeth)
  - point at which it is crossed by left main bronchus (28 cm from incisor teeth)
  - termination (43 cm from upper incisor teeth).
- In the lower oesophagus there is a site of portosystemic anastomosis; between the azygos vein (systemic) and the oesophageal tributary of the left gastric vein

(portal). Oesophageal varices may arise at this site in portal hypertension.

- Left atrial enlargement owing to mitral stenosis may be noted on a barium swallow, which shows marked backwards displacement of the oesophagus by the dilated atrium.

Stomach

- Approximately 'J' shaped.
- Two surfaces: anterior and posterior.
- Two curvatures: greater and lesser curve.
- Two orifices: cardia and pylorus.
- Initially projects to the left, the dome-like gastric fundus projecting above the level of the cardia.
- In the erect living subject, the vertical part of the 'J' shape of the stomach represents the upper two-thirds of the stomach.
- Lesser curve of stomach is vertical in its upper two-thirds but then turns upwards and to the right where it becomes the pyloric antrum.
- Junction of body with pyloric antrum marked along the lesser curve by a notch—the incisura angularis.
- Body of stomach lies between cardia and pylorus.
- Pyloric antrum is a narrow area immediately before the pylorus.
- Left margin of stomach is the greater curvature.
- In the erect subject, this may reach or lie below the umbilicus.
- Greater curvature then passes upwards to the right as the lower margin of the pyloric antrum.
- The lesser omentum is attached to the lesser curvature of the stomach.
- The greater omentum is attached to the greater curvature of the stomach.
- The thickened pyloric sphincter surrounds the pyloric canal.
- Junction of pylorus with duodenum is marked by a constant prepyloric vein of Mayo, which crosses it vertically.

Relations

- Anteriorly: from left to right, the diaphragm, abdominal wall and left lobe of the liver.
- Posteriorly: separated from diaphragm, aorta, pancreas, spleen, left kidney and suprarenal gland, transverse mesocolon and colon by lesser sac of peritoneum.

Blood Supply

The blood supply (Fig. 2.17) is via:

- the left gastric artery, which is derived from the coeliac axis and runs along the lesser curvature of the stomach where it anastomoses with the right gastric branch of the hepatic artery
- the right gastric artery from the hepatic artery
- the right gastroepiploic artery: arises from the gastroduodenal branch of the hepatic artery and anastomoses along the greater curve with the left gastroepiploic artery
- left gastroepiploic artery arises from splenic artery
- the short gastric arteries arise from the splenic artery
- venous drainage follows the arteries

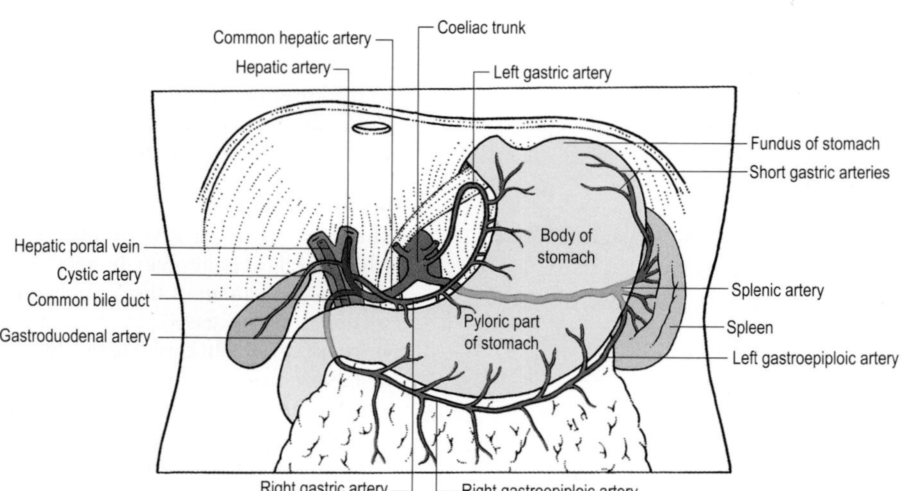

Fig. 2.17 The arterial blood supply of the stomach.

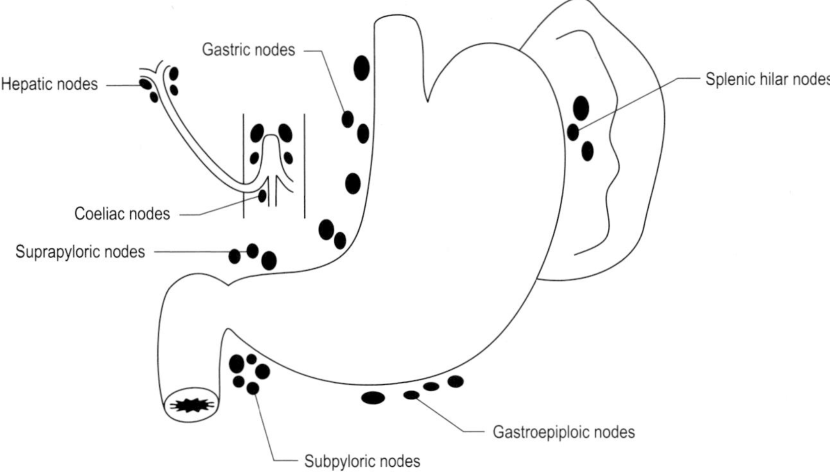

Fig. 2.18 The lymphatic drainage of the stomach.

- venous drainage is into the portal system
- stomach has such a rich blood supply that ligation of three of the four main arteries does not compromise its blood supply.

Lymphatic Drainage (Fig. 2.18)

- Area of stomach supplied by splenic artery drains via lymphatics accompanying that artery to lymph nodes at the hilum of the spleen, and then to those situated along the upper border of the pancreas and eventually to the coeliac nodes.
- Cardiac area of the stomach drains along the left gastric artery to reach the coeliac nodes.
- The remainder of the stomach drains as follows:
  - via branches of the hepatic artery through nodes along the lesser curve to the coeliac nodes
  - through nodes along the right gastroepiploic vessels to the subpyloric nodes and then to the coeliac nodes.
- Retrograde spread of carcinoma may occur into the hepatic lymph nodes at the porta hepatis—enlargements of these nodes may cause external compression of the bile ducts with obstructive jaundice.
- Extensive and complex lymphatic drainage of stomach creates problems in dealing with gastric cancer—involvement of nodes around coeliac axis may render growth incurable.

Nerve Supply

- Anterior and posterior vagus nerves enter the abdomen through the oesophageal hiatus.
- Anterior vagus nerve lies close to wall of oesophagus but posterior nerve is at a little distance from the wall of the oesophagus.
- Anterior vagus gives off hepatic branch and pyloric branch to the pyloric sphincter.
- Posterior vagus nerve gives off coeliac branch passing to coeliac axis before sending a gastric branch to the posterior surface of the stomach.
- Gastric divisions of both anterior and posterior vagi reach the stomach at the cardia and descend along the lesser curve between the anterior and posterior peritoneal attachments of the lesser omentum.
- These nerves are referred to as the anterior and posterior nerves of Latarjet.
- Nerve supply of stomach has become largely of historical interest, as operations to divide the vagus nerve are rarely carried out nowadays following the advent of H_2 receptor antagonists, proton pump inhibitors and the discovery of the role of *Helicobacter pylori* in the aetiology of peptic ulceration.

Structure of the Gastric Mucosa (Fig. 2.19)

- The surface of the gastric mucosa is covered by columnar epithelial cells that secrete mucus and alkaline fluid that protect the epithelium from mechanical injury and from gastric acid.
- The gastric mucosa can be divided into three areas:
  - cardiac gland area via gastro-oesophageal junction containing principally mucus-secreting cells
  - acid-secreting region (oxyntic gland area) containing parietal (oxyntic cells) and chief (zymogen) cells

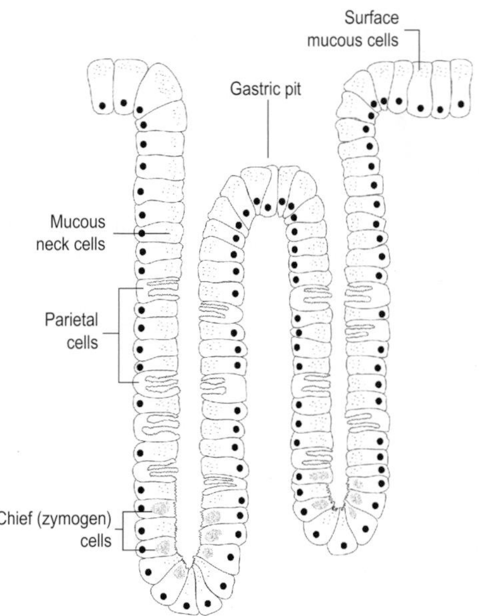

Fig. 2.19 A gastric gland and its cells.

- pyloric end area constituting the distal 30% of the stomach: contains 'G' cells that produce gastrin together with mucus-secreting cells.
- Histological features of the mucosa in the oxyntic gland area are shown in Fig. 2.19.

Clinical Points

- An ulcer on the lesser curve of the stomach may erode into either the right or left gastric arteries, resulting in haematemesis and melaena.
- A posterior gastric ulcer or carcinoma may erode the pancreas, giving rise to pain referred to the back.

Duodenum

- 'C' shaped.
- Curves round the head of the pancreas and is approximately 25 cm (10 inches) long.
- Divided into four parts.

First Part

- Approximately 5 cm long.
- Ascends from the pylorus, being directed superiorly, posteriorly and to the right.
- First 2–3 cm has a complete investment of visceral peritoneum.
- Relations:
  - anteriorly: liver and gall bladder
  - posteriorly: portal vein, common bile duct, gastroduodenal artery; behind these is the IVC.

Second Part

- Descends as a curve around the head of the pancreas.
- Approximately 7.5 cm long.
- Bile ducts and main pancreatic ducts enter the second part of the duodenum together at the duodenal papilla on its posteromedial side.
- Point of entry marks junction of foregut and midgut.
- Accessory pancreatic duct of Santorini opens into the duodenum a little above the papilla.
- The second part of the duodenum is crossed by the transverse colon and lies anteriorly to the right kidney and ureter.

Third Part

- Approximately 10 cm long.
- Runs horizontally to left.
- Crosses the IVC, the aorta and third lumbar vertebra.
- Crossed anteriorly by the root of the mesentery and superior mesenteric vessels.

Fourth Part

- Approximately 2.5 cm long.
- Ascends vertically to end by turning abruptly anteriorly to the left to continue as the jejunum.
- At the DJ flexure, the small intestine leaves the posterior abdominal wall and acquires a mesentery.
- At surgery the DJ flexure may be identified by the presence of the suspensory ligament of Treitz—a peritoneal fold descending from the right crus of the diaphragm to the termination of the duodenum.

Blood Supply of the Duodenum

- Superior pancreaticoduodenal artery arising from the gastroduodenal artery.
- Inferior pancreaticoduodenal artery originating from the superior mesenteric artery.
- These two arteries lie in the curve between the duodenum and head of the pancreas, supplying both the duodenum and head of the pancreas.

Clinical Point

- The relationship of the gastroduodenal artery to the first part of the duodenum is important because erosion of posterior duodenal ulcers into the gastroduodenal artery will cause haematemesis and melaena.

Small Intestine

- Variable in length, averaging some 6 m.
- Upper half is termed the jejunum, the remainder the ileum, although the distinction between the two is not sharply defined.
- Jejunum and ileum lie in free edge of mesentery.

- The mesentery of the small intestine is about 15 cm long and attached across the posterior abdominal wall.
- Commences at DJ flexure to the left of the second lumbar vertebra and passes obliquely downwards to the right sacroiliac joint.
- From left to right the root of the mesentery crosses anterior to the following structures:
  - third part of the duodenum
  - aorta
  - IVC
  - right psoas major muscle
  - right ureter
  - right gonadal vessels
  - right iliacus muscle.
- Mesentery contains:
  - the superior mesenteric vessels, which enter the mesentery anterior to the third part of the duodenum
  - lymph nodes draining the small intestine
  - autonomic nerve fibres.
- At surgery the following factors serve to distinguish the jejunum from the ileum:
  - the jejunum has a thicker wall owing to circular folds of mucosa (valvulae conniventes or plicae circulares), which are larger and more numerous than in the ileum
  - the jejunum is of greater diameter than the ileum
  - in the mesentery of the jejunum, the arteries form one or two arcades some distance from the free edge of the mesentery, and long straight branches from these arcades run to supply the jejunum. In the ileum, the arterial supply forms several rows of arcades in the mesentery, and the final straight arteries to the ileum are shorter and more numerous than in the jejunum
  - the mesentery becomes thicker and more fat-laden from above downwards
  - in general, the jejunum is most likely to be found at or above the level of the umbilicus while the ileum tends to lie below the level of the umbilicus in the hypogastrium and pelvis.

Large Intestine

The large intestine extends from the ileocaecal junction to the anus. It is approximately 1.5 m in length in average. It is divided into:

- caecum with the vermiform appendix
- ascending colon
- hepatic flexure
- transverse colon
- splenic flexure
- descending colon
- sigmoid colon
- rectum
- anal canal.

Caecum

- Dilated blind-ended pouch situated in the right iliac fossa.
- Usually completely covered by peritoneum.
- Ileocaecal valve lies on the left side of the junction between caecum and ascending colon.
- Appendix rises from the posteromedial aspect of the caecum about 2.5 cm below the ileocaecal valve.

Ascending Colon

- Extends from the caecum to the undersurface of the liver where, at the hepatic flexure, it turns left to become the transverse colon.
- Covered on anterior and lateral aspects by peritoneum.
- Posterior relations include:
  - iliacus
  - quadratus lumborum
  - perirenal fascia over lateral aspect of kidney.

Transverse Colon

- Passes to the left where it becomes the descending colon at the splenic flexure.
- Attached to the anterior border of the pancreas by the transverse mesocolon.
- Relations:
  - superiorly: liver, gall bladder, greater curvature of stomach and spleen
  - inferiorly: coils of small intestine
  - anteriorly: anterior layers of the greater omentum
  - posteriorly: right kidney, second part of duodenum, pancreas, small intestine and left kidney.

Descending Colon

- Passes from splenic flexure to sigmoid colon.
- Peritoneum covers its anterior and lateral surfaces.
- Between the splenic flexure and diaphragm is a fold of peritoneum, the phrenicocolic ligament.
- Relations:
  - posteriorly: left kidney, quadratus lumborum and iliacus
  - anteriorly: coils of small intestine.

Sigmoid Colon

- Commences at pelvic brim and extends to rectosigmoid junction.
- Has a mesentery which is occasionally extensive, allowing sigmoid colon to hang down into pelvis.
- Root of sigmoid colon crosses the external iliac vessels and left ureter.

- The sigmoid loop rests on the bladder in the male and is related to the uterus and posterior fornix of the vagina in the female.

Taenia Coli

- Three flattened bands of longitudinal muscle which pass from the caecum to rectosigmoid.
- Converge at the base of the appendix.
- The taenia are shorter than the length of the bowel, hence the sacculated appearance of the large bowel.
- There are no taenia coli on the appendix or rectum.

Appendices Epiploicae

- Fat-filled tags scattered over the surface of the colon.
- Most numerous in the sigmoid colon.
- Absent on the appendix, caecum and rectum.

Appendix

- Attached to posteromedial aspect of the caecum below the ileocaecal valve.
- Variable in length but usually 5–10 cm.
- Position is variable:
  - 75% lies behind the caecum or colon, i.e. retrocaecal or retrocolic
  - 20% pelvic
  - 5% preileal or retroileal.
- Bears a mesentery containing the appendicular artery, which is a branch of the ileocolic artery.
- Appendix mesentery descends behind the ileum as a triangular fold containing the appendicular artery in its free edge.

Clinical Points

- The appendicular artery is an end-artery and therefore, in acute appendicitis, if it thromboses there is a consequent rapid development of gangrene with perforation of the appendix.
- The lumen of the appendix is relatively wide in infancy and often obliterated in the elderly. Since obstruction of the appendicular lumen is a usual precipitating cause of acute appendicitis, it is therefore uncommon at the extremes of life.
- A long pelvic appendix may hang down and irritate the bladder, giving rise to frequency of micturition, simulating cystitis.

Rectum

The rectum is about 12 cm (5 inches) long, commencing anterior to the third segment of the sacrum and ending about 2.5 cm in front of the coccyx, where it bends sharply backwards to become the anal canal.

- Peritoneal coverings:
  - extraperitoneal on its posterior aspect
  - upper third: covered by peritoneum on its front and sides
  - middle third: covered by peritoneum only on its anterior aspect
  - lower third: completely extraperitoneal, lying below the pelvic peritoneum.
- Curved to follow the contour of the sacral hollow.
- Three lateral inflexions projected to the left, right and left again from above downwards.
- Each inflexion is capped by a valve of Houston.

Relations

- Anteriorly:
  - in the male lie the rectovesical pouch, base of bladder, seminal vesicles and prostate
  - a layer of fascia (of Denonvilliers) lies in front of the rectum, separating it from the prostate
  - in the female lie the rectouterine pouch (of Douglas) and posterior wall of the vagina
  - the upper two-thirds of the rectum is covered with peritoneum anteriorly and related to coils of small bowel and the sigmoid colon in the rectovesical or rectouterine pouch.
- Posteriorly: sacrum, coccyx, lower sacral nerves, middle sacral artery.
- Laterally: below peritoneal reflexion lie the levator ani and coccygeus.

Blood Supply of the Large Intestine (Fig. 2.20)

- Supplied by branches of both the superior and inferior mesenteric artery.
- The branches of the superior mesenteric artery are:
  - the ileocolic artery, supplying the caecum and commencement of the ascending colon
  - the right colic artery, supplying the ascending colon
  - the middle colic artery, supplying the transverse colon.
- The branches of the inferior mesenteric artery supplying the colon are:
  - the left colic artery, supplying the descending colon
  - the sigmoid branches, supplying the sigmoid colon
  - the superior rectal artery, supplying the rectum.
- Each branch of the superior and inferior mesenteric artery anastomoses with its neighbour above and below, establishing a continuous chain of anastomosis along the length of the colon known as the marginal artery (of Drummond).
- The superior rectal artery supplies the whole of the rectum and the upper half of the canal, while the inferior rectal artery supplies the lower half of the anal canal.

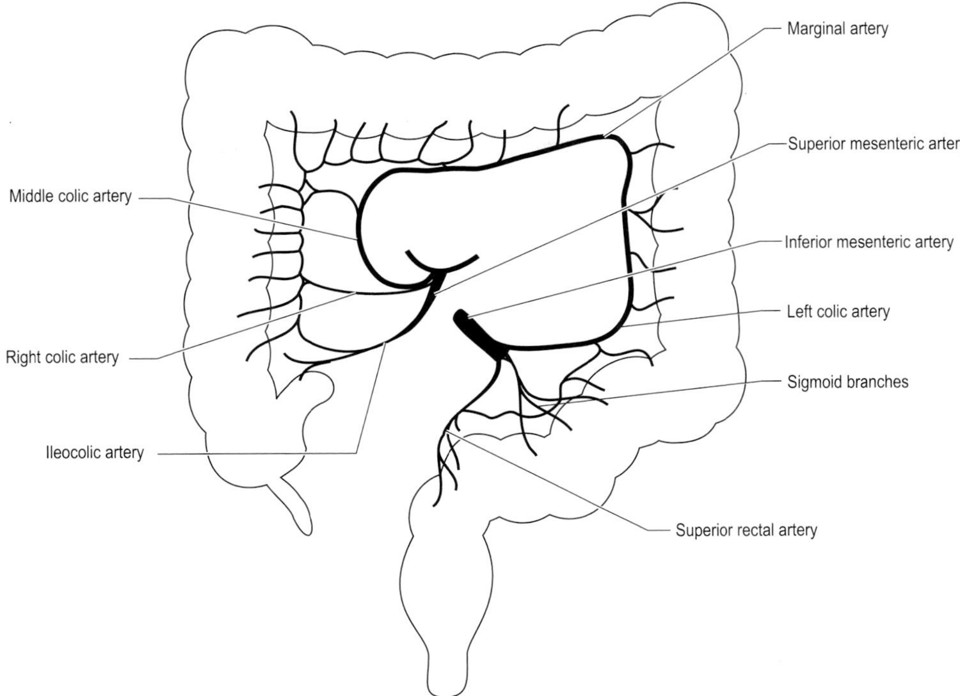

Fig. 2.20 The arterial blood supply of the large intestine.

- The middle rectal artery is small and supplies only the muscle coats of the rectum.
- When the superior rectal artery reaches the rectum, it first divides into two branches, which run either side of the rectum, then the right branch divides into two further branches. These branches descend to the level of the anal valves, where they anastomose with branches of the inferior rectal artery.
- They are accompanied by tributaries of the superior rectal vein draining into the portal system.
- The position of these vessels, one on the left and two on the right, explain why haemorrhoids occur at 3, 7 and 11 o'clock when the anal canal is viewed with the patient in the lithotomy position.

Clinical Points

- The marginal artery is weakest and sometimes deficient where the superior and inferior mesenteric artery distributions meet just proximal to the splenic flexure. Diminution of the blood supply in this region may lead to the condition known as ischaemic colitis.
- The marginal artery is also important in allowing the surgeon to transpose large segments of colon as far as the neck or thorax to replace segments of oesophagus, the bowel depending on the marginal artery for its blood supply.

Lymphatic Drainage of the Large Intestine

- Lymphatics drain to small lymph nodes lying near to or even on the bowel wall.
- These drain to further groups lying along the blood vessels.
- These then drain to nodes near the origins of the superior and inferior mesenteric arteries.
- Efferent vessels from these join to drain into the cisterna chyli.
- The field of lymphatic drainage of each segment of bowel corresponds more or less to its arterial blood supply.
- High ligation of the vessels to the involved segment of bowel with the removal of a wide surrounding segment of mesocolon and bowel wall will result in the removal of lymph nodes draining that particular area, e.g. division of the inferior mesenteric artery and resection of sigmoid mesocolon would be performed for carcinoma of the sigmoid colon.

Anal Canal

The anal canal is about 4 cm long and passes downwards and backwards.

- Surrounded by a complex arrangement of sphincters consisting of smooth and striated muscle.
- At the midpoint of the canal there is a series of vertical columns in the mucosa (the columns of Morgagni).
- At the distal end of the vertical columns are some valve-like folds (the anal valves of Ball).
- Behind these valves are the anal sinuses into which open the anal glands.
- The upper half of the anal canal is lined with columnar epithelium.
- The lower half is lined with stratified squamous epithelium transforming into skin near the anal verge.
- The boundaries between these zones are not clear-cut.
- The upper half of the anal canal is derived from endoderm; the lower half is derived from ectoderm. There are some important anatomical facts with clinical significance resulting from this derivation of the anal canal. They are as follows:
  - the upper half is lined by columnar epithelium and the lower half with stratified squamous epithelium; consequently, carcinoma of the upper anal canal is adenocarcinoma while that of the lower part is a squamous cell carcinoma
  - the upper half of the anal canal is supplied by the autonomic nervous system; the lower part has somatic innervation from the inferior rectal nerve. The lower part of the anal canal is sensitive to pinprick sensation while the upper part is not. This is an important factor when injecting haemorrhoids
  - the upper half of the anal canal drains into the portal venous system whereas the lower half drains into the systemic venous system. This therefore is an important site of portosystemic anastomosis in portal hypertension
  - the lymphatic drainage of the upper half of the anal canal is along the superior rectal vessels to the abdominal nodes; whereas below this site, drainage is to the inguinal nodes. This is clinically important as a carcinoma of the rectum which invades the lower anal canal may metastasize to inguinal lymph nodes.

Anal Sphincters

- The anal canal is surrounded by a complex arrangement of muscles.
- The internal anal sphincter is composed of smooth muscle continuous above with the circular muscle of the rectum. It surrounds the upper two-thirds of the canal and is supplied by sympathetic nerves.
- The external anal sphincter is composed of striated muscle, which surrounds the internal anal sphincter but extends further distally (Fig. 2.21).
- The external anal sphincter is divided into three parts:
  - subcutaneous
  - superficial, which is attached to the coccyx behind and the perineal body in front
  - deep, which is continuous with the puborectalis part of levator ani.
- The deep part of the external sphincter where it blends with levator ani together with the internal anal sphincter is termed the anorectal ring.
- The anorectal ring is palpable with a finger in the anal canal where it forms a ring, immediately above which the finger enters the ampulla of the rectum.
- The subcutaneous part of the external anal sphincter is traversed by a fan-shaped expansion of longitudinal muscle fibres of the anal canal.

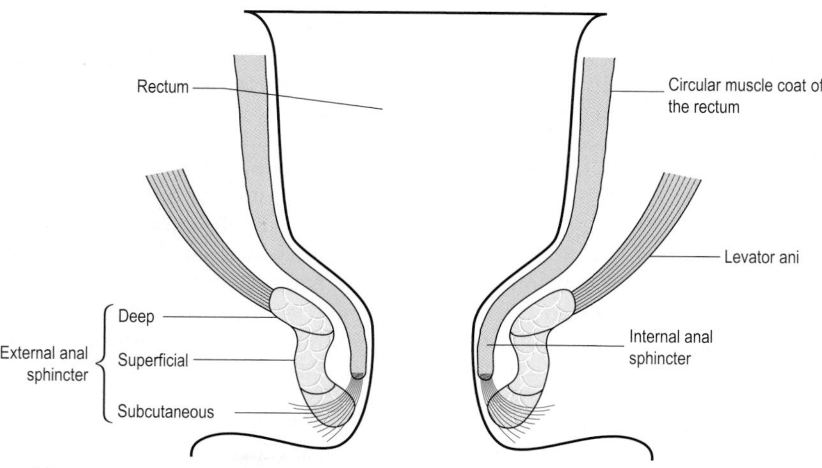

Fig. 2.21 The anal sphincters.

- The nerve supply of the external sphincter is via the inferior rectal branch and the pudendal nerve (S2, S3) and the perineal branch of S4.

Rectal Examination

The following structures can be palpated by the finger passed per rectum in the normal patient.

- Both sexes:
  - anorectal ring
  - coccyx
  - sacrum
  - ischiorectal fossae
  - ischial spines.
- Male:
  - prostate
  - rarely, the seminal vesicles.
- Female:
  - perineal body
  - cervix
  - occasionally, the ovaries.

The following abnormalities can also be detected.

- Lumen:
  - faecal impaction
  - foreign bodies.
- In the wall:
  - rectal tumours
  - rectal strictures
  - thrombosed haemorrhoids (haemorrhoids are not palpable unless thrombosed).
- Outside rectal wall:
  - prostatic abnormalities
  - abnormalities of the uterine cervix
  - ovarian enlargement
  - masses in the pouch of Douglas
  - tenderness in the pouch of Douglas with peritonitis
  - pelvic bony tumours
  - foreign bodies in the vagina, e.g. tampon, pessary or others.

Liver

The liver is the largest organ in the body. It lies across the right hypochondrium, epigastrium and left hypochondrium. It is divided into two unequal lobes by a fold of peritoneum, the falciform ligament. It has the following features.

- Superior surface: dome-shaped; related to the diaphragm, which separates it from the pleura, lungs, pericardium and heart.
- Posteroinferior surface is related to the abdominal oesophagus, stomach, duodenum, hepatic flexure of the colon, right kidney and right suprarenal gland.
- The posteroinferior surface is covered with peritoneum except where the gall bladder is attached and at the porta hepatis and the fissure for the ligamentum venosum.
- The posterior surface is connected to the diaphragm over the right lobe of the liver by the coronary ligament, between the two layers of which is a non-peritonealized area, i.e. the bare area.
- To the left of the bare area is the caudate lobe, which bounds the lesser sac in front.
- The anatomical right and left lobes of the liver are separated anteriorly and superiorly by the falciform ligament, and posteroinferiorly by the H-shaped arrangement of the fossae (Fig. 2.22).

Porta Hepatis

- Gateway to and from the liver.
- Contains the following structures:
  - common hepatic duct anteriorly
  - hepatic artery in the middle
  - portal vein posteriorly.
- Contains lymph nodes which, when enlarged by malignancy, may compress the bile ducts and cause obstructive jaundice.

Peritoneal Relations of the Liver (Fig. 2.23)

- The liver is almost completely covered by peritoneum, except for the bare area in which the IVC is embedded.
- Bare area is between upper and lower leaves of coronary ligament.
- Upper and lower leaves of coronary ligament fuse to form the right triangular ligament.
- Falciform ligament passes upwards from umbilicus to right of midline, the ligamentum teres running in its free border.
- Falciform ligament passes over dome of liver and separates, its right part joining the upper leaf of the coronary ligament, while the left part forms part of the left triangular ligament, the latter being attached to the peritoneum on the undersurface of the diaphragm.
- The left triangular ligament, when traced to the right and posteriorly, joins the lesser omentum in the fissure for the ligamentum venosum.
- The left triangular ligament contains no major blood vessels and therefore may be divided safely so that the left lobe of the liver may be retracted to expose the oesophagus.
- The lesser omentum arises from the fissure for the ligamentum venosum and porta hepatis and passes as a sheet to be attached along the lesser curve of the stomach.
- The free edge of the lesser omentum contains the common bile duct to the right, the hepatic artery to the left and the portal vein posteriorly.

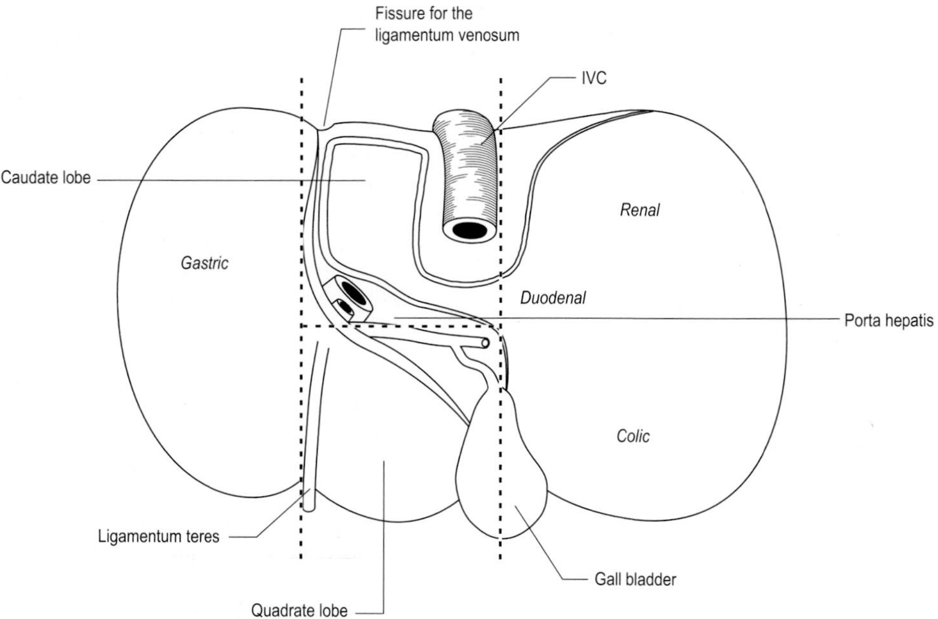

Fig. 2.22 The inferior aspect of the liver. The H-shape (dotted line) demonstrates the various fissures, the groove for the inferior vena cava (IVC) and the fossa for the gall bladder. The sites of impressions of the various relations are indicated in italics.

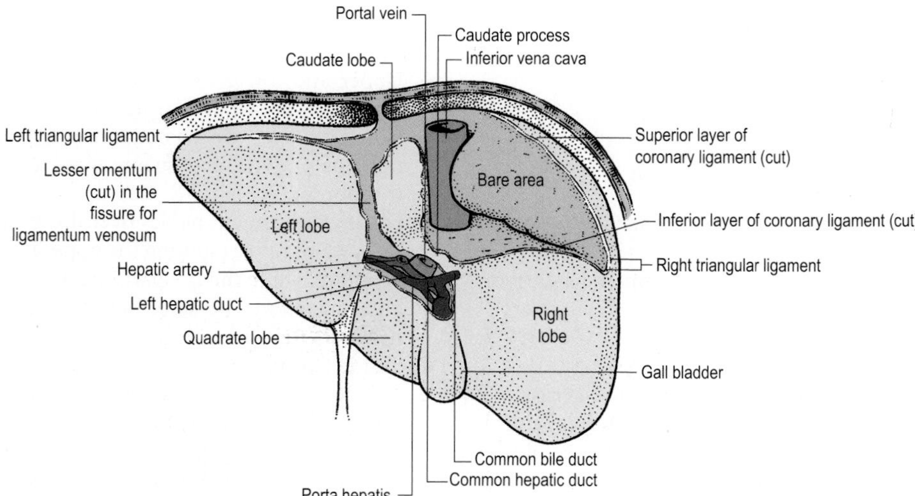

Fig. 2.23 The liver—posterior view.

Functional Anatomy of the Liver

- The gross anatomical division of liver into right and left lobes demarcated by falciform ligament anteriorly and fissure for ligamentum teres and ligamentum venosum posteroinferiorly is not pertinent to understanding of the surgical anatomy of the liver.
- Functional anatomy is based on the description of hepatic segmentation, which divides the liver into

segments according to the distribution of portal pedicles and location of hepatic veins.

- Functional division of liver into right and left lobes is not demarcated by any visible line on the surface of the liver.
- The division is through a plane which passes through the gall bladder fossa and fossa for the IVC.
- Each of these two functional lobes has its own arterial and portal venous blood supply and its own biliary drainage.
- Surgical division of the right hepatic artery and the right branch of the portal vein is followed by a clear demarcation on the liver surface running anteroposterior from the gall bladder fossa to the IVC in the principal vascular plane.
- These two functional lobes are further subdivided into segments, each lobe being divided into four segments (Fig. 2.24).

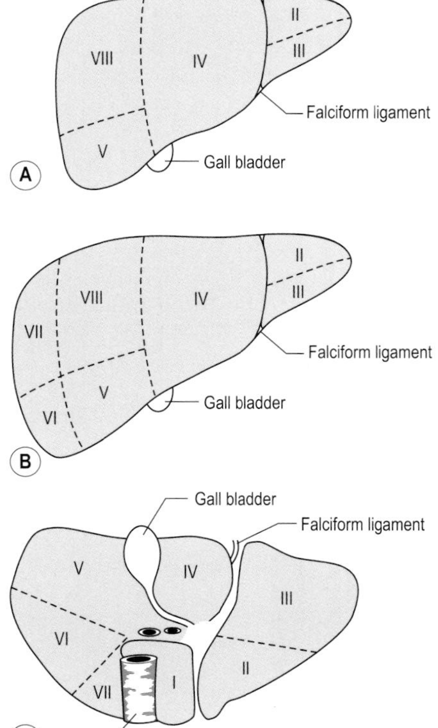

Fig. 2.24 The functional division of the liver into segments. (A) Anterior view, as seen in the patient. (B) Anterior view with the liver 'flattened' in the ex-vivo position (note that segments VI and VII may now be seen—in vivo they appear more laterally and posteriorly). (C) Inferior view.

Hepatic Veins

- There are three main hepatic veins:
  - right
  - central
  - left.
- They pass backwards and upwards from the substance of the liver, draining into the IVC at the superior limit of the liver.
- The caudate lobe of the liver has independent hepatic veins which drain directly into the IVC.
- Three main hepatic veins divide the liver into four sectors, each of which receives a portal pedicle, with an alternation between hepatic veins and portal pedicles (Fig. 2.25).
- The middle hepatic vein lies at the line of the principal plane of the liver between its right and left functional lobes.
- Terminology in liver resection is based on function and segmental anatomy.
- A right hemihepatectomy would involve segments V, VI, VII and VIII.
- A left hemihepatectomy would involve segments II, III and IV.
- Excision of the anatomical left lobe of the liver would involve only segments II and III.
- Excision of the functional left lobe of the liver would involve segments II, III, IV and possibly I.

Extrahepatic Biliary System (Fig. 2.26)

Right and left hepatic ducts join at the porta hepatis to form the common hepatic duct.

- Common hepatic duct is joined by cystic duct to form bile duct (common bile duct).
- Bile duct is about 9 cm long, commencing approximately 4 cm above the duodenum then passing behind it.
- Bile duct runs in a groove on the posterior aspect of the head of the pancreas before opening into the medial aspect of the second part of the duodenum.
- In 90% of individuals, the main pancreatic duct joins the common bile duct to form a common dilated channel, i.e. the ampulla of Vater.
- The opening of the ampulla of Vater into the duodenum is guarded by the sphincter of Oddi (periampullary sphincter).
- Occasionally bile duct and pancreatic ducts open separately into the duodenum.
- There may be an additional duct, which receives ducts from the lower part of the head of the pancreas, known as the accessory pancreatic duct. It opens into the medial wall of the second part of the duodenum about 2 cm proximal to the main duodenal papilla (endoscopists should be aware of these anatomical variations).

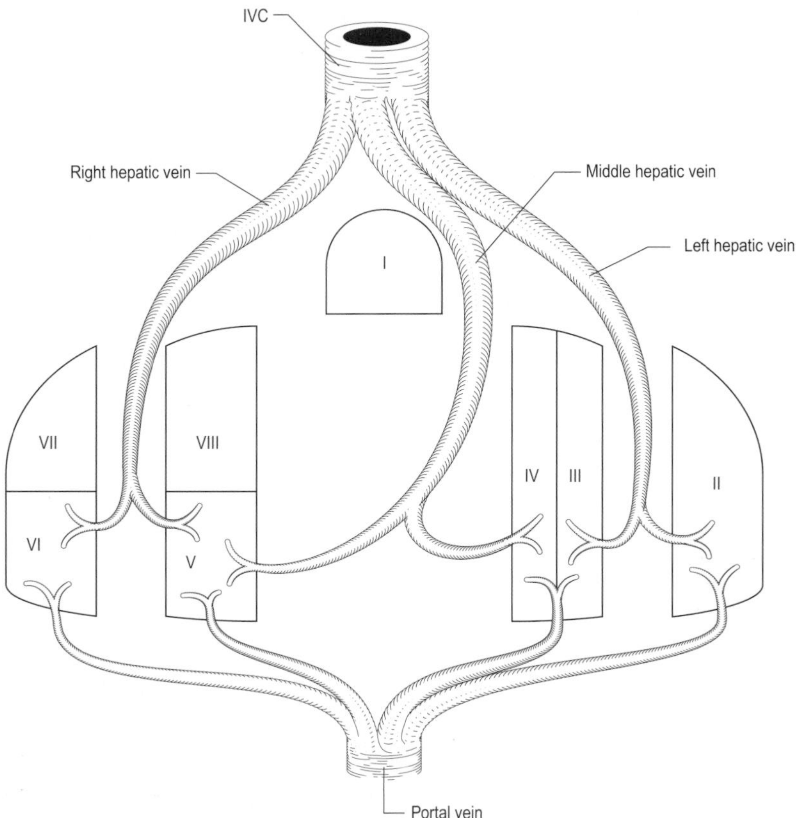

Fig. 2.25 A schematic representation of the functional anatomy of the liver. The three main hepatic veins divide the liver into four sectors, each of which receives a portal pedicle.

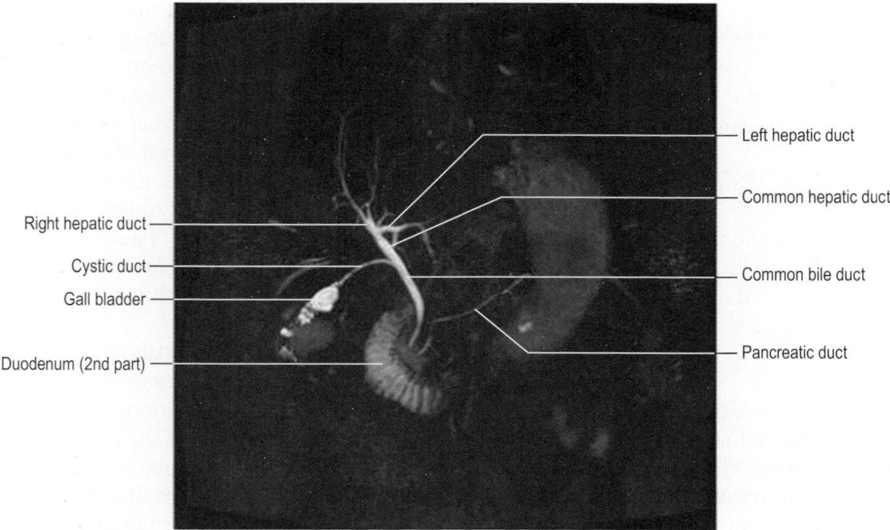

Fig. 2.26 Magnetic resonance cholangiopancreatogram (MRCP).

- The common hepatic duct and supraduodenal part of the common bile duct lie in the free edge of the lesser omentum. Their relations are as follows:
  - bile duct: anteriorly to the right
  - hepatic artery: anteriorly to the left
  - portal vein: posterior
  - IVC, posteriorly: separated from the portal vein by the epiploic foramen.

Gall Bladder

- Pear-shaped organ adherent to the undersurface of the liver, lying in a fossa which separates the morphological right and left lobes.
- Acts as a reservoir for bile, which it also concentrates.
- Holds about 50 mL of bile when physiologically distended.
- The gall bladder consists of:
  - fundus
  - body
  - neck: the neck opens into the cystic duct, which conveys bile to and from the common bile duct.
- The lumen of the cystic duct contains a spiral mucosal valve (of Heister).
- The gall bladder is related inferiorly to the duodenum and transverse colon.
- A small pouch may be present on the ventral aspect of the gall bladder just proximal to the neck (Hartmann's pouch); a stone may lodge in the pouch.

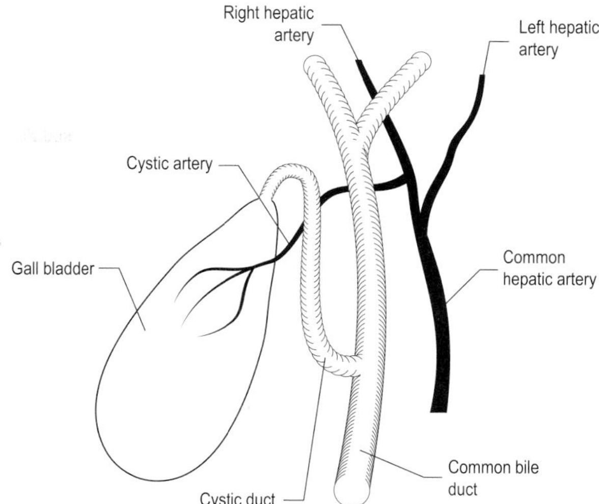

Fig. 2.27 The gall bladder and its arterial supply.

Blood Supply (Fig. 2.27)

- Via the cystic artery (usually a branch of the right hepatic artery).
- Cystic artery lies in a triangle made up of the liver, the cystic duct and the common hepatic duct, i.e. Calot's triangle.
- Cystic artery passes behind the common hepatic duct and cystic duct to gain the upper surface of the neck of the gall bladder.
- Occasionally the cystic artery arises from the main hepatic artery and crosses in front of or behind the (common) bile duct or common hepatic duct.
- Gall bladder also obtains a blood supply directly from arteries in the bed of the liver.
- Venous drainage is via small veins draining directly into the bed of the liver.

Clinical Points

- Variations in the anatomy of the extrahepatic biliary system are not uncommon (Fig. 2.28).
- The close relationship between the fundus of the gall bladder and duodenum may result in inflamed gall bladder ulcerating into the duodenum, causing a cholecystoduodenal fistula and subsequent gallstone 'ileus'.
- Haemorrhage during cholecystectomy or from liver trauma may be controlled by compressing the hepatic artery and portal vein in the free edge of the lesser omentum (Pringle's manoeuvre).
- Gangrene of the gall bladder is rare because, even if the cystic artery thromboses, it gets a second blood supply directly from the liver bed.
- The wall of the gall bladder and cystic duct contains smooth muscle. This is virtually absent in the bile duct, hence little pain from a gallstone in the bile duct.
- The mucosa is lined throughout by columnar cells and bears a considerable number of mucus-producing goblet cells.
- When the neck of the gall bladder is obstructed, bile is absorbed and the goblet cells produce mucus, resulting in a mucocele of the gall bladder.

The Portal Venous System (Fig. 2.29)

- A portal system is one that has capillaries at each end.
- The portal venous system drains blood from:
  - the abdominal part of the alimentary canal (excluding the lower part of the anus)
  - spleen
  - pancreas
  - gall bladder.

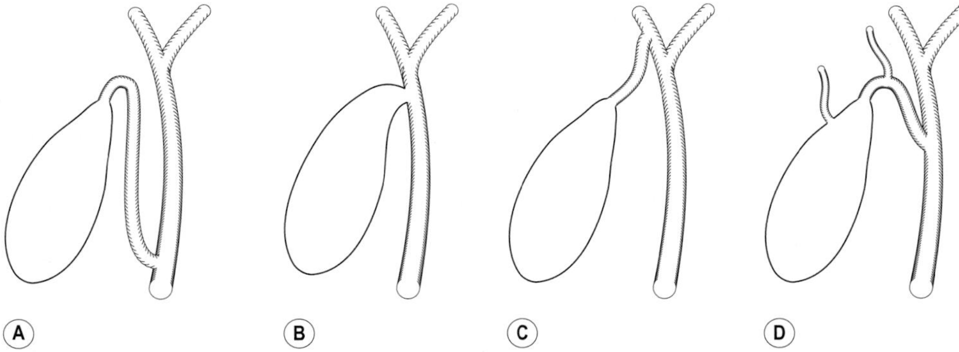

Fig. 2.28 Variations in the extrahepatic biliary anatomy. (A) A long cystic duct joins the common hepatic duct behind the duodenum. (B) The cystic duct is short or absent, the gall bladder opening directly into the common hepatic duct. (C) The cystic duct enters the right hepatic duct. (D) Accessory hepatic ducts may open into the gall bladder or cystic duct.

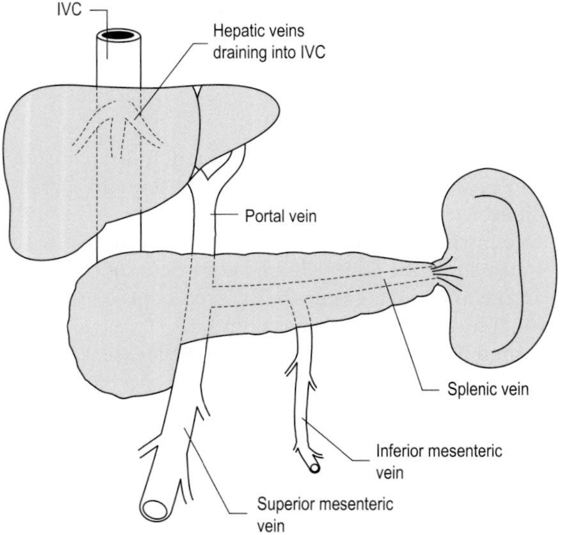

Fig. 2.29 The portal venous system.

- Portal vein is formed by the junction of the splenic vein and superior mesenteric vein behind the neck of the pancreas.
- Inferior mesenteric vein ascends above the point of origin of its artery to enter the splenic vein behind the body of the pancreas.
- Portal vein ascends behind first part of duodenum, entering the free edge of the lesser omentum in the anterior wall of the foramen of Winslow.
- At this point it lies immediately posterior to bile duct and hepatic artery.
- Portal vein ascends to porta hepatis where it divides into right and left hepatic branches, breaking up into capillaries running between the lobules of the liver.
- These capillaries drain into the radicles of the hepatic vein, eventually emptying into the IVC.
- There are no valves in the portal system so that obstruction, e.g. due to cirrhosis of the liver, causes a rise in pressure throughout the system.
- To escape, the blood passes through any anastomosis between portal and systemic system and the anastomotic veins become dilated and may bleed.
- Sites of anastomosis between portal and systemic venous system are:
  - between the oesophageal branch of the left gastric vein (portal) and the oesophageal tributaries of the azygos system (systemic); in the presence of portal hypertension oesophageal varices will develop that may be the source of severe haematemesis
  - between the superior rectal branch of the inferior mesenteric vein (portal) and the inferior rectal veins (systemic); this may give rise to dilated veins in the anal canal which bleed
  - between the portal tributaries in the mesentery and retroperitoneal veins (systemic), resulting in retroperitoneal varices
  - between the portal veins in the liver and the veins of the abdominal wall (systemic) via veins passing along the falciform ligament to the umbilicus; this may result in the formation of a group of dilated veins radiating out from the umbilicus known as a caput medusae
  - between portal branches in the liver and the veins of the diaphragm (systemic) in relation to the bare area of the liver.

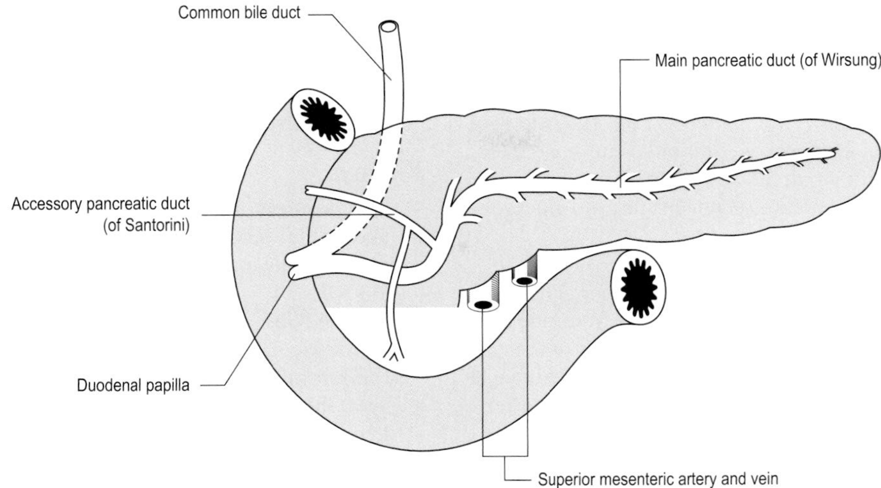

Fig. 2.30 The pancreas and duodenum, showing the common bile duct and pancreatic ducts with their orifices.

Clinical Point

- Surgery on patients with portal hypertension may be very complicated and very bloody. This is because of dilated veins in the abdominal wall, in the mesentery and in the retroperitoneal area. Pressure in these veins may be extremely high, resulting in considerable portal venous bleeding.

Pancreas

The pancreas lies retroperitoneally in the upper abdomen in the transpyloric plane. It is divided into:

- head
- uncinate process
- neck
- body
- tail.

The head of the pancreas lies in the C-shape of the duodenum and is continuous with the uncinate process below, which passes posterior to the superior mesenteric vessels as they in turn pass from behind the head of the pancreas and into the root of the mesentery (Fig. 2.30).

Relations

- The head of the pancreas is adherent to the medial aspect of the C-shaped portion of the duodenum and lies in front of the IVC, renal vessels and superior mesenteric vessels.
- The uncinate process lies behind the superior mesenteric vessels.
- The common bile duct passes through a groove on the posterior aspect of the head of the pancreas.
- The stomach and first part of the duodenum lie partly in front of the head of the pancreas, separated from it by the lesser sac.
- Behind the neck of the pancreas lies the junction of the superior mesenteric vein and splenic vein, forming the portal vein.
- The body of the pancreas is in contact posteriorly with the aorta, the left crus of the diaphragm, and the suprarenal gland and left kidney.
- The tail of the pancreas lies at the splenic hilum.
- The tortuous splenic artery runs along the superior border of the pancreas.
- The splenic vein runs behind the pancreas.
- The transverse mesocolon is attached along the anterior aspect of the pancreas.
- Below the attachment of the transverse mesocolon, the DJ flexure, the left flexure of the colon and the small intestine lie in relation to the gland.
- The main pancreatic duct (of Wirsung) passes along the gland from the tail to the head, joining the common bile duct before entering the medial aspect of the second part of the duodenum at the ampulla of Vater.
- The accessory duct (of Santorini) passes from the lower part of the head in front of the main duct, usually communicating with it, and, if present, opens into the duodenum approximately 2 cm proximal to the ampulla of Vater.

Structure

- Gland encapsulated by fibrous capsule sending septae into the gland, forming lobules.

- Lobules composed of acini of serous cells, which secrete pancreatic enzymes.
- Ducts lined by cuboidal epithelium drain secretions into pancreatic ducts.
- Scattered throughout the pancreas are the islets of Langerhans, which appear as spheroidal clusters of pale-staining cells with a rich blood supply.
- Cells of islets of Langerhans secrete insulin and glucagon.

Blood Supply

- From splenic artery via arteria pancreatica magna.
- Supply to head and uncinate process is from superior pancreaticoduodenal artery, which is a branch of the gastroduodenal artery, and the inferior pancreaticoduodenal artery, which is a branch of the superior mesenteric artery.

Lymphatics

- These drain into:
  - nodes along the upper border of the pancreas
  - nodes related to the medial aspect of the duodenum and head of the pancreas
  - nodes in the root of the mesentery.

Spleen

- About the size of the patient's clenched fist.
- Lies in the left hypochondrium.
- Forms the left lateral extremity of the lesser sac.
- The gastrosplenic ligament connects it to the greater curvature of the stomach (carries the short gastric and left gastroepiploic vessels).
- The lienorenal ligament connects it to the posterior abdominal wall (carries the tail of the pancreas and the splenic vessels).

Relations

- Anteriorly: the stomach.
- Posteriorly: the left part of the diaphragm separating it from the pleura, left lung and 9th, 10th and 11th ribs.
- Inferiorly: the splenic flexure of the colon.
- Medially: the left kidney.

Blood Supply

- Via the splenic artery, which is a branch of the coeliac axis.
- The splenic vein is joined by the superior mesenteric vein to form the portal vein.
- The splenic artery and vein, lymph nodes and the tail of the pancreas are enclosed in the lienorenal ligament.

Clinical Points

- Trauma to the left lower chest wall and left upper abdomen may result in damage to the spleen; look particularly for fractures of the left lower ribs.
- Accessory spleens (splenunculi) occur near the hilum, tail of the pancreas, omentum, small bowel mesentery; if left behind they may hypertrophy and result in persistence of symptoms following splenectomy, e.g. for thrombocytopenic purpura.

Kidneys

- The kidneys lie retroperitoneally on the posterior abdominal wall. The right kidney lies lower than the left owing to downward displacement by the liver.

Relations (Figs. 2.31 and 2.32)

- At the medial aspect of the kidney there is a vertical slit, the hilum, which transmits from backwards the renal vein, the renal artery and the pelvis of the ureter.
- Lymphatics and nerves also enter at the hilum.

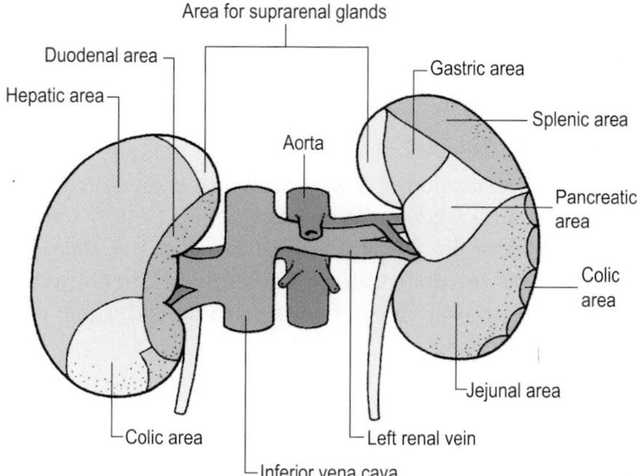

Fig. 2.31 The anterior surfaces of the kidneys and their relations.

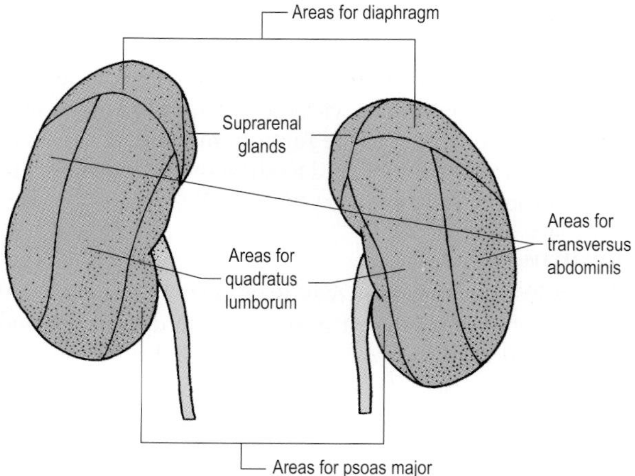

Fig. 2.32 The posterior relations of the kidneys.

- The kidney lies in a fatty cushion (perinephric fat) contained within the renal fascia.
- Above, the renal fascia blends with the fascia over the diaphragm, leaving a separate compartment for the suprarenal gland (it is therefore easily separated from the kidney and left behind during a nephrectomy).
- Medially, the fascia blends with the sheaths of the aorta and IVC.
- Laterally, it is continuous with transversalis fascia.
- It remains open inferiorly.
- The kidney has three capsules:
  - fascial (renal fascia)
  - fatty (perinephric fat)
  - a true fibrous capsule, which strips readily from the kidney surface.

Blood Supply

- From the renal artery directly from the aorta.
- The renal vein drains into the IVC.
- The left renal vein (which is longer than the right and receives two tributaries), the adrenal and gonadal vein (which passes in front of the aorta immediately below the origin of the superior mesenteric artery).
- The right renal artery passes behind the IVC.
- Aberrant vessels are common.

Lymphatic Drainage

- Lymph drains directly to the para-aortic lymph nodes.

Clinical Points

- Hypermobility of the kidney may occur (floating kidney): the kidney can be moved up and down in its fascial compartment, but not from side to side.
- Blood from a traumatic rupture of the kidney or pus in a perinephric abscess will distend the renal fascia and then take the line of least resistance, tracking down within the fascial compartment to the pelvis.
- Anatomy of surgical exposure of the kidney via a loin approach:
  - an oblique incision is made halfway between the 12th rib and iliac crest, extending forwards from the lateral border of erector spinae to the lateral border of rectus abdominis
  - latissimus dorsi and serratus posterior inferior are divided
  - the free posterior border of external oblique is identified and split along the line of its fibres
  - internal oblique and transversus are then divided, revealing peritoneum anteriorly
  - the peritoneum is swept forwards
  - the renal fascial capsule is opened
  - the subcostal nerve and vessels are usually encountered and are preserved
  - if more room is required, the lateral edge of quadratus lumborum is divided and part of the 12th rib excised, being careful not to damage the pleura which descends below the medial half of the rib.

Ureter

- Conveys urine from kidneys to bladder.
- Each ureter is 25–30 cm long and approximately 3 mm in diameter.
- The ureter is a hollow muscular tube which commences at the renal pelvis and terminates at its entry into the bladder.
- The upper end of each ureter is expanded at the pelvis, which is divided into two parts called major calyces. These are subdivided into about 12 minor calyces.
- Papillae project into the calyces, the latter being the apices of the renal pyramids.
- The ureter is divided into three parts:
  - abdominal
  - pelvic
  - intravesical.
- Relations of the ureter in the abdomen:
  - anterior: peritoneum, colic vessels, testicular or ovarian vessels, ileum and mesentery (right side), sigmoid colon and sigmoid mesocolon (left side)
  - posteriorly: psoas major, psoas minor tendon (occasionally), genitofemoral nerve and bifurcation of common iliac artery
  - the right ureter lies close to the lateral side of the IVC.
- Relations in the pelvis:
  - In the male:
    - each ureter enters the pelvis by crossing the bifurcation of the common iliac artery; runs down to ischial spine, crossing the obturator nerve and the anterior branches of the internal iliac artery; turns medial to reach the bladder and passes below the vas deferens just before entering the bladder.
  - In the female:
    - course as above for male, but ureter crosses close to the lateral fornix of the vagina below the uterine artery and posterior part of bladder, and ends as in male.
- Narrowest parts of ureter are:
  - pelviureteric junction
  - at the brim of the pelvis
  - at entry to bladder.
- Calculus may impact at one of these three areas.

Blood Supply

- The ureter receives a rich segmental blood supply from:

- renal arteries (may receive a considerable contribution from a lower polar artery)
- testicular or ovarian artery
- internal iliac artery
- inferior vesical arteries.

Clinical Points

- Ureter readily identified at operation as it strips up with the peritoneum and worm-like movements can be noticed in its wall, particularly if it is stimulated by the tip of a pair of forceps.
- A ureteric stone on a plain radiograph may be seen along the course of the ureter projected onto the bony skeleton:
  - runs along the tips of the transverse processes
  - crosses in front of the sacroiliac joint
  - swings out on the pelvic wall and crosses the ischial spine
  - passes medially to bladder.

Suprarenal Glands

- Asymmetrical.
- Right is pyramidal and embraces the upper pole of the right kidney.
- Left is crescentic and embraces the medial border of the left kidney above the hilum.

Relations

- Anteriorly: right side—liver, IVC; left side—stomach across the lesser sac.
- Posteriorly: the diaphragm.
- Inferiorly: the upper pole of the kidney.

Blood Supply

- A branch from the aorta.
- A branch from the inferior phrenic artery.
- A branch from the renal artery.
- Venous drainage on the right is via a short vein directly into the IVC.
- Venous drainage on the left is by a longer vein into the left renal vein.

Structure

- Comprises a cortex and a medulla.
- Medulla derived from neural crest (ectoderm).
- Cortex derived from mesoderm.
- Medulla receives preganglionic sympathetic fibres from the greater splanchnic nerve and secretes adrenaline and noradrenaline.
- The cortex secretes mineralocorticoids (from zona glomerulosa), glucocorticoids (from zona fasciculata) and sex hormones (from the zona reticularis).

Bladder

The bladder is a distensible reservoir with muscular walls. It lies in the true pelvis posterior to the symphysis pubis. It does not rise above the pubis until it is very full. When fully distended, the adult bladder projects from the pelvic cavity into the abdomen, lifting the peritoneum upwards from the abdominal wall as it distends.

Relations

- Anteriorly: the pubic symphysis.
- Superiorly: covered by peritoneum with coils of small intestine and sigmoid colon resting on it. The relationship between the sigmoid colon and bladder is important in diverticular disease when a colovesical fistula may arise. In the female the body of the uterus lies superior to the bladder.
- Posteriorly: in the male, the rectum and seminal vesicles; in the female, the vagina and supravaginal part of the cervix.
- Laterally: the bladder is separated from levator ani and obturator internus muscle by loose connective tissue.
- The neck of the bladder fuses with the prostate in the male.
- In the female it lies directly on the pelvic fascia surrounding the short urethra.

Blood Supply

- Superior and inferior vesical arteries, which are branches of the anterior division of the internal iliac artery.
- Rich venous plexus around the bladder, draining into the internal iliac veins.

Lymphatic Drainage

- Drainage along the vesical vessels to the internal iliac nodes and then to the para-aortic nodes.

Nerve Supply

- Efferent parasympathetic fibres from S2, S3, S4 accompany the vesical arteries to the bladder and carry motor fibres to muscles of bladder wall and inhibitory fibres to internal sphincter.
- Sympathetic efferent fibres carry inhibitory fibres to bladder muscles and motor fibres to its sphincter.
- The external sphincter is made up of striated muscle supplied by the pudendal nerve.
- Sensory fibres, stimulated by distension, are conveyed in both sympathetic and parasympathetic nerves.

Cystoscopy

- Inspection of the interior of the bladder and three orifices, i.e. the internal meatus and both ureters.

- Submucosa and mucosa of most of bladder are only loosely adherent to underlying muscles, and are thrown into folds when bladder is empty.
- Over the trigone, the mucosa is adherent and remains smooth even in the empty bladder.
- Between the ureters there is a raised fold of mucosa called the interureteric ridge.

Prostate

The prostate surrounds the prostatic urethra. There are two principal components to the prostate:

- glandular component
- smooth muscle component.

Approximately 25% of the normal prostate is composed of smooth muscle. The majority of the prostate lies on the lateral and posterior aspect of the urethra with little anterior prostatic tissue.

Relations

- Anteriorly: the pubic symphysis separated by the extraperitoneal fat of the retropubic space (cave of Retzius).
- Posteriorly: the rectum separated by the fascia of Denonvilliers.
- Superiorly: the prostate is continuous with the neck of the bladder.
- Inferiorly: the apex of the prostate rests on the external urethral sphincter within the deep perineal pouch.
- Laterally: levator ani.

Clinically, the prostate is divided into lobes:

- the posterior lobe lies posterior to the urethra and inferior to the plane defined by the course of the ejaculatory ducts
- a median lobe lies between the ejaculatory ducts and posterior to the urethra
- two lateral lobes (right and left lobes) are separated by a shallow posterior median groove, which can be felt on rectal examination
- anterior to the urethra there is a narrow isthmus only, consisting of mainly fibromuscular tissue.

Normally there are two prostatic capsules but, with benign prostatic hypertrophy, a third develops.

- True capsule: a thin, fibrous sheath surrounding the prostate.
- The false capsule: condensed extraperitoneal fascia continuous with the fascia surrounding the bladder and with the fascia of Denonvilliers posteriorly—the prostatic venous plexus lies between the true and false capsules.
- Pathological capsule: benign prostatic hypertrophy compresses the normal peripheral part of the gland, creating a capsule.
- In enucleation of the prostate for benign prostatic hypertrophy, it is the plane between the adenomatous mass and the pathological capsule that is entered.

Blood Supply

- Via the inferior vesical artery, which is a branch of the internal iliac artery.
- Venous drainage is via the prostatic venous plexus, which drains into the internal iliac vein on each side.
- Some venous blood drains posteriorly around the rectum to the valveless vertebral veins of Batson—this may explain why prostatic carcinoma metastasizes early to the bones of the lumbar spine and pelvis.

Seminal Vesicles

- Lie one on each side in the interval between the base of the bladder anteriorly and the rectum posteriorly.
- Lie lateral to the termination of vas deferens.
- Each seminal vesicle has a common drainage with its neighbouring vas via the common ejaculatory duct.
- The normal vesicles are usually impalpable on rectal examination; however, if they are enlarged by infection, e.g. tuberculosis, they become palpable.

Uterus (Fig. 2.33)

The uterus is a pear-shaped organ, which is approximately 7 cm long, 5 cm from side to side at its widest point and 3 cm anteroposteriorly. It is composed of:

- fundus
- body
- cervix.

The fallopian tubes enter into each supralateral angle, which lie above the fundus.

Relations

- Anteriorly: the body of the uterus is related to the uterovesical pouch of peritoneum and lies on either the superior surface of the bladder or occasionally on coils of intestine. The part of the cervix lying outside of the vagina is related directly to the bladder, whereas the infravaginal cervix has the anterior fornix as an immediate anterior relation.
- Posteriorly: lies the rectouterine pouch (of Douglas), which is directly related to coils of intestine lying in the pouch.
- Laterally: lies the broad ligament; the ureter lies superiorly and lateral to the supravaginal cervix.

Blood Supply (Fig. 2.34)

- The uterine artery (from the internal iliac artery) runs in the base of the broad ligament, and about 2 cm lateral to the cervix, it passes anterior and superior to the ureter, reaching the uterus at the level of the internal os.

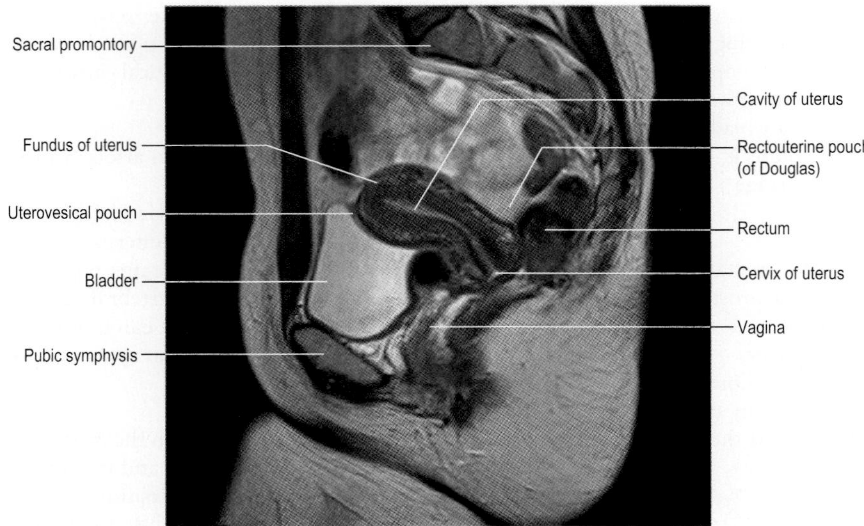

Fig. 2.33 Sagittal MRI through the female pelvis showing the uterus and its relations.

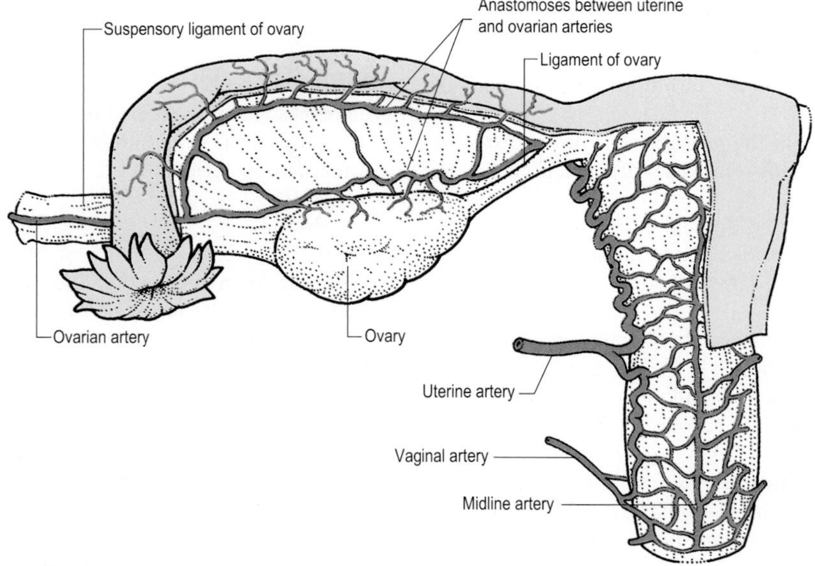

Fig. 2.34 The arterial supply of the ovary, uterine tube, uterus and vagina.

- The uterine artery then ascends in a tortuous manner, running up the lateral side of the body of the uterus before turning laterally and inferiorly to the uterine tube (fallopian tube), where it terminates by anastomosing with the terminal branches of the ovarian artery.
- The uterine artery also gives off a descending branch, which supplies the cervix and upper vagina.
- Uterine veins accompany the arteries, draining to the internal iliac vein.

Lymphatic Drainage

Lymphatics from the uterus drain as follows.

- The fundus:
  - drains along the ovarian vessels to the para-aortic nodes

- some drains with lymphatics, which pass via the round ligament to the inguinal nodes
- metastases from the fundus of the uterus therefore may occur in the inguinal nodes.
- Body drains via lymphatics in the broad ligament to the iliac lymph nodes.
- The cervix drains in three directions:
  - laterally via the broad ligament to the external iliac nodes
  - posteriorly in the uterosacral fold to the sacral lymph nodes
  - posterolaterally along the uterine vessels to the internal iliac nodes.

Fallopian Tubes

The fallopian or uterine tubes are 10–12 cm long and run from the lateral side of the body of the uterus to the pelvic wall, where they end by opening near the ovary. The opening of the fallopian tube is called the ostium. The broad ligament of the peritoneum is draped over the fallopian tube like a sheet over a washing line.

- Each tube comprises the following parts:
  - the infundibulum: this is the trumpet-shaped extremity which opens into the peritoneal cavity at the ostium. Its opening is fimbriated and overlies the ovary
  - the ampulla, which is wide, thin-walled and tortuous
  - the isthmus, which is narrow, straight and thick-walled
  - the intramural part.
- The fallopian tube:
  - is covered by peritoneum except for the intramural part
  - contains a muscular coat of outer longitudinal and inner circular fibres
  - is lined by mucosa in the form of columnar–ciliated cells and lies in longitudinal ridges, each of which is thrown into numerous folds
  - functions to propel ova along the lumen to the uterus, accompanied by muscular contraction, ciliary action and the production of lubricating fluid.
- A fertilized ovum may occasionally implant ectopically in the tube—this gives rise to ectopic pregnancy, which may cause rupture of the tube with intraperitoneal haemorrhage.
- The distal end of the tube is open into the peritoneal cavity, providing direct communication between the peritoneum and the outside, and is therefore a potential pathway for infection.

Broad Ligament

- A fold of peritoneum which connects the lateral margin of the uterus with the side wall of the pelvis. The broad ligament contains or attaches to the following structures:
  - the fallopian tube in its free edge
  - the round ligament
  - the ovarian ligament
  - the uterine vessels and branches of the ovarian vessels
  - the mesovarium attaching the ovary to its posterior aspect
  - lymphatics.
- In the base of the broad ligament, the ureter passes forwards to the bladder lateral to and then immediately above the lateral fornix of the vagina.

Vagina

- A muscular tube approximately 7 cm in length.
- The cervix opens into the anterior wall superiorly, bulging into the vaginal lumen.
- The vagina forms a ring around the cervix and, although this ring is continuous, it is divided into anterior, posterior and lateral fornices.
- It surrounds the cervix of the uterus and then passes downwards and forwards through the pelvic floor to open into the vestibule (the area enclosed by the labia minora and containing the urethral orifice lying immediately behind the clitoris).

Relations

- Anteriorly: cervix enters the vagina above, and below this is the base of the bladder and the urethra, which is embedded in the anterior vaginal wall.
- Posteriorly: the posterior fornix is covered by peritoneum in the rectouterine pouch (of Douglas). Below this, the anterior wall of the rectum is immediately posterior to the vagina, and below that, the anal canal is separated from it by the perineal body.
- Superiorly: the ureter lies superior and lateral to the lateral fornix.
- Laterally: levator ani and pelvic fascia.

Blood Supply

- The arterial blood supply is derived from several sources on each side:
  - the vaginal artery
  - the uterine artery
  - the middle rectal artery
  - the internal pudendal artery supplying the lower third.
- Venous drainage is via a plexus of veins in the connective tissue around the vagina draining into the internal iliac vein.

Lymphatic Drainage

- From the upper and middle third drain into the external iliac nodes.
- From the lower third drains into the superficial inguinal nodes.

Ovary

- Size and shape of an almond.
- Attached to the posterior aspect of the broad ligament by the mesovarium.
- The superior pole is attached to a prominent fold of peritoneum, the suspensory ligament of the ovary, which passes upwards over the pelvic brim and external iliac vessels to merge with the peritoneum over psoas major.
- Ovarian artery gains access to the ovary through the mesovarium and suspensory ligament.
- A further ligament, the ovarian ligament, runs within the broad ligament to the cornu of uterus.

Relations

- Extremely variable in position.
- Lies on the side wall of the pelvis in a shallow ovarian fossa surrounded by the external iliac vessels in front and the ureter and internal iliac vessels behind.
- Fascia over obturator internus forms the floor of this fossa and obturator nerve is close by.
- Ovary is very variable in position and may prolapse into the pouch of Douglas.
- Relations of the ovary are of considerable importance clinically. They may be divided into:
  - structures within the broad ligament
  - structures on the lateral wall of the pelvis
  - abdominal and pelvic viscera.

Blood Supply

- From the ovarian artery, which is a branch of the aorta arising at the level of the renal artery.
- The right ovarian vein drains into the IVC.
- The left ovarian vein drains into the left renal vein.

Lymphatic Drainage

- Follows the ovarian arteries to the para-aortic nodes.

Vaginal examination

- Inspection of the introitus while the patient strains detects uterine prolapse and stress incontinence.
- Anteriorly, the urethra, bladder and pubis may be felt.
- Posteriorly, the rectum may be felt and the presence of invasion of the posterior vaginal wall by a rectal neoplasm assessed; abnormalities may be felt in the pouch of Douglas, e.g. ovarian lesions, malignant deposits.
- Laterally, the ovary, tube and side wall of the pelvis may be felt; rarely a stone may be palpated in the ureter via the lateral fornix.
- At the apex, the cervix is felt projecting back from the anterior wall of the vagina. In the normal anteverted uterus the anterior lip of the cervix presents first; in retroversion either cervical os or posterior lip are felt first; cervical neoplasia can be felt.
- Bimanual examination assesses pelvic size, size of uterus, position of uterus, enlargement of ovary, abnormalities of uterine tube.

OSCE SCENARIOS

OSCE Scenario 2.1

A 19-year-old male presents with a history of vague central abdominal pain of 8 h duration. He has now developed a sharp pain in the right iliac fossa which is exacerbated by moving and coughing. He has a temperature of 37.4°C and a white cell count of 15×10^9/L. He is tender with rebound in the right iliac fossa. A provisional diagnosis is made of acute appendicitis and he elects for an open appendicectomy.

1. Explain the anatomical basis for the two types of pain he has experienced.
2. Describe the structures encountered in a gridiron incision for appendicectomy.
3. What variations in position of the appendix may be encountered when attempting to locate the appendix?

OSCE Scenario 2.2

A 40-year-old male presents with severe pain in the right loin radiating into the right groin. A diagnosis of right ureteric colic is made and a plain abdominal radiograph is requested.

1. Where would you look for the course of the ureter projected onto the bony skeleton?
2. At which points along the course of the ureter is a stone likely to impact?
3. How would you identify the ureter during an extraperitoneal approach?
4. What is the blood supply of the ureter and why, when removing a kidney for transplantation, is it important to leave abundant connective tissue around the ureter?

OSCE Scenario 2.3

A 40-year-old female has had two attacks of acute cholecystitis and has recently had an attack of biliary colic. She has been admitted for laparoscopic cholecystectomy.

1. Describe biliary colic. What causes it?
2. What is Calot's triangle?
3. Why is a knowledge of the structures in the free edge of the lesser omentum important while performing gall bladder surgery?
4. What may result from the close relationship between the fundus of the gall bladder and the duodenum?
5. Gangrene of the gall bladder with perforation is rare, even if the cystic artery has thrombosed. Why?

OSCE 2.4

A 78-year-old male is brought into the Accident and Emergency department with a history of a sizeable fresh blood haematemesis. He has a history of peptic ulcer disease. He is hypotensive and tachycardic.

1. Describe your initial management of this patient?
2. What are the potential options for treating bleeding duodenal ulcers?
3. Which vessel is most commonly involved in bleeding duodenal ulcers—describe its anatomy?
4. Name three other causes of upper GI bleeding.

OSCE 2.5

A 62-year-old male presents to his GP with weight loss, abdominal pain, jaundice and a palpable gallbladder. He has dark urine and pale stools.

1. What are three potential causes for his jaundice?
2. What is Courvoisier's Law?
3. What would you expect to see on the liver function tests?

Answers in Appendix pages 433–436

Please check your eBook at https://studentconsult.inkling.com/ for more self-assessment questions. See inside cover for registration details.

3

The Upper Limb and Breast

THE PECTORAL GIRDLE

The pectoral girdle consists of two bones:

- Clavicle.
- Scapula.

These are joined to:

- The axial skeleton at the sternoclavicular joint.
- Each other at the acromioclavicular joint.

THE BONES OF THE UPPER LIMB

Scapula (Fig. 3.1)

- Extends from the second to the seventh ribs posteriorly (when arm is by the side).
- Spine, acromion and coracoid process are easily palpable.
- The glenoid fossa laterally contributes to the shoulder joint.
- Rotation of the scapula is required in full abduction of the limb.
- Strong muscular coverings protect the scapula and fracture is rare, requiring direct and severe violence.

Clavicle

- Medial two-thirds convex anteriorly and circular in cross section.
- Lateral third convex posteriorly and flattened in cross section.
- Articulates medially at the sternoclavicular joint (articular disc in joint).
- Attached to the first costal cartilage by the costoclavicular ligament.
- Articulates laterally with acromion at the acromioclavicular joint (incomplete articular disc in joint).
- Attached to the coracoid process by tough coracoclavicular ligament.
- It has no medullary cavity.
- It is the first bone to ossify in the fetus.
- It is the only long bone to develop in membrane.
- It may be pierced by the supraclavicular nerves.

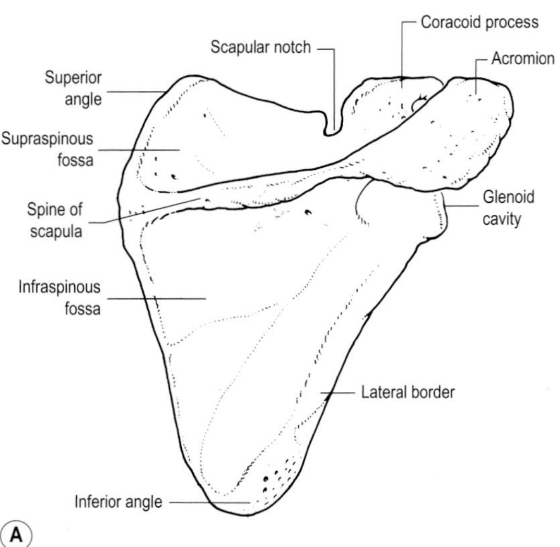

Fig. 3.1 The scapula. (A) Posterior view. (B) Anterior view.

- It transmits forces from the upper limb to the axial skeleton.
- It acts as a strut to hold the arm free from the trunk.
- It is the most commonly fractured bone in the body, the fracture usually occurring at the junction of the middle and outer thirds.

Humerus (Fig. 3.2)

- The head is third of a sphere and faces medially, upwards and backwards.
- The head is separated from the greater and lesser tubercles by the anatomical neck.
- The tubercles are separated from one another by the bicipital groove (containing the tendon of the long head of the biceps).
- The upper end and shaft meet at the surgical neck, around which lies the axillary nerve and circumflex humeral vessels.
- The shaft is circular in the section above and flattened lower down.
- The spiral groove lies posteriorly on the shaft and is related to the radial nerve, which winds round it between the medial and lateral head of triceps.
- The lower end bears the rounded capitulum laterally for articulation with the radial head, and the trochlea medially for articulation with the trochlear notch of the ulna.
- Medial and lateral epicondyles are extracapsular. The ulnar nerve lies in a groove on the posterior aspect of the medial epicondyle.
- Fractures of the humerus are common and important in view of the close relationship of the axillary, radial and ulnar nerves.

Radius and Ulna (Fig. 3.3)

- Considered together as they are complementary in the makeup of the forearm.
- Radius consists of head, neck, shaft and expanded distal end.
- Ulna consists of the olecranon, trochlear fossa, coronoid process with its radial notch (for articulation with the radial head), shaft and small distal head (for articulation with the medial aspect of the distal radius).

The Carpus (Figs. 3.4 and 3.7)

- Made up of two rows of four bones.

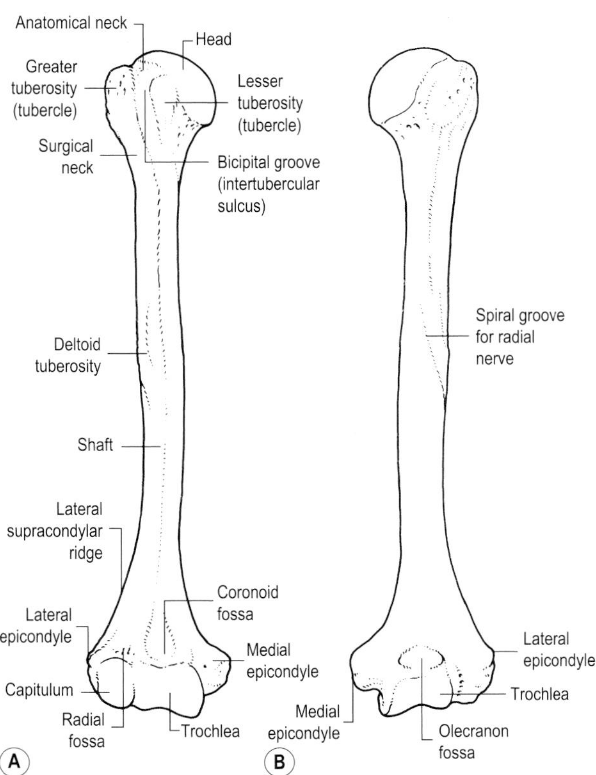

Fig. 3.2 The humerus. (A) Anterior view. (B) Posterior view.

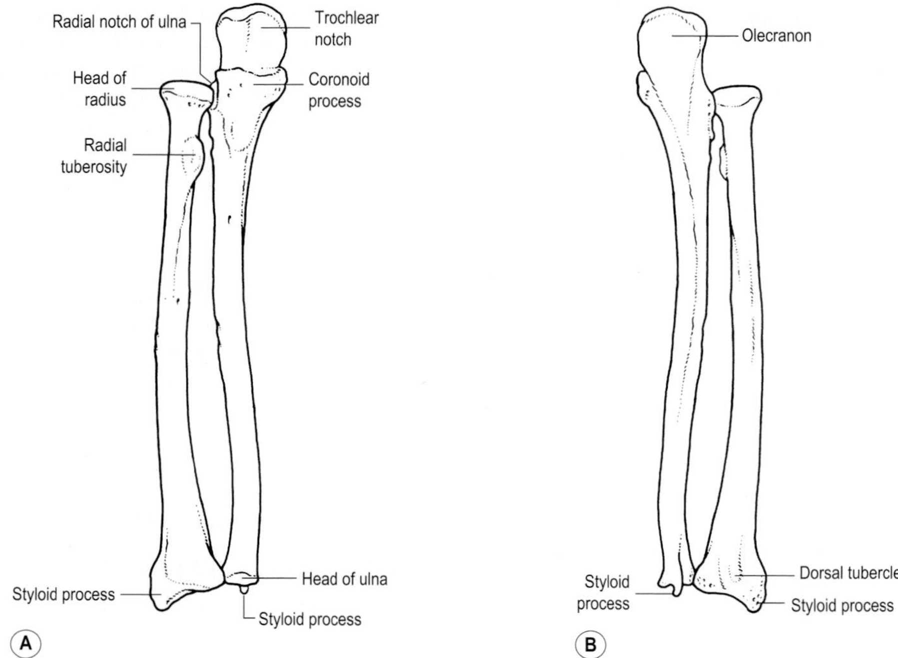

Fig. 3.3 The radius and ulna. (A) Anterior view. (B) Posterior view.

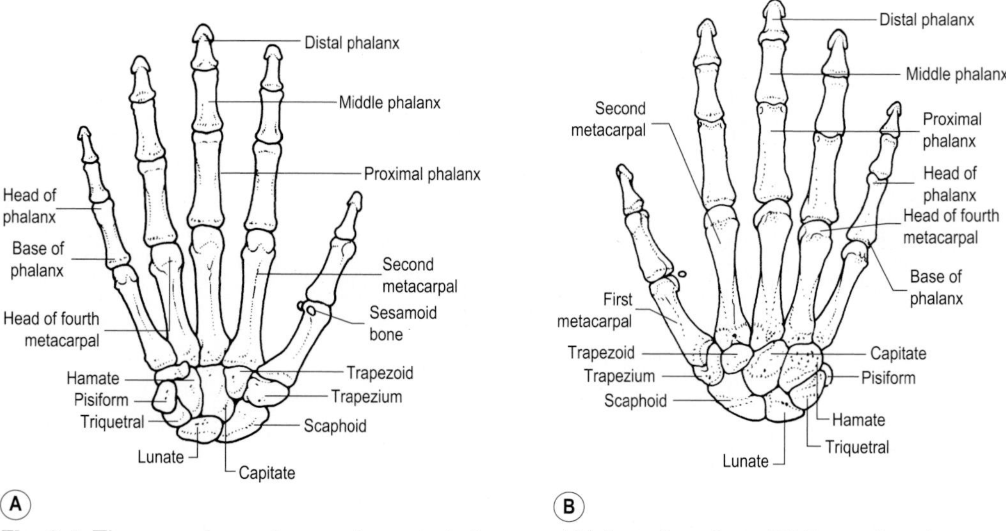

Fig. 3.4 The carpals, metacarpals and phalanges. (A) Anterior view. (B) Posterior view.

- Proximally, lateral to medial—scaphoid, lunate, triquetral (plus attached pisiform).
- Distally, lateral to medial—trapezium, trapezoid, capitate, hamate.
- Carpus is arched transversely, the palmar aspect being concave.
- Arch is maintained by individual bones, which are broader posteriorly than anteriorly (except the lunate).

- Arch is also maintained by the flexor retinaculum passing from the scaphoid and trapezium laterally to the pisiform and hook of the hamate medially.

Metacarpals and Phalanges

- First metacarpal is important because of the mobility of its carpometacarpal joint, which is responsible for opposition of the thumb.
- Second metacarpal articulates with three carpal bones: trapezium, trapezoid and capitate.
- Capitate articulates with three metacarpals: second, third and fourth.

JOINTS OF THE UPPER LIMB

Shoulder Joint (Fig. 3.5)

- Ball-and-socket joint.
- Articular surfaces: head of humerus with shallow glenoid fossa of scapula (deepened somewhat by the labrum glenoidale—a cartilaginous ring).
- Capsule: lax and attached around epiphyseal line of glenoid and humeral head. Extends down to diaphysis on the medial aspect of the neck of the humerus. Capsule lined by synovial membrane along tendon of long head of biceps, which passes through joint. Synovium communicates with subcapsular bursa beneath tendon of subscapularis.
- Stability depends largely on strength of surrounding muscles:
    - rotator cuff
    - long head of biceps
    - deltoid, pectoralis major, latissimus dorsi, teres major, long head of biceps.

Muscles Acting on Shoulder Joint

- Abductors: supraspinatus, deltoid.
- Adductors: pectoralis major, latissimus dorsi.
- Flexors: anterior fibres of deltoid, pectoralis major, coracobrachialis.
- Extensors: latissimus dorsi, teres major, posterior fibres of deltoid.
- Medial rotators: pectoralis major, latissimus dorsi, teres major, subscapularis, anterior fibres of deltoid.
- Lateral rotators: infraspinatus, teres minor, posterior fibres of deltoid.

The Shoulder Girdle

Movements of the shoulder joint itself cannot be separated from those of the shoulder girdle as a whole.

Sternoclavicular Joint

- Articular surfaces: medial end of clavicle and sternum, intra-articular disc.
- Ligaments: costoclavicular ligament passes from clavicle to first costal cartilage. This forms a fulcrum so that when the outer end of the clavicle is raised, e.g. shrugging the shoulders, the medial end is depressed.

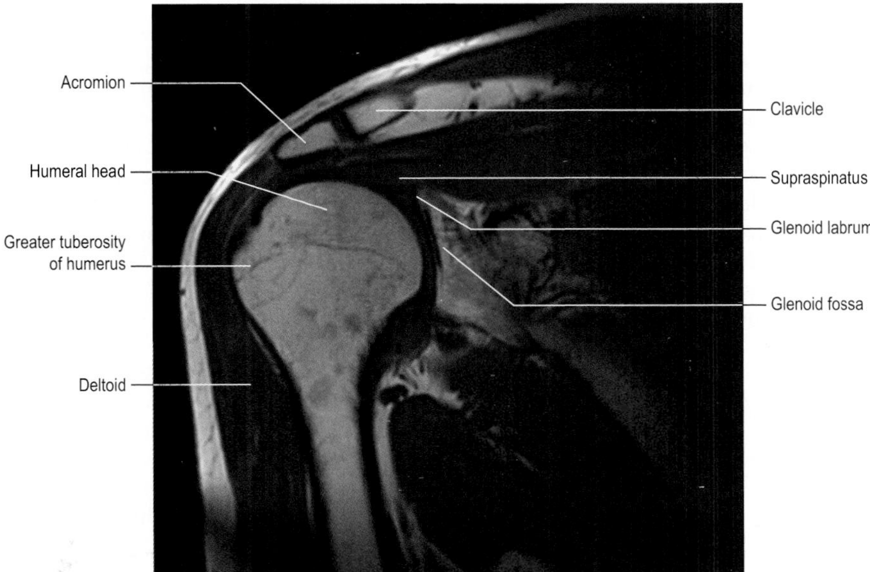

Fig. 3.5 Coronal MRI right shoulder joint.

Acromioclavicular Joint

- Articular surfaces: lateral end of clavicle and the acromion, incomplete articular disc.
- Ligaments: coracoclavicular (conoid and trapezoid ligaments).
- Movements: induced passively by scapular movement.
- Dislocation of the outer end of the clavicle at the joint is easily reduced; maintenance of reduction is difficult, owing to inclination of joint surfaces.

Rotator Cuff

- Sheath of tendons of short muscles of the shoulder which surround and blend with all but the inferior aspect of the joint.
- Consists of supraspinatus, infraspinatus and teres minor, which are inserted from above down into the greater tuberosity of the humerus, and subscapularis, which is inserted into the lesser tuberosity.
- All the above muscles originate from the scapula.
- Supraspinatus is important in initiation of abduction of the shoulder joint.
- Supraspinatus passes over the apex of the shoulder beneath the acromion and coracoacromial ligament, from which it is separated by the subacromial bursa.

Movements of Shoulder Girdle

- All but very slight glenohumeral movements are always accompanied by movements of the scapula on the clavicle and of the clavicle on the manubrium.
- Abduction is initiated by supraspinatus (15°).
- Deltoid then abducts to 90°.
- Further movement to 180° is brought about by rotation of the scapula by trapezius and serratus anterior.
- As soon as abduction commences at the shoulder joint, rotation of the scapula begins.
- Movements of the scapula occur with reciprocal movements of the sternoclavicular joint, i.e. elevate the shoulder and the joint is depressed; move the shoulder forwards and the joint moves backwards.
- The scapula can be elevated (shrugging the shoulders) and depressed. Trapezius and levator scapulae elevate; gravity, pectoralis major and pectoralis minor depress.
- The scapula can be protracted (moved forwards round the chest wall) and retracted. Serratus anterior and pectoralis minor protract; rhomboids and middle fibres of trapezius retract.
- Rotation of the scapula upwards is carried out by trapezius and serratus anterior.

Clinical Points

- In fractures of the clavicle, trapezius is unable to support the weight of the arm. The patient therefore supports the upper limb with the opposite hand. The lateral fragment is depressed and drawn medially by the shoulder adductors and the broken ends overlap. Slight elevation of the medial fragment occurs due to sternocleidomastoid.
- Rupture of the tendon of supraspinatus results in inability to actively initiate abduction of the shoulder. The patient develops a trick movement of tilting the body to the injured side so gravity allows the limb to swing away from the trunk. Deltoid then comes into action.
- Supraspinatus tendinitis results in a painful arc of shoulder movement between 60° and 120°. It is during this range of movement that the tendon impinges against the overlying acromion and coracoacromial ligament.
- Serratus anterior, which protracts the scapula and keeps it applied to the chest wall, is supplied by the long thoracic nerve of Bell, C5, C6 and C7. Damage to this nerve (neck, breast or axillary surgery) results in winging of the scapula.

Elbow Joint (Fig. 3.6)

Consists of three articulations and one synovial cavity.

- Humeroulnar: trochlea of humerus and trochlear notch of ulna (hinge joint).
- Humeroradial: capitulum and radial head (ball-and-socket joint).
- Proximal radioulnar: head of radius and radial notch of ulna (pivot joint).
- Capsule: thin and lax anteriorly and posteriorly; thickened at sides to form medial and lateral collateral ligaments. The lateral ligament is attached to annular ligament, which holds the head of the radius in place. The medial and lateral epicondyles are extracapsular.
- Movement: flexion and extension. Pronation and supination occur at proximal radioulnar joint (with distal radioulnar joint).
- Muscles acting on joint are:
  - flexors: biceps, brachialis, brachioradialis, forearm flexors
  - extensors: triceps, anconeus
  - pronators: pronator teres, pronator quadratus
  - supinators: biceps, supinator.

Wrist Joint (Fig. 3.7)

- Articular surfaces: distal radius and head of ulna, the latter separated from the carpus by an articular disc. Proximal articular surfaces of scaphoid, lunate, triquetral.
- Condyloid joint: allows flexion, extension, adduction, abduction and circumduction.
- Movements are:
  - flexion: all muscles crossing the anterior aspect of the joint

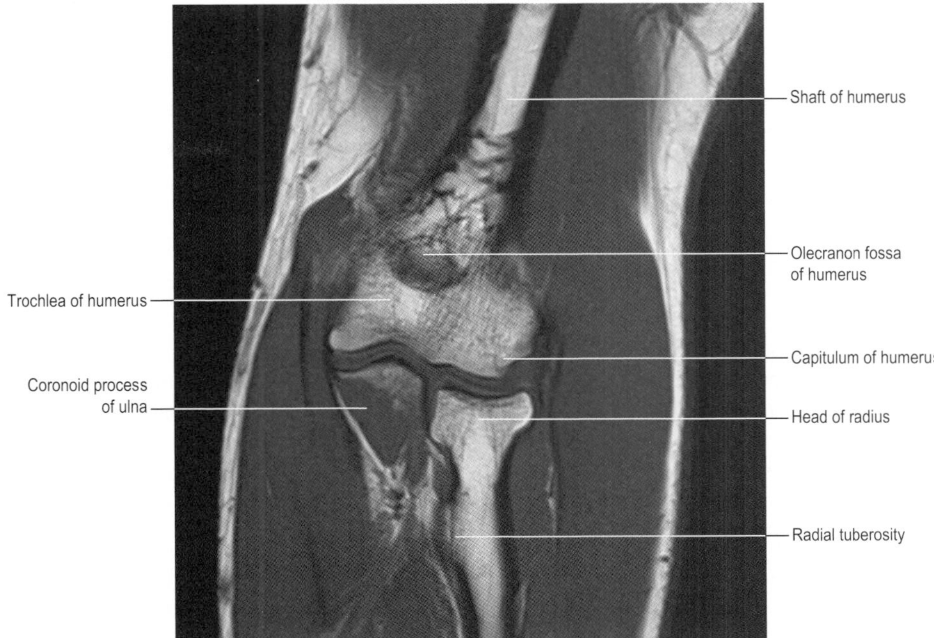

Fig. 3.6 Coronal MRI left elbow joint.

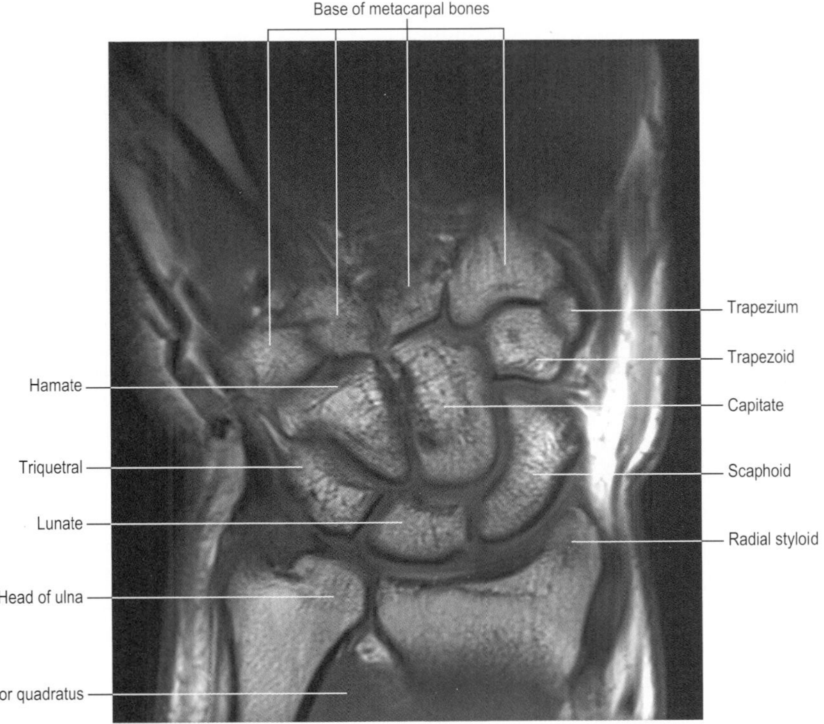

Fig. 3.7 Coronal MRI left wrist joint.

- extension: all muscles crossing the posterior aspect of the joint
- adduction: flexor carpi ulnaris, extensor carpi ulnaris
- abduction: flexor carpi radialis, extensor carpi radialis longus, abductor pollicis longus, extensor pollicis longus.

Joints of the Hand

Carpometacarpal Joint

Thumb

- Saddle joint.
- Flexion, extension, abduction, adduction, opposition.
- Flexion/extension in plane parallel to palm.
- Abduction/adduction in plane at right angle to palm.
- Opposition: thumb opposes to little finger.
- Other carpometacarpal joints have limited gliding movement only.

Metacarpophalangeal Joints

- 60° range of flexion/extension at metacarpophalangeal joint of thumb.
- 90° at other metacarpophalangeal joints, together with abduction, adduction and circumduction.
- Abduction and adduction are impossible with the metacarpophalangeal joints flexed.
- Metacarpophalangeal joints of fingers (not thumb) are joined by deep transverse ligaments which prevent them spreading during a firm grip.

Interphalangeal Joints

- Hinge joints.
- Flexion/extension only.
- Collateral ligaments lax in extension and taut in flexion.

Muscles Controlling the Hand

Long Flexors

- Flexor digitorum profundus: inserted into base of distal phalanx.
- Flexor digitorum superficialis: inserted into sides of middle phalanx.
- Profundus tendon pierces superficialis tendon over proximal phalanx.
- Profundus flexes the distal phalanx.
- Superficialis flexes the middle phalanx.
- Both muscles flex the fingers and the wrist.

Long Extensors

- Extensor digitorum longus inserted into the extensor expansion.
- Extensor indicis inserted into the medial side of the extensor digitorum longus to index finger.
- Extensor digiti minimi inserted into the medial side of extensor digitorum longus to the little finger.
- They extend the fingers and wrist.

Extensor Expansion (Fig. 3.8)

- Covers the dorsum of the proximal phalanx and sides of its base.
- Attaches by central slip into the base of the middle phalanx and two lateral slips into the base of the distal phalanx.
- Receives the insertion of the interossei and lumbricals.

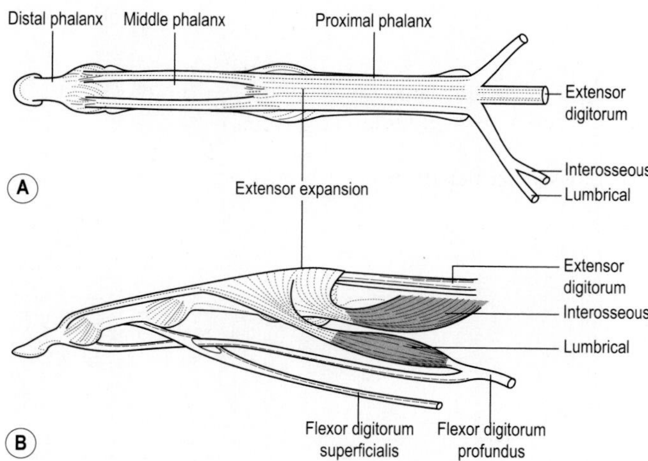

Fig. 3.8 The extensor expansion and tendons of a finger. (A) Dorsal view. (B) Lateral view.

Small Muscles of the Hand

Interossei

- Arise from the sides and front of metacarpals.
- Abduct and adduct the fingers.
- Insert into the extensor expansion.
- Flex the metacarpophalangeal joints.
- Extend the interphalangeal joints.

Lumbricals

- Arise from the four profundus tendons.
- Insert into the extensor expansion.
- Flex the metacarpophalangeal joints.
- Extend the interphalangeal joints.

Muscles of the Thumb

Long muscles

- Flexor pollicis longus: inserted into distal phalanx.
- Extensor pollicis longus: inserted into the distal phalanx.
- Extensor pollicis brevis: inserted into proximal phalanx.
- Abductor pollicis longus: inserted into the first metacarpal.

Short muscles (thenar eminence)

- Adductor pollicis: inserted into base of proximal phalanx.
- Flexor pollicis brevis: inserted into base of proximal phalanx.
- Abductor pollicis brevis: inserted into base of proximal phalanx.
- Opponens pollicis: inserted along the first metacarpal.

Muscles of the Little Finger (Hypothenar Eminence)

- Abductor digiti minimi.
- Opponens digiti minimi.
- Flexor digiti minimi.

Muscle Actions

- Flexor digitorum profundus flexes the distal phalanx.
- Flexor digitorum superficialis flexes the middle phalanx.
- Profundus and superficialis acting together flex the fingers and wrist.
- The interossei and lumbricals flex the metacarpophalangeal joints and extend the interphalangeal joints.
- The interossei plus abductor digiti minimi abduct and adduct the fingers.
- Extensor digitorum has a weak abduction action.
- The long flexors have a weak adduction action.
- The abductor/adductor actions of extensor digitorum and the long flexors are eliminated by placing the hand flat on a table. Abduction/adduction then become the actions of the intrinsic muscles only.
- The above can be tested by gripping a card between the fingers (tests T1 and partly ulnar nerve integrity).

VEINS OF THE UPPER LIMB

- Important in cannulation.
- Important in creation of arteriovenous fistula for dialysis.

Superficial Veins

- Commence as dorsal venous network on dorsum of hand.
- Dorsal venous network drains into lateral cephalic vein and dorsal basilic vein.

Cephalic Vein

- Lies subcutaneously just behind the radial styloid, where it is very constant in position.
- Runs up the anterior aspect of the forearm.
- Lies in groove along the lateral border of biceps in the upper arm.
- Passes to the deltopectoral triangle.
- Pierces the clavipectoral fascia to enter the axillary vein.
- Is superficial until it reaches the deltopectoral triangle.

Basilic Vein

- Runs along the posteromedial aspect of the forearm.
- Passes to the anterior aspect of the elbow on the medial side.
- Runs in the groove along the medial border of biceps.
- Pierces the deep fascia at the middle of the upper arm.
- Joins venae comitantes of brachial artery, eventually forming the axillary vein.

Veins at the Elbow

- Variable pattern.
- Median cubital vein connects the cephalic and basilic veins.
- The veins are separated from the underlying brachial artery by the tough bicipital aponeurosis.

Clinical Points

- The cephalic vein at the wrist is very constant and available for cannulation and for the formation of radiocephalic (Cimino–Brescia) fistulae for dialysis (the radial artery is in close proximity).
- Avoid injection of irritant drugs into the veins at the elbow. There is a risk of accidentally entering the brachial artery or a superficially placed aberrant ulnar artery. Drug addicts are not aware of these anatomical relations!

Deep Veins

- Venae comitantes (accompanying the arteries).
- Usually in pairs or multiple.

- Nuisance value when exposing deep arteries, to which they are closely applied.

ARTERIES OF THE UPPER LIMB (Fig. 3.9)

- Axillary.
- Brachial.
- Radial.
- Ulnar.

Axillary

- Commences at the lateral border of the first rib as the continuation of the subclavian artery.
- Ends at the lower border of teres major to become the brachial artery.
- Divided into three parts by pectoralis minor:
  - First part gives off one branch:
    - superior thoracic artery.
  - Second part gives off two branches:
    - acromiothoracic artery
    - lateral thoracic artery.
  - Third part gives off three branches:
    - subscapular artery
    - anterior circumflex humeral artery
    - posterior circumflex humeral artery.
- Relations: brachial plexus cords surround the artery, i.e. the lateral, medial and posterior cords.

Brachial Artery

- Commences at the lower border of teres major as a continuation of the axillary artery.
- Terminates at the level of the neck of the radius where it divides into the radial and ulnar artery.
- It lies immediately below the deep fascia in most of its course where it is readily accessible, e.g. for brachial embolectomy.
- It is crossed superficially from the lateral to medial side by the median nerve at the level of the midhumerus.
- High bifurcation of the artery is not unusual.

Radial Artery

- Commences at the level of the radial neck lying on the tendon of biceps (frequently bifurcation may be higher).
- Overlapped by brachioradialis in its upper half.
- In the distal forearm it lies between brachioradialis and flexor carpi radialis where it can be palpated at the wrist.
- It is closely related to the radial nerve in the middle of the forearm.
- Distal to the wrist the branches given off contribute to the superficial palmar arch.
- Passes deep to tendons of abductor pollicis longus and extensor pollicis brevis to enter the anatomical snuffbox where it is palpable.
- Pierces first dorsal interosseous and adductor pollicis to contribute to deep palmar arch.

Ulnar Artery

- Commences at level of neck of radius (frequently bifurcation may be higher).
- Passes deep to muscles from common flexor origin.
- Lies on flexor digitorum profundus, overlapped by flexor carpi ulnaris.
- Crossed superficially by the median nerve separated from it by the deep head of pronator teres.
- Distally in the forearm it becomes superficial between the tendons of the flexor carpi ulnaris and flexor digitorum profundus.

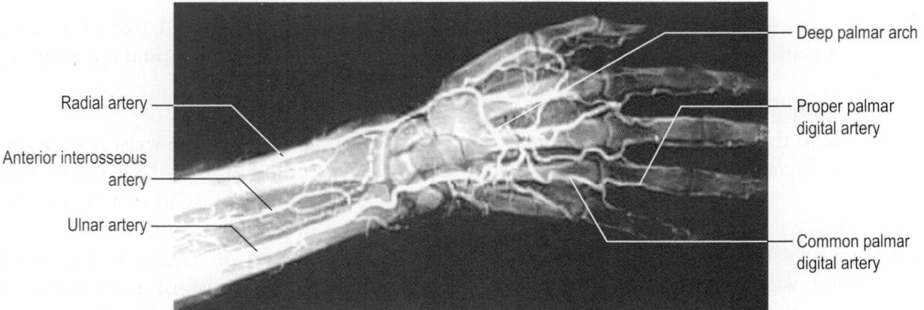

Fig. 3.9 MRA left forearm and hand. (© University of Michigan Medical School, with kind permission of Thomas R. Gest PhD.)

- Crosses in front of the flexor retinaculum to form the superficial palmar arch with the superficial branch of the radial artery.
- The ulnar nerve accompanies the artery on its medial side in the distal two-thirds of the forearm and across the flexor retinaculum.

BRACHIAL PLEXUS (Fig. 3.10)

Partly in the neck and partly in axilla, the plexus is composed as follows:
- Roots: between scalenus anterior and scalenus medius.
- Trunks: in the posterior triangle of the neck.
- Divisions: behind the clavicle.
- Cords: in the axilla.

Roots (5)

- Anterior primary rami of C5, 6, 7, 8, T1.

Trunks (3)

- Upper (C5, 6).
- Middle (C7).
- Lower (C8, T1).

Divisions (6)

- Each trunk divides into anterior and posterior divisions.

Cords (3)

- Lateral: fused anterior divisions of upper and middle trunks.
- Medial: anterior division of lower trunk.
- Posterior: fusion of all three posterior divisions.

Nerves

From the continuation of the cords:
- Musculocutaneous nerve: from the lateral cord.
- Ulnar nerve: from the medial cord.
- Radial nerve: from the posterior cord.
- Axillary nerve: from the posterior cord.
- Median nerve: from a cross-communication between lateral and medial cords.

Branches of the Brachial Plexus

Roots
- Nerve to rhomboids.
- Nerve to subclavius.
- Nerve to serratus anterior (long thoracic nerve of Bell, C5, 6, 7).

Trunks
- Suprascapular: upper trunk; supplies supraspinatus and infraspinatus.

Cords:

Lateral
- Musculocutaneous.
- Lateral pectoral.
- Lateral root of median.

Medial
- Medial pectoral nerve.
- Medial cutaneous nerve of the arm and forearm.
- Ulnar nerve.
- Medial root of median.

Posterior
- Thoracodorsal nerve (to latissimus dorsi).
- Subscapular nerve.
- Axillary nerve.
- Radial nerve.

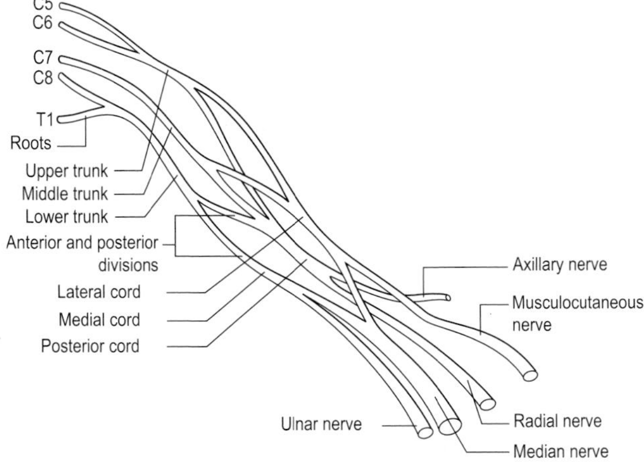

Fig. 3.10 The brachial plexus.

The brachial plexus can be pre-fixed or post-fixed on rare occasions. A pre-fixed plexus has a contribution from C4; a post-fixed from T2.

Nerves of the Upper Limb

- Axillary.
- Radial.
- Musculocutaneous.
- Median.
- Ulnar.

Axillary Nerve

- Root value C5, 6.
- Arises from posterior cord.
- Winds round surgical neck of humerus.
- Accompanied by circumflex humeral arteries.
- Muscular branches to deltoid, teres minor.
- Cutaneous branch supplying sensation to skin over deltoid.

Radial Nerve

- Root value C5, 6, 7, 8, T1.
- Arises from the posterior cord.
- Lies initially behind the axillary artery.
- Passes posteriorly between the long and medial head of the triceps.
- Accompanied by profunda brachii artery.
- Lies in the spiral groove of the humerus.
- Pierces the lateral intermuscular septum at the lower third of the humerus and enters the anterior compartment.
- Lies between brachialis and brachioradialis.
- Gives off posterior interosseous nerve at level of lateral epicondyle.
- Radial nerve continues as superficial branch to brachioradialis.
- Above wrist emerges posteriorly from under brachioradialis and supplies sensation by cutaneous branches to posterior aspect of radial three-and-a-half digits.
- Main radial nerve supplies triceps, anconeus, brachioradialis, extensor carpi radialis longus and part of brachialis.
- Posterior interosseous branch supplies supinator, abductor pollicis longus and all remaining extensor muscle.
- Cutaneous supply is to the back of the arm, the flexor and radial aspects of the dorsum of the hand.

Musculocutaneous Nerve

- Root value C5, 6, 7.
- Continuation of lateral cord of brachial plexus.
- Pierces coracobrachialis and runs between biceps and brachialis.
- Supplies biceps, brachialis and coracobrachialis.
- Innervates the skin of the lateral forearm.

Median Nerve

- Root value C6, 7, 8, T1.
- Arises from the joining of branches of the medial and the lateral cord of the plexus.
- Lies initially anterior to the third part of the axillary artery.
- Continues along the lateral aspect of the brachial artery.
- Crosses superficial (occasionally deep) to the brachial artery at midhumeral level to lie on the medial side of the brachial artery.
- Enters the forearm between the heads of pronator teres.
- At this level it gives off the anterior interosseous branch.
- The median nerve then lies on the deep aspect of flexor digitorum superficialis.
- Superficial at the wrist lying to the ulnar side of flexor carpi radialis in the midline.
- Gives off palmar cutaneous branch at the wrist, which passes superficial to the flexor retinaculum and supplies the palmar skin over the thenar eminence.
- It then passes deep to the flexor retinaculum, giving a branch to the thenar muscles beyond the distal skin crease.
- Supplies in its course all muscles of the flexor aspect of the forearm (except flexor carpi ulnaris and the ulnar half of flexor digitorum profundus), the muscles of the thenar eminence and the radial two lumbricals.
- Supplies sensation to the radial three-and-a-half digits and skin of the radial side of the palm.

Ulnar Nerve

- Root value C7, 8, T1.
- Formed by the medial cord of the plexus.
- Lies medial to the axillary and brachial artery to midhumerus.
- Pierces the medial intermuscular septum, descending on the anterior surface of the triceps.
- Passes behind the medial epicondyle (where it is palpable).
- Descends between flexor carpi ulnaris and flexor digitorum profundus and then lies superficial on the radial side of the tendon of flexor carpi ulnaris.
- Accompanies ulnar artery in distal two-thirds of forearm, which lies to its radial side.
- Gives off a dorsal cutaneous branch 5 cm above the wrist, which is sensory to the dorsal aspect of the ulnar one-and-a-half fingers.
- Crosses the flexor retinaculum superficially.

- Supplies:
  - flexor carpi ulnaris
  - medial half of flexor digitorum profundus
  - hypothenar muscles
  - interossei
  - medial two lumbricals
  - adductor pollicis.

ANATOMY OF NERVE LESIONS

Brachial Plexus

Erb's (Erb–Duchenne) Paralysis

- Forced downward traction on arm during birth.
- Fall on side of head and shoulder, forcing the two apart.
- Root C5, C6 affected.
- Paralysis of deltoid, supraspinatus, infraspinatus, brachialis, biceps.
- Arm hangs limply by side (abductors paralysed) with forearm pronated (brachialis and biceps flex and supinate) and palm facing backwards (waiter's tip position).

Klumpke's paralysis

- Upward traction on arm may damage T1 (e.g. breech delivery).
- Intrinsic muscles of hand paralysed.
- Claw hand:
  - unopposed action of long flexors and long extensors
  - extensors extend metacarpophalangeal joints
  - flexors flex the interphalangeal joints
  - use of the intrinsic muscles is lost; therefore, they cannot extend the interphalangeal joints, and hence clawing occurs owing to unopposed action of the long flexors.
- Associated area of numbness along inner and upper arm and forearm centred on elbow joint level.
- May be associated with Horner's syndrome due to traction on sympathetic chain.
- Wasting of small muscles of hand; 'channels' between metacarpals, wasting of first dorsal interosseus.
- Similar lesions may occur with Pancoast's tumour or a cervical rib.

Axillary Nerve

- Damaged in fracture of surgical neck of humerus or anterior dislocation of the shoulder joint.
- Deltoid paralysed, therefore abduction lost.
- Small patch of anaesthesia over the insertion of deltoid ('badge area').

Radial Nerve

- Damaged in fractures of midshaft of humerus, or compression of nerve against humerus when a drunk falls asleep with the arm over the back of a hard chair, trapping the nerve between the chair and the humerus ('Saturday night palsy'). Also pressure from crutch, but axillary weightbearing crutches are rare nowadays.
- Posterior interosseous may be damaged in fractures or dislocations of the radial head or in the surgical approach to the radial head.
- Results in wrist drop if main nerve is damaged.
- Damage to posterior interosseous branch allows extension of the wrist (due to extensor carpi radialis longus, which is supplied by the main radial nerve before the posterior interosseous branch is given off).
- Small area of anaesthesia on the skin on dorsum of first web space.

Median Nerve

- Damaged in lacerations at the wrist and supracondylar fractures of the humerus.
- Damage at the elbow results in:
  - loss of forearm pronation
  - weakness of wrist flexion with ulnar deviation (flexion depends on flexor carpi ulnaris and the medial half of flexor digitorum profundus)
  - loss of sensation on the lateral palm and radial three-and-a-half digits.
- Damage at wrist results in:
  - paralysis of the thenar muscles (except adductor pollicis)
  - paralysis of radial two lumbricals
  - loss of sensation over radial three-and-a-half digits.
- Damage of the nerve at both sites causes loss of accurate opposition, and the loss of cutaneous innervation makes this a serious injury with loss of tactile response.

Ulnar Nerve

- Damage at medial epicondyle, e.g. fracture of the medial epicondyle or dislocations of the elbow; lacerations at wrist.
- Damage at the wrist results in:
  - clawing of the hand similar to Klumpke's paralysis, except less clawing in second and third digits because of median nerve supply to lumbricals, which is intact
  - sensory loss over medial one-and-a-half fingers.
- Damage at the elbow results in:
  - similar lesion to wrist except less clawing in fourth and fifth fingers, as flexor digitorum profundus to those fingers is paralysed

  - flexor carpi ulnaris is paralysed, therefore a tendency to radial deviation at the wrist.
- Damage to ulnar nerve leaves a remarkably efficient hand. Confirmation of the diagnosis is by testing for lack of sensation of the medial one-and-a-half digits, and loss of abduction and adduction of the fingers with the hand flat on a table (excludes trick movements of long flexors and extensors).

SPACES OF THE HAND

Pulp Spaces of Fingers (Fig. 3.11)

- Pulp space is fat packed between fibrous septa from skin to periosteum.
- Blood vessels have to pass through this space, except the proximal branch to the base of the distal phalanx.
- Pulp space infection increases the pressure in the space. This may result in arterial thrombosis and necrosis of the distal phalanx with the exception of its base, which is spared because of the proximal branch.

Bursae of the Hand and Synovial Tendon Sheaths (Fig. 3.12)

- Flexor tendons traverse a fibro-osseous tunnel for each digit.
- The fibrous sheaths end at insertion of flexor digitorum profundus.
- The fibrous sheaths are lined by synovial membrane.
- Second, third and fourth fingers have synovial sheaths that close proximally at the metacarpal head.
- Synovial sheaths of thumb and little finger extend proximally into the palm.

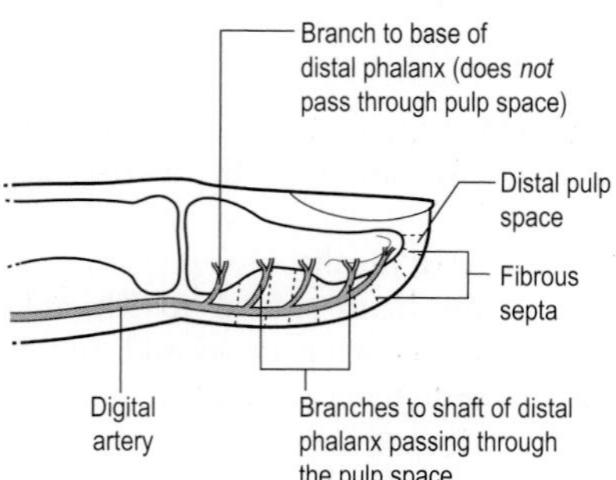

Fig. 3.11 Distal pulp space of a finger showing the blood supply to the distal phalanx. (From Easterbrook P Basic Medical Sciences for MRCP Part 1, 2nd edn. Churchill Livingstone, Edinburgh, 1999, with permission.)

- Synovial sheath of long flexor of the thumb extends through the palm deep to the flexor retinaculum to 2.5 cm proximal to wrist (radial bursa).
- Synovial sheath of fifth finger forms the ulnar bursa, which encloses all finger tendons in the palm and extends proximally deep to the flexor retinaculum for 2.5 cm above the wrist.
- The radial and ulnar bursae may communicate.
- Infection of the synovial sheath to the second, third and fourth digits is confined to the finger. However, infection of the first and fifth sheaths may spread into the palm or from one bursa to another.

Palmar Spaces

Midpalmar Space

- Behind the flexor tendons and ulnar bursa.
- In front of the third, fourth and fifth metacarpals.
- First and second metacarpals are cut off by adductor pollicis, which arises from the shaft of third metacarpal.

Thenar Space

- Superficial to second and third metacarpals and adductor pollicis.
- Separated from midpalmar space by fibrous partition.
- Infection in spaces is usually from a direct penetrating injury or neglected tendon sheath infection.
- Infection rare in spaces, due to antibiotics.

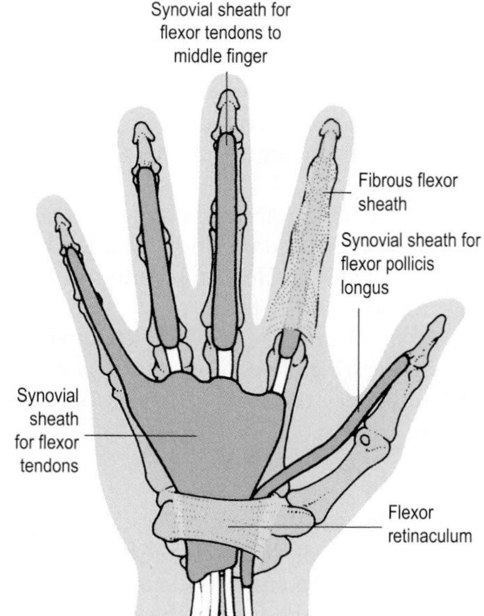

Fig. 3.12 The synovial sheaths of the wrist and hand, anterior view.

Palmar infections may result in marked dorsal oedema. This is caused by the thick palmar skin being firmly bound down to the underlying palmar aponeurosis. In contrast, the skin of the dorsum of the hand is loose and fluid can readily collect deep into it.

Palmar Aponeurosis

- Part of the deep fascia of the hand.
- Blends with the fibrous flexor sheath of the fingers.
- Attached to sides of proximal and middle phalanges.
- Dupuytren's contracture results in thickening and contraction of the palmar fascia with flexion of the metacarpophalangeal joints and proximal interphalangeal joints. The distal interphalangeal joint is not involved.

SPECIALIZED AREAS OF THE ARM

Axilla

The axilla is a pyramidal space through which structures from the head, neck and thorax pass into the arm, and structures from the arm pass into the thorax. Being pyramidal it has a base, four walls and an apex.

- Base: skin and fascia of the armpit.
- Medial wall: rib cage covered by serratus anterior.
- Lateral wall: bicipital groove of the humerus.
- Anterior wall: pectoralis major and pectoralis minor.
- Posterior wall: latissimus dorsi, teres major and, more superiorly, supscapularis.
- Apex is bounded anteriorly by the clavicle, first rib medially, and the acromion and superior border of the scapula posteriorly.
- Contents:
    - brachial plexus
    - axillary artery
    - axillary vein
    - lymph nodes
    - fat.

Antecubital Fossa

- Bounded by pronator teres medially and brachioradialis laterally.
- Its floor is formed by brachialis and supinator.
- The roof is formed by skin, superficial fascia and deep fascia augmented by the bicipital aponeurosis.
- Contents include the brachial artery and medial to it, the median nerve.

Carpal Tunnel (Fig. 3.13)

- The flexor retinaculum forms the roof of a tunnel, the floor and walls of which are formed by the concavity of the carpal bones.
- Within this tunnel are the tendons of flexor digitorum superficialis, flexor digitorum profundus, flexor pollicis longus and flexor carpi radialis (the latter tendon is in its own separate osseofascial compartment).
- The most important structure to pass through the tunnel is the median nerve. Any lesion diminishing the size of the tunnel may result in compression of the median nerve (carpal tunnel syndrome).
- The superficial palmar branch of the nerve is given off proximal to the flexor retinaculum, and therefore there is no sensory impairment on the lateral side of the palm if the nerve is compressed in the carpal tunnel.

Anatomical Snuffbox

- Medial border formed by tendon of extensor pollicis longus.
- Lateral border formed by the tendons of abductor pollicis longus and extensor pollicis brevis.
- Contents include the base of the metacarpal of the thumb, the trapezium, the scaphoid, the radial styloid and the dorsal branch of the radial artery.
- Important clinically as tenderness can be felt in the anatomical snuffbox with fractures of the scaphoid.

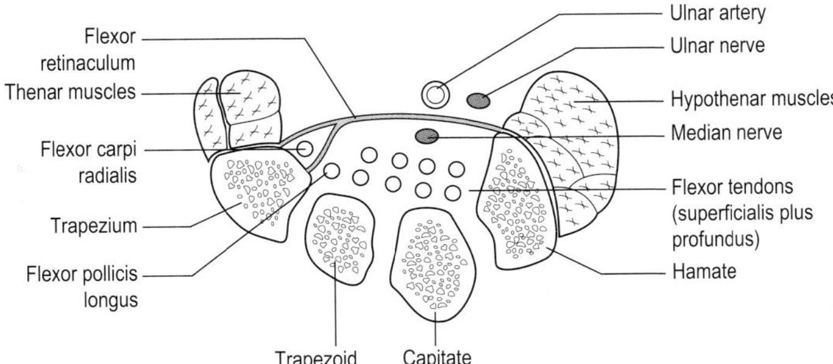

Fig. 3.13 Transverse section through carpal tunnel at level of distal carpal bones, showing the relations of structures to the flexor retinaculum.

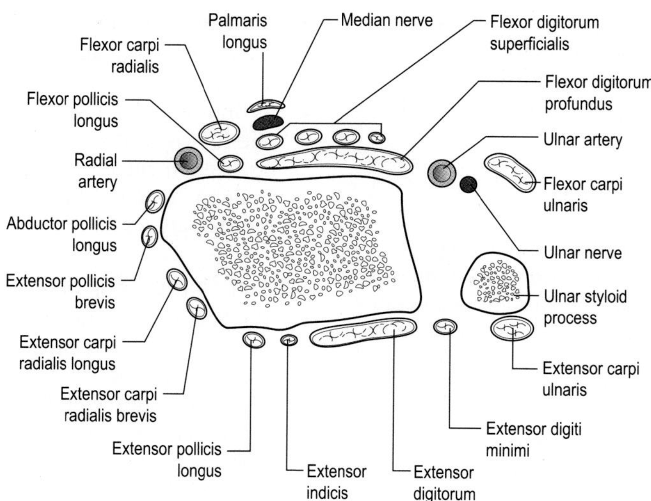

Fig. 3.14 Relations around the wrist. Transverse section through distal right radius and ulna styloid, made with hand and forearm in full supination and viewed from distal aspect.

- Dorsal branch of the radial artery lies close to the cephalic vein and therefore this is an appropriate site for creating arteriovenous fistulae for dialysis.

Structures Around the Wrist Joint

These are shown in Fig. 3.14.

LYMPHATICS OF THE UPPER LIMB

- Superficial and deep lymphatics. Superficial lymphatics accompany the veins and the deep lymphatics accompany the arteries.
- Few superficial lymph nodes in the upper limbs: chiefly the epitrochlear nodes.
- Efferents from epitrochlear nodes pierce the deep fascia and end in the axillary nodes.

Axillary Lymph Nodes

- Drain the following:
  - the breast
  - the pectoral region
  - the upper abdominal wall down to the umbilicus
  - the skin of the back down to the iliac crest
  - the upper limb.
- Arranged in five groups, although these are not distinct:
  - lying deep to pectoralis major along the lower border of pectoralis minor
  - posterior: along the subscapular vessels
  - lateral: along the axillary vein
  - central: in the axillary fat
  - apical: immediately behind the clavicle at the apex of the axilla above pectoralis minor, and arranged along the axillary vein (all other axillary nodes drain through this group).
- From these nodes the subclavian lymph trunk emerges.
- Surgical anatomy of the axillary lymph nodes is important in relation to breast surgery. From this point of view they are classified into three levels:
  - level 1 nodes: present below and lateral to the inferolateral border of pectoralis minor
  - level 2 nodes: behind pectoralis minor
  - level 3 nodes: above the upper border of pectoralis minor.

Distribution of Dermatomes and Cutaneous Nerves in the Upper Limb

These are shown in Fig. 3.15 (dermatomes) and Fig. 3.16 (cutaneous nerves).

THE BREAST

- The female breast is made up of:
  - fat
  - fibrous tissue
  - glandular tissue.
- Fat predominates in the non-lactating breast.
- Contains 15–20 lobules of glandular tissue.
- Lobules separated by fibrous septa running from the subcutaneous tissues to the fascia of the chest wall (the ligaments of Astley Cooper).

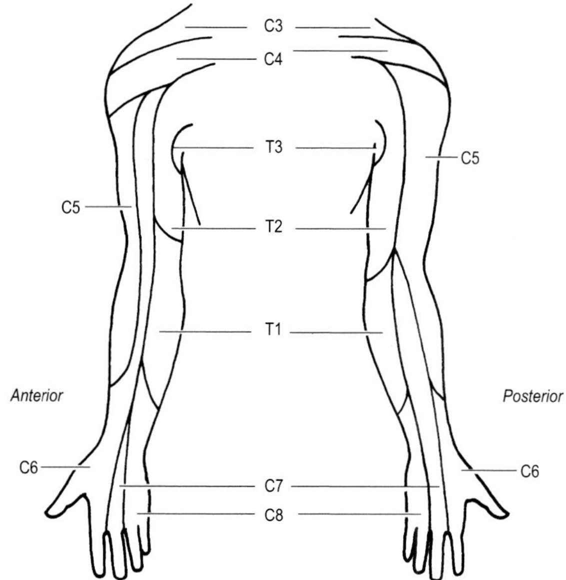

Fig. 3.15 Dermatomes of the upper limb.

- Each gland drains into a lactiferous duct, which converges towards the nipple, and each becomes dilated to form a lactiferous sinus beneath the areola.
- The areola is lubricated by the glands of Montgomery—large modified sebaceous glands.

Blood Supply

- The axillary artery via lateral thoracic and acromiothoracic branches.
- The internal mammary (thoracic) artery via its perforating branches.
- From the intercostal arteries via the lateral perforating branches.
- Venous drainage is to the corresponding veins.

Lymphatic Drainage

- Along tributaries of the axillary vessels to the axillary lymph nodes.
- Along tributaries of the internal mammary vessels to the internal mammary chain.
- Although there is free communication between the lymphatic vessels lying between the lobules of the breast,

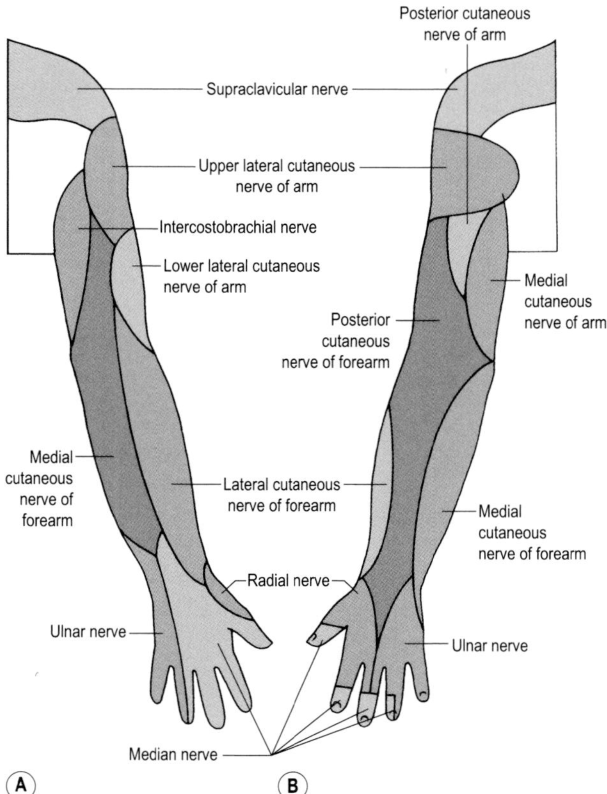

Fig. 3.16 The territories of supply of the cutaneous nerves of the upper limb. (A) Anterior view. (B) Posterior view.

there is a tendency for the lateral part of the breast to drain towards the axilla and the medial part to drain to the internal mammary chain.

Anatomical Classification

- Axillary nodes are arranged into five groups:
  - anterior—lying along the inferolateral border of pectoralis major related to the lateral thoracic artery
  - posterior—lying along the subscapular vessels
  - lateral—lying along the axillary vein
  - central—lying in the axillary fat
  - apical—lying immediately behind the clavicle at the apex of the axilla superior to pectoralis minor.

Surgical Classification

- Level 1 nodes—lying inferior to the inferolateral border of pectoralis minor, usually comprising the lateral, anterior and posterior nodes.
- Level 2 nodes—consisting of those nodes posterior to pectoralis minor, comprising the central nodes and some of the apical nodes.
- Level 3 nodes—consisting of those nodes beyond the superior border of pectoralis minor, comprising the apical nodes and the infraclavicular nodes.

Male Breast

- Rudimentary.
- Small, primitive ducts may be present, supported by fibrous tissue and fat.
- Carcinoma may occur.

Clinical Points

- When spread of a carcinoma of the breast has infiltrated normal pathways of lymphatic drainage, it may spread by other routes to:
  - lymphatics of the opposite breast
  - contralateral axillary lymph nodes
  - inguinal lymph nodes
  - cervical lymph nodes.
- Incisions in the breast are made radially, to avoid cutting across the line of the ducts.
- A blocked duct may become dilated during lactation to form a galactocele.
- Glands of Montgomery become enlarged in pregnancy to form Montgomery's tubercles.
- Dimpling of the skin over a carcinoma of the breast is the result of malignant infiltration and contraction of Cooper's ligaments.
- The nipple may fail to evert and it is important to know if this has been present since birth or is a recent event, as the latter may indicate carcinoma or duct ectasia.
- Supernumerary nipples may be present along the 'milk line' (line of mammary gland of primitive mammals).

OSCE SCENARIOS

OSCE Scenario 3.1

A patient attempts suicide by slashing the flexor aspect of his wrists in a radial to ulnar direction.

1. Which tendons are likely to be divided and how would you test their integrity?
2. Which nerves are likely to be affected?
3. How would you test the integrity of these nerves?

OSCE Scenario 3.2

A patient with chronic renal failure is being assessed for construction of a radiocephalic arteriovenous fistula on the left wrist.

1. Where would you palpate the radial and ulnar pulses to assess their integrity?
2. The ulnar pulse is not readily palpable. What test would you use to assess the integrity of the circulation to the hand and how would you perform it?

OSCE Scenario 3.3

A 30-year-old male is taken to the Accident and Emergency department, having fallen from a horse and landed on the point of his right shoulder. On examination, any attempt to move the shoulder is painful.

1. Describe the anatomy of the upper end of the humerus.
2. X-ray shows a fracture of the surgical neck of the humerus. Which nerve is likely to have been damaged?
3. Describe the distribution of the nerve and how you would test for damage to the nerve.

OSCE Scenario 3.4

A 30-year-old motorcyclist is brought to the Accident and Emergency department after a road traffic accident. Following application of the ATLS protocol, secondary survey revealed significant soft tissue injury to the right shoulder and axillary areas. He was unable to abduct his arm and you suspect he has shoulder dislocation with tear to the rotator cuff muscles and possible injury to the brachial plexus.

1. What muscles make up the rotator cuff?
2. What muscles are involved in abduction of the shoulder joint?
3. The patient is noted to have his arm hanging adducted by his side, medially rotated while the elbow is extended

and pronated. Which part of the brachial plexus is affected and what is this injury called?

4. Where does the long thoracic nerve originate from? What muscle does it supply? How can you test for potential injury to it after axillary dissection?

OSCE Scenario 3.5

A 63-year-old female attends breast clinic after feeling a left breast lump. On examination, she had a 3×3 cm palpable hard lump in the upper outer quadrant, and you noticed skin puckering with arm elevation. Axillary examination demonstrated palpable enlarged lymph nodes.

1. What is the blood supply to the breast?
2. What is the lymph drainage to the breast?
3. How do you classify axillary lymph nodes anatomically and surgically?

Answers in Appendix pages 436–438

Please check your eBook at https://studentconsult.inkling.com/ for more self-assessment questions. See inside cover for registration details.

4

The Lower Limb

THE PELVIC GIRDLE

The pelvis is made up of:
- innominate (hip) bones
- the sacrum
- the coccyx.

These bones are bound to one another by strong ligaments.

The Hip Bone (Os Innominatum) (Fig. 4.1)

This consists of three fused bones:
- ilium
- pubis
- ischium.

Ilium

- Anterosuperiorly is a broad, thin blade for muscle attachment and visceral protection.
- Posteroinferiorly is a thick, weight-transmitting bar with an articular surface at each end (laterally for the head of the femur; medially for the sacrum).
- Iliac crest runs superiorly between the anterior and posterior superior iliac spines; below each of these lies the corresponding inferior iliac spine.
- Posterior border of ilium curves inferiorly between the sacroiliac joint and the ischial spine, forming the greater sciatic notch.
- The glutei and tensor fasciae latae muscles attach to the outer aspect of the blade of the ilium, producing well-defined ridges.
- The three-layered abdominal wall muscles attach to the anterior two-thirds of the crest.
- Latissimus dorsi and erector spinae attach posteriorly to the crest.
- The inguinal ligament attaches laterally to the anterior superior iliac spine.

Pubis

- Shaped like a rotated L.
- Comprises a body and superior and inferior pubic ramus.
- Superior ramus connects the acetabulum and symphyseal articular surfaces of the pubis.
- The inferior ramus extends downwards from the tubercle to its point of fusion with the ischium.
- The inguinal ligament attaches to the pubic tubercle.
- The adductors, perineal muscles and perineal membrane attach to the inferior ramus.

Ischium

- J-shaped bone with a massive body posteriorly bearing the ischial component of the acetabulum.
- Inferiorly is the ischial tuberosity, which bears the weight of the sitting trunk.
- Anteriorly is the ramus uniting with the pubis.
- The posterior border of the body bears the ischial spine, separating the greater sciatic notch superiorly from the lesser sciatic notch inferiorly.
- The hamstrings and short hip rotators (except piriformis) attach to the outer aspect of the tuberosity and the lower body.
- The ischium and pubis together form the circumference of the obturator foramen.
- All three bones fuse together at the acetabulum and form a socket for the femoral head. The acetabulum consists of about one-fifth pubis and two-fifths each of ilium and ischium.

Sacrum (Fig. 4.2)

- Made up of five fused vertebrae and roughly triangular in shape.
- Anterior border of upper part forms the sacral promontory.
- The anterior aspect comprises:
  - a central mass
  - a row of four anterior sacral foramina on each side (transmitting the upper four sacral anterior primary rami)
  - the lateral masses of the sacrum.
- The superior aspect of the lateral mass on each side forms the ala.
- Posteriorly lies the sacral canal (the continuation of the vertebral canal), surrounded by short pedicles, strong laminae and small spinous processes.

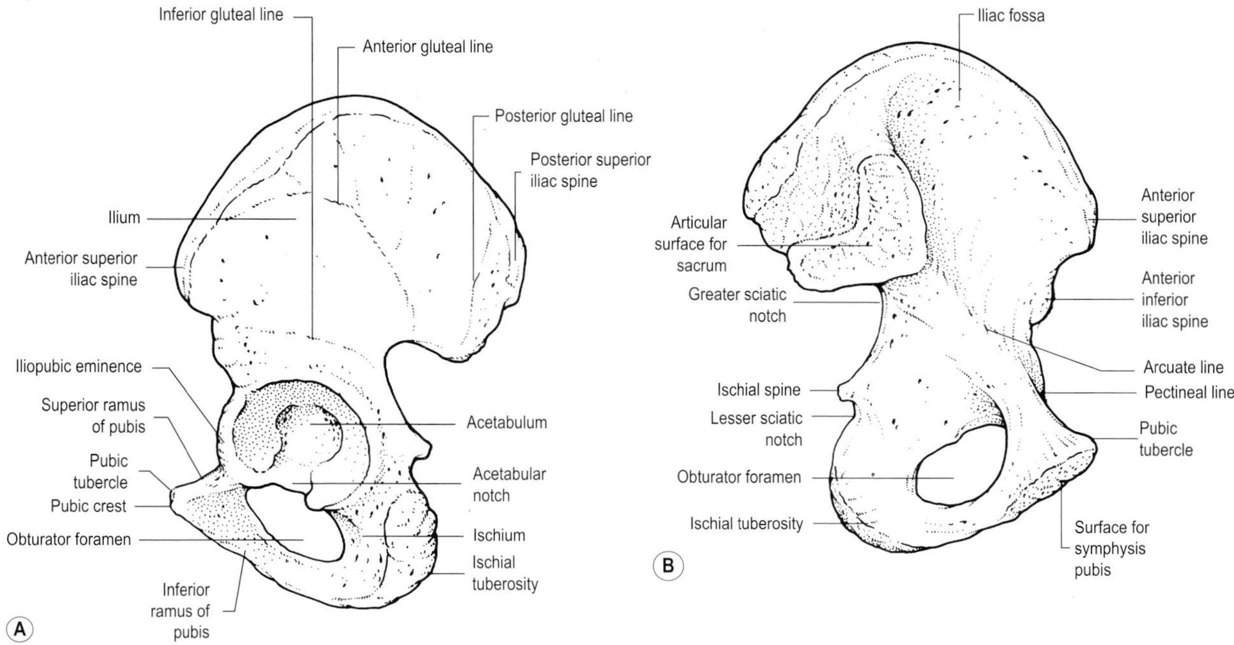

Fig. 4.1 The innominate bone. (A) Lateral view. (B) Medial view.

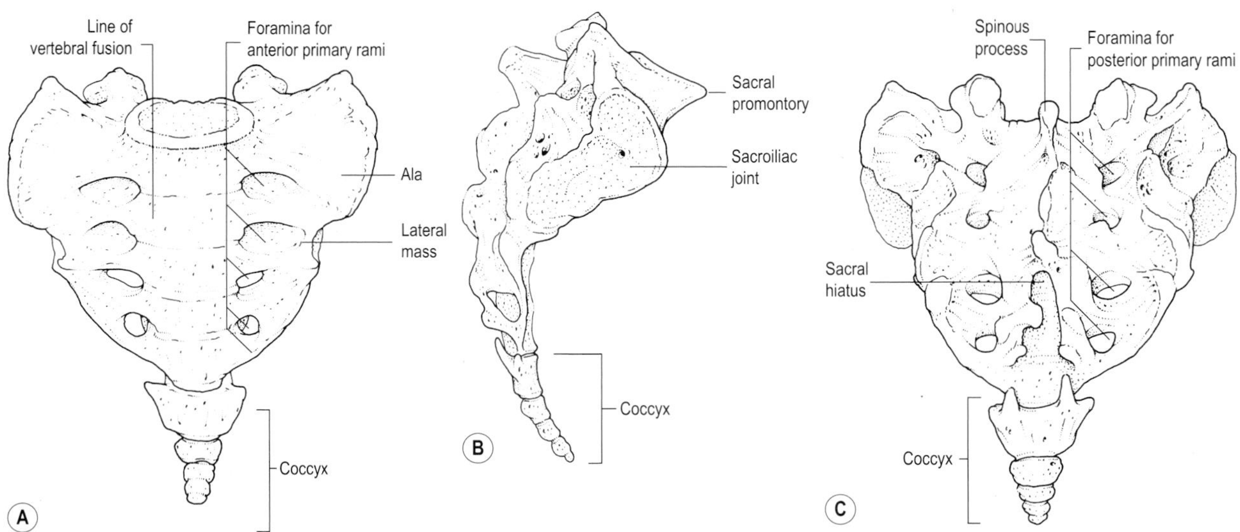

Fig. 4.2 The sacrum and coccyx. (A) Ventral surface. (B) Lateral surface. (C) Dorsal surface.

- Extending from the sacral canal is a row of four posterior sacral foramina on each side.
- Inferiorly, the vertebral canal terminates in the sacral hiatus, which transmits the fifth sacral nerve.
- On either side of the hiatus lies the sacral cornu.
- On the lateral aspect of the sacrum is a large facet for articulation with the corresponding surface of the ilium.

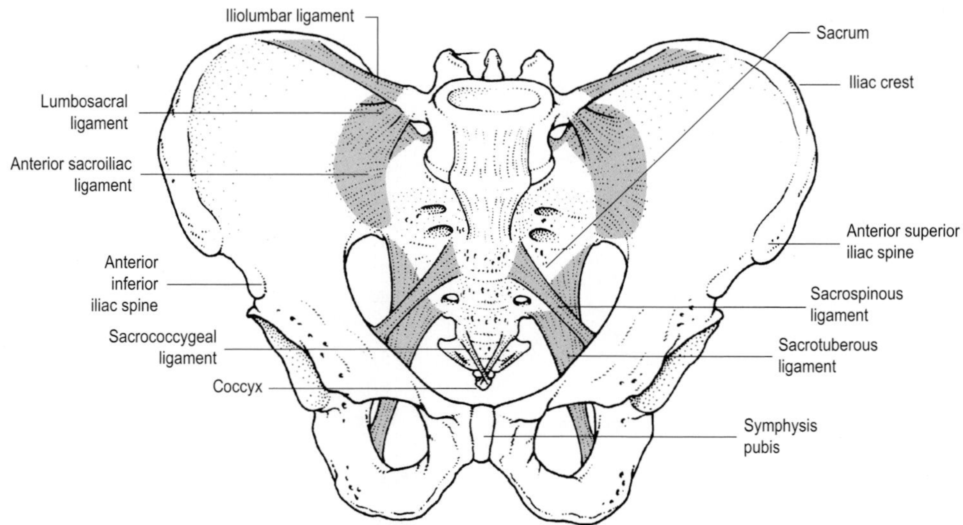

Fig. 4.3 The male pelvis showing the major ligaments, viewed from the front and slightly above.

- Occasionally the fifth lumbar vertebra fuses with the sacrum.
- The dural sheath terminates distally at the second piece of the sacrum.
- Beyond this the sacral canal contains the extradural space, the cauda equina and the filum terminale.

Coccyx

- Made up of three to five fused vertebrae, which articulate with the sacrum.

JOINTS AND LIGAMENTS OF THE PELVIS (Figs. 4.3 and 4.4)

Symphysis Pubis

- Like all symphyses it lies in the median plane and comprises a disc of fibrocartilage firmly fixed between two articular surfaces of hyaline cartilage.
- Surrounded and strengthened by fibrous ligaments.
- A nonsynovial cavity often appears in the disc of fibrocartilage in adult life.

Sacroiliac Joints

- Large and very stable joints connecting the girdle proper with the axial skeleton.
- Joints change in character with age:
  - in the very young they are synovial, with almost plane surfaces
  - in the elderly they are almost entirely fibrous, with irregular surfaces.

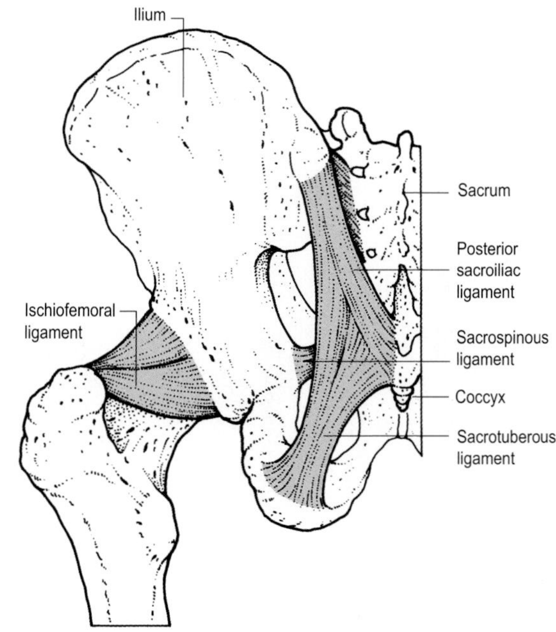

Fig. 4.4 The ligaments of the pelvis and femur, posterior view.

- Stability of the sacroiliac joints is dependent on powerful ligaments:
  - posterior sacroiliac ligaments, which oppose the tendency for downwards and backwards displacement of the sacrum between the hip bones

    - the iliolumbar ligaments attaching to the transverse processes of L5 and the iliac crest.
- The sacrotuberous and sacrospinous ligaments attach the sacrum to the ischium and oppose downwards rotation of the sacrum in the sagittal plane.
- The sacrotuberous ligament passes from the ischial tuberosity to the side of the sacrum and coccyx.
- The sacrospinous ligament passes from the ischial spine to the side of the sacrum and coccyx.
- The sacrospinous and sacrotuberous ligaments define two important exits from the pelvis:
    - the greater sciatic foramen, formed by the sacrospinous ligament and the greater sciatic notch
    - the lesser sciatic foramen, formed by the sacrotuberous ligament and the lesser sciatic notch.
- Major anatomical relations include:
    - sacroiliac joints: the internal iliac vessels pass anteriorly
    - pubic symphysis: urethra and deep dorsal vein of the penis pass inferiorly.

GLUTEAL REGION (Fig. 4.5)

- The muscles of the gluteal region are:
    - gluteus maximus
    - gluteus medius
    - gluteus minimus
    - piriformis
    - obturator internus
    - superior and inferior gemelli
    - quadratus femoris
    - tensor fasciae latae.

  The glutei form the mass of the buttock.

Gluteus Maximus

Origin

- Ilium above and behind posterior gluteal line.
- Sacrum and coccyx.
- Sacrotuberous ligament.

Insertion

- Iliotibial tract: three-quarters.
- Gluteal tuberosity of femur: one-quarter.

Nerve Supply

- Inferior gluteal nerve (L5, S1, 2).

Actions

- Extension of the thigh.
- Lateral rotator of the thigh.
- Balances pelvis on thigh (with psoas and iliacus).
- Steadies femur on knee joint on standing (via iliotibial tract).

General Points

- Large, coarse muscle with small nerve supply and therefore not capable of fine or precise movements.
- Covers posterior part of gluteus medius.
- Covers all short muscles around hip joints, the sciatic nerve, the proximal part of hamstrings, both sciatic foramina and the structures passing through them.
- Lower border overlaps ischial tuberosity on standing (but not sitting) and the sacrotuberous ligament.
- Its lower border does *not* correspond to the gluteal fold.

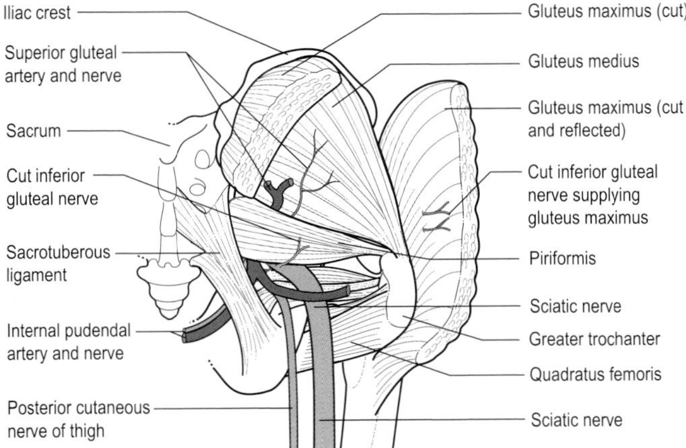

Fig. 4.5 The gluteal region.

Gluteus Medius

Origin

- Outer surface of ilium between anterior and posterior gluteal lines.

Insertion

- Lateral side of greater trochanter of femur.

Nerve Supply

- Superior gluteal (L4, 5, S1).

Action

- Abduction of thigh.
- Tilting upwards of opposite side of pelvis.
- Gluteus medius of limb that is on the ground during walking supports the pelvis and prevents it from tilting to the other side.

Gluteus Minimus

Origin

- Outer aspect of ilium between anterior and inferior gluteal lines.

Insertion

- Anterior aspect of greater trochanter.

Nerve Supply

- Superior gluteal nerve (L4, 5, S1).

Action

- Abduction of thigh.
- Medial rotation of thigh.
- Assists gluteus medius in walking to prevent pelvis tilting.

Tensor Fasciae Latae

Origin

- Anterior part of iliac crest posterior to the anterior superior iliac spine.

Insertion

- Iliotibial tract.

Nerve Supply

- Superior gluteal nerve (L4, 5, S1).

Action

- Assists gluteus maximus in tightening the iliotibial tract.

Piriformis

Origin

- Anterior surface of sacrum.

Insertion

- Passes out of greater sciatic foramen to upper border of greater trochanter.

Nerve Supply

- Directly from second and third sacral nerves.

Action

- This and the following three small muscles cause lateral rotation of the thigh.

Obturator Internus

Origin

- Obturator membrane and surrounding bone.

Insertion

- Tendon leaves by lesser sciatic foramen to insert into the greater trochanter on its medial surface.

Nerve Supply

- Nerve to obturator internus (L5, S1, 2).

Gemelli (Superior and Inferior)

Origin

- Upper and lower margins of lesser sciatic notch.

Insertion

- Sides of tendon of obturator internus.

Nerve Supply

- Superior by nerve to obturator internus.
- Inferior by nerve to quadratus femoris.

Quadratus Femoris

Origin

- Outer border of tuberosity of ischium.

Insertion

- Quadrate tubercle of upper part of trochanteric crest.

Nerve Supply

- Nerve to quadratus femoris (L4, 5, S1).

Greater and Lesser Sciatic Foramina

Sacrotuberous and sacrospinous ligaments convert the sciatic notches into foramina.

Greater Sciatic Foramen

Boundaries

- Superior and anterior: greater sciatic notch.
- Posterior: sacrotuberous ligament.

- Inferior: sacrospinous ligament and ischial spine.

Structures passing through the foramen include

- Piriformis.
- Above piriformis:
  - superior gluteal vessels
  - superior gluteal nerve.
- Below piriformis:
  - inferior gluteal vessels
  - inferior gluteal nerve
  - internal pudendal vessels
  - internal pudendal nerves
  - sciatic nerve
  - posterior cutaneous nerve of thigh
  - nerve to quadratus femoris
  - nerve to obturator internus.

Lesser Sciatic Foramen

Boundaries

- In front: body of ischium and sacrospinous ligament.
- Behind: sacrotuberous ligament.

Structures passing through the foramen include

- tendon of obturator internus
- nerve to obturator internus
- internal pudendal vessels
- pudendal nerve.

Clinical Points

- The buttock is a common site for intramuscular injections.
- It is important to remember that the buttock extends upwards as far as the iliac crest and laterally as far at the greater trochanter. It does not just include the aesthetically pleasing mound.
- The surface marking of the sciatic nerve is represented by a curved line joining the midpoint between the posterior superior iliac spine and ischial tuberosity, with the midpoint between the ischial tuberosity and the greater trochanter. Injections into the upper and outer quadrant of the buttock will therefore avoid accidental injection into the sciatic nerve (see Fig. 4.17).

BONES OF THE LEG AND FOOT

The Femur (Fig. 4.6)

- The largest bone in the body, being about 45 cm long.
- Upper end of femur consists of the rounded head, the neck and two processes, the greater and lesser trochanters.
- Head forms two-thirds of a sphere, facing upwards medially and slightly forwards.
- It is covered with cartilage, except at the central fovea where the ligamentum teres is attached.
- The neck is 5 cm long and lies at an angle of 125° to the shaft (in the female the angle is slightly smaller).
- The greater trochanter is a massive process which can be palpated as the most lateral bony point in the region of the hip.
- The lesser trochanter is much smaller and it is situated most posteriorly on the femur.
- The junction between neck and shaft is marked anteriorly by the intertrochanteric line, laterally by the greater trochanter, medially and posteriorly by the lesser trochanter and posteriorly by the trochanteric crest, which joins the two trochanters.
- The femoral shaft is roughly circular in section at its centre but is flattened posteriorly at each extremity.
- The posterior surface carries a rough raised line in its middle third, i.e. the linea aspera. In the upper and lower thirds, this line splits into two diverging lines.
- Inferiorly the two diverging lines, i.e. the medial and lateral supracondylar ridges, mark the medial and lateral boundaries of a smooth, flattened area, i.e. the popliteal surface of the femur.
- The medial supracondylar line ends distally in the adductor tubercle.
- The lower end of the femur bears prominent condyles, which are separated by a deep intercondylar notch posteriorly and join anteriorly to form the articular surface for the patella.
- The lateral condyle is more prominent than the medial and acts as a buttress to prevent lateral displacement of the patella.

Blood Supply of the Femoral Head

- This is from:
  - vessels from the hip capsule where this is reflected onto the neck in longitudinal bands or retinacula (retinacular vessels)
  - vessels travelling up the diaphysis
  - an artery in the ligamentum teres, which is a negligible source in the adult.
- The chief source is from the retinacular vessels.

Clinical Points

- Fractures of the femoral neck completely interrupt the blood supply from the diaphysis. If the retinacula are torn, avascular necrosis of the femoral head will occur. Avascular necrosis of the femoral head is much more likely to occur with intracapsular fractures than extracapsular fractures because intracapsular fractures are more likely to disrupt the retinacular blood flow.
- Fractures of the femoral neck result in shortening, external rotation and adduction of the affected limb. Shortening is because of the strength of the longitudinally lying muscles, especially quadriceps and hamstrings. The adductors pull the limb superomedially.

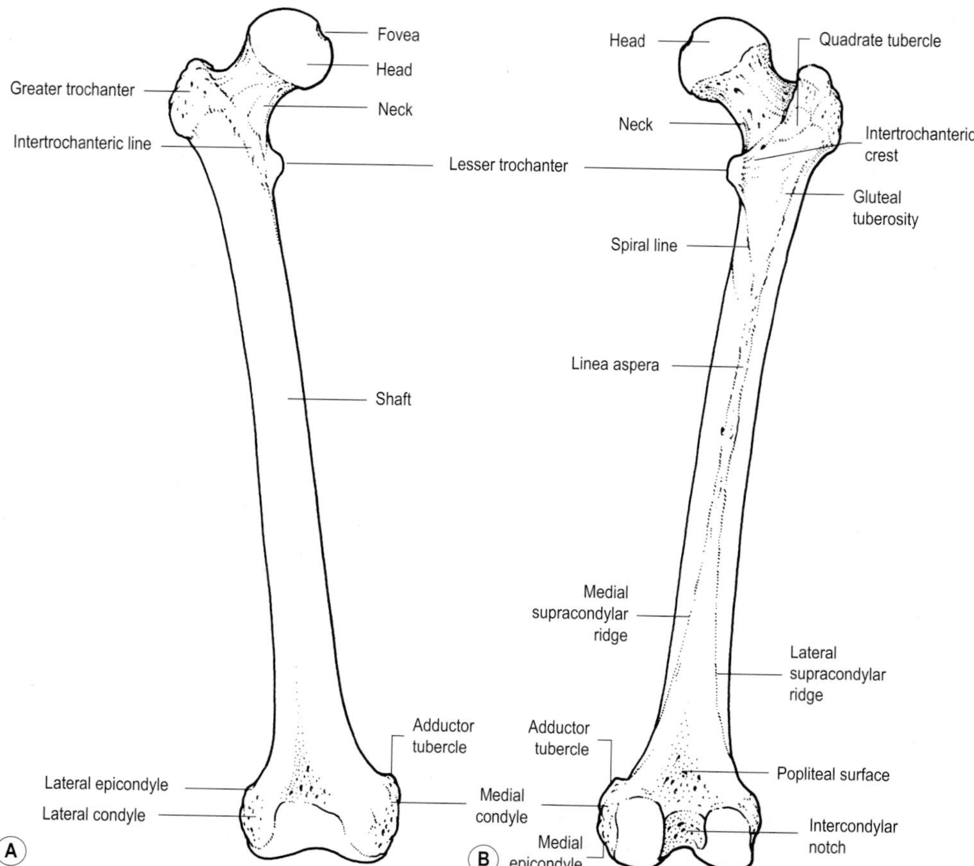

Fig. 4.6 The right femur. (A) Anterior view. (B) Posterior view.

Instead of rotating about an axis between hip and knee, the femur now rotates about the axis of its shaft. Because of this, iliopsoas now acts as an external rotator.

- Fractures of the femoral shaft are accompanied by considerable bleeding due to damage of the perforating branches of the profunda femoris artery, which are in close relation to the shaft.
- Fractures of the femoral shaft are also accompanied by considerable shortening owing to contractions of the powerful surrounding muscles:
  - the proximal segment is flexed by iliopsoas and abducted by gluteus medius and minimus
  - the distal segment is pulled medially by the adductor muscles.
- The popliteal artery is closely related to the popliteal surface of the femur. Supracondylar fractures of the femur may damage the popliteal artery. This is because gastrocnemius tilts the distal fragment posteriorly and the sharp proximal edge of this fragment impinges upon the popliteal artery.

The Patella

- Largest sesamoid bone in the body. Developed in the expansion of the quadriceps tendon, which continues from the apex of the patella as the ligamentum patellae.
- Anterior surface is roughened for the attachment of part of the quadriceps tendon.
- Posterior surface is smooth and covered with hyaline cartilage for articulation with the corresponding areas of the femur.
- The lateral facet is the larger (this explains how you can 'side' a patella—if placed on a flat surface with the apex pointing away from you, it will fall to the side to which it belongs).

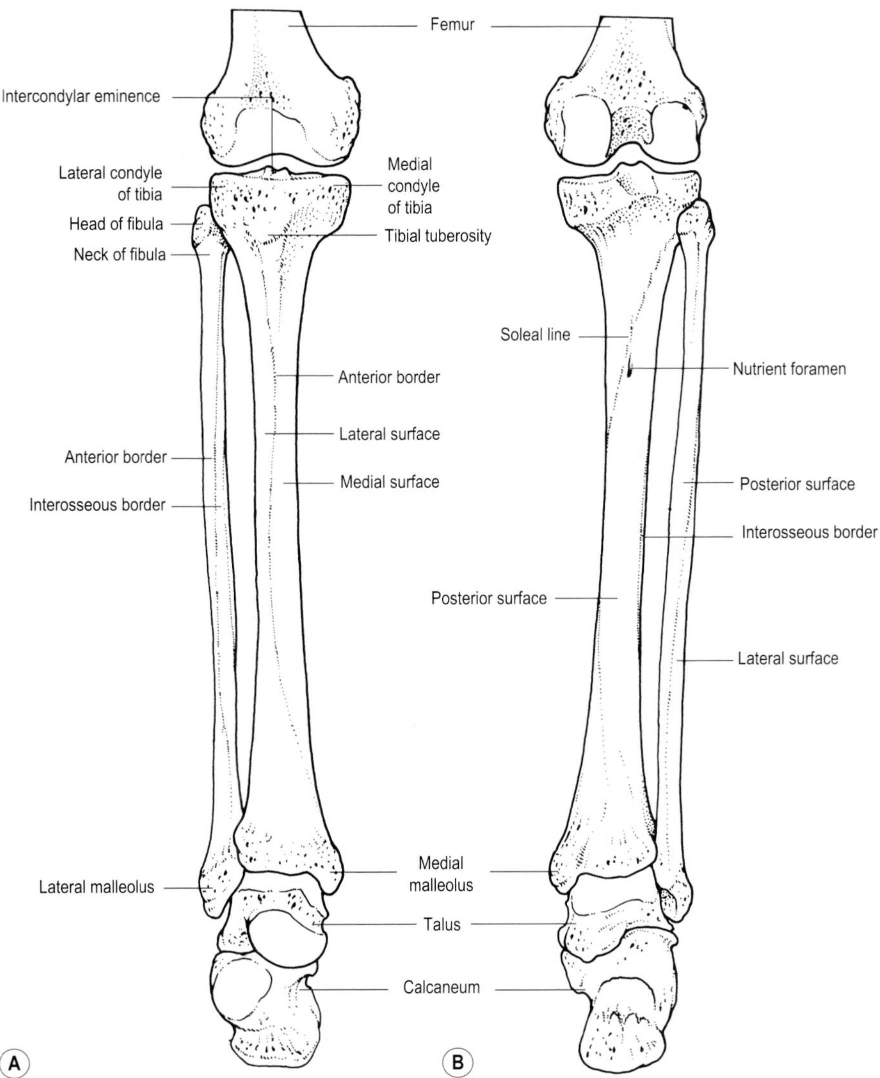

Fig. 4.7 The lower end of the femur, tibia, fibula, talus and calcaneum. (A) Anterior view. (B) Posterior view.

Clinical Points

- Lateral dislocation of the patella is resisted by the more prominent lateral femoral condyle and by the pull of the lowermost fibres of vastus medialis, which insert almost horizontally along the medial margin of the patella. Recurrent dislocation of the patella may occur if the lateral condyle of the femur is underdeveloped.
- Direct trauma to the patella may shatter it into several fragments. These are not avulsed because the quadriceps expansion remains intact.

The Tibia (Fig. 4.7)

- The more medial bone of the lower leg. Comprises a shaft and an expanded upper and lower end. It alone articulates with the femur at the knee joint, the fibula being excluded.
- The upper end is expanded into the medial and lateral condyles, the medial having the greater surface area of the two.
- Between the condyles is the intercondylar area, which bears the intercondylar eminence. The cruciate

ligaments are attached to the intercondylar area, as are the horns of the medial and lateral menisci.

- The tuberosity of the tibia is at the upper end of the anterior border of the shaft and gives attachment to the ligamentum patellae.
- The shaft of the tibia is triangular in cross section, its anterior border and anteromedial surface being subcutaneous throughout its length.
- The posterior surface of the shaft has the soleal line at its upper end, which marks the origin of soleus.
- The interosseous border is on the lateral side and gives attachment to the interosseous membrane, which runs upwards to the shaft of the fibula.
- The lower end of the tibia expands from the triangular shaft into a quadrilateral mass of bone from the medial surface of which the medial malleolus projects downwards and medially.
- The medial malleolus is grooved posteriorly by the tendon of tibialis posterior.
- The inferior surface of the lower end of the tibia is smooth, being covered with hyaline cartilage and forms, with the malleoli, the upper articular surface of the ankle joint.

Clinical Points

- The shaft of the tibia is subcutaneous anteromedially throughout its course. Being so exposed, it is not surprising that the tibia is the most commonly fractured long bone and sustains most compound injuries.
- Lacerations over the subcutaneous surface of the tibia heal poorly because of lack of vascularity in the subcutaneous tissues as only the periosteum supports the skin.

The Fibula (Fig. 4.7)

- The fibula is a long, thin bone with a small head at its upper end and an expanded lateral malleolus distally.
- The upper end has a head which articulates with the tibia, below which is a neck around which winds the common peroneal nerve.
- The shaft is slender and bears an attachment for the interosseous membrane, the fibres of which run downwards and medially towards the tibia.
- The lower end of the fibula is expanded to form the lateral malleolus, which bears an articular facet medially for articulation with the talus.
- The posterior aspect of the lateral malleolus is grooved by the tendons of peroneus longus and peroneus brevis.

Clinical Points

- The common peroneal nerve winds round the neck of the fibula. Damage to the nerve at this point, e.g. fractures of the neck of the fibula owing to car-bumper injuries, or tight below-knee plasters, will result in foot drop.

Bones of the Foot (Fig. 4.8)

These consist of the tarsal bones, metatarsals and phalanges.

The Tarsal Bones

- These consist of a proximal row and a distal row. The proximal row is made up of:
  - talus
  - calcaneum
  - navicular bone.
- The distal row is made up of:
  - the cuboid bone
  - the three cuneiform bones.

Talus

- Bears a large facet on the upper surface for articulation with the tibia.
- Bears facets on the medial and lateral sides for the medial and lateral malleoli, respectively.

The superior articular surface is wider in front than behind such that, when the foot is dorsiflexed, the talus is wedged between the malleoli, but in plantarflexion there is a little play so that a minor degree of tilting can occur at this joint (this is not inversion and eversion, which occurs at the subtalar joints).

- The talus is grooved posteriorly for the tendon of flexor hallucis longus.
- There are no muscular or tendinous attachments to the talus but a number of ligaments are attached to it (see arches of the foot).

Calcaneum

- Medial side easily recognized because of sustentaculum tali (which is cantilevered out to support the head of the talus).
- There are two facets for talocalcaneal joints.
- The posterior surface can be divided into three areas:
  - the middle, roughened area is for the insertion of tendo calcaneus
  - the upper, smooth area is a site of the bursa between tendo calcaneus and the bone
  - the lower area is covered by a fibro–fatty pad that forms the heel.
- The undersurface has medial and lateral tubercles, of which the former is the larger and is the weightbearing part of the heel.
- The anterior surface consists of an almost plane facet for the cuboid.

Cuboid

- Articulates with the anterior facet on the calcaneum.
- Grooved on its undersurface by the tendon of peroneus longus.

Navicular

- Articulates with the head of the talus behind and with the three cuneiforms in front.

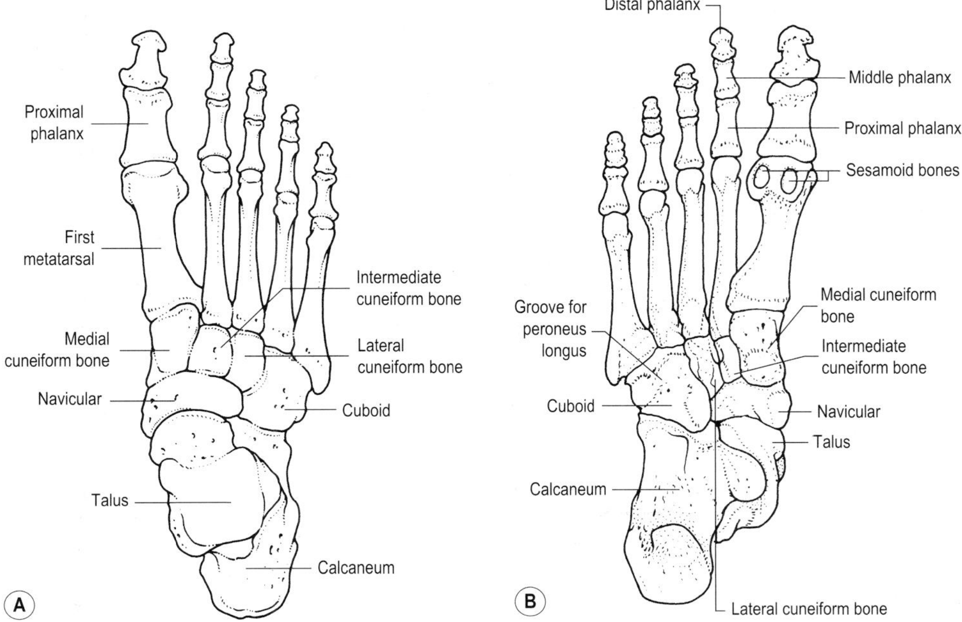

Fig. 4.8 The bones of the foot. (A) Superior view. (B) Inferior view.

- Bears a tuberosity for the insertion of tibialis posterior.
- The spring ligament passes from the sustentaculum tali of the calcaneum to the tuberosity of the navicular.

Cuneiforms

- Cuneus means wedge. The wedge-shaped bones help maintain the transverse arch of the foot.

Metatarsals

- The first metatarsal is thickest and sturdiest, bearing on its undersurface two depressions lined with articular cartilage for two sesamoid bones in the tendon of flexor hallucis brevis.
- The second metatarsal is the longest and thinnest and in the event of fatigue is liable to break (march fracture).
- The fifth metatarsal has a tuberosity on its base for insertion of peroneus brevis.
- In the standing position the metatarsal heads are in contact with the ground.

FEMORAL TRIANGLE (Fig. 4.9)

Boundaries

- Above: inguinal ligament.
- Medially: medial border of adductor longus.
- Laterally: medial border of sartorius.

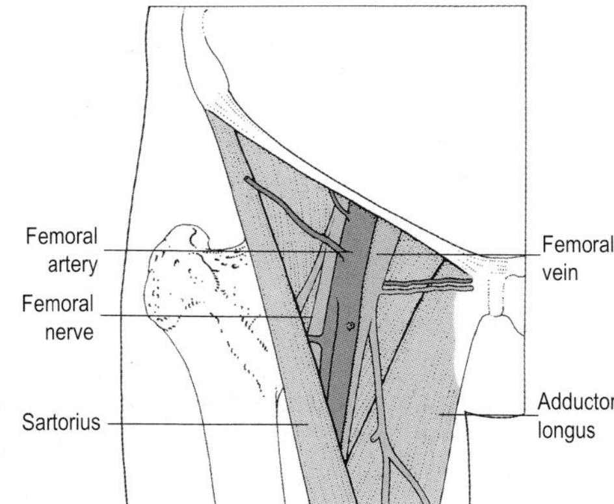

Fig. 4.9 The femoral triangle.

Floor

- Iliacus.
- Psoas major tendon.
- Pectineus.
- Adductor longus.

Roof

- Skin.
- Superficial fascia.

- Superficial inguinal lymph nodes.
- Great saphenous vein.
- Deep fascia of thigh (fascia lata).
- Cribriform fascia (part of fascia lata).
- Pierced by great saphenous vein and lymphatics at saphenous opening.

Contents

- Femoral canal.
- Femoral vein.
- Femoral artery.
- Femoral nerve.
- Deep inguinal lymph nodes.

Femoral Sheath

- Prolongation of fascia derived from transversalis fascia (anteriorly) and fascia over iliacus (posteriorly).
- Contains the femoral canal medially, the femoral vein in the middle and the femoral artery laterally.

Femoral Canal

- Medial compartment of the femoral sheath.
- Entered via the femoral ring.
- Contains fat and lymph nodes (Cloquet's node).

Femoral Ring

This is the entry to the femoral canal. Its relations are:

- anteriorly: inguinal ligament
- medially: the lacunar ligament (may contain an abnormal obturator artery in its free edge)
- posteriorly: the pectineal ligament
- laterally: the femoral vein.

Inguinal Lymph Nodes

These are divided as follows.

- Superficial group:
  - horizontal: below and parallel to inguinal ligament
  - vertical: around the termination of the great saphenous vein.
- Deep group:
  - medial to femoral vein and in femoral canal (Cloquet's node).
- Sites draining to the inguinal nodes include:
  - lower limb
  - buttock
  - lower trunk and back below the level of the umbilicus
  - perineum, scrotal skin and penis
  - vulva and lower third of vagina
  - abdominal wall below and including the umbilicus
  - lower half of the anal canal
  - fundus of the uterus (lymphatics follow the round ligament).

The Adductor Canal (Subsartorial Canal, Hunter's Canal)

This passes from the apex of the femoral triangle to the popliteal fossa. Its relations are:

- Posteriorly: adductor longus and adductor magnus.
- Anteromedially: sartorius forming the roof of the canal.
- Anterolaterally: vastus medialis.
- Contents:
  - femoral artery
  - femoral vein (behind the artery)
  - saphenous nerve.

The Popliteal Fossa (Fig. 4.10)

This is a diamond-shaped space behind the knee. Its relations and contents are as follows.

- Above and medial: semimembranosus and semitendinosus.
- Above and lateral: biceps femoris tendon.
- Below and lateral: lateral head of gastrocnemius.
- Below and medial: medial head of gastrocnemius.
- Roof:
  - skin
  - superficial fascia
  - deep fascia (pierced by the small saphenous vein).
- Floor (from above down):
  - posterior surface of femur
  - posterior aspect of knee joint
  - popliteus muscle covering the upper surface of the tibia.
- Contents:
  - popliteal artery (deepest structure)
  - popliteal vein
  - sciatic nerve above
  - common peroneal nerve below
  - tibial nerve below
  - lymph nodes (draining the lateral side of foot and heel)
  - fat
  - bursae.

ARTERIES OF THE LOWER LIMB (Figs. 4.11 and 4.12)

Femoral Artery

- Continuation of external iliac artery below the inguinal ligament.
- Passes to the apex of the femoral triangle.
- Enters adductor canal.
- Terminates by passing through the hiatus in adductor magnus to become the popliteal artery.

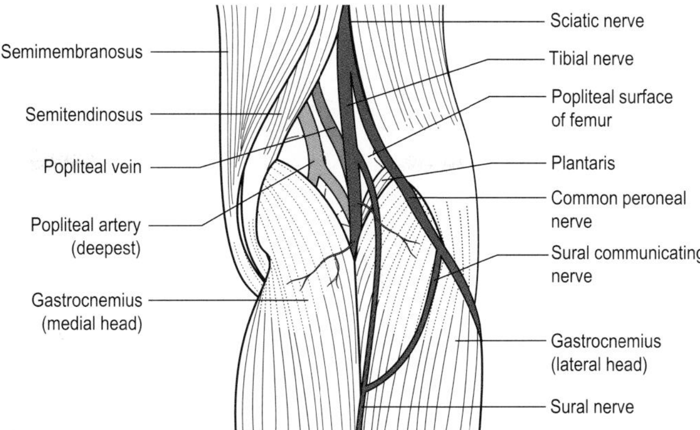

Fig. 4.10 The right popliteal fossa.

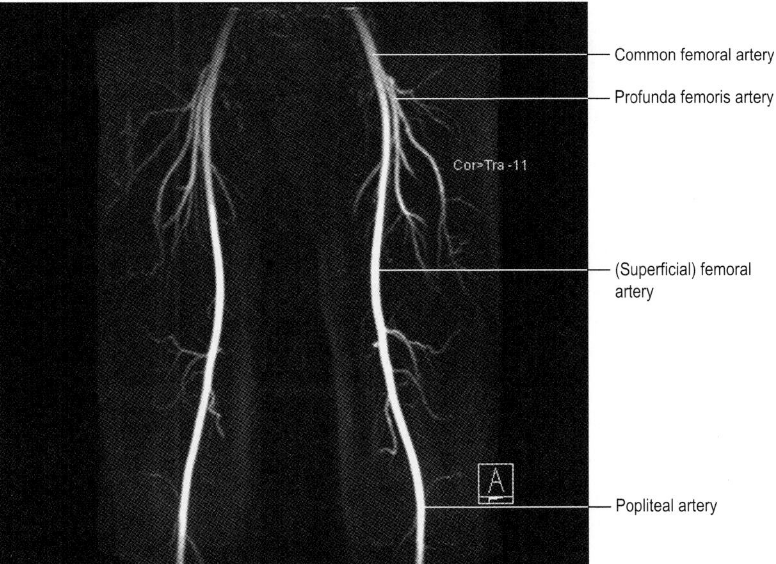

Fig. 4.11 MRA of thigh showing the (common) femoral artery and its branches.

- Relations:
  - anteriorly: skin, superficial fascia, deep fascia, femoral branch of genitofemoral nerve, sartorius, saphenous nerve
  - posteriorly: psoas tendon, profunda vessels, pectineus, adductor longus, femoral vein (at apex of femoral triangle and in subsartorial canal), tendon of adductor magnus
  - medially: femoral vein (in femoral triangle), adductor longus
  - laterally: femoral nerve, sartorius (in femoral triangle), vastus medialis.
- Branches include:
  - superficial epigastric artery
  - superficial circumflex iliac artery
  - superficial external pudendal artery
  - deep external pudendal artery
  - profunda femoris artery.

Profunda Femoris

- Arises posterolaterally from femoral artery, 5 cm distal to the inguinal ligament.
- Passes distally in femoral triangle lying on iliacus, psoas, pectineus, adductor brevis and adductor magnus.

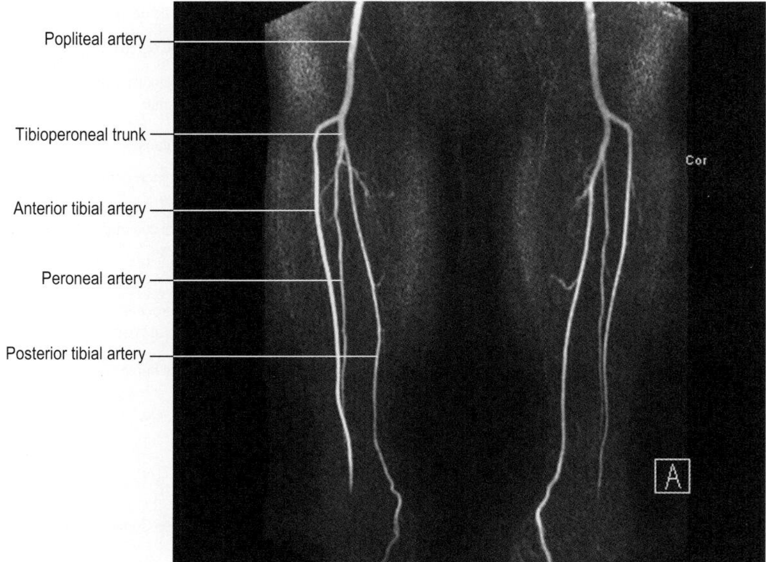

Fig. 4.12 MRA of popliteal artery and its branches.

- Adductor longus passes superficial to it.
- Separated from femoral artery by femoral vein and profunda veins and adductor longus.
- Terminates in the lower third of the thigh by perforating adductor magnus.
- Branches include:
  - lateral circumflex artery
  - medial circumflex artery
  - four perforating branches.
- Branches supply the muscles of the thigh.
- Acts as collateral channels linking the arterial anastomoses around knee and hip.

Popliteal Artery

- Continuation of femoral artery at hiatus in adductor magnus.
- Passes to lower border of popliteus where it divides into anterior and posterior tibial arteries.
- Relations include:
  - overlapped by semimembranosus in upper part of fossa
  - covered below by gastrocnemius and plantaris
  - lies deep within the fossa, covered superficially by the popliteal vein and more superficially by the tibial nerve.
- Branches include:
  - muscular
  - geniculate to the knee joint
  - anterior tibial artery
  - posterior tibial artery.

Posterior Tibial Artery

- Terminal branch of popliteal artery.
- Extends from lower border of popliteus to the lower margin of the flexor retinaculum at the ankle, where it divides into medial and lateral plantar arteries.
- Relations include:
  - upper two-thirds covered by soleus and gastrocnemius
  - lower third lies superficially between medial border of tendo calcaneus and medial border of tibia
  - tibial nerve is at first medial but soon crosses posteriorly to reach lateral side
  - lies on tibialis posterior, flexor digitorum longus, tibia and back of ankle joint
  - accompanied by venae comitantes and tibial nerve.
- Branches include:
  - peroneal artery (the artery of lateral compartment): arises 2.5 cm below popliteus, runs on posterior aspect of fibula, supplies adjacent muscles, gives a nutrient branch to the fibula, gives a perforating branch, which pierces interosseous membrane and anastomoses with arteries on dorsum of foot
  - medial plantar artery
  - lateral plantar artery.

Anterior Tibial Artery

- Terminal branch of popliteal artery.
- Arises at lower border of popliteus.
- Extends in front of ankle joint where it becomes dorsalis pedis artery.
- Artery of the anterior compartment.
- Relations include:
  - lies deeply on interosseous membrane
  - becomes superficial just above ankle between tendons of extensor hallucis longus and tibialis anterior
  - crossed superficially by tendon of extensor hallucis longus just proximal to ankle joint.
- Branches include:
  - small branches, which form collaterals with vessels around the knee joint and ankle joint
  - dorsalis pedis, which runs from front of ankle to first interosseous space; plunges deeply between first and second metatarsals to anastomose with lateral plantar artery to form plantar arch supplying plantar aspect of toes
  - lies between tendons of extensor hallucis longus and extensor digitorum longus on dorsum of foot.

Clinical Points

- The femoral artery may be palpated at the midinguinal point—halfway between the anterior superior iliac spine and the pubic symphysis.
- Arterial puncture for blood gases and arteriography is often performed at this site.
- A venous sample may be obtained from the femoral vein, which lies immediately medial to the femoral artery.
- The femoral artery is quite superficial in the femoral triangle where it may be easily injured, e.g. butchers, bullfighters, stabbings in the groin.
- The popliteal artery may be palpated in the lower part of the popliteal fossa by compressing it against the posterior surface of the upper end of the tibia. It cannot be palpated easily in the upper part of the fossa as it is pushed into the intercondylar notch.
- The relation of the popliteal artery to the lower end of the femur makes it vulnerable in supracondylar fractures.
- A popliteal artery aneurysm may cause pressure on adjacent structures, e.g. vein (leading to DVT), tibial and common peroneal nerve (leading to pain and nerve palsies).
- The posterior tibial artery is palpable behind the medial malleolus midway between the latter and the tendo calcaneus.
- The dorsalis pedis artery is palpable on the dorsum of the foot lying between the tendon of extensor hallucis longus (medial) and extensor digitorum longus to the second toe (lateral).
- There is a rich anastomosis between the femoral artery and its branches, which is important in the development of collaterals in arteriosclerotic disease.

THE VEINS OF THE LOWER LIMB

These are divided into superficial and deep. The deep veins accompany the major arteries of the limb. Superficial veins are the great and small saphenous veins.

Great (Long) Saphenous Vein

- Commences on the medial side of the dorsal venous arch of the foot.
- Ascends immediately in front of the medial malleolus (accompanied by the saphenous nerve).
- Passes a hand's breadth behind the medial border of the patella.
- Ascends obliquely up the medial aspect of the thigh, piercing the deep fascia to terminate in the femoral vein at the saphenous opening 4 cm inferolateral to the pubic tubercle.
- Tributaries include:
  - superficial epigastric vein
  - superficial circumflex iliac vein
  - superficial external pudendal vein
  - lateral accessory vein, which joins the main vein at midthigh.

Small (Short) Saphenous Vein

- Commences on the lateral side of the dorsal venous arch of the foot.
- Passes behind the lateral malleolus.
- Courses up the back of the thigh, perforating the deep fascia over the popliteal fossa to enter the popliteal vein.
- Accompanied in its course by the sural nerve.
- Communicates with the deep veins of the foot and the great saphenous vein.

Clinical Points

- The relationship of the great saphenous vein to the medial malleolus is constant. It may therefore be used for life-saving cannulation.
- The saphenous nerve is immediately adjacent to the vein and may be caught in a ligature while doing a cutdown or during varicose vein surgery.
- The tributaries of the great saphenous vein at the saphenofemoral junction are important when carrying out a high tie during varicose vein surgery. Failure to ligate all tributaries may result in recurrence. Patterns of these veins are variable.

LEG COMPARTMENTS

Thigh

The deep fascia (fascia lata) of the thigh surrounds muscles and sends septa in between the principal groups. The thigh is divided into compartments as follows.

- Anterior compartment of the thigh, containing:
  - quadriceps muscles: vastus lateralis, vastus intermedius, vastus medialis, rectus femoris
  - sartorius.
- Medial compartment of the thigh, containing:
  - obturator externus, adductor magnus, adductor brevis, adductor longus, pectineus, gracilis.
- Posterior compartment of the thigh, containing:
  - hamstring muscles: semitendinosus, semimembranosus, biceps femoris.

Lower Leg

- The deep fascia of the leg divides it into three compartments:
  - anterior compartment
  - posterior compartment
  - lateral compartment.

Anterior Compartment

- Contains the following:
  - tibialis anterior
  - extensor hallucis longus
  - extensor digitorum longus
  - peroneus tertius.
- All muscles are supplied by the deep peroneal nerve.
- The artery of this compartment is the anterior tibial artery.

Posterior Compartment

- Contains the following:
  - gastrocnemius
  - soleus
  - plantaris
  - popliteus
  - flexor hallucis longus
  - flexor digitorum longus
  - tibialis posterior.
- All muscles are supplied by the tibial nerve.
- The artery of this compartment is the posterior tibial artery.

Lateral Compartment (Peroneal Compartment)

- Contains the following:
  - peroneus longus
  - peroneus brevis.
- The nerve of this compartment is the superficial peroneal nerve.
- The artery of this compartment is the peroneal artery.

The Nerves of the Lower Limb

These are derived from the lumbar and sacral plexuses.

LUMBAR PLEXUS (Fig. 4.13)

- Formed from the anterior primary rami of L1–4 (with a contribution from T12).
- Formed in the substance of psoas major.
- Trunks emerge from lateral border of psoas with the exception of the obturator nerve (medial border) and the genitofemoral nerve (anterior aspect).
- The principal branches of the lumbar plexus are:
  - femoral nerve
  - obturator nerve
  - ilioinguinal nerve
  - lateral cutaneous nerve of thigh
  - genitofemoral nerve.

Femoral Nerve

- Root value L2–4.
- Passes through substance of psoas major, emerging on lateral aspect.
- Passes under inguinal ligament lateral to femoral artery lying on iliopsoas.
- About 5 cm below inguinal ligament breaks up into its terminal branches.
- Branches include:
  - muscular: quadriceps, sartorius, pectineus
  - cutaneous: medial cutaneous nerve of thigh, intermediate cutaneous nerve of thigh, saphenous nerve
  - articular branches to hip and knee.

Obturator Nerve

- Root value L2–4.
- Emerges from medial aspect of psoas.
- Runs downwards and forwards deep to internal iliac vessels to reach the upper part of the obturator foramen.
- Enters the thigh through the obturator foramen accompanied by the obturator vessels.
- Branches include:
  - anterior branch: descends in front of the adductor brevis, behind pectineus and adductor longus; supplies gracilis, adductor longus, adductor brevis and skin over medial aspect of thigh and hip joint
  - posterior branch: passes through the obturator externus and behind adductor brevis; supplies adductor magnus, obturator externus, knee joint and occasionally adductor brevis.

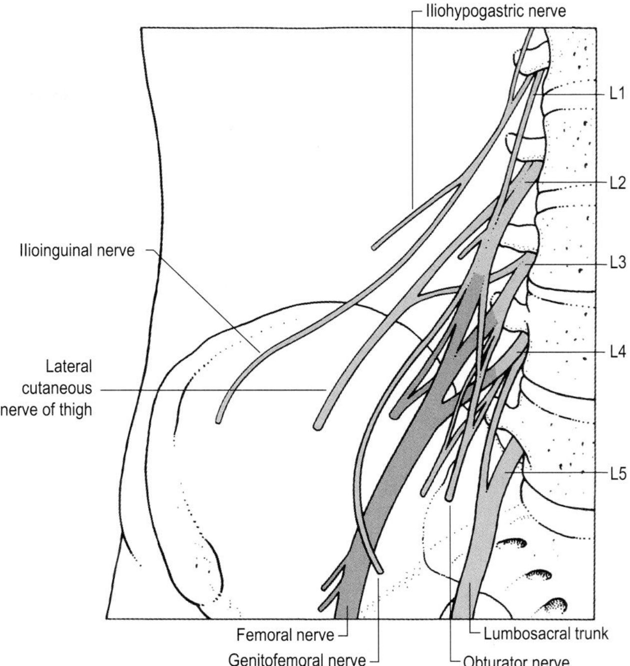

Fig. 4.13 The lumbar plexus.

Other Branches of Lumbar Plexus

- Ilioinguinal nerve: enters the inguinal canal and is important in hernia surgery. It supplies the skin of the groin and the anterior part of the scrotum.
- Lateral cutaneous nerve of thigh: arises directly from lumbar plexus and enters thigh deep to inguinal ligament. Occasionally it pierces the inguinal ligament. May be trapped by inguinal ligament, resulting in pain and numbness in its distribution (meralgia paraesthetica).
- Genitofemoral nerve:
  - formed within psoas major from L1, 2
  - emerges on anterior surface of psoas major
  - runs inferiorly passing posteriorly to the ureter
  - divides into genital and femoral branches
  - in the male, the genital branch enters the deep inguinal ring in company with the vas deferens and supplies the cremaster muscle
  - emerging from the superficial inguinal ring, it supplies the skin of the scrotum
  - in the female, it ends in supplying the skin of the labium majus
  - femoral branch passes deep to the inguinal ligament within the femoral sheath to supply the skin just inferior to the ligament.

SACRAL PLEXUS (Fig. 4.14)

- Formed from the anterior primary rami of L4–5, S1–4.
- Sacral nerves emerge from the anterior sacral foramina and unite in front of piriformis, where they are joined by the lumbosacral trunk (L4, 5).

Branches

Muscular

- Piriformis.
- Obturator internus.
- Quadratus femoris.
- Gemelli.

Superior Gluteal

- L4, 5, S1.
- Passes out of the greater sciatic foramen above piriformis.
- Accompanies superior gluteal vessels.
- Supplies gluteus medius, gluteus minimus and tensor fascia lata.

Inferior Gluteal

- L5, S1, 2.
- Passes out of the pelvis below piriformis.
- Supplies gluteus maximus.

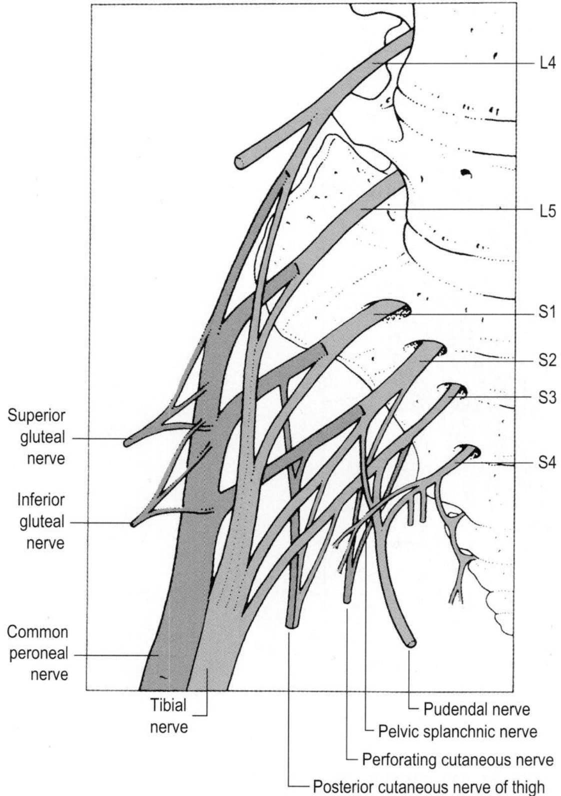

Fig. 4.14 The sacral plexus. The anterior division has lighter shading.

Pudendal Nerve

- Root value S2, 3, 4.
- Passes out of the greater sciatic foramen between piriformis and coccygeus.
- Lies medial to sciatic nerve.
- Winds over sacrospinous ligament medial to internal pudendal artery.
- Re-enters pelvis through lesser sciatic foramen.
- Enters pudendal canal in obturator fascia (accompanied by vessels) on the lateral wall of the ischiorectal fossa and divides into three branches: inferior rectal (haemorrhoidal), perineal, dorsal nerve of penis.

Sciatic Nerve

- Root value L4, 5, S1, 2, 3.
- Largest nerve in the body.
- Nerve emerges from the greater sciatic foramen below piriformis.
- Covered by gluteus maximus.
- Crosses posterior surface of ischium.
- Descends on adductor magnus lying deep to the hamstrings.
- Crossed by the long head of biceps femoris.
- Divides into tibial nerve and common peroneal nerve.
- The level of division is variable and the nerves may be separate entities even at their origin from the sacral plexus.
- Branches include:
  - muscular to biceps femoris, semimembranosus, semitendinosus and part of adductor magnus (also supplied by the obturator nerve)
  - tibial nerve
  - common peroneal nerve.

Tibial Nerve

- Root value L4, 5, S1, 2, 3.
- Larger terminal branch of sciatic nerve.
- Traverses popliteal fossa superficial to popliteal vein and artery, crossing from lateral to medial side of artery.
- Descends deep to soleus in calf.
- Accompanied by posterior tibial vessels.
- Passes behind medial malleolus.
- Divides into medial and lateral plantar nerves.
- Branches include:
  - in the popliteal fossa:
    - muscular: gastrocnemius, popliteus, soleus
    - cutaneous: sural nerve (accompanies small saphenous vein)
    - articular: knee joint.
  - in the leg and foot:
    - muscular: the flexor hallucis longus; flexor digitorum longus; tibialis posterior; intrinsic muscles of the foot
    - cutaneous: skin of the sole of the foot; lateral plantar nerve supplies lateral part and lateral one-and-a-half toes; medial plantar nerve supplies medial half and medial three-and-a-half toes (compare median nerve and ulnar nerve in hand).

Common Peroneal Nerve

- Root value L4, 5, S1, 2.
- Smaller terminal branch of sciatic nerve.
- Enters popliteal fossa lateral to tibial nerve.
- Passes along medial border of biceps tendon.
- Winds round neck of fibula deep to peroneus longus, where it divides into superficial and deep peroneal nerves.

Deep Peroneal Nerve

- Pierces extensor digitorum longus.
- Descends (accompanied by anterior tibial vessels) over the anterior interosseous membrane and across the ankle joint.
- Branches:

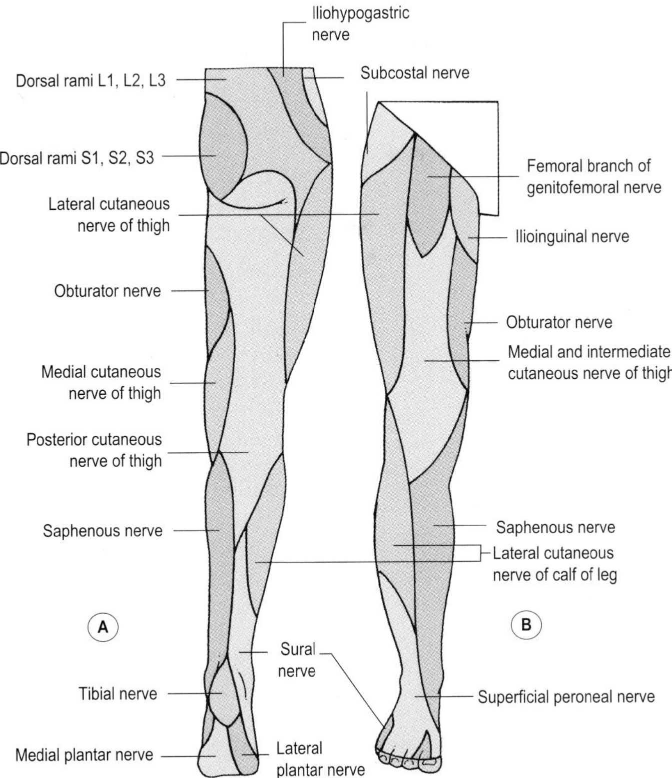

Fig. 4.15 The cutaneous nerve supply of the lower limb. (A) Posterior view. (B) Anterior view.

- muscular: tibialis anterior, extensor hallucis longus, extensor digitorum longus, extensor digitorum brevis, peroneus tertius
- cutaneous: to the skin of the web space between first and second toes.

Superficial Peroneal Nerve

- Muscular: peroneus longus, peroneus brevis.
- Cutaneous: distal two-thirds of the lateral aspect of the leg, the dorsum of the foot (except the first web space).

Cutaneous Nerve Supply of the Leg

(Fig. 4.15)

Dermatomes of the Leg

(Fig. 4.16)

Tendon Reflexes of the Lower Limb

- Knee: quadriceps (L3, 4 via femoral nerve).
- Ankle: gastrocnemius (S1 via sciatic nerve—tibial branch).

Clinical Points

- Nerve supply to the hip joint and knee joint involves the same nerves (femoral, obturator, sciatic). Pain from hip disease therefore may be referred to the knee.
- An obstructed or strangulated obturator hernia may press on the obturator nerve at the obturator foramen. This may cause pain in its cutaneous distribution on the medial aspect of the thigh. Intestinal obstruction associated with pain in the cutaneous distribution of the obturator nerve may indicate obturator hernia.
- The relationship of the pudendal nerve to the ischial spine is important in obstetrics. The ischial spine can be palpated per vaginam and a needle directed to the nerve to deliver local anaesthetic. Bilateral block of the pudendal nerve leads to loss of anal reflex, relaxation of muscles of pelvic floor and loss of sensation to vulva and lower third of vagina.
- Sciatic nerve injury may result from posterior dislocation of the hip, direct penetrating injuries or inappropriately placed injections (Fig. 4.17). Nerve injuries to the lower limb are dealt with below.

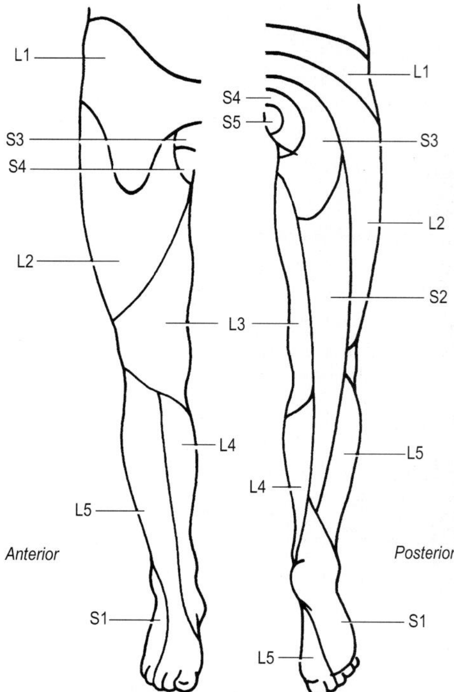

Fig. 4.16 Dermatomes of the lower limb.

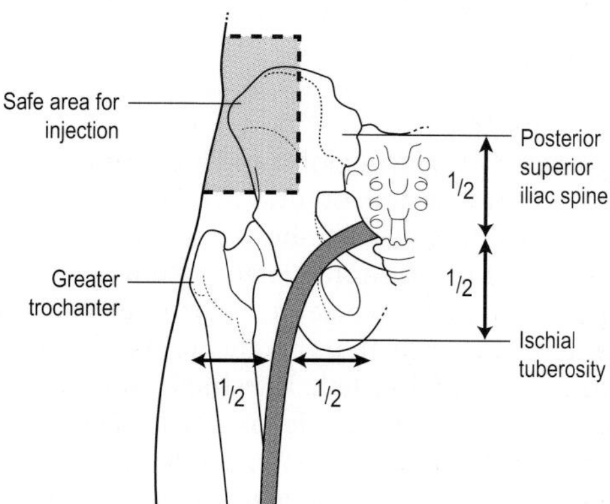

Fig. 4.17 Surface marking of the sciatic nerve in the buttock, showing the safe area for injection.

- An artery accompanies the sciatic nerve running in its substance (arteria comitans nervi ischiadici). Bleeding can be troublesome when the nerve is divided in an above-knee amputation. It must be carefully teased out and ligated in isolation to avoid ligation of nerve fibres with subsequent pain and neuroma formation.
- The common peroneal nerve may be damaged where it winds round the neck of the fibula. Car-bumper injuries, below-knee plasters and the Lloyd–Davies position for abdominoperineal resection of the rectum may compromise the nerve.

NERVE INJURIES

Sciatic Nerve

- Paralysis of hamstrings and all muscles of leg and foot supplied by nerve.
- All movement is lost below the knee joint, with foot drop (see below).
- All sensation is lost below the knee except that supplied by the saphenous nerve (branch of femoral), i.e. over medial malleolus and medial border of foot to great toe.

Tibial Nerve

- Isolated injury of this nerve is rare and likely to be caused by penetrating injury.
- Loss of active plantarflexion.
- Loss of sensation over the sole of the foot.

Common Peroneal Nerve

- Injury is not uncommon.
- Foot drop results.
- Components of foot drop include:
  - failure of dorsiflexion owing to paralysis of anterior compartment muscles (deep peroneal nerve)
  - failure of eversion owing to paralysis of lateral compartment muscles (superficial peroneal nerve)
  - patient exaggerates flexion of hip and knee when walking to lift foot well clear of ground to prevent scuffing toe of shoe
  - loss of sensation over lower lateral leg, dorsum of foot except medial aspect (saphenous nerve) and lateral aspect (sural nerve).

JOINTS

Hip Joint (Fig. 4.18)

- Largest joint in the body.
- Ball-and-socket joint.

Articular Surfaces

- Femoral head: two-thirds of a sphere.
- Acetabulum deepened by the fibrocartilaginous labrum acetabulare.
- Non-articular acetabular notch is closed by the transverse acetabular ligament.
- Ligament teres passes from this notch to the fovea of the femoral head.

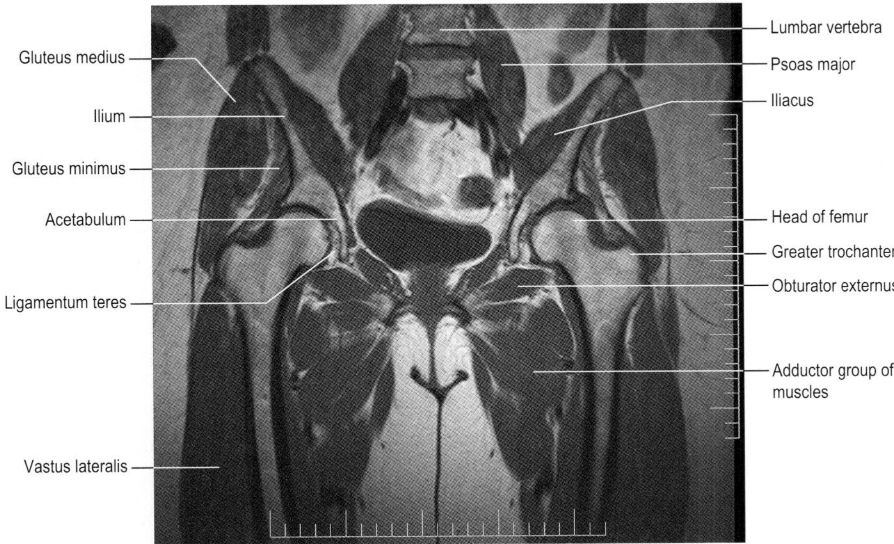

Fig. 4.18 Coronal MRI of hip joint and its relations.

Capsule

- Attached proximally to acetabulum and transverse acetabular notch.
- Attached distally along the intertrochanteric line, the bases of greater and lesser trochanters and posterior to the femoral neck about 1.2 cm from the trochanteric crest. Capsular fibres are reflected from the distal attachment onto the femoral neck, i.e. retinacular fibres.

Ligaments

- Iliofemoral: from anterior inferior iliac spine, bifurcating to attach at each end of the trochanteric line (inverted Y—strongest of the three ligaments).
- Pubofemoral: from iliopubic junction to blend with medial aspect of the capsule.
- Ischiofemoral: from ischium to attach to base of greater trochanter.

Synovium

- Covers the nonarticular surfaces.
- May form or connect with a bursa anteriorly beneath psoas tendon, where this crosses the anterior aspect of the joint.

Nerve Supply

- Obturator.
- Sciatic.
- Femoral.

Movements

- Flexion: iliacus, psoas major, rectus femoris, sartorius, pectineus.
- Extension: gluteus maximus, biceps, semimembranosus, semitendinosus.
- Adduction: adductor longus, adductor brevis, adductor magnus, gracilis, pectineus.
- Abduction: gluteus medius, gluteus minimus, tensor fasciae latae.
- Lateral rotation: gluteus maximus (chiefly), obturator internus, obturator externus, gemelli, quadratus femoris.
- Medial rotation: tensor fasciae latae, anterior fibres of gluteus medius and gluteus minimus.

Relations

- Anterior: iliacus, psoas, pectineus, femoral artery, femoral vein.
- Posteriorly: obturator internus tendon and gemelli, quadratus femoris, sciatic nerve, and gluteus maximus overlying these.
- Laterally: tensor fasciae latae, gluteus medius, gluteus minimus.
- Superiorly: reflected head of rectus femoris.
- Inferiorly: obturator externus passing back to be inserted into the trochanteric fossa.

Clinical Points

- The sciatic nerve is a close posterior relation of the hip and is in danger in dislocation of the hip.

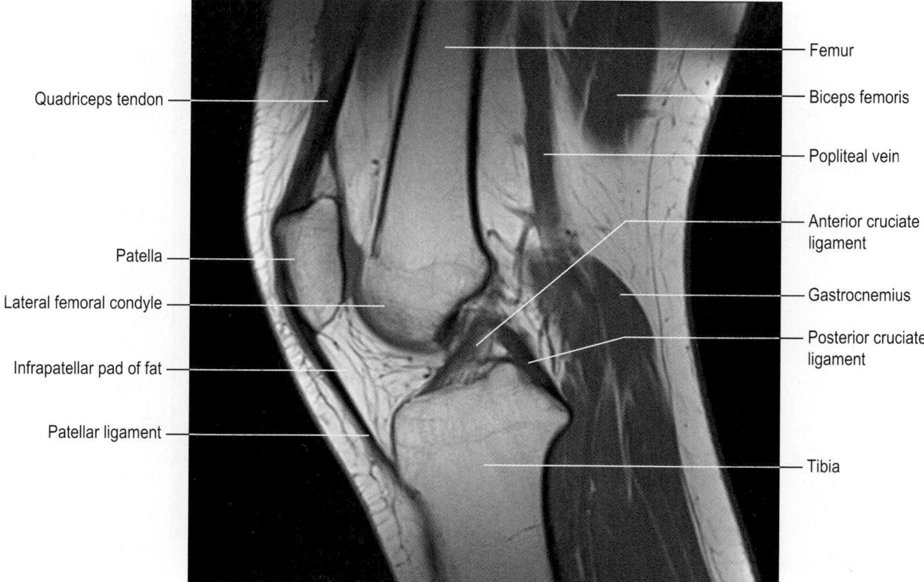

Fig. 4.19 Sagittal MRI of right knee joint through medial aspect of lateral femoral condyle.

- Surgical exposure of the hip joint may be carried out in three ways.
  1. Lateral approach: involves splitting the fibres of tensor fasciae latae, gluteus medius and gluteus minimus to reach the femoral neck. If further access is required, the greater trochanter may be detached with its gluteal insertions.
  2. Anterior approach: between gluteus medius and minimus laterally and sartorius medially—the reflected head of rectus femoris is then divided to expose the anterior aspect of the hip joint.
  3. Posterior approach: through an angled incision commencing at the posterior superior iliac spine passing to the greater trochanter and then extended vertically downwards. Gluteus maximus is split in the line of its fibres and incised along its tendinous insertion. Gluteus medius and gluteus minimus are detached from their insertions into the greater trochanter.

Knee Joint (Figs. 4.19 and 4.20)

- Hinge joint.

Articular Surfaces

- Lower end of femur (condyles).
- Upper end of tibia (condyles).
- Patella.

Capsule

- Attached to margins of articular surfaces.
- Communicates with suprapatellar bursa (between lower part of femur and quadriceps).
- Communicates posteriorly with bursa on the medial head of gastrocnemius.
- Often communicates with bursa under semimembranosus.
- Capsule perforated posteriorly by popliteus.

Ligaments

- Medial collateral ligament: passes from medial epicondyle of femur to tibia (posterior fibres attached to the medial meniscus).
- Lateral collateral ligament: passes from lateral epicondyle of femur to head of fibula; it is free from the capsule.
- Ligamentum patellae and retinacula:
  - continue through the patella with the quadriceps tendon
  - strong and thick and strengthen capsule anteriorly
  - attached to tibial tuberosity
  - retinacula are expanded parts of quadriceps tendon going to the tibia and reinforcing the ligamentum patellae.
- Oblique ligament: expansion of semimembranosus tendon blending with the joint capsule posteriorly.

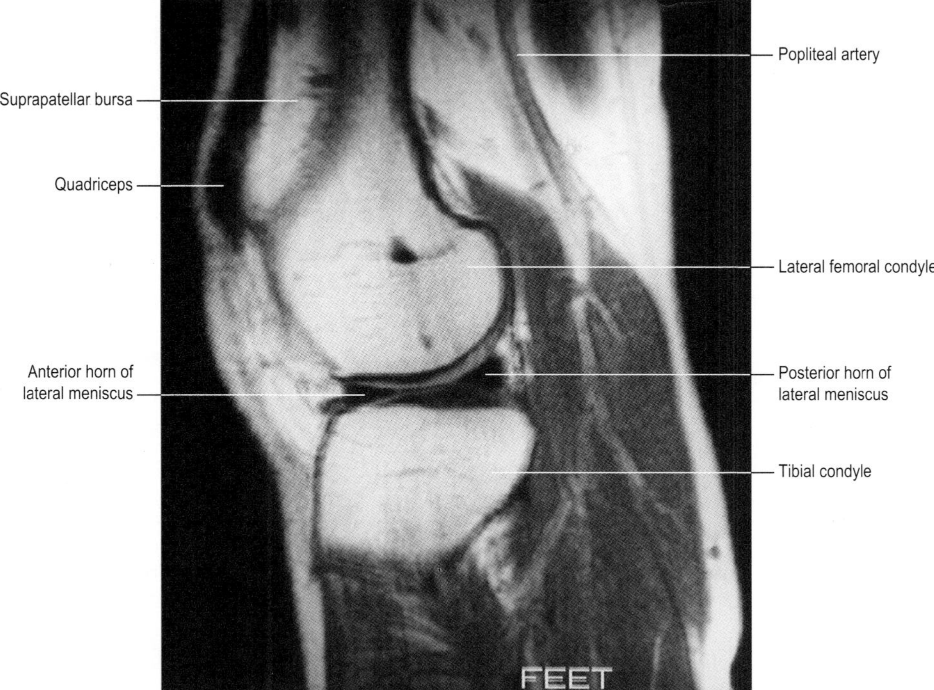

Fig. 4.20 Sagittal MRI through lateral part of the right knee joint, showing lateral meniscus. (From Jacob S: Atlas of Human Anatomy. Churchill Livingstone 2002, with permission.)

Synovium

- Lines the capsule.
- Surrounds the cruciate ligaments.
- Communicates with suprapatellar bursa.
- In adult, menisci are not covered by synovial membrane.

Intra-articular Structures

- Cruciate ligaments:
  - strong connections between femur and tibia
  - take their names from the tibial origins
  - anterior cruciate: from the front of the intercondylar area of the tibia obliquely upwards to the intercondylar notch of the femur
  - posterior cruciate: from the posterior aspect of the intercondylar area of the tibia upwards to the front of the intercondylar notch of the femur
  - anterior cruciate ligament resists forwards displacement of tibia on femur—taut in hyperextension of the knee
  - posterior cruciate ligament resists backwards displacement of tibia on femur and is taut in hyperflexion.
- Semilunar cartilages (menisci) (Fig. 4.21):
  - crescentic in shape
  - triangular in cross-section
  - medial larger than lateral
  - attached by extremities to intercondylar notch
  - attached at periphery to capsule
  - popliteus inserts into posterior aspect of lateral cartilage.
- Infrapatellar fat pad:
  - fills space between ligamentum patellae and femoral intercondylar notch
  - synovium covering pad projects into knee joint, raising folds on each side of it (the alar folds).

Nerve Supply

- Femoral, obturator, sciatic (according to Hilton's law).

Movements

- Flexion: hamstrings, gracilis, gastrocnemius, sartorius.
- Extension: quadriceps femoris.
- Rotation: when the knee is flexed, medial rotation is possible (via popliteus).
- Full extension of the knee is accompanied by slight lateral rotation of the tibia (medial rotation of the femur if the foot is on the ground). This 'locks' the joint.

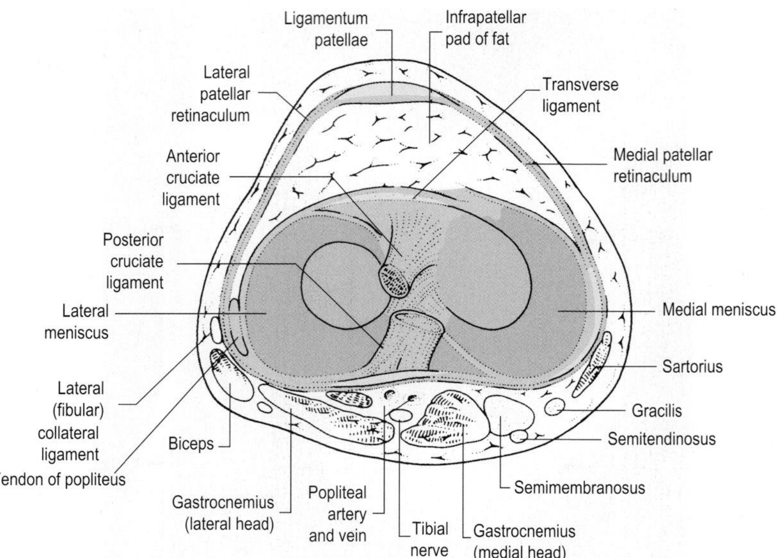

Fig. 4.21 The left knee joint, transverse section. The meniscus, cruciate ligaments and the relations of the joint are shown.

- Flexion from full extension is initiated by popliteus, which rotates the femur laterally or the tibia medially and is said to 'unlock' the joint.

Clinical Points

- Because of the incongruity of the articular surfaces, stability of the knee depends on the surrounding muscles and ligaments. Quadriceps femoris is important and, if this is strong, the knee will function satisfactorily even with considerable ligamentous damage.
- The semilunar cartilages can tear only when the knee is flexed and able to rotate.
- The collateral ligaments are taut in full extension of the knee and therefore liable to injury in this position. The medial ligament is liable to damage with a violent abduction strain, whereas an adduction strain will damage the lateral ligament. The anterior cruciate ligament, which is taut in extension, may be torn in hyperextension injuries of the knee or in anterior dislocation of the tibia on the femur. The posterior cruciate ligament may be damaged in posterior dislocations.
- Stability depends on muscles and ligaments. The power of quadriceps is most important, especially in ligamentous damage. If quadriceps wastes, failure of reconstructed ligament is likely.

Tibiofibular Joint

- Superior tibiofibular joint: between head of fibula and lateral condyle of tibia.
- Interosseous membrane: fibres directed downwards and medially from tibia to fibula.
- Crossed by anterior tibial vessels above and perforated by peroneal artery below.
- Inferior tibiofibular joints (syndesmosis) between each bone just above ankle joint.

Ankle Joint (Fig. 4.22)

- Hinge joint.

Articular Surfaces

- Mortice formed between lower ends of tibia and fibula and body of talus.

Capsule

- Thin.
- Attached round margins of articular surfaces.
- Reinforced medially and laterally by collateral ligaments.

Ligaments

- Lateral: three parts—anterior talofibular, calcaneofibular, posterior talofibular.
- Medial: strong and triangular; runs from medial malleolus to medial aspect of body of talus.

Movements

- Dorsiflexion: tibialis anterior, extensor hallucis longus, extensor digitorum longus, peroneus tertius.

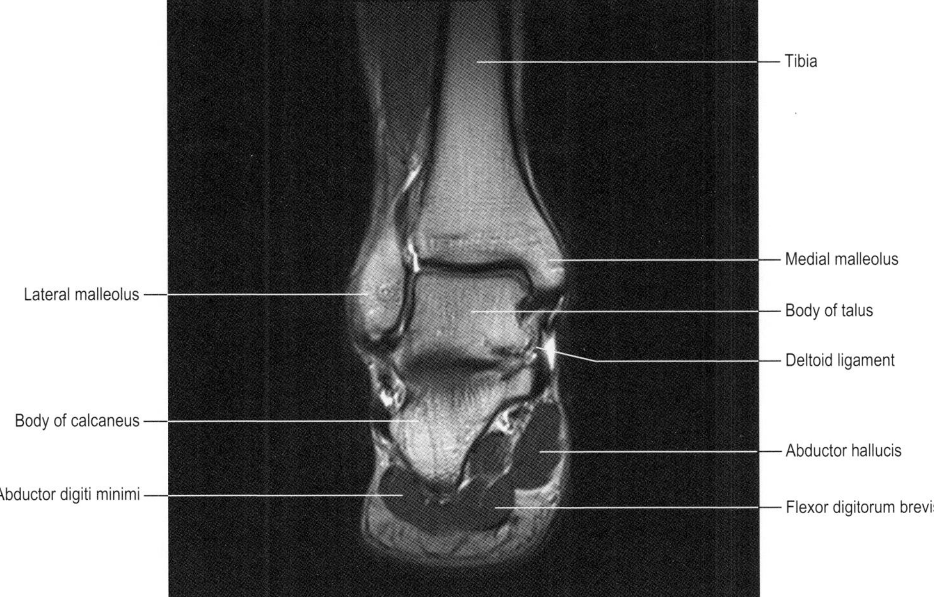

Fig. 4.22 Coronal MRI through right ankle joint.

- Plantarflexion: gastrocnemius and soleus, tibialis posterior, flexor hallucis longus, flexor digitorum longus.

Relations

- Shown in Fig. 4.23.

Clinical Point

- Forced abduction or adduction injuries sprain or tear the collateral ligaments—more commonly, the lateral. If the ligament is completely torn, the talus can be tilted in its mortice.

Foot Joints

- Inversion and eversion occur at the subtalar joints.
- Inversion is caused by tibialis anterior and tibialis posterior, aided by extensor hallucis longus and flexor hallucis longus.
- Eversion is caused by peroneus longus and peroneus brevis.

ARCHES OF THE FOOT

The bones of the foot are arranged in the form of two longitudinal arches (medial and lateral) and a transverse arch. They are formed as follows.

- Longitudinal:
  - medial: calcaneum, talus, navicular, three cuneiforms, medial three metatarsals
  - lateral: calcaneum, cuboid, lateral two metatarsals.
- Transverse:
  - bases of metatarsals
  - each foot is really half an arch—lateral side on ground, medial side at upper limit of arch.
- Factors maintaining the arches include:
  - shape of interlocking bones
  - muscles
  - ligaments.

Medial Longitudinal Arch (Fig. 4.24)

This is supported as follows.

- Muscular:
  - flexor hallucis longus
  - flexor digitorum longus
  - tibialis anterior
  - tibialis posterior
  - flexor digitorum brevis.
- Ligaments:
  - spring ligament
  - interosseous ligaments.

Lateral Longitudinal Arch

This is maintained by:

- Muscular:
  - peroneus longus
  - flexor digitorum longus to the fourth and fifth toes
  - flexor digitorum brevis.

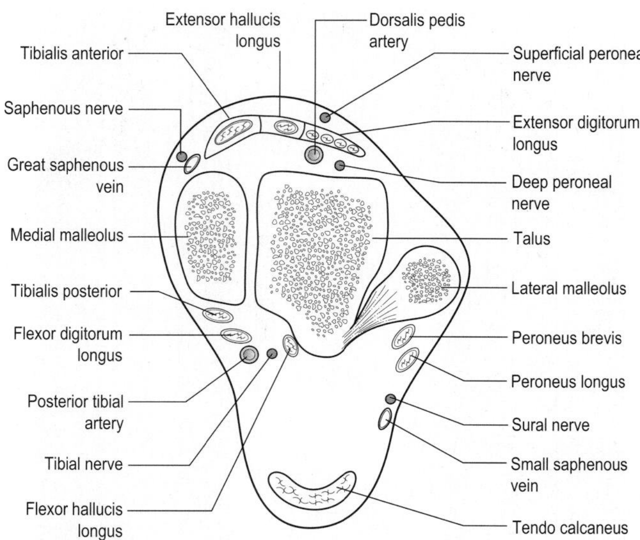

Fig. 4.23 Transverse section through lower part of the talocrural joint, showing relations of the ankle joint.

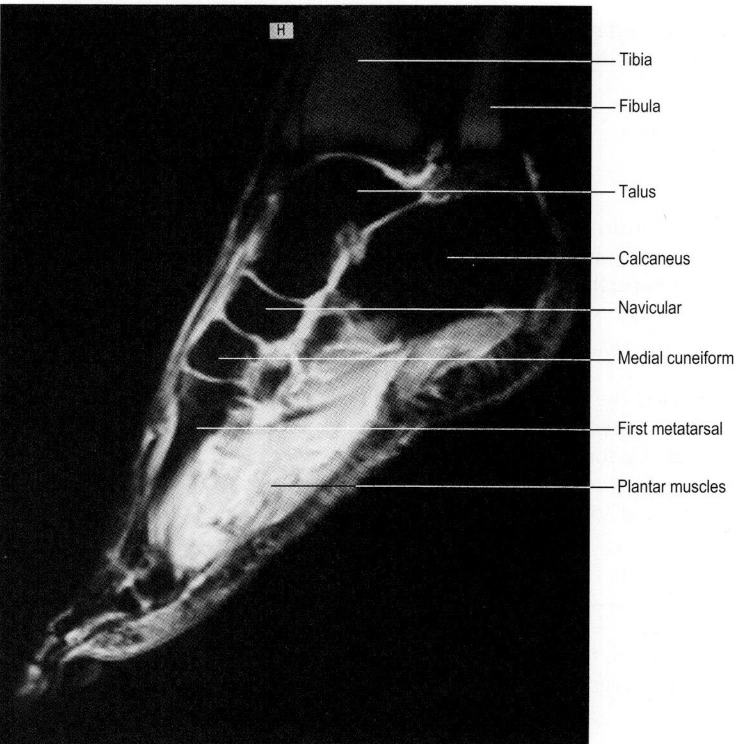

Fig. 4.24 Sagittal MRI of the foot, showing medial longitudinal arch. (From Jacob S: Atlas of Human Anatomy. Churchill Livingstone 2002, with permission.)

- Ligaments:
  - long plantar ligament
  - short plantar ligament.

Transverse Arch

This is supported by:

- Muscular:
  - peroneus longus.
- Ligaments:
  - interosseous.

Ligaments

- Short plantar ligament:
  - from plantar surface of calcaneum to cuboid.
- Long plantar ligament:
  - from calcaneum to base of second, third and fourth metatarsals
  - covers short plantar ligament
  - forms a tunnel for the tendon of peroneus longus with the cuboid bone.
- Spring ligament:
  - sustentaculum tali of calcaneum to tuberosity of navicular.
  - Action of all ligaments reinforced by plantar aponeurosis.

OSCE SCENARIOS

OSCE Scenario 4.1

An 85-year-old female trips over the edge of a carpet at home. She cannot get up from the floor. On arrival at hospital she complains of pain in the right groin. On examination the right leg is externally rotated, shortened and adducted.

1. Classify fractures of the neck of the femur.
2. Explain the anatomical basis for external rotation, shortening and adduction.
3. What is the blood supply of the head of the femur?
4. Explain why some fractures require a dynamic hip screw while others require a hemiarthroplasty.

OSCE Scenario 4.2

You are asked to examine the pulses in a patient's lower limb.

1. Describe the anatomical landmarks you would use to locate the peripheral pulses in the lower limb.

OSCE Scenario 4.3

A 60-year-old female presents with a swelling in the right groin.

1. What are the boundaries of the femoral triangle?
2. On examination, the lump is below the inguinal ligament. Based on your knowledge of the contents of the femoral triangle, with the exception of lymphadenopathy, what pathological conditions may arise from the contents of the triangle?
3. On examination, you believe that the lump is a lymph node. Which structures drain to the inguinal lymph nodes?

OSCE 4.4

A 27-year-old male is impaled on a metal pole after falling from some scaffolding. It has entered his right buttock. You are asked to see him on the ward several days after recovering from surgery. The nurse looking after him is concerned he has a nerve injury.

1. What is the likely nerve to be injured in a penetrating injury to the buttock?
2. What are the roots of this nerve?
3. If he has a nerve injury, what are the likely clinical signs and why?

OSCE 4.5

A 52-year-old male has been hit by a car on the outside of his left leg as he crossed the road. It is obvious he has a nasty fracture of his lower leg. The plain X-ray has shown a nasty comminuted proximal fibular fracture and a tibial fracture.

1. What is the likely nerve to have been injured and what would be the examination findings?
2. What other nerves are injured in fractures/dislocations?
3. He is placed in a plaster cast but just after midnight the nurse on the ward calls to tell you he is in tremendous pain and his leg feels 'odd'. What is the likely diagnosis and what would be the treatment?

Answers in Appendix pages 438–440

Please check your eBook at https://studentconsult.inkling.com/ for more self-assessment questions. See inside cover for registration details.

5

The Head, Neck and Spine

DEVELOPMENT

Branchial Arches

Branchial arches lie in the side walls and floor of the fetal pharynx. They support the lateral walls of the cranial part of the foregut or primitive pharynx. The arches are separated from one another by ectodermal branchial clefts or grooves. On the inside of the primitive pharynx are five endodermal pharyngeal pouches. Each arch has a mesodermal core covered by ectoderm and an internal layer of endoderm.

A typical branchial arch contains:

- a skeletal element (cartilaginous bar), which will form bones and ligaments
- an artery
- a nerve
- striated muscle supplied by the nerve of that arch.

The derivatives of the pharyngeal pouches and branchial arches are shown in Box 5.1 and Table 5.1.

The Tongue

A nodule, the tuberculum impar, develops in the floor of the pharynx.

- This is covered by two lingual swellings, which arise from each side of the first branchial arch to fuse in the midline and form the anterior two-thirds of the tongue (nerve supply V—trigeminal).

BOX 5.1 Derivatives of Pharyngeal Pouches

Arch	Structures
First	Eustachian tube, middle ear, mastoid antrum
Second	Tonsillar fossa (palatine tonsil)
Third	Thymus, inferior parathyroid
Fourth	Superior parathyroid, part of thyroid

TABLE 5.1 Derivatives of the Branchial Arches

Arch	Nerve	Skeletal Structures	Muscles	Ligaments
First (mandibular)	V	Incus and malleus (Meckel's cartilage)	Mastication Mylohyoid Anterior belly of digastric Tensor tympani Tensor palati	Sphenomandibular Anterior ligament of malleus
Second (hyoid)	VII	Stapes Styloid process Upper part of body of hyoid Lesser cornu of hyoid	Facial expression Posterior belly of digastric Stylohyoid Stapedius	Stylohyoid
Third	IX	Lower part of body of hyoid Greater cornu of hyoid	Stylopharyngeus	–
Fourth–sixth	X (recurrent laryngeal, superior laryngeal)	Thyroid cartilage Arytenoid cartilage Corniculate cartilage Cuneiform cartilage	Muscles of pharynx, larynx, palate	–

- A part of the second branchial arch contributes to the anterior two-thirds of the tongue (nerve supply VII—chorda tympani).
- The posterior third of the tongue develops largely from the third branchial arch (nerve supply IX—glossopharyngeal).
- The tongue musculature is derived from migrating occipital myotomes dragging their nerve supply with them (XII—hypoglossal).

The tongue therefore develops from the first, second and third branchial arches and receives nerve contributions from each:

- lingual nerve (V): anterior two-thirds—general sensation
- chorda tympani (VII): anterior two-thirds—taste
- glossopharyngeal (IX): posterior third—general sensation and taste.

Development of the Face

The face develops around the primitive mouth, i.e. stomodaeum, as follows.

- Frontonasal process grows down from the cranium and forms:
  - nose
  - nasal septum
  - nostril
  - philtrum (midline depression on upper lip)
  - premaxilla (bearing four incisor teeth).
- The maxillary processes fuse with the frontonasal processes and form:
  - cheeks
  - upper lip (except philtrum)
  - upper jaw
  - palate (except premaxilla).
- Mandibular processes meet in the midline to form:
  - lower jaw.

Abnormalities may arise from abnormalities of fusion of the above elements. These include:

- abnormalities of closure of the stomodaeum, e.g. macrostoma (too big), microstoma (too small)
- cleft lip
- cleft palate
- inclusion dermoids.

Cleft Lip ('Hare' Lip; Fig. 5.1)

- On one or both sides of philtrum, occurring as failure of fusion of maxillary and frontonasal processes.
- May extend into nostril or alongside nose as far as orbit.
- May be associated with cleft palate.
- Median cleft is rare; occurs with failure of development of philtrum from frontonasal process.

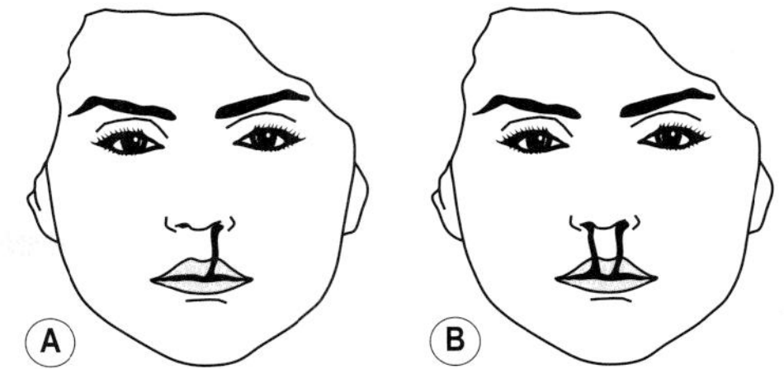

Fig. 5.1 Cleft lip. (A) Unilateral. (B) Bilateral.

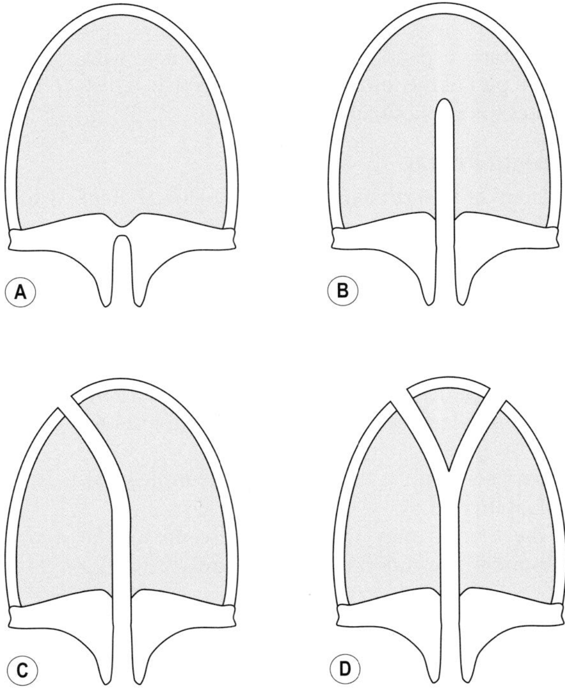

Fig. 5.2 Types of cleft palate. (A) Cleft of soft palate. (B) Partial cleft palate. (C) Unilateral complete cleft palate. (D) Bilateral complete cleft palate.

Cleft Palate (Fig. 5.2)

- Fusion occurs between primary palate (anterior section of premaxilla and attached four teeth) and secondary palate (hard and soft palate).
- Failure of fusion of segments may result in:
  - cleft of soft palate (bifid uvula)
  - partial cleft involving posterior part of hard palate
  - unilateral complete cleft: running the full length of the maxilla and then alongside one aspect of the premaxilla
  - bilateral complete cleft: running full length of maxilla and on both aspects of premaxilla, separating it completely.

Inclusion Dermoids

- May form along lines of facial fusion.
- Commonest is at the lateral extremity of the eyebrow, i.e. external angular dermoid.

Development of the Thyroid

- Develops as diverticulum from floor of embryonic pharynx just caudal to the tuberculum impar (site of developing tongue); site of origin remains as foramen caecum of tongue.
- Grows caudally superficial to branchial arches and hence to hyoid and larynx to its definitive position.
- As lobes expand, they come into contact with the ventral part of the fourth pharyngeal pouch, which contributes the parafollicular (C) cells.

Clinical Points

- Stem of diverticulum, the thyroglossal duct, usually disappears, although traces may remain as thyroglossal cysts.
- Thyroglossal duct attaches to body of hyoid bone and the latter must be excised when dealing with the thyroglossal ducts surgically; or when dealing with a thyroglossal cyst, which is adherent to the body of the hyoid bone.
- Aberrant thyroid tissue may appear anywhere between the foramen caecum of the tongue and the normal site of the gland.
- Thyroid tissue at the foramen caecum is known as lingual thyroid.
- The thyroid may sometimes descend too far and be found in the superior mediastinum.

Parathyroids

- Superior parathyroids develop from the fourth pharyngeal pouch.
- Inferior parathyroids develop from the third pharyngeal pouch in company with the thymus.
- The inferior parathyroid may be dragged beyond the thyroid into the superior mediastinum and be found in association with (or even within) the thymus.

Development of the Spine

A dorsal groove appears on the surface of the embryo: the neural groove.

- Neural groove becomes closed off, forming the neural canal, which becomes separated from the ectodermal covering of the body.
- Anterior to the neural canal is a solid cord of cells: the notochord.
- Vertebral bodies develop around the notochord, each vertebra ossifying from three primary centres: one for each side of the arch and one for the body.
- The two halves of the arch fuse initially in the thoracic region, and this spreads up and down the column.
- Failure of the two arches to fuse posteriorly results in spina bifida, which is most common in the lumbar region.

Types of Spina Bifida

Spina bifida occulta

- Vertebral anomaly: failure of arches to fuse exists in isolation.
- The cord and meninges are intact.
- There may be an overlying dimple or tuft of hair at the site.

Spina Bifida Manifesta

There are two types:

- Meningocele, where the meninges herniate through the bony defect and are covered by skin of variable quality.
- Meningomyelocele, where there is a failure of closure of the neural tube. The defect is formed by exposed neural tissue.

Hydrocephalus frequently accompanies meningomyelocele. The likely reason for this is:

- the spinal cord is tethered at the site of the lesion
- differential growth between spinal cord and vertebral column pulls the hindbrain into the foramen magnum (Arnold–Chiari malformation)
- this interferes with circulation of cerebrospinal fluid (CSF).

Growth of Spinal Cord and Vertebral Column

- In the embryo the spine is curved in a gentle C-shape.
- As the infant lifts its head the cervical spine develops a curvature concaved posteriorly, i.e. cervical lordosis.
- As the child learns to walk the lumbar spine develops a curvature concaved posteriorly, i.e. lumbar lordosis.
- Up to the third month of fetal life the spinal cord occupies the full length of the vertebral canal.
- Vertebral growth then occurs more rapidly than that of the spinal cord.
- At birth the cord reaches the level of the third lumbar vertebra.
- By adolescence the cord is at its definitive position at the level of the disc between the first and second lumbar vertebrae.

Clinical Points

- Lumbar puncture must be performed well clear of the termination of the cord.
- A line joining the iliac crests passes through the fourth lumbar vertebra, and therefore the intervertebral space above and below this landmark can be safely used for lumbar puncture (below is safer in babies and young children).

HEAD

Face

The facial skeleton is shown in Figs. 5.3 and 5.4. The skeleton surrounds cavities at three levels:

- paired orbits housing the eyes
- paired nasal cavities: the openings of the respiratory tract and organs of smell
- single buccal (oral) cavity: the opening of the alimentary tract.

The facial skeleton is braced against the base of the skull by three pairs of struts, all meeting the cranial skeleton at the level of the middle cranial fossa:

- the zygomatic arches defining the temporal fossae on each side
- the pterygoid plates of the sphenoid forming the posterior walls of the pterygopalatine fossae
- the vertical rami of the mandible: meeting the base of the skull at the temporomandibular joints.

Mandible

- The body of the mandible is the horizontal part bearing the alveolar process and the lower teeth.
- Posteriorly, at the angle, the body joins the ramus, which is almost vertical.
- The ramus bears an anterior coronoid and a posterior condyloid process or head.
- Between the coronoid and condyloid processes is the mandibular notch.
- On the medial aspect of the ramus is the mandibular foramen for the inferior alveolar branch of the mandibular division of the trigeminal nerve.
- The inferior alveolar branch of the mandibular nerve traverses the body of the mandible within the mandibular canal and emerges as the mental nerve through the mental foramen on the lateral surface of the body.
- The mandibular foramen is shielded by a projecting process, the lingula.
- A small groove runs inferiorly and forwards from the mandibular foramen, i.e. the mylohyoid groove, in which lie the nerve and vessels of the same name.
- Above this groove is a prominent ridge, the mylohyoid line, which gives attachment to the mylohyoid muscle.
- The upper border of the body bears the alveolar border with 16 dental sockets or alveoli.

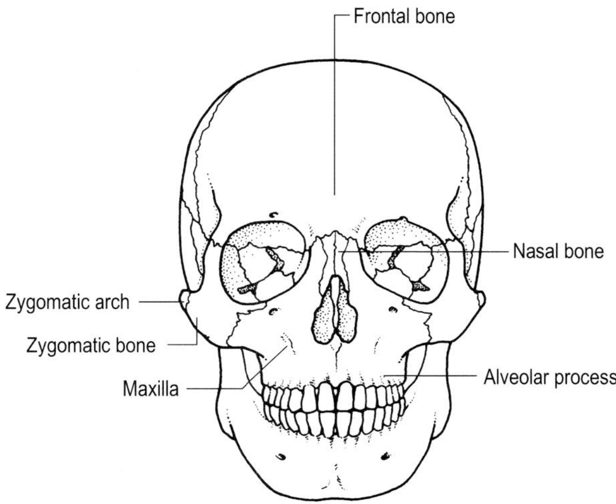

Fig. 5.4 External view of the skull from the front.

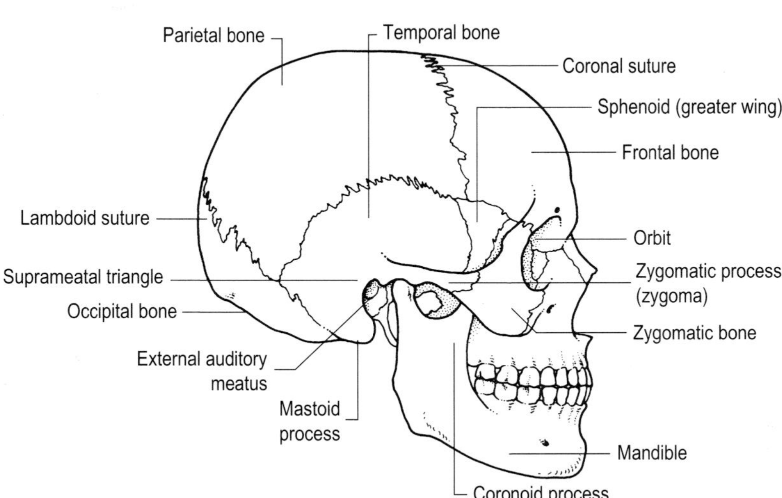

Fig. 5.3 External view of the skull from the side.

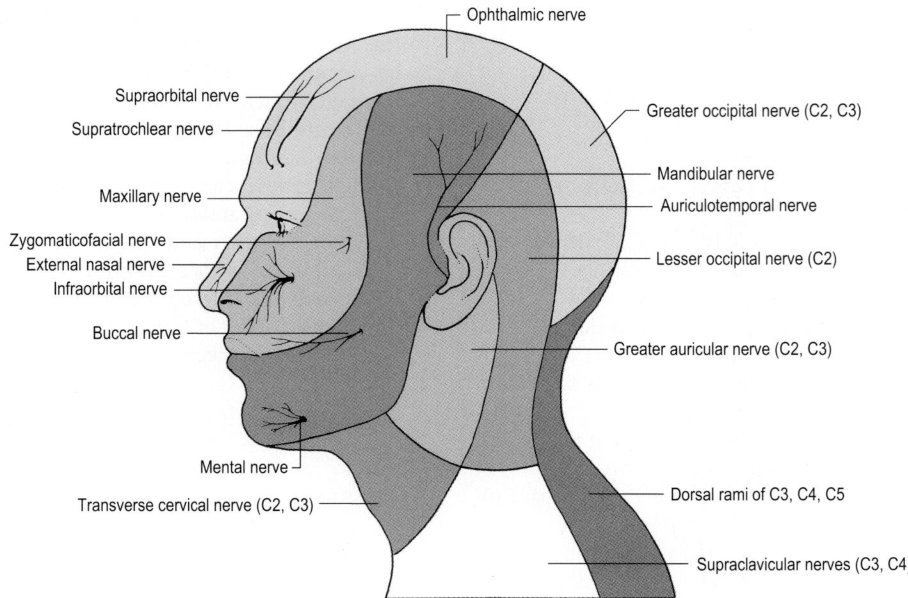

Fig. 5.5 The sensory innervation of the head and neck.

- The lateral surface is roughened by muscle attachment on the angle and ramus.
- Masseter is inserted at the lateral surface.
- The midline of the mandible is often referred to as the symphysis menti, which is a joint up to the second year of life, after which fusion takes place.

Sensory Nerve Supply of the Face (Fig. 5.5)

This is via the trigeminal nerve, except for a small area over the parotid, which is supplied by the greater auricular nerve, a branch of the cervical plexus. The distribution of the nerves is as follows:

- ophthalmic: nose, orbital region, frontal region of scalp
- maxillary: upper jaw, including teeth
- mandibular: lower jaw and associated structures, including the anterior two-thirds of the tongue.

The nerve supplied is carried by three major branches, one of each division of the following nerves.

- Supraorbital nerve:
  - branch of ophthalmic division
  - passes through the supraorbital foramen
  - travels back as far as the vertex of the skull
  - supplies the skin of the scalp as far back as the vertex, the skin of the forehead, the skin of the upper eyelid, the skin of the front of the nose, the cornea.
- Infraorbital nerve:
  - a branch of maxillary nerve
  - emerges from the infraorbital foramen
  - supplies the skin of the cheek, side of the nose, mucous membrane of the inside of the corresponding part of the cheek, outer surface of the gum.
- Mental nerve:
  - a branch of mandibular nerve
  - supplies skin of chin, mucous membrane of lower lip, outer surface of gums.

These three nerves are supplemented by a number of smaller nerves, whose distribution is shown in Fig. 5.5.

Dermatomes of the Head and Neck (Fig. 5.6)

- Anterior to the auricle, the scalp is supplied by the three branches of the trigeminal nerve.
- Posterior to the auricle, the scalp is supplied by the spinal cutaneous nerves from the neck.

Facial Musculature

There are two groups of muscles on the face.

- Muscles of mastication, supplied by the mandibular division of the trigeminal nerve.
- The muscles of facial expression, supplied by the facial nerve.

The muscles of mastication

- Temporalis can be seen in the temporal region, covered by the tough temporal fascia.
- Masseter is on the side of the face and its anterior border can be palpated when the teeth are clenched.

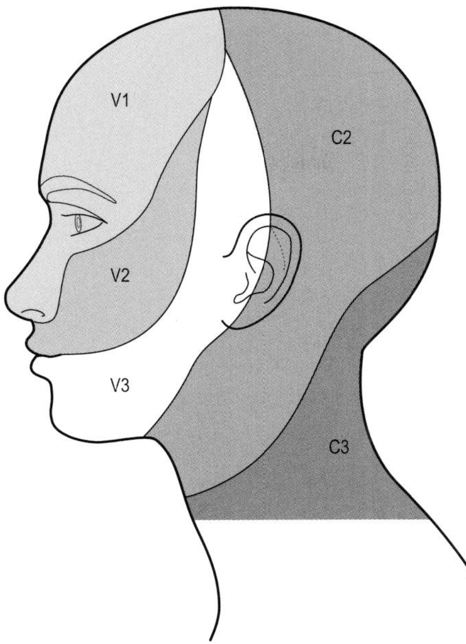

Fig. 5.6 Dermatomes of the head and neck. V1, ophthalmic division of trigeminal nerve; V2, maxillary division of trigeminal nerve; V3, mandibular division of trigeminal nerve.

Muscles of facial expression

- Superficial muscles that can move the skin and superficial fascia in various directions, thus altering facial expression.
- Orbicularis oculi surrounds the eye. The palpebral part is in the eyelid and closes the eye as in sleep; the orbital part surrounds the orbit and forcibly closes the eye, e.g. when dust blows in the face.
- Orbicularis oris surrounds the mouth. In gentle contraction it closes the lips, in powerful contraction it protrudes the lips, as in whistling and kissing.
- Buccinator is the main muscle of the cheek. It keeps the cheek in contact with the gums so that food does not accumulate in the vestibule.
- Occipitofrontalis elevates the eyebrows as in a look of surprise.

Clinical Points

- To test the integrity of the facial nerve one can ask the patient to screw up the eyes, to smile or to whistle.
- Loss of muscle tone causes the normal skin folds to disappear on the side of the lesion.
- Paralysis of the palpebral part of orbicularis oculi causes the lower eyelid to fall away from the eye, with tears draining over the cheek.
- Loss of orbicularis oris can cause dribbling of saliva.
- Paralysis of buccinator may lead to food accumulating in the vestibule of the mouth.

Blood Vessels of the Face

Arteries

- Main arterial supply to face is facial artery (branch of the external carotid).
- Enters face by passing over lower border of mandible with anterior border of masseter, in close relation to the submandibular gland.
- Has a tortuous course.
- Anastomoses between facial artery and other small arteries on the same side and on the other side of the face are common.
- The face is therefore very vascular and cuts bleed considerably but heal quickly.
- Superficial temporal artery (branch of the external carotid artery) can often be seen over the temporal area.
- Pulsation can be felt just in front of tragus of ear.
- Becomes more noticeable in age when it becomes tortuous.
- Wide anastomosis between superficial temporal artery and facial artery.

Veins

- The main vein draining the face is the facial vein.
- Communicates freely with deeper veins such as those of the pterygoid venous plexus.
- Communicates with veins of orbit and then with the cavernous sinus.
- Central area of the face is sometimes known as the 'dangerous area', as infection can spread via the veins to the cavernous sinus.

The Scalp

The scalp consists of five layers:

- S: skin
- C: connective tissue
- A: aponeurosis
- L: loose areolar tissue
- P: periosteum.
- Skin:
  - rich in sebaceous glands
  - scalp common site for sebaceous cysts.
- Subcutaneous connective tissue:
  - lobules of fat between tough fibrous septae
  - has richest cutaneous blood supply of body
  - haemorrhage from scalp laceration is therefore profuse
  - blood vessels of the scalp lie in this layer
  - divided vessels retract between fibrous septae and cannot be picked up individually by artery forceps in the usual way.

- Aponeurotic layer:
  - part of occipitofrontalis, which is fibrous over the vertex of the skull but muscular in the occipital and frontal areas.
- Loose connective tissue:
  - skin of scalp very mobile under underlying tissue
  - 'scalping' occurs through this layer
  - wounds gape when aponeurosis is torn owing to the 'pull' of occipitalis and frontalis.
- Periosteum:
  - adherent to suture lines of skull
  - collections of blood beneath this layer are therefore limited by suture lines, e.g. cephalohaematoma.

CRANIAL CAVITY

The cranium consists of the cranial cavity and the facial skeleton. Most bones of the cranial cavity are flat bones and have:
- two plates of compact bone separated by a thin layer of trabecular bone or diploë
- inner and outer surfaces are lined by periosteum
- inner periosteum is the endosteal layer of the dura mater.

The bones of the cranial cavity are:
- frontal
- occipital
- sphenoid
- ethmoid
- paired temporal bones
- parietal bones.

The cranial cavity consists of:
- cranial vault
- base of cranium containing three cranial fossae.

Cranial Vault (Fig. 5.7)

- Roof of the cranial cavity.
- Formed by:
  - frontal bone anteriorly
  - paired parietal bones laterally
  - occipital bone posteriorly.
- A midline sagittal groove marks the position of the superior sagittal sinus.
- Falx cerebri is attached along the lips of the groove.
- Irregular depressions along the groove lodge the arachnoid granulations.
- Sagittal suture separates two parietal bones in midline.
- Coronal suture divides the frontal from parietal bones.
- The lambdoid suture divides the two parietal bones from the occipital bone and the temporal bones.
- Posterior to the coronal suture, the middle meningeal vein accompanied by the middle meningeal artery groove the vault of the skull.

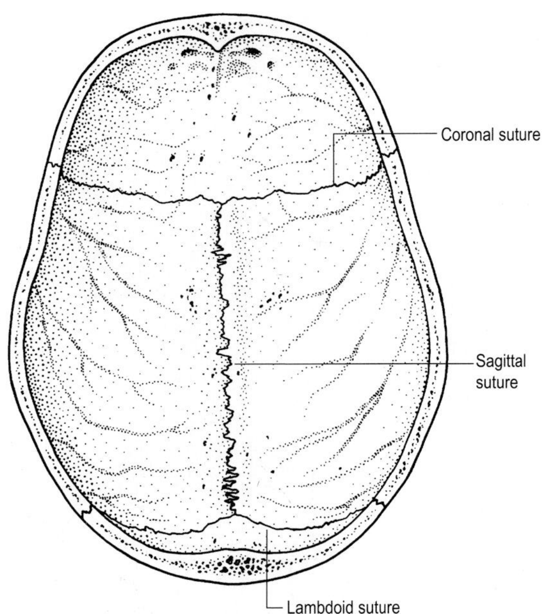

Fig. 5.7 The vault of the skull from below.

- The lambda is the junction between the lambdoid suture and the sagittal suture (it is the area of the posterior fontanelle in the infant).
- The bregma is the junction between the coronal and sagittal suture (it is the area of the anterior fontanelle in infants).
- The glabella is the prominence above the nasion, which is the depression between the two supraorbital margins.
- The pterion is the thin part of the skull at the junction of the parietal, frontal and temporal bones, and the greater wing of the sphenoid in the temporal region of the skull.
- The anterior branch of the middle meningeal artery traverses the pterion.

Cranial Fossae (Fig. 5.8)

There are three cranial fossae:
- anterior
- middle
- posterior.

Anterior Cranial Fossa

- Overlies the orbit and nasal cavities.
- Formed by the orbital plate of the frontal bones supplemented posteriorly by the lesser wing of the sphenoid.
- The ethmoid bone with its cribriform plate and the crista galli occupies the gap between the two orbital plates.
- Orbital plates separate anterior cranial fossa from orbit.

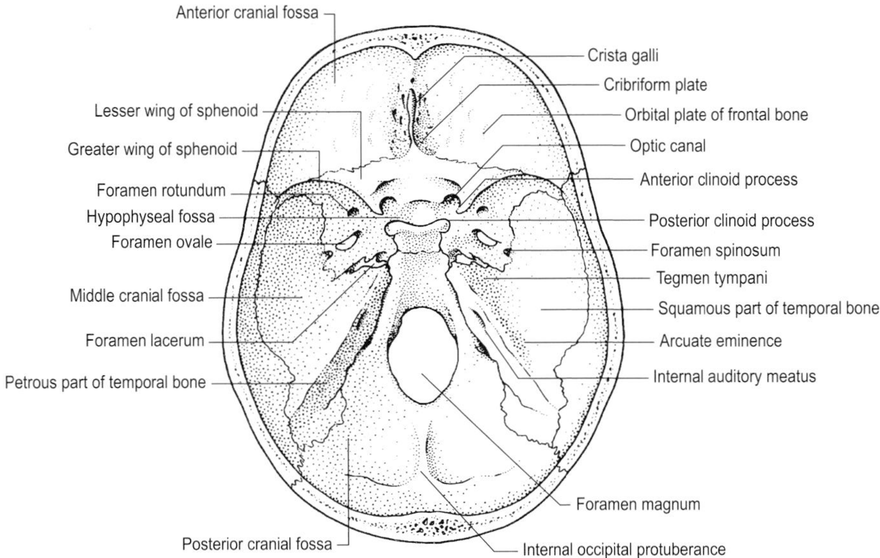

Fig. 5.8 The floor of the cranial cavity.

- The frontal lobe of the brain lies in the anterior cranial fossa.
- The cribriform plate roofs the nasal cavities.
- The following structures pass between the anterior cranial fossa and the nasal cavity:
  - olfactory nerves: pass through cribriform plate and enter olfactory bulb, which lies in cribriform plate
  - emissary veins: connecting cerebral veins in nasal cavity also pass through cribriform plate
  - anterior ethmoidal nerves and arteries accompanied by veins: pass through the anterior part of the cribriform plate into the nasal cavities.
- Fracture of anterior cranial fossa may cause bleeding into the nose and/or orbit and CSF rhinorrhoea. Bleeding into the orbit may manifest as subconjunctival haemorrhage. Fractures involving the cribriform plate will affect the sense of smell (see Ch. 6 section on Olfactory Nerve).

Middle Cranial Fossa

- Body of sphenoid forms floor of pituitary fossa.
- Laterally are the greater wings of the sphenoid and the squamous parts of the temporal bones.
- Petrous part of the temporal bone contains the middle and inner ear.
- Pituitary fossa is bounded in front and behind by the anterior and posterior clinoid processes.
- The middle cranial fossa contains the following foramina:
  - optic canal
  - superior orbital fissure
  - foramen rotundum
  - foramen ovale
  - foramen spinosum
  - foramen lacerum.

Structures passing through the various foramina are detailed in Table 5.2.

- Fractures of the middle cranial fossa are common as the bone is weakened by the foramina and canals:
  - fracture involving the tegmen tympani results in bleeding into the middle ear
  - excessive bleeding into the middle ear can rupture the tympanic membrane, resulting in bleeding from the ear
  - CSF otorrhoea may occur
  - cranial nerves VII and VIII may also be involved, as they run in the petrous temporal bone.

Posterior Cranial Fossa

- Anterior wall formed by petrous temporal bone laterally and body of sphenoid and basilar part of occipital bone medially.
- Latter two form the clivus, which extends from the foramen magnum to the dorsum sellae.
- Occipital bone forms most of the floor and lateral walls of the fossa.
- Internal occipital protuberance is in the midline on the posterior wall.
- Above the internal occipital protuberance the skull is grooved by the superior sagittal sinus.

TABLE 5.2 **Skull Foramina and Contents**

Fossa	Foramina	Contents
Anterior cranial fossa	Cribriform plate (multiple small foramina)	olfactory nerve emissary veins arteries and veins
Middle cranial fossa	Optic canal	optic nerve ophthalmic artery
	Superior orbital fissure	oculomotor nerve trochlear nerves abducens nerve ophthalmic division of trigeminal nerve ophthalmic veins sympathetic nerves
	Foramen rotundum	maxillary division of trigeminal nerve
	Foramen ovale	mandibular division of trigeminal nerve accessory meningeal artery
	Foramen spinosum	middle meningeal artery meningeal branch of mandibular nerve
	Foramen lacerum	internal carotid artery
Posterior cranial fossa	Foramen magnum	medulla oblongata, continuing into spinal cord accessory nerves vertebral arteries
	Jugular foramen	internal jugular vein (continuation of sigmoid sinus) glossopharyngeal, vagus and accessory nerves inferior petrosal sinus
	Hypoglossal canal	hypoglossal nerve meningeal branch of ascending pharyngeal artery
	Internal auditory meatus	facial nerve vestibulocochlear nerve labyrinthine artery (Facial nerve exits the base of the skull via the stylomastoid foramen)

- Transverse sinuses run anterolaterally on either side of the internal occipital protuberance, continuing down beneath the petrous temporal bone as the sigmoid sinus.
- The posterior cranial fossa contains the following foramina:
  - jugular foramen
  - hypoglossal canal
  - foramen magnum
  - internal acoustic meatus.
- Fractures of the posterior cranial fossa may involve the basilar part of the occipital bone, which separates the pharynx from the posterior cranial fossa. Bleeding may occur into the pharynx. More lateral fractures can bleed into the back of the neck.

Base of the Skull

The bones of the base of the skull and the various foramina are shown in Fig. 5.9.

ORBIT AND EYEBALL

The Bony Orbit (Fig. 5.10)

The function of the orbit is to:

- protect the eye against external blows
- maintain the constant distance between the pupils necessary for binocular vision.

Contraction of the external ocular muscles must rotate the eye and not displace it. The margins of the orbit are

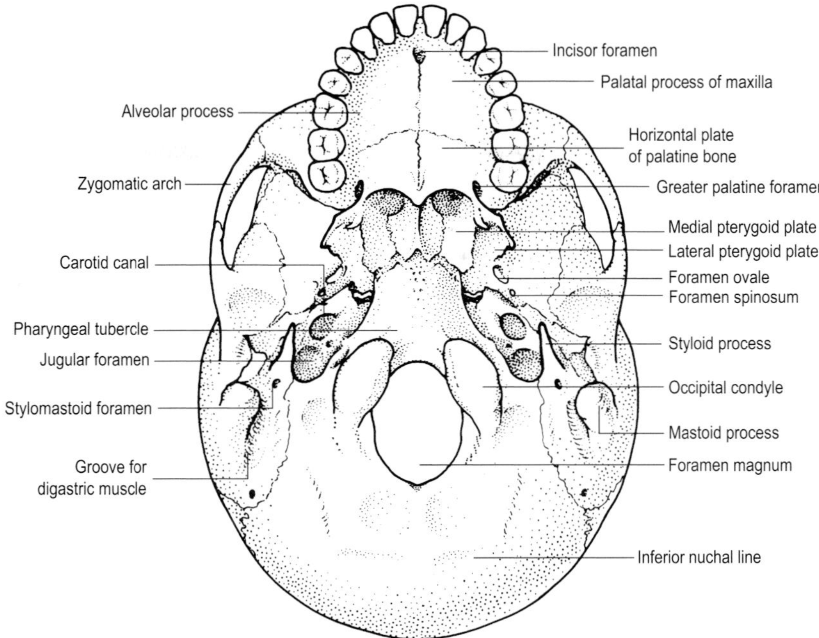

Fig. 5.9 The base of the skull from below.

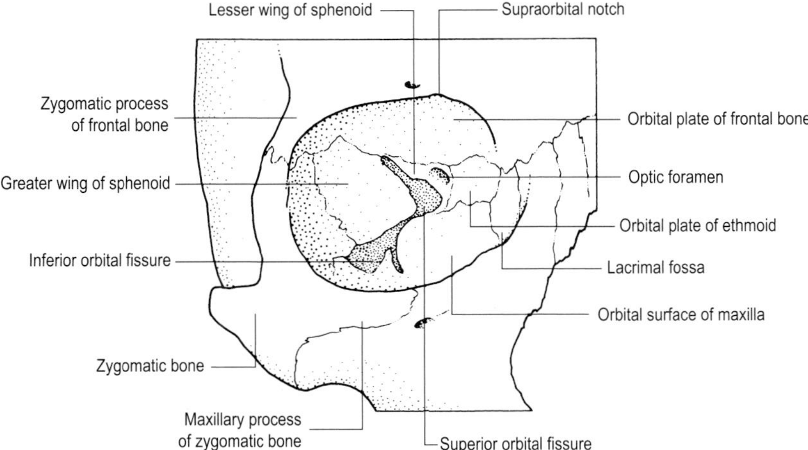

Fig. 5.10 The bony orbit.

formed by the frontal, maxillary and zygomatic bones. The more precise boundaries are as follows.

- Roof:
  - frontal bone anteriorly
  - lesser wing of sphenoid posteriorly.
- Lateral wall:
  - frontal process of zygomatic bone
  - zygomatic process of frontal bone.
- Floor:
  - maxillary process of zygomatic bone laterally
  - maxilla medially.
- Medial wall:
  - frontal process of maxilla
  - frontal bone

- lacrimal bone
- orbital plate of ethmoid bone
- body of the sphenoid.

Structures Entering and Leaving the Orbit

Passing through the optic foramen are:

- the optic nerve
- the ophthalmic artery.

Passing through the superior orbital fissure are:

- the three cranial nerves supplying the external ocular muscles:
  - oculomotor nerve
  - trochlear nerve
  - abducens nerve
- the ophthalmic division of the trigeminal nerve
- the ophthalmic veins draining back into the cavernous sinus.

Passing through the inferior orbital fissure are:

- the infraorbital nerve, the major branch of the maxillary division of the trigeminal nerve
- veins draining orbital structures into the veins of the pterygopalatine fissure and infratemporal fossa.

Passing through the nasolacrimal canal is:

- nasolacrimal duct.
- Passing through the anterior and posterior ethmoidal foramina are:
- anterior and posterior ethmoidal vessels.

THE CONTENTS OF THE ORBIT

The contents of the orbit are:

- eyeball
- extraocular muscles.

The Eyeball (Fig. 5.11)

The eyeball is spherical and contained within the orbit. It is formed by segments of two spheres with the segment of the smaller sphere, corresponding to the cornea, superimposed anteriorly. It consists of three coats enclosing three refractive media. The coats are:

- fibrous: sclera, cornea
- vascular: choroid, ciliary body, iris
- neural: retina.

The refractive media are:

- aqueous humour
- vitreous body
- lens.

Fibrous Coat

- Transparent anterior part: cornea.
- Opaque posterior part: sclera.

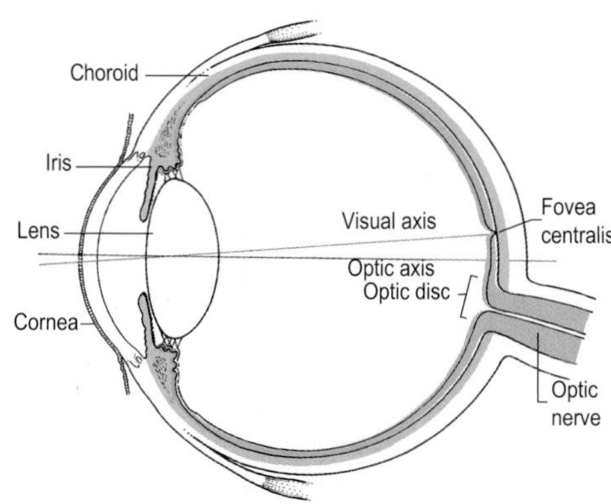

Fig. 5.11 Horizontal section of the eyeball, showing the optic and visual axes.

- Cornea is continuous with the sclera at the sclerocorneal junction.
- Sclera is tough fibrous membrane which maintains the shape of the eyeball and receives insertion of the extraocular muscles.
- Sclera is continuous posteriorly with the dural sheath of the optic nerve.
- Posteriorly the sclera is pierced by the optic nerve 3 mm to the medial side of the optical axis (posterior pole).

Vascular Coat

This is composed of:

- choroid
- ciliary body
- iris.

Choroid

- Thin, highly vascular membrane lying in a surface of sclera.
- Pierced posteriorly by optic nerve.
- Connected anteriorly to iris by ciliary body.

Ciliary body

The ciliary body includes:

- ciliary ring: a fibrous ring continuous with the choroid
- ciliary processes: approximately 70 folds arranged radially between the ciliary ring and the iris, and connected posteriorly to the suspensory ligament of the lens
- ciliary muscles: outer radial and inner circular layer of smooth muscle responsible for changes in the convexity of the lens in accommodation.

Iris

- Coloured membrane suspended in the aqueous humour behind the cornea and in front of the lens.

- In its centre is a circular aperture, the pupil.
- Connected to the circumference of the ciliary body.
- Consists of four layers:
  - anterior mesothelial layer
  - connective tissue stroma containing pigment cells
  - smooth muscle: radial (dilator pupillae), circular (sphincter pupillae)
  - posterior layer of pigmented cells.

Neural

- Retina is the expanded termination of the optic nerve.
- Consists of an outer pigmented and an inner nervous layer.
- Lies between the choroid and hyaloid membrane of the vitreous body.
- Anteriorly is an irregular edge, the ora serrata.
- Posteriorly, the surface nerve fibres join to form the optic nerve.
- The inner surface contains (Fig. 5.12):
  - macula lutea (yellow spot) situated at the posterior pole on the optical axis
  - fovea centralis: a depression in the macula
  - optic disc (medial to the macula), where the optic nerve enters
  - central vessels of the retina coursing over the optic disc
  - central artery of the retina emerging from the optic disc and dividing into upper and lower branches, e.g. dividing into a nasal and temporal branch.
- The retina consists of:
  - rods and cones: inner receptor cell layer
  - intermediate bipolar neurons
  - layer of ganglion cells whose axons form the superficial layer of optic nerve fibres.

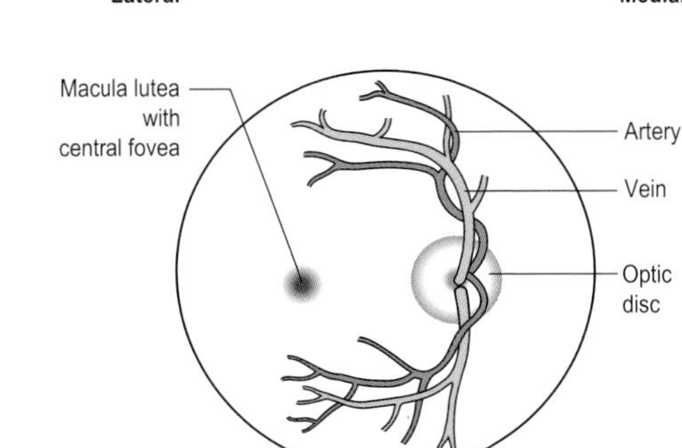

Fig. 5.12 The right fundus as seen by ophthalmoscopy.

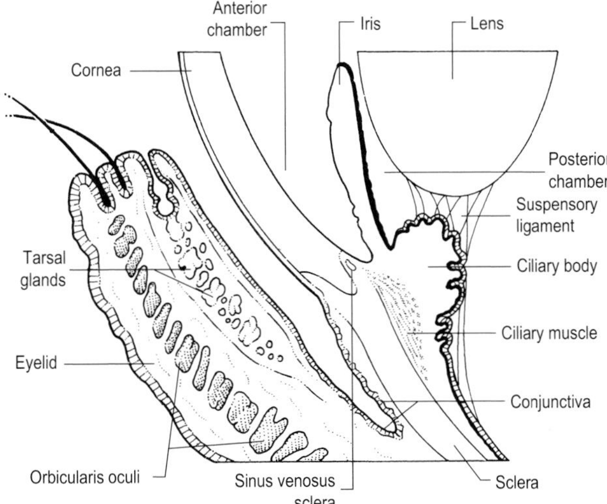

Fig. 5.13 The sclerocorneal junction.

Contents of the Eyeball (Fig. 5.13)

Lens

- Biconvex.
- Enclosed in lens capsule.
- Lies between vitreous and aqueous humour just behind iris.
- Surrounded by suspensory ligament connecting it to ciliary processes.

Aqueous humour

- Filtrate of plasma secreted by vessels of iris and ciliary body into space between lens and iris (posterior chamber of eye).
- Passes through pupillary aperture into area between cornea and iris (anterior chamber of the eye).
- Reabsorbed into ciliary veins via canal of Schlemm (sinus venosus sclerae).

Vitreous body

- Occupies posterior four-fifths of eyeball.
- Soft gelatinous substance contained within the hyaloid membrane.
- Hyaloid membrane passes forwards in front where it is thickened, receiving the attachments from the ciliary processes and giving rise to the suspensory ligament of the lens.
- The hyaloid canal (containing lymph) passes forwards through the vitreous from the optic disc as far as the capsule of the lens.

ORBITAL MUSCLES

The orbital muscles are:

- levator palpebrae superioris which elevates the upper eyelid

- medial, lateral, superior, inferior recti
- superior and inferior oblique.

Four Recti

- Originate from tendinous ring around optic nerve and medial part of superior orbital fissure.
- Insert into sclera anterior to equator of eyeball.

Superior Oblique

- Originates just above tendinous ring.
- Inserts via a tendon which loops around a fibrous pulley on the medial part of the roof of the orbit, into the sclera, just lateral to the insertion of superior rectus behind the equator of the eyeball.

Inferior Oblique

- Originates from the medial part of the floor of the front of the orbit.
- Inserts by passing on the undersurface of the eye, into the sclera between superior and lateral recti behind the equator of the eyeball.

Nerve Supply

- Lateral rectus: abducens (VI).
- Superior oblique: trochlear (IV).
- All others: oculomotor (III).

Movements of the Eyeball

- Elevation.
- Depression.
- Adduction.
- Abduction.
- Rotation.
- Medial recti: adduction—move eyeball in one axis only.
- Lateral recti: abduction—move eyeball in one axis only.
- Superior rectus: elevation, adduction, medial rotation.
- Inferior rectus: depression, adduction, lateral rotation.
- Superior oblique: depression, abduction, medial rotation.
- Inferior oblique: elevation, abduction, lateral rotation.
- Superior rectus and inferior oblique acting together: pure elevation.
- Inferior rectus and superior oblique acting together: pure depression.

Eyelids

- Upper is larger and more mobile.
- Upper contains levator palpebrae superioris.
- Each eyelid consists of following layers from without in:
  - skin
  - connective tissue
  - orbicularis oculi
  - tarsal plates (fibrous tissue)
  - tarsal glands
  - conjunctiva.
- Eyelashes arise at mucocutaneous junction (infection of hair follicle here results in a stye).

Meibomian glands (large sebaceous glands) open behind eyelashes and, if blocked, produce Meibomian cysts.

Conjunctiva

- Mucous membrane lining the inner surface of the lids.
- Reflected over anterior part of sclera to cornea.
- Thick and highly vascular over eyelids, thin over sclera, and single layer of cells only over cornea.
- Lines of reflection from lid to sclera are called the fornices.

Lacrimal Apparatus

- Lacrimal gland lies in depression at superolateral angle of orbit.
- Twelve to fourteen ducts open into the superior conjunctival fornix.
- Tears are drained away by lacrimal canaliculi, which pass medially to open into the lacrimal sac.
- Lacrimal sac lies in a small depression on the medial surface of the orbit.
- Lacrimal sac drains via nasolacrimal duct into the anterior part of the inferior meatus of the nose.

THE EAR

The ear is composed of three parts:

- external
- middle
- internal.

External Ear

This is composed of:

- auricle
- external auditory meatus.

Auricle (Fig. 5.14)

- Plate of elastic cartilage covered with skin.
- It has numerous ridges and depressions.

External Auditory Meatus

- Extends inwards to tympanic membrane.
- Approximately 3.5 cm long.
- Formed partly by cartilage and partly bone.
- Passes medially upwards and forwards, then medially and backwards, and finally medially forwards and downwards.
- Lined by skin with hairs and ceruminous glands, which secrete wax.

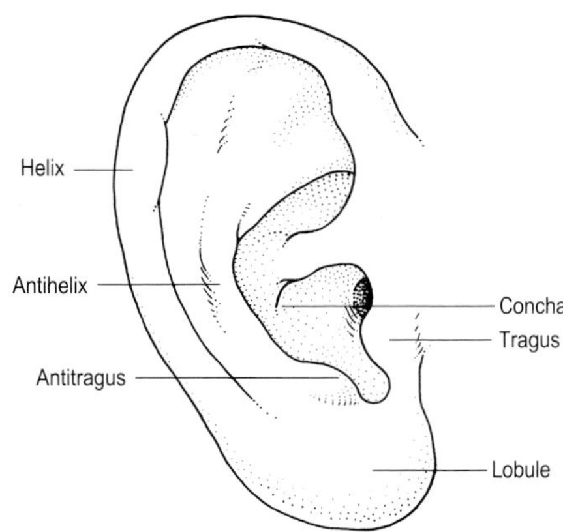

Fig. 5.14 The auricle.

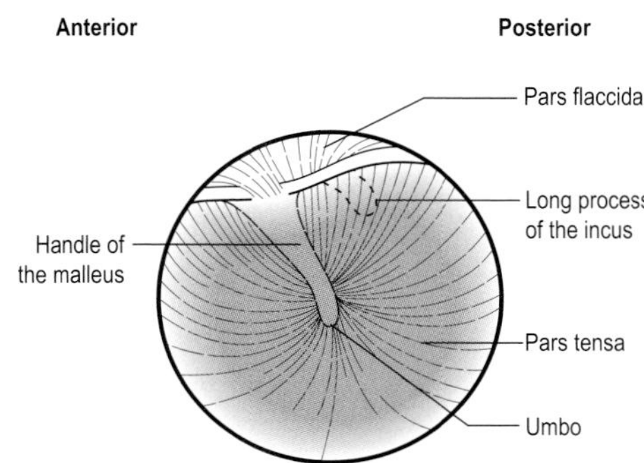

Fig. 5.15 The tympanic membrane as seen through an auroscope.

Middle Ear

- Narrow slit-like cavity contained in the petrous temporal bone (tympanic cavity).
- Contains a chain of bones (ossicles) which transmit sound vibrations from tympanic membrane to internal ear.
- Communicates with pharynx via auditory or pharyngotympanic (Eustachian) tube.

Tympanic Cavity

The tympanic cavity has four walls, a roof and a floor.

Lateral Wall

- Tympanic membrane separating it from the external auditory meatus.

Medial Wall

- Separates the cavity from the inner ear.
- Presents the following features:
  - fenestra vestibuli (oval window): occupied by the base of the stapes
  - promontory below the fenestra vestibuli: formed by the projection of the first turn of the cochlea
  - fenestra cochleae (round window): lies at the bottom of a funnel-shaped depression behind the promontory; closed by the secondary tympanic membrane
  - prominence caused by the underlying canal for the facial nerve.

Posterior Wall

- Carries a small pyramidal projection at the level of the fenestra vestibuli, which houses stapedius muscle.
- Posterior wall continues into mastoid process and mastoid air cells.

Anterior Wall

- Contains openings of canal for tensor tympani and of the auditory canal.
- Below these, a thin plate of bone separates the cavity from the canal for the internal carotid artery.

Floor

- Thin plate of bone separating the cavity from the bulb of the jugular vein.

Roof

- Thin sheet of bone: the tegmen tympani.
- Tegmen tympani separates the epitympanic recess (which extends laterally superior to the tympanic membrane) from the floor of the middle cranial fossa and the temporal lobe of the brain.

Tympanic Membrane (Eardrum) (Fig. 5.15)

- Separates middle ear from external auditory meatus.
- Consists of three layers:
  - outer stratified squamous epithelium
  - middle layer of fibrous tissue
  - inner mucous layer facing the tympanic cavity and continuous with the mucoperiosteum of the cavity.
- Faces laterally downwards and forwards.
- Bulges into middle ear, making lateral surface concave.
- Upper part is thin and loose: pars flaccida; the remainder is taut: pars tensa.
- Translucent except at its margins: it is possible to see the underlying malleus and part of the incus through it.
- The point of greatest concavity is the umbo, marking the attachment of the handle of the malleus to the membrane.

The Ossicles

These are:

- malleus

- incus
- stapes.

They form an interconnecting chain of bones conducting sound through the middle ear.

- Malleus is the largest and has:
  - a handle attached to tympanic membrane
  - a head articulating with the incus
  - a lateral process from which the malleolar folds radiate.
- Incus has:
  - a body which articulates with the malleus
  - a short process attached to the posterior wall of the middle ear
  - a long process articulating with the stapes.
- Stapes has:
  - a head for articulation with the incus
  - a base fixed to the membrane closing the fenestra vestibuli (oval window)
  - two muscles which serve to dampen high-frequency vibrations are associated with the ossicles:
    - stapedius: attached to the neck of the stapes and supplied by the facial nerve
    - tensor tympani: inserted into the handle of the malleus and supplied by the mandibular division of the trigeminal nerve.

Auditory Tube (Eustachian Tube)

- Passes downwards, forwards and medially from the anterior part of the tympanic cavity to the lateral wall of the nasopharynx.
- It is 35 mm long, the first part being bony and the rest cartilaginous.
- Lined by columnar ciliated epithelium.
- Its nasopharyngeal opening is surrounded by lymphoid tissue, the tubal tonsil, which may swell with infection, blocking the tube and predisposing to middle ear infection.

Inner Ear (Fig. 5.16)

The inner ear or labyrinth is divided into two parts:

- bony labyrinth
- membranous labyrinth.

The membranous labyrinth lies within the bony labyrinth. The bony labyrinth comprises:

- vestibule
- semicircular canals
- cochlea.

The membranous labyrinth comprises:

- semicircular ducts
- utricle } within the
- saccule } vestibule
- duct of the cochlea (within the cochlea).

Features of the inner ear

- The membranous labyrinth contains a fluid: endolymph.
- The bony labyrinth contains perilymph surrounding the membranous labyrinth.
- The vestibulocochlear nerve divides into:
  - a vestibular division supplying utricle, saccule and semicircular ducts
  - a cochlear division running up the central canal of the cochlea and supplying the organ of Corti in the cochlear duct.

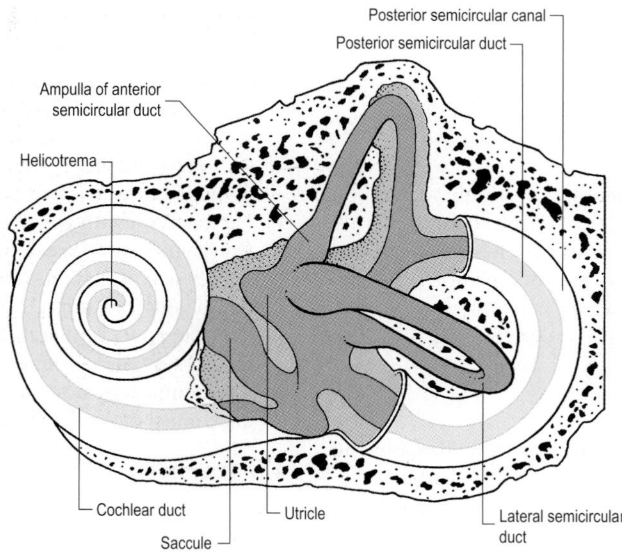

Fig. 5.16 The membranous labyrinth superimposed on the osseous labyrinth.

- The function of the semicircular ducts is to convey a sense of motion in any direction, i.e. they tell you where you are going.
- The function of the utricle and saccule is to convey a sense of position in space, i.e. they tell you where you are.
- Each component of the membranous labyrinth has specialized receptors to achieve their function(s):
  - maculae of the utricle and saccule
  - ampullary crests of semicircular canals
  - spiral organ of Corti in the cochlea.
- The disposition of the semicircular canals in three planes at right angles to each other renders this part of the labyrinth well suited to signal changes in position of the head.
- The organ of Corti is adapted to record sound vibrations transmitted by the stapes at the oval window as follows:
  - sound waves set up vibrations in the tympanic membrane
  - transmission occurs through the ossicles and the stapes is pushed backwards and forwards in the oval window, setting up vibrations in the perilymph
  - these travel up the scala vestibuli (filled with perilymph) in the cochlea, through the helicotrema and down through the scala tympani to the secondary tympanic membrane (Fig. 5.17).
- This sets up vibrations in the basilar membrane, and these are transformed into nerve impulses.

THE NOSE AND PARANASAL AIR SINUSES

The Nose

The nose comprises:

- external nose
- nasal cavity.

External Nose (Fig. 5.18)

- Bony and cartilaginous framework overlaid by skin and fibro–fatty tissue.

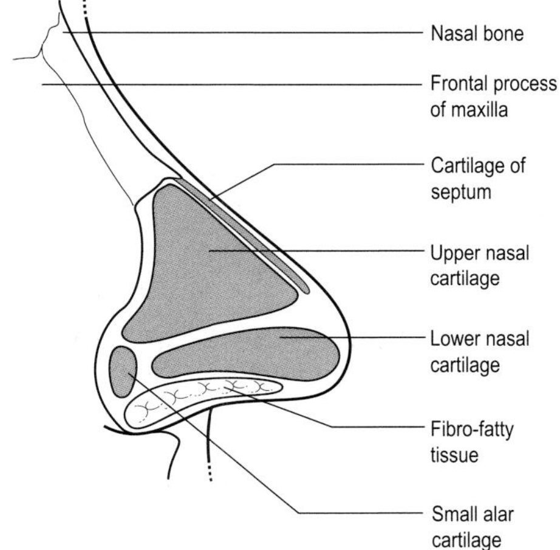

Fig. 5.18 The bones and cartilage of the lateral aspect of the right side of the nose.

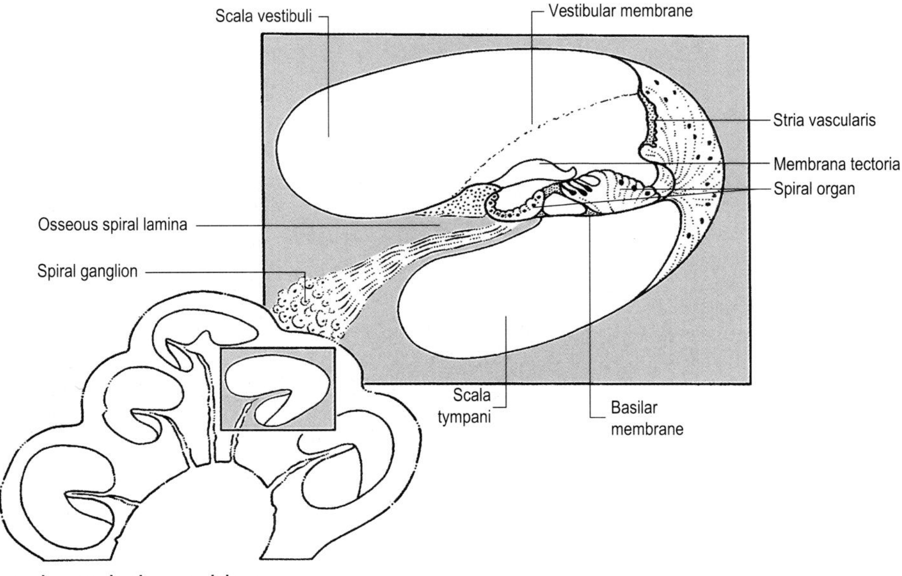

Fig. 5.17 Section through the cochlea.

- Bony margins are the two nasal bones and the frontal process of maxilla.
- Margins completed by nasal cartilages, supported by septal cartilage.
- Ala is movable and contains small cartilages, but is composed solely of fatty tissue at its lower free edge.

Nasal Cavity

The nasal cavities are separated from one another by the septum—open in front by the nostrils, and behind by the posterior apertures opening into the nasopharynx. Each cavity possesses:

- roof
- floor
- medial wall
- lateral wall.

Roof

- Highly arched.
- Formed by:
  - nasal bones
  - nasal spine of frontal bone
  - cribriform plate of ethmoid
  - undersurface of body of sphenoid
  - alae of vomer
  - sphenoidal process of palatine bone.

Floor

- Corresponds to roof of mouth.
- Formed by:
  - palatine process of maxilla
  - horizontal plate of palatine bone.

Medial wall (nasal septum)

- Cartilage of septum.
- Crest of nasal bones.
- Perpendicular plate of ethmoid.
- Vomer.

Lateral wall

- Very irregular due to projections of three conchae.
- Formed by:
  - frontal process of maxilla
  - lacrimal bone
  - ethmoid bone
  - nasal surface of maxilla
  - perpendicular plate of palatine bone
  - medial pterygoid plate of sphenoid.

The features of the lateral wall are shown in Fig. 5.19.

Conchae

- Three conchae project into nasal cavity from its lateral wall:
  - superior concha
  - middle concha
  - inferior concha.

Meatuses

- Conchae divide lateral wall into four recesses:
  - sphenoethmoidal recess above superior concha
  - superior recess below superior concha
  - middle recess below middle concha
  - inferior recess below inferior concha.

Openings

- Sphenoethmoidal recess: sphenoidal sinus.
- Superior meatus: posterior ethmoidal air cells.
- Middle meatus:
  - bulla of ethmoid (middle ethmoidal air cells open onto it)

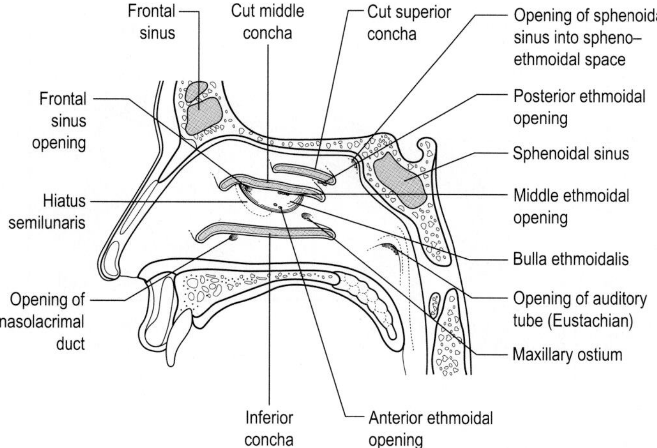

Fig. 5.19 The lateral wall of the nasal cavity.

- hiatus semilunaris: receives infundibulum of frontal sinus and anterior ethmoidal air cells in front and maxillary ostium behind.
- Inferior meatus: nasolacrimal duct.

Mucous Membrane

- Olfactory:
  - superior concha
  - upper part of middle concha
  - corresponding part of septum
  - roof of nose.
- Respiratory:
  - lines remainder of nasal cavity.

The epithelium of the various parts of the nose is as follows:

- olfactory region: columnar epithelium
- respiratory region (and paranasal sinuses): columnar ciliated epithelium with mucous cells
- vestibule: stratified squamous epithelium.

Olfactory Nerve

- Passes from the olfactory mucosa.
- Passes through holes in the cribriform plate to reach the olfactory bulb.

Blood Supply

- Upper part of nasal cavity: ethmoidal branches of ophthalmic artery.
- Lower part of nasal cavity: sphenopalatine branch of maxillary artery.
- Septal branch of facial artery anastomoses with sphenopalatine branch of maxillary artery on the anteroinferior part of septum (Little's area); nosebleeds occur from this area.
- Venous drainage:
  - downwards into facial vein
  - backwards to ethmoidal tributaries of ophthalmic veins, and hence ultimately to cavernous sinus.

PARANASAL AIR SINUSES

Paranasal air sinuses are a complex series of air-filled cavities opening into the nasal cavity on each side. They are effectively extensions of the nasal cavity. They are lined by columnar ciliated epithelium. The sinuses are:

- maxillary sinus opening into the middle meatus
- ethmoidal air cells (sinuses), which are variable in number, in three groups: the anterior, middle and posterior. The anterior and middle cells open into the middle meatus; the posterior air cells into the superior meatus
- the frontal sinus opening into the middle meatus via the infundibulum
- the sphenoidal sinus opening into the sphenoethmoidal recess.

Maxillary Sinus

- Largest of the paranasal sinuses.
- The medial wall is composed of thin and delicate bones on the lateral wall of the nasal cavity. The opening of the sinus into the hiatus semilunaris lies high on the medial wall just below the floor of the orbit. As the ostium is high on the wall, drainage depends on ciliary action and not gravity.
- The roof of the sinus is the floor of the orbit. The canal for the infraorbital nerve produces a ridge into the sinus from the roof.
- The posterior wall faces the pterygopalatine fossa and infratemporal fossa.
- The anterior wall is comparatively thick and lies between the infraorbital margin and the premolar teeth.
- The floor is a narrow cleft between the posterior and anterior wall in the alveolar process of the maxilla overlying the second premolar and first molar teeth. The canine and all molars may be included in the floor if the sinus is large. The roots of these teeth may produce projections into the sinus or occasionally perforate the bone. A tooth abscess may rupture into the sinus. The floor of the maxillary sinus is at a more inferior level than the floor of the nasal cavity.

Clinical Points

- For maxillary sinus washout a cannula is inserted into the sinus via the inferior meatus of the nasal cavity.
- In the Caldwell–Luc operation for maxillary sinusitis the anterior bony wall of the maxillary sinus is removed, the mucosa is stripped and a permanent drainage hole is made into the nose through the inferior meatus.
- Carcinoma of the maxillary sinus may invade the palate and cause dental problems. It may block the nasolacrimal duct, causing epiphora.
- Spread of the tumour into the orbit causes proptosis.
- Posterior spread may involve the palatine nerves and produce severe pain referred to the teeth of the upper jaw.

Nerve Supply

- The maxillary division of the trigeminal nerve via infraorbital and superior dental nerves. Pain due to sinusitis may often manifest itself as toothache.

Lymphatic Drainage

- To the upper deep cervical nodes.

Ethmoidal Air Cells (Sinuses)

- Group of 8–10 air cells within the lateral mass of the ethmoid.
- Lie between the side walls of the upper nasal cavity and the orbits.
- Above they lie on each side of the cribriform plate and are related to the frontal lobes of the brain.
- Anterior and middle air cells open into middle meatus. Posterior air cells open into the superior meatus.

Frontal Sinus

- Contained in frontal bone.
- Varies greatly in size and shape.
- Absent until end of first year.
- Separated from one another by bony septum.
- Each sinus drains into the anterior part of the middle meatus via the infundibulum into the hiatus semilunaris.

Sphenoidal Sinus

- Very small at birth.
- Lies within the body of the sphenoid.
- Pituitary gland lies above it and cavernous sinus laterally.
- Opens into the sphenoethmoidal recess above the superior concha.

THE MUSCLES OF MASTICATION

The muscles of mastication are:
- masseter
- temporalis
- lateral pterygoid
- medial pterygoid.

They are all developed from the mandibular arch, and therefore supplied by the mandibular division of the trigeminal nerve.

Masseter

Origin

- Anterior two-thirds of lower border of zygomatic arch, posterior third of lower border and whole of deep surface of arch.

Insertion

- Outer surface of ramus of mandible from mandibular notch to angle.

Action

- Closes the jaw.

Temporalis

Origin

- From the temporal fossa.

Insertion

- The coronoid process of the mandible.

Action

- Closes the jaw; the most posterior fibres, being horizontal, retract the jaw.

Lateral Pterygoid

Origin

- By two heads: lower head from lateral surface of lateral pterygoid plate; upper head from the interior surface of the greater wing of the sphenoid.

Insertion

- Passes horizontally backwards to insert into the anterior surface of the disc of the temporomandibular joint and into the neck of the mandible.

Action

- Aids in opening the mouth by sliding the condyle forwards, and also protrudes the jaw. One muscle acting alone pulls the chin over to the opposite side.

Medial Pterygoid

Origin

- Medial side of lateral pterygoid plate with a small slip from the tubercle of the maxilla.

Insertion

- Fibres pass downwards, backwards and laterally to the medial surface of the mandible in the roughened area near the angle.

Action

- Closes the jaw. One muscle acting alone pulls the chin over to the opposite side. Medial pterygoids are chewing muscles for molar teeth grinding.

TEMPOROMANDIBULAR JOINT

- Synovial joint.
- Articular surfaces: head of mandible articulates with mandibular fossa and articular eminence of temporal bone.
- Articular surfaces are covered by fibrocartilage (not hyaline), and there is also a fibrocartilaginous articular disc dividing the joint cavity into upper and lower compartments.
- Capsule: attached to neck of mandible around head; above it is attached just anterior to the articular eminence in front and to the squamotympanic fissure behind.

- Articular disc attached around its periphery to joint capsule.
- Anteriorly the disc is attached to the lateral pterygoid muscle, and posteriorly to the temporal bone.
- The posterior attachment of the disc is elastic, allowing forwards movement of the disc with the mandible by contraction of lateral pterygoid during opening of the mouth.
- Capsule of joint is reinforced by the lateral temporomandibular ligament, the sphenomandibular ligament and the stylomandibular ligament.
- Movements of the joint are:
  - depression
  - elevation
  - protrusion
  - retraction
  - side-to-side movements of the mandible.

The muscles affecting these movements are:

- elevation: masseter, temporalis, medial pterygoid
- depression: lateral pterygoid together with digastric, mylohyoid and geniohyoid; gravity also allows the jaw to open during sleep
- retraction: posterior fibres of temporalis
- protraction (protrusion): lateral pterygoid
- side-to-side: lateral and medial pterygoids together, acting alternately on each side.

Clinical Points

- The muscles of mastication and their nerve supply are tested clinically by asking the patient:
  - to clench the teeth; contraction of the masseter and temporalis can be felt
  - to move the chin from side to side, testing the activity of the pterygoid muscles.
- Dislocation of the mandible occurs in a forwards direction, where the condyloid process of the mandible slides forwards onto the articular eminence and then into the infratemporal fossa. This can be reduced by pressing down the mandible on the molar teeth to stretch the masseter and temporalis which are in spasm and then pulling up the chin to lever the condyle back into the mandibular fossa.

FLOOR OF THE MOUTH AND TONGUE (Fig. 5.20)

Floor of the Mouth

- Formed by the mylohyoid, which separates the oral cavity from the neck.
- Mylohyoid muscles of both sides meet along a midline raphe.
- Mylohyoids are reinforced superiorly by geniohyoids.
- Anterior part of tongue rests on mucosa covering the floor of the mouth.
- In the midline the frenulum of the tongue is seen on the floor connecting the tongue to the mandible.
- On either side of the frenulum is the sublingual papilla on which the submandibular gland duct opens.
- Lateral to this is the sublingual fold produced by the sublingual gland.
- More posteriorly between mylohyoid and tongue lies the hyoglossus muscle.
- A number of important structures in the floor of the mouth lie on hyoglossus. These are, from above downwards:
  - lingual nerve
  - deep part of submandibular gland and submandibular duct
  - hypoglossal nerve.

Lingual Nerve

- Branch of mandibular division of trigeminal nerve.
- Runs forwards above mylohyoid.

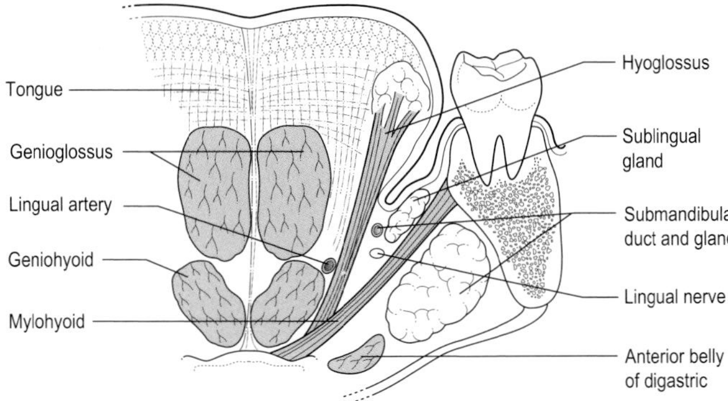

Fig. 5.20 Coronal section of the floor of the mouth.

- Gives off gingival branch, which supplies the whole of the lingual gingiva and the mucous membrane of the floor of the mouth.
- Winds round submandibular duct before being distributed to the mucosa of the anterior two-thirds of the tongue.
- Submandibular ganglion is suspended from lingual nerve as it lies on hyoglossus.
- Preganglionic fibres in the chorda tympani synapse in submandibular ganglion.
- Before reaching the floor of the mouth, the lingual nerve lies against the periosteum of the alveolar process closely related to the third molar tooth. The nerve can be damaged here during dental extraction.

Hypoglossal Nerve

- Descends between internal jugular vein and internal carotid artery.
- Supplies the superior limb of the ansa cervicalis (C1) to innervate the infrahyoid muscles.
- Reaches the surface of the hyoglossus by passing deep to the posterior belly of digastric.
- On hyoglossus, breaks up into branches to supply all muscles of the tongue except palatoglossus.

THE TONGUE

- Buccal and pharyngeal parts separated by V-shaped groove, sulcus terminalis, at the apex of which is the foramen caecum.
- Larger vallate papillae lie immediately in front of sulcus terminalis.
- Median frenulum lies on inferior surface of tongue. The lingual veins can be seen on either side of the frenulum.
- On either side of the base of the frenulum are the orifices of the submandibular ducts.

Structure

- Covered by thick stratified squamous epithelium bearing papillae on the anterior two-thirds. Papillae carry taste buds.
- Posterior third has no papillae but has numerous lymphoid nodules.
- Tongue is divided by a median septum, on either side of which are the intrinsic and extrinsic muscles of the tongue.
- Intrinsic muscles are longitudinal, vertical and transverse; they alter the shape of the tongue.
- Extrinsic muscles move the tongue as a whole:
  - genioglossus: protrudes the tongue
  - styloglossus: retracts the tongue
  - hyoglossus: depresses the tongue.

Blood Supply

- Lingual branch of the external carotid artery.
- Little cross-circulation across the midline, therefore a relatively avascular plane.

Lymphatic Drainage

- Tip drains to submental nodes.
- Anterior two-thirds drain to submental and submandibular nodes and then to lower deep cervical nodes; little cross-communication between drainage of two sides of tongue.
- Posterior third drains to upper deep cervical nodes; extensive cross-communication, therefore tumours may spread to contralateral nodes.

Nerve Supply

- Anterior two-thirds: sensory supply from lingual branch of cranial nerve V. Taste fibres pass in lingual nerve (from chorda tympani of cranial nerve VII).
- Posterior third: sensation and taste (including vallate papillae) from nerve IX.
- Motor supply from the hypoglossal nerve, except for palatoglossus.

Clinical Points

- Hypoglossal nerve damage results in wasting of the tongue on the same side. Deviation to the paralysed side on protrusion.
- In the unconscious patient, when the tongue has dropped back, causing laryngeal obstruction, pushing the mandible forwards by pressure on the angle of the jaw on each side will pull the tongue forwards with the jaw, owing to attachment of genioglossus to the lower jaw.

SALIVARY GLANDS

Parotid Gland (Serous Gland)

The parotid gland is the largest salivary gland.

Relations

- Anteriorly: mandible and masseter.
- Medially: internal jugular vein, internal carotid artery, IX, X, XI and XII nerves, and lateral wall of pharynx separated by styloid process and its muscles.
- Superiorly: external auditory meatus and temporomandibular joint.
- Inferiorly: posterior belly of digastric.

Traversing the gland from superficial to deep are:

- facial nerve
- retromandibular vein
- external carotid artery, dividing into the superficial temporal and maxillary branches.

Parotid Duct (Stensen's Duct)

- Arises from the anterior part of the gland.
- Passes over masseter muscle (can be palpated over the tensed masseter a finger's breadth below the zygomatic arch).
- Pierces buccinator opening opposite the upper second molar tooth.
- The gland is traversed by the facial nerve, which emerges from the stylomastoid foramen.
- Nerve divides into two main divisions resulting in five branches:
  - temporal and zygomatic
  - buccal, mandibular and cervical.
- Cross-communications occur between the branches in the gland, which are not important and can be divided safely.
- The mandibular division is the longest, thinnest and therefore most vulnerable branch.

Submandibular Gland (Mixed Serous and Mucous Gland)

The submandibular gland has a large superficial, and a small, deep lobe connecting with each other around the posterior border of mylohyoid.

Relations

- Superficial:
  - platysma
  - marginal mandibular branch of facial nerve
  - cervical branch of facial nerve
  - facial vein.
- Deep:
  - mylohyoid
  - hyoglossus
  - lingual nerve
  - hypoglossal nerve.
- Separated posteriorly from parotid gland by stylomandibular ligament.
- The facial artery grooves the superficial aspect of a gland, ascending onto the face.
- The submandibular duct (Wharton's duct) arises from the deep part of the gland. It runs forwards and opens at the side of the frenulum of the tongue. It is crossed from superficial to deep by the lingual nerve, which passes from the lateral side of the duct, below and then medial to it; it 'double-crosses' it.
- Submandibular lymph nodes lie between the gland and mandible. Occasionally they are embedded in the gland.

Clinical Points

- The mandibular branch of the facial nerve descends below the angle of the mandible before arching upwards onto the face. To avoid this branch, the incision to approach the gland should be made more than 2.5 cm below the angle of the mandible.
- The gland (and a stone in the duct) can be palpated bimanually in the floor of the mouth.

The Sublingual Gland (Mucous Gland)

- Almond-shaped salivary gland lying immediately below the mucosa of the floor of the mouth.
- Lies immediately in front of the deep part of the submandibular gland.
- Medially, it is separated from the base of the tongue by the submandibular duct and the lingual nerve.
- Laterally, it rests against the sublingual groove of the mandible.
- Opens separately into the floor of mouth by a series of ducts.
- Part of it also opens into the submandibular duct.

THE NECK

The Fascial Compartments of the Neck

Consist of a 'cylinder' around the neck (investing layer) and a complex system of septae between the neck muscles and other structures. The fascia of the neck is divided into:

- Superficial fascia.
- Deep fascia, which is divided into a further three layers:
  - investing layer (enveloping)
  - prevertebral fascia
  - pretracheal fascia.

Investing Fascia

- Invests the muscles of the neck.
- Attached to all the bony landmarks at the upper and lower margins of the neck.
- Above to the mandible, zygomatic arch, mastoid process and superior nuchal line.
- Below to the manubrium, clavicle, acromion and scapular spine.
- Splits to enclose the trapezius, sternocleidomastoid, strap muscles and parotid and submandibular glands.
- External jugular vein pierces the investing fascia below omohyoid, just above the midpoint of the clavicle (if the vein is divided here, the deep fascia holds it open, air is drawn into the veins on inspiration and air embolism occurs).

Prevertebral Fascia

- Passes across the vertebrae and prevertebral muscles.
- Oesophagus, pharynx and great vessels lie in front.
- Forms a base upon which the pharynx, oesophagus and carotid sheath slide in swallowing and neck movements.

- Laterally, covers the cervical and brachial plexuses and muscles in the floor of the posterior triangle.
- Brachial plexus and subclavian artery are covered with a sheath formed from the prevertebral fascia, which becomes the axillary sheath.

Pretracheal Fascia

- Extends from hyoid bone above to fibrous pericardium below.
- Encloses larynx, trachea, pharynx, oesophagus and thyroid gland.

Carotid Sheath

- Separate tube of fascia, strong over carotid arteries and weak over jugular vein (to allow for expansion of latter).
- Contains:
  - carotid artery
  - internal jugular vein
  - vagus nerve.

THE TRIANGLES OF THE NECK (Fig. 5.21)

- Anterior triangle bounded by:
  - in front, the midline of the neck
  - above, the ramus of the mandible
  - behind, the anterior border of sternocleidomastoid.
- Posterior triangle bounded by:
  - in front, the posterior border of the sternocleidomastoid
  - below, the middle third of the clavicle
  - behind, the anterior margin of trapezius.

Anterior Triangle

The anterior triangle contains, among other structures:

- thyroid and parathyroid glands
- submandibular gland
- carotid sheath
- trachea and larynx
- pharynx and oesophagus
- deep cervical lymph nodes
- suprahyoid and infrahyoid groups of muscles.

The anterior triangle can be further divided into four smaller triangles:

- submental
- submandibular
- carotid
- muscular.

Muscles Attached to the Hyoid Bone

- These are in two groups:
  - suprahyoid
  - infrahyoid.
- The suprahyoids consist of:
  - stylohyoid
  - mylohyoid
  - digastric
  - geniohyoid.
- The suprahyoid muscles:
  - elevate the hyoid and pull it forwards during swallowing.
- The infrahyoids are active in opening the mouth against resistance.
- Infrahyoids consist of:
  - sternohyoid
  - sternothyroid
  - thyrohyoid
  - omohyoid.
- The thyroid gland, larynx and trachea lie deep to the infrahyoids.

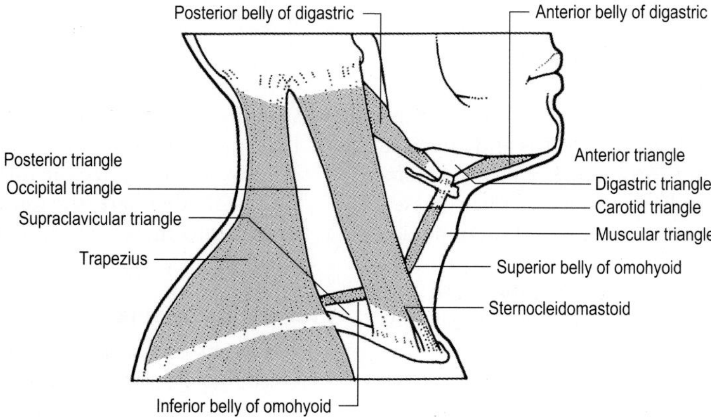

Fig. 5.21 The triangles of the neck.

- The infrahyoids or the strap muscles are supplied by the ansa cervicalis (C1, 2, 3), which is a nerve loop on the internal jugular vein.
- The branches enter the muscles in their lower half; therefore, during exposure of a large goitre, the strap muscles are cut in their upper half to preserve the nerve supply from the ansa cervicalis.

Blood Vessels of the Anterior Triangle (Fig. 5.22)

Common carotid artery

- On the right side it is a branch of the brachiocephalic trunk.
- On the left side it arises from the arch of the aorta.
- Bifurcates into external and internal carotid arteries at the upper border of the thyroid cartilage (level of third cervical vertebra).
- Enclosed in carotid sheath with the internal jugular vein lateral to it and the vagus nerve between the artery and the vein posteriorly.

Internal carotid artery

- Passes vertically upwards as a continuation of common carotid without giving any branches in the neck.
- Enclosed in carotid sheath.
- Separated from external carotid artery by:
  - styloid process
  - stylopharyngeus muscle
  - glossopharyngeal nerve
  - pharyngeal branch of vagus.
- At base of skull, enters the carotid canal.
- Intracranial part supplies the brain and the eye.

External carotid artery

- Extends from point of bifurcation of common carotid to a point midway between the angle of the mandible and the mastoid process.
- Upper part of artery enters parotid gland, where it divides into its two terminal branches, the maxillary artery and the superficial temporal artery.
- At its commencement it is anteromedial to the internal carotid artery and can be distinguished from the internal carotid artery by the presence of branches (the internal carotid has no branches in the neck).
- The branches of the external carotid artery are:
  - superior thyroid artery
  - lingual artery
  - facial artery
  - occipital artery
  - posterior auricular artery
  - ascending pharyngeal artery
  - maxillary artery
  - superficial temporal artery.

Internal jugular vein

- Formed at the jugular foramen as a continuation of the sigmoid sinus.
- At its commencement, lies behind the internal carotid artery.

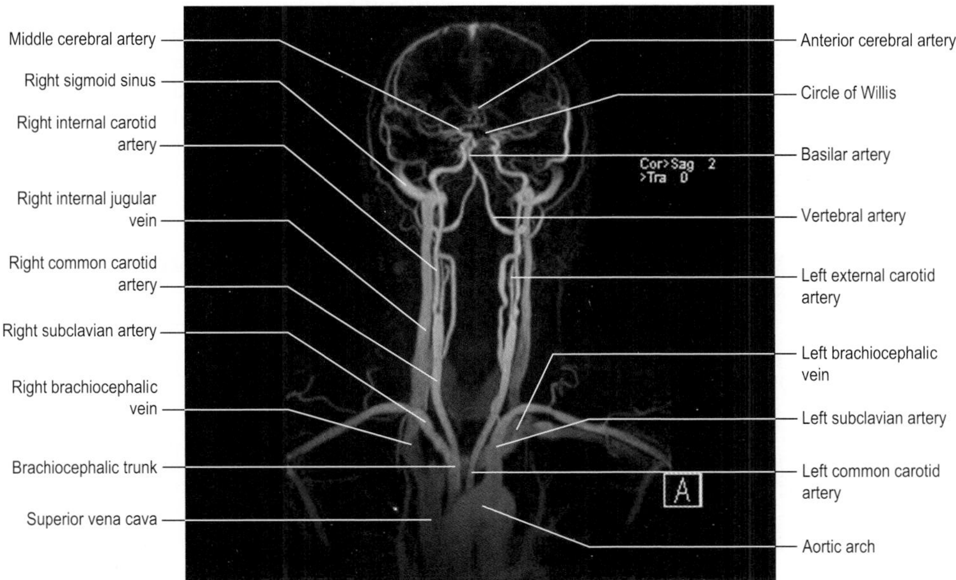

Fig. 5.22 MRA showing the blood vessels of the neck and formation of the circle of Willis.

- As it descends, occupies a position lateral to the internal carotid artery and the common carotid artery.
- Contained within the carotid sheath, which is thinner over the vein, allowing it to distend.
- The deep cervical chain of lymph nodes is found along the internal jugular vein.
- In block dissection of the neck, the internal jugular vein is removed to facilitate removal of the nodes.
- At the root of the neck, the internal jugular vein lies behind the gap between the sternal and clavicular heads of sternocleidomastoid.
- The vein terminates by joining the subclavian vein to form the brachiocephalic vein.

Internal jugular vein cannulation

- Usually carried out on right side as the right vein is in a straight line with the right brachiocephalic vein and superior vena cava.
- High approach: vein is palpated lateral to common carotid artery pulsation deep to anterior border of sternocleidomastoid at the level of C6 vertebra.
- Low approach: the needle is inserted near the apex of the triangular gap between the sternal and clavicular heads of the sternocleidomastoid.

THE THYROID GLAND

The thyroid gland is composed of:

- isthmus: overlying second and third tracheal rings
- lateral lobes: extending from lateral aspect of thyroid cartilage to level of sixth tracheal ring
- inconstant pyramidal lobe extending up from isthmus.

Relations (Fig. 5.23)

- Anteriorly:
  - strap muscles
  - sternocleidomastoid
  - enclosed in pretracheal fascia.
- Posteriorly:
  - larynx
  - trachea
  - pharynx
  - oesophagus.
- Laterally:
  - carotid sheath.
- Recurrent laryngeal nerve runs in groove between trachea and oesophagus.
- External branch of superior laryngeal nerve lies deep to upper pole.

Blood Supply

Arterial

- Superior thyroid artery from external carotid passes to upper pole; closely related to external branch of superior laryngeal nerve.
- Inferior thyroid artery from thyrocervical trunk of first part of subclavian; related to the recurrent laryngeal nerve close to gland.
- Thyroidea ima, from aortic arch; inconstant.

Venous

- Superior thyroid vein drains upper pole to internal jugular vein.
- Middle thyroid vein drains to internal jugular vein.
- Inferior thyroid vein drains lower pole to brachiocephalic veins.

Clinical Points

- Enlargement of the thyroid gland may compress or displace any of its close relations, e.g. trachea, resulting in breathing difficulties and difficult intubation for anaesthetist; oesophagus, resulting in dysphagia.
- Carcinoma of the thyroid may invade the recurrent laryngeal nerve, producing hoarseness of voice.

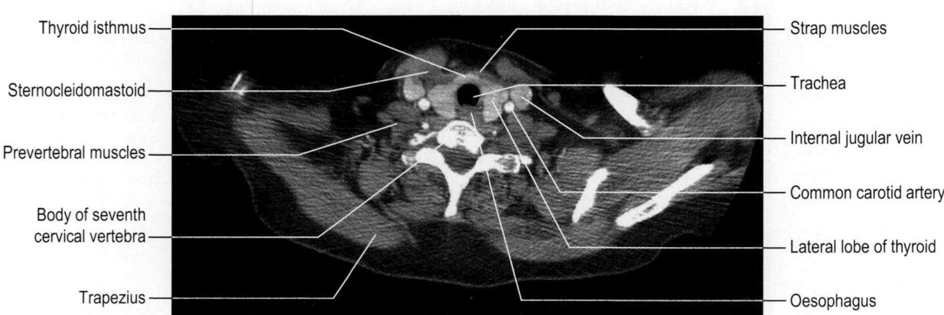

Fig. 5.23 CT scan passing through the body of the seventh cervical vertebra showing the thyroid gland and its relations.

- Thyroidectomy is carried out through a transverse incision in a skin crease two fingers' breadth above the supersternal notch.
- Structures encountered are:
  - platysma
  - investing fascia, which is opened longitudinally between the strap muscles and between the anterior jugular veins
  - strap muscles, which may be divided in their upper half to preserve their nerve supply from the ansa cervicalis, which is into their lower half.
- Pretracheal fascia is then divided, exposing the thyroid gland.
- Care must be taken in dividing the superior thyroid artery (close to the gland, to avoid the external branch of the superior laryngeal nerve) and the inferior thyroid artery (far away from the gland, to avoid the recurrent laryngeal nerve).

PARATHYROID GLANDS

- Four in number, superior and inferior on each side.
- Superior glands are usually constant in position and lie at the middle of the posterior border of the lobe of the thyroid above the level at which the inferior thyroid artery crosses the recurrent laryngeal nerve.
- Inferior glands are subject to variation, but are normally on the posterior part of the lower pole of the thyroid.
- Variations of the inferior parathyroid glands are common, and may be found in the carotid sheath and in the superior mediastinum in company with the thymus. Rarely, they may be found behind the oesophagus or even in the posterior mediastinum.
- They are supplied by the posterior branches of the superior and inferior thyroid arteries.

Clinical Points

- Because of their aberrant sites, searching for them may be difficult at surgery.
- Occasionally they may be removed or rendered ischaemic during thyroid surgery, resulting in tetany due to hypocalcaemia.

THE LARYNX (Fig. 5.24 and 5.25)

The larynx consists of:

- epiglottis
- thyroid cartilage
- cricoid cartilage
- arytenoid cartilages.

Epiglottis

- Leaf-shaped elastic cartilage.
- Attached to body of hyoid and back of thyroid cartilage.
- Sides connected to arytenoids by aryepiglottic folds, which form the margins of the aditus to the larynx.

Thyroid Cartilage

- Two lateral plates meeting in the midline at the laryngeal prominence.
- Cricoid cartilage.
- Signet ring–shaped; deepest posteriorly.
- Complete ring of cartilage.
- Attached to trachea by cricotracheal membrane.

Arytenoid cartilages

- Attached to each side of the 'signet' of cricoid cartilage.

Corniculate Cartilage

- Small nodule.
- Lies at apex of arytenoids.

Cuneiform Cartilage

- Lies at margin of aryepiglottic fold.

Cricothyroid Membrane (Cricovocal Membrane)

- Sheet of elastic yellow tissue.
- The anterior attachment of the upper edges is to the posterior surface of the thyroid cartilage and posteriorly to the vocal process of the arytenoids.
- Upper edge forms the vocal ligament.
- Anteriorly, the membrane thickens to form the cricothyroid ligament.

Vestibular Fold

- Upper fold of mucosa passing forwards from arytenoids to back of thyroid cartilage.
- Forms the false vocal cord.

Vocal Cord

- Lower fold of mucosa passing forwards from arytenoids to the back of the thyroid cartilage.
- Contains the vocal ligaments.
- There is no submucosa over the vocal ligament.

Rima Glottidis

- Space between the vocal cords.

Three Compartments of the Larynx

- Supraglottic (vestibule), above the false cords.
- Glottic, between false and true cords.
- Subglottic, between true cords and first tracheal ring.

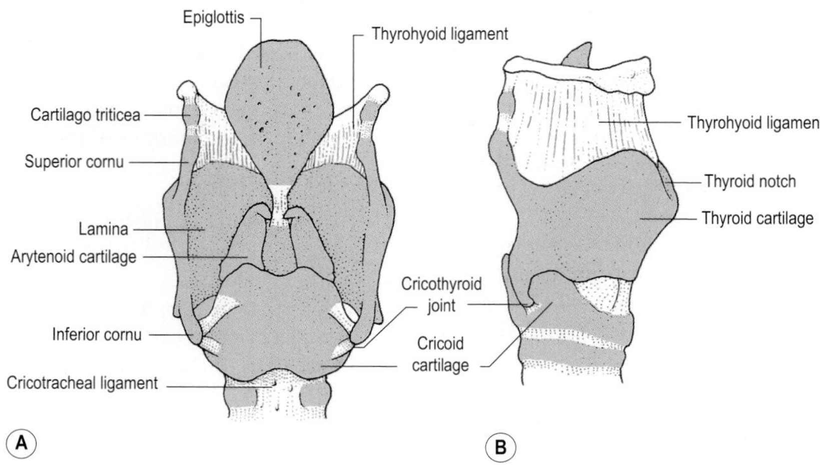

Fig. 5.24 The cartilages of the larynx and the hyoid bone. (A) Posterior view. (B) Lateral view.

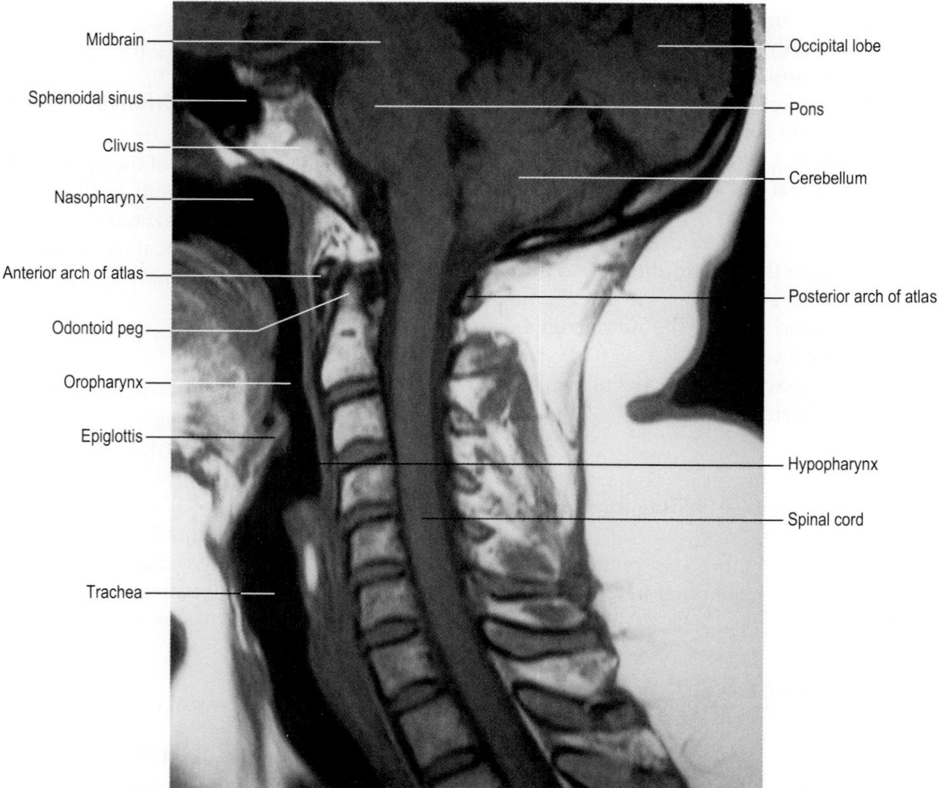

Fig. 5.25 Sagittal MRI scan of neck showing the pharynx, larynx and trachea. (From Jacob S: Atlas of Human Anatomy. Churchill Livingstone 2002, with permission.)

Piriform Fossa

- A recess on either side of the larynx where foreign bodies may lodge.

Muscles of the Larynx

Functions of muscles of the larynx are to:

- open the glottis in inspiration
- close the glottis in swallowing
- alter the tension of the vocal cords in phonation.

Actions

These include:

- cricothyroid tenses the vocal cord
- posterior cricoarytenoid abducts the cords
- all other muscles adduct the cords, i.e. sphincter action.

Blood Supply

- Superior and inferior laryngeal arteries.
- Accompany the superior laryngeal nerve and the recurrent laryngeal nerves, respectively.

Lymphatic Drainage

- Above the vocal cords to the upper deep cervical nodes.
- Below the vocal cords to the lower deep cervical nodes.
- Vocal cords separate the two areas of drainage anteriorly but posteriorly there is cross-communication.

Nerve Supply

Superior laryngeal nerve

- Branch of vagus.
- Internal branch pierces thyrohyoid membrane and supplies laryngeal mucosa down to the level of the vocal cords.
- External laryngeal branch is motor to the cricothyroid (extrinsic muscle).

Recurrent laryngeal nerve

- Branch of vagus.
- Supplies all the intrinsic muscles of the larynx.
- Supplies the mucosa below the vocal cords.

Clinical Points

- The laryngeal nerves are at risk during thyroidectomy. The external branch of the superior laryngeal nerve is close to the superior thyroid artery and may be damaged when ligating the vessel. The recurrent laryngeal nerve is related to the inferior thyroid artery close to the gland. To avoid injury it should be ligated well laterally.
- Damage to the superior laryngeal nerve results in a change of pitch of the voice owing to loss of innervation of cricothyroid muscle, which is a tensor of the vocal cord.
- Damage to recurrent laryngeal nerve results in the cord on the affected side being paralysed in a position between abduction and adduction. The voice may be hoarse. Bilateral damage results in loss of voice with difficulty in breathing through the partially open glottis.
- The larynx can be inspected either directly by means of a laryngoscope, or indirectly through a laryngeal mirror. The following structures may be seen (Fig. 5.26):
    - base of the tongue
    - valleculae
    - epiglottis
    - aryepiglottic folds
    - piriform fossa
    - false cords, which are red and wide apart
    - pearly white true cords.

PHARYNX (Fig. 5.25)

The pharynx is a muscular tube attached to the base of the skull and extends below as far as the sixth cervical vertebra, where it continues as the oesophagus. It has three parts:

- nasopharynx, opening anteriorly into the nasal cavities
- oropharynx, opening into the oral cavity
- laryngopharynx, opening into the larynx and continuing downwards as the oesophagus.

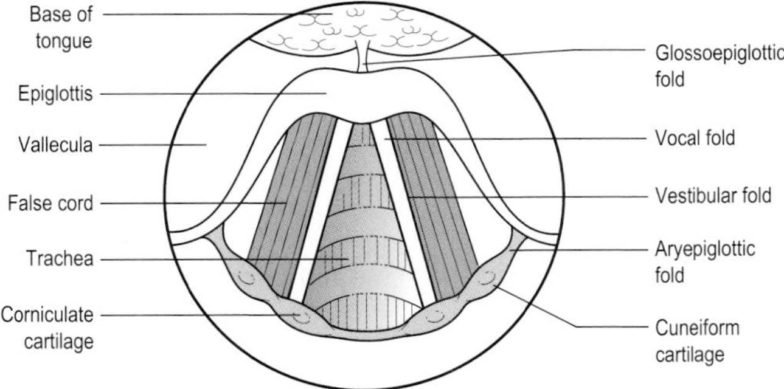

Fig. 5.26 View of the larynx as seen by laryngoscope.

Nasopharynx

- Lies above the soft palate, which cuts it off from the remainder of the pharynx during deglutition, therefore preventing regurgitation of food into the nose.
- The nasopharynx contains:
  - the nasopharyngeal tonsil (adenoids)
  - the orifice of the Eustachian tube (auditory tube), which connects the pharynx to the middle ear.

Examination of the nasopharynx can be performed by placing a small, angled mirror in the oropharynx. The following structures can be visualized:

- opening of the Eustachian tube
- tubal elevation
- pharyngeal recess
- adenoids
- posterior choanae
- posterior end of the inferior concha.

Oropharynx

The most important structure in the oropharynx is the palatine tonsil (tonsil).

- Lies in the tonsillar fossa bounded by the anterior and posterior pillars of the fauces.
- Anterior pillar is the palatoglossal arch produced by palatoglossus muscle.
- Posterior pillar is the palatopharyngeal arch formed by the palatopharyngeus muscle.
- Floor is the superior constrictor.
- Pharyngobasilar fascia, lining the inner surface of the constrictor, forms the capsule of the tonsil, and lies between the tonsil and the muscle.
- Capsule is normally separated from muscle by loose areolar tissue.
- Tonsil is accumulation of lymphoid tissue.
- Oral surfaces are lined by mucous membrane, having stratified squamous epithelium.
- Tonsillar crypts are clefts on inner surface.

Blood Supply

- Tonsillar branch of facial artery, which pierces superior constrictor to enter lower pole of tonsil.
- Additional branches from lingual, ascending palatine and ascending pharyngeal arteries.
- Venous drainage passes to the pharyngeal plexus of veins.
- A paratonsillar vein extends from the soft palate to lie on the lateral surface of the tonsil before piercing the superior constrictor. It may be a troublesome cause of bleeding during tonsillectomy.

Lymphatic Drainage

- To the jugular digastric lymph node situated behind the angle of the mandible.
- This node is often palpable in chronic tonsillitis.

Clinical Points

- Tonsillectomy involves removal of the tonsil and the fascial capsule separating it from the loose areolar tissue clothing the superior constrictor.
- The tonsil is dissected clear until it remains attached only by a pedicle of vessels near its lower pole, which is divided.
- A quinsy is suppuration in the peritonsillar tissue.

Laryngopharynx (Hypopharynx)

- Extends from the level of the tip of the epiglottis to the termination of the pharynx into the oesophagus at level of the sixth cervical vertebra.
- Inlet of the larynx, which is vertical, is bounded by the epiglottis, aryepiglottic fold and the arytenoids.
- Anterolateral to the inlet is a recess known as the piriform fossa.
- The piriform fossa is a common site for lodging of foreign bodies.
- The piriform fossa has a rich lymphatic drainage and is a 'silent' area for tumours, which spread rapidly into the deep cervical nodes.

Structure of the Pharynx

The pharyngeal wall consists of:

- mucosa
- submucosa
- pharyngobasilar fascia
- muscle
- buccopharyngeal fascia (areolar tissue).

Mucosa

- Pseudostratified columnar ciliated epithelium in the nasopharynx.
- Stratified squamous epithelium in the rest of the pharynx.

Muscles of the Pharynx

The main muscles of the pharynx are three fan-shaped constrictor muscles:

- superior constrictor
- middle constrictor
- inferior constrictor.

These are reinforced by smaller longitudinal muscles:

- stylopharyngeus
- salpingopharyngeus
- palatopharyngeus.

The Constrictor Muscles

Each constrictor muscle starts from a limited origin anteriorly, and broadens out laterally and posteriorly to be inserted into a posterior midline raphe.

- Each constrictor overlaps the one above posteriorly.

- There are gaps laterally:
  - between upper border of superior constrictor and base of skull, which is bridged by pharyngobasilar fascia. The Eustachian tube enters the pharynx through this gap
  - between the middle and superior constrictor, where the stylopharyngeus muscle accompanied by the glossopharyngeal nerve enters the pharynx
  - between the inferior and middle constrictor, which is occupied by the thyrohyoid ligament and associated structures.
- The inferior constrictor has two parts:
  - thyropharyngeus: fan-shaped and attached to the lamina of the thyroid cartilage
  - cricopharyngeus: circular and acts like a sphincter.
- The weakest area of the pharyngeal wall is the gap between thyropharyngeus and cricopharyngeus in the midline posteriorly. This is Killian's dehiscence, a common site for pharyngeal pouches.

Innervation of the Pharynx

- Motor innervation: all the muscles of the pharynx except stylopharyngeus are supplied by pharyngeal branches of the vagus nerve. Stylopharyngeus is supplied by the glossopharyngeal nerve.
- Sensory innervation:
  - nasopharynx: maxillary division of trigeminal nerve
  - oropharynx: glossopharyngeal nerve
  - laryngopharynx: internal laryngeal branch of the vagus.

Posterior Triangle

The boundaries are:

- anterior: posterior border of sternocleidomastoid
- posterior: anterior border of trapezius
- apex: meeting points of the upper attachment of trapezius and sternocleidomastoid
- base: middle third of clavicle
- roof: investing layer of deep cervical fascia extending between trapezius and sternocleidomastoid
- floor: from above downwards, splenius capitis, levator scapulae, scalenus medius, scalenus anterior; all covered by prevertebral fascia
- the skin over the anterior triangle has platysma only in its anterior part.

Contents

- Subclavian artery (third part).
- Transverse cervical artery.
- Suprascapular artery.
- Occipital artery.
- External jugular vein courses in the superficial fascia obliquely, pierces the deep fascia just above the clavicle and drains into the subclavian vein.
- The most important structure in the posterior triangle is the spinal accessory nerve:
  - exits from jugular foramen
  - passes deep to sternocleidomastoid and enters posterior triangle
  - lies superficially embedded in deep cervical fascia of roof
  - enters under surface of trapezius
  - supplies sternocleidomastoid and trapezius.

Surface Marking of Accessory Nerve

- Draws a line connecting the junction between the upper third and lower two-thirds of the posterior border of sternocleidomastoid to a point joining the lower third and upper two-thirds of trapezius.
- It lies on the levator scapulae.

Clinical Points

- The accessory nerve may be damaged during biopsy of a lymph node in the posterior triangle of the neck or as a result of a penetrating injury.
- This will result in paralysis of trapezius, causing inability to shrug the shoulder on the affected side.

CERVICAL PLEXUS (Fig. 5.27)

The first four anterior primary rami contribute to the cervical plexus. The ascending branch of the first cervical nerve joins the hypoglossal nerve and this arrangement gives rise to two sets of branches:

- superficial, supplying the skin over the head and neck
- deep, supplying muscles.

Superficial Branches

The superficial branches of the cervical plexus are:

- lesser occipital nerve
- greater auricular nerve
- transverse cervical nerve
- supraclavicular nerve.

Deep Branches

The deep branches of the cervical plexus supply muscles derived from the flexor compartment of the neck:

- prevertebral muscles
- infrahyoid muscles
- diaphragm.

Infrahyoid Muscles

- Supplied by the ansa cervicalis.

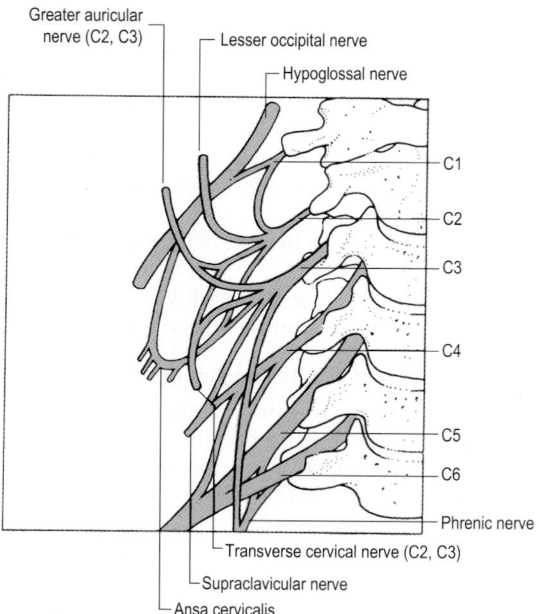

Fig. 5.27 The cervical plexus.

- Ansa cervicalis is a loop formed anterior to the carotid sheath by a branch of C1 after it has joined the hypoglossal nerve, and a branch from the union of C2 and C3.

The Phrenic Nerve

- The most important branch of the cervical plexus.
- Each nerve supplies:
  - all of the muscles in its own half of the diaphragm
  - sensory fibres to the mediastinal and diaphragmatic pleura
  - sensory fibres to the parietal pericardium
  - sensory fibres to the diaphragmatic peritoneum (sensation at the periphery of the diaphragm is supplied by the intercostal nerves).

Course of the Phrenic Nerve

- Formed at the lateral border of scalenus anterior, passing inferiorly on its anterior surface lateral to the internal jugular vein.
- Leaves the neck by passing between subclavian artery posteriorly and subclavian vein anteriorly, traversing the thoracic inlet in contact with the mediastinal pleura.
- As it descends through the thorax it lies anteriorly to the root of the lung in contact with the mediastinal pleura.
- Right phrenic nerve:
  - anterior to right vagus nerve
  - on lateral surface of superior vena cava and superior mediastinum
  - runs vertically down the right surface of the pericardium to pierce the diaphragm in company with the inferior vena cava.
- Left phrenic nerve:
  - in the superior mediastinum it lies between the left subclavian artery posteriorly and the left common carotid artery anteriorly
  - crosses left side of arch of aorta to pass anteriorly to root of lung
  - travels down on the left surface of the pericardium to pierce the diaphragm.

ROOT OF NECK (Fig. 5.28)

Knowledge of the anatomy of the root of the neck is essential to perform procedures such as subclavian vein catheterization or brachial plexus block, and to understand the effect of a Pancoast tumour. The root of the neck is the junctional area between the thorax and neck, and contains all the structures going from thorax to neck and vice versa. Important structures of the root of the neck are:

- suprapleural membrane (Sibson's fascia)
- subclavian artery
- subclavian vein
- brachial plexus
- thoracic duct
- stellate ganglion.

Suprapleural Membrane (Sibson's Fascia)

- Attached to the inner border of the first rib and to the transverse process of the sixth cervical vertebra.
- Prevents the lung and pleura rising further into the neck during inspiration.
- Subclavian artery, subclavian vein and brachial plexus lie on suprapleural membrane.

Subclavian Artery

- Arches laterally over cervical pleura and Sibson's fascia and apex of lung to reach surface of first rib.
- Lies posterior to insertion of scalenus anterior on first rib.
- Root and trunks of brachial plexus lie behind subclavian artery on the first rib between scalenus anterior and scalenus medius.
- Continues beyond the first rib into the axilla as axillary artery.
- Pulse of subclavian artery can be felt at the medial third of the clavicle near the lateral border of sternocleidomastoid on deep palpation against first rib.

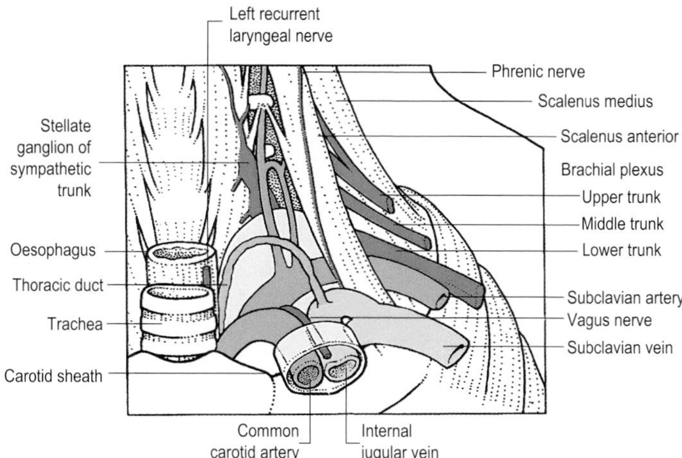

Fig. 5.28 The structures of the thoracic inlet. The carotid sheath and contents are cut and reflected to show the deep structures in the neck.

- The branches of the subclavian artery are as follows:
  - vertebral artery
  - internal mammary (thoracic) artery
  - thyrocervical trunk
  - costocervical trunk.

Subclavian Vein

- Follows course of subclavian artery in neck but lies in front of scalenus anterior on the first rib.
- Veins accompanying branches of subclavian artery drain into the external jugular, the subclavian or its continuation, the brachiocephalic vein.

Brachial Plexus

This is described in the section on the upper limb (see Chapter 3).

Thoracic Duct

The thoracic duct carries lymph from the whole body, except from the right side of the thorax, right upper limb, and right side of head and neck, which drains into the right lymph duct. The course of the thoracic duct is as follows:

- Commences at the cisterna chyli between the abdominal aorta and right crus of the diaphragm.
- Passes upwards through aortic opening to become thoracic duct.
- Ascends behind the oesophagus, inclining to the left at the level of T5.
- At root of neck it arches laterally, lying between carotid sheath and vertebral artery, and enters the junction between the internal jugular and subclavian veins.

Clinical Point

- Inadvertent puncture or laceration of the thoracic duct will cause escape of lymph into the surrounding tissues and occasionally into the chest (chylothorax).

Stellate Ganglion

- First thoracic ganglion frequently fuses with the inferior cervical ganglion to form the stellate ganglion.
- The stellate ganglion lies at the root of the neck against the neck of the first rib.

Clinical Points

- Damage to the stellate ganglion or invasion of it in a Pancoast tumour will result in Horner's syndrome:
  - constriction of the pupil
  - slight ptosis
  - anhidrosis on the side of the lesion.

LYMPH NODES OF THE HEAD AND NECK

These are divided into superficial and deep groups.

Superficial Nodes

- Anterior cervical nodes along the anterior jugular vein.
- Superficial cervical nodes along the external jugular vein.
- These nodes drain from the superficial tissues of the regions drained by the veins along which they lie. Efferents drain to the deep cervical nodes.

Deep Lymph Nodes

These are arranged in a vertical chain along the internal jugular vein, and a circular chain.

Vertical Chain

- Constitutes the terminal group for all lymph nodes in the head and neck.
- Lies within the fascia of the carotid sheath closely related to the internal jugular vein.
- Divided into:
  - superior deep cervical nodes
  - inferior deep cervical nodes.
- Superior group lies in region where posterior belly of digastric crosses internal jugular vein, and here they are also known as the jugulodigastric nodes. They drain:
  - tonsils
  - tongue (posterior third).
- The lower group lies where the omohyoid crosses the internal jugular vein, and hence is sometimes referred to as the jugulo-omohyoid group. These nodes drain:
  - tongue (anterior two-thirds)
  - oral cavity
  - trachea
  - oesophagus
  - thyroid gland.
- A few nodes in the deep cervical group extend into the posterior triangle of the neck. They may be palpated in the supraclavicular region.
- An example is Virchow's node associated with intra-abdominal malignancy (Troisier's sign).

Circular Chain

The circular chain of lymph nodes consists of the following.

- Submental nodes, which drain:
  - tip of tongue
  - floor of mouth
  - central part of lower lip.
- Submandibular nodes, which drain:
  - side of nose
  - upper lip
  - lateral part of lower lip
  - cheeks
  - gums
  - anterior two-thirds of margin of the tongue.
- Parotid nodes, which drain:
  - eyelids
  - front of scalp
  - external and middle ear
  - pinna of ear
  - parotid gland.
- Posterior auricular nodes, which drain:
  - back of scalp
  - back of auricle
  - external auditory meatus.
- Occipital nodes, which drain:
  - back of scalp.

In addition, there are other groups.

- Retropharyngeal nodes, which lie between pharynx and prevertebral fascia and drain:
  - back of nasal cavity, nasopharynx and Eustachian tube.
- Pretracheal and prelaryngeal nodes, which drain:
  - adjacent viscera.

Clinical Points

In block dissection of the neck all the lymph nodes in the anterior and posterior triangles of the neck, along with the associated structures, are removed *en bloc*.

- Block dissection of the neck extends from the mandible above to the clavicle below and the midline anteriorly to the anterior border of trapezius posteriorly.
- All structures from platysma to pretracheal fascia are removed, leaving only the carotid arteries, the vagus nerve, the sympathetic trunks, and the lingual and hypoglossal nerves.
- Sternocleidomastoid, posterior belly of digastric and omohyoid are all removed, along with the internal jugular and external jugular veins, submandibular gland and lower part of the parotid gland.
- The accessory nerve, to which lymph nodes are related in the posterior triangle, is also sacrificed.

SPINE

Vertebral Column

The vertebral column is made up of 32–34 vertebrae:

- seven cervical vertebrae
- twelve thoracic vertebrae
- five lumbar vertebrae
- sacrum (five fused vertebrae)
- coccyx (three to five fused vertebrae).

Basic vertebral pattern (Fig. 5.29)

The basic vertebral pattern consists of a body and a neural arch surrounding a vertebral canal.

Neural Arch

- Composed of a pedicle on either side, supporting a lamina which meets its opposite posteriorly in the midline.
- Pedicle bears a notch above and below, with which its neighbour forms the intervertebral foramen.
- Each arch bears:
  - posterior spine
  - lateral transverse processes
  - upper and lower articular facets.
- The intravertebral foramina transmit the segmental spinal nerves as follows:

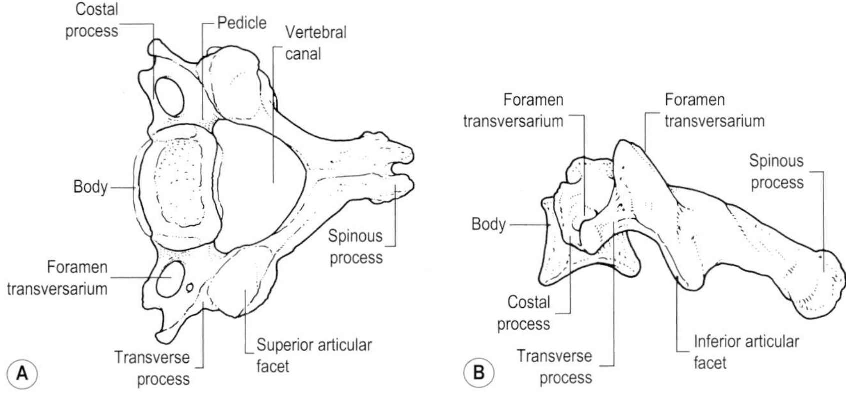

Fig. 5.29 A typical cervical vertebra, C5. (A) Superior view. (B) Lateral view.

- C1–7 pass over the superior aspects of their corresponding cervical vertebrae
- C8 passes through the foramen between C7 and T1
- all subsequent nerves pass between the vertebra of their own number and the one below.

- Pedicles and lamina serve to protect neural and vascular tissue.

Body

- Bears the major part of the weight transmitted by the vertebra.
- Adapted to resist compressive forces, being composed of interlocking plates of cancellous bone, the trabeculae being arranged mainly at right angles to one another.
- Contain red marrow; erythropoiesis continues throughout life in the axial skeleton.
- Articulate with one another via strong intervertebral discs.

Vertebrae from individual regions have distinguishing features.

Cervical Vertebrae (Fig. 5.30)

- Contain foramen transversarium perforating the transverse processes.
- Foramen transversarium transmits vertebral artery, vertebral vein and sympathetic fibres (artery does not pass through the foramen of the seventh cervical vertebra).
- Spines small and bifid, except C1 and C7, which are single.
- Articular facets horizontal.
- The atlas (C1):
  - has no body
  - bears a kidney-shaped superior articular facet on a thick, lateral mass, which articulates with the occipital condyles of the skull
  - posterior to this facet the upper part of the posterior arch is grooved by the vertebral artery.
- The axis (C2):
  - bears the dens (odontoid process) on the superior aspect of its body (represents the detached centrum of C1)
  - nodding (agreement) and lateral flexion occur at the atlanto-occipital joint
  - rotation of the skull (disagreement) occurs at the atlantoaxial joint.
- Vertebra prominens (C7)—so called because it is the first clearly palpable spine of the vertebral column (T1 below it is in fact the most prominent one).
- Occasionally foramen transversarium is absent on C7 (does not transmit the vertebral artery).

Thoracic Vertebrae (Fig. 5.31)

- Characterized by demifacets on sides of body for articulation with heads of ribs.
- Characterized by facets on their transverse processes for the rib tubercles (apart from lower two thoracic vertebrae).
- Characterized by long and downward-sloping spines.
- Articular facets relatively vertical.

Lumbar Vertebrae (Fig. 5.32)

- Large with strong, square, horizontal spines.
- Articular facets lie in the sagittal plain.
- L5 has a massive transverse process, which connects with the whole of the lateral aspect of its pedicle and encroaches on the body.

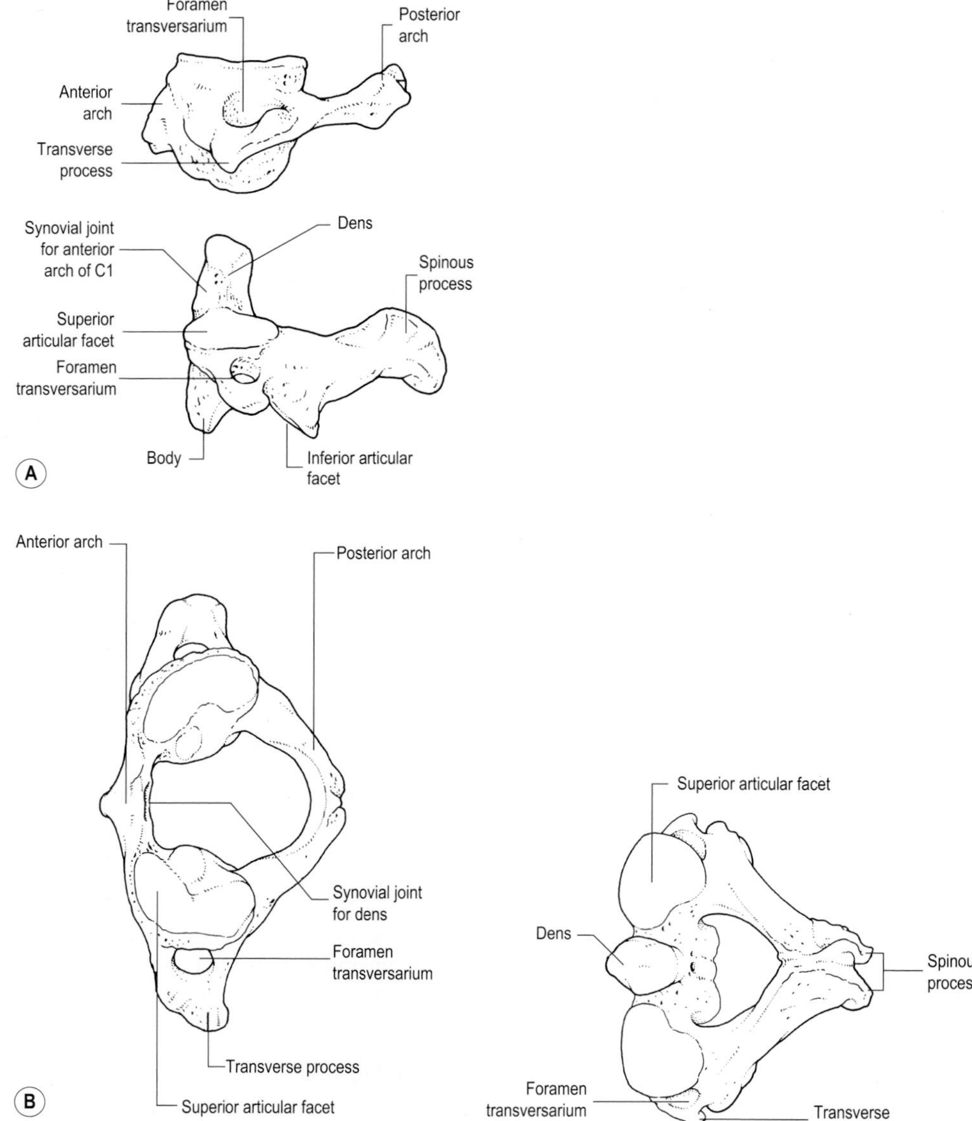

Fig. 5.30 The atlas and the axis, C1 and C2. (A) Lateral views. (B) Superior views.

- Transverse processes of the lumbar vertebrae attach solely to the junction of pedicle with lamina.

Sacrum and Coccyx

Described with pelvic girdle (see Chapter 4).

Intervertebral Joints (Fig. 5.33)

- Vertebral laminae linked by the ligamentum flavum of elastic tissue.
- Vertebral spines linked by the tough supraspinous and weak interspinous ligaments.
- Articular facets linked by articular ligaments around synovial joints.
- Tough anterior and posterior longitudinal ligaments run the whole length of the vertebral bodies along anterior and posterior aspects, respectively.
- Vertebral bodies joined by strong, intervertebral discs.

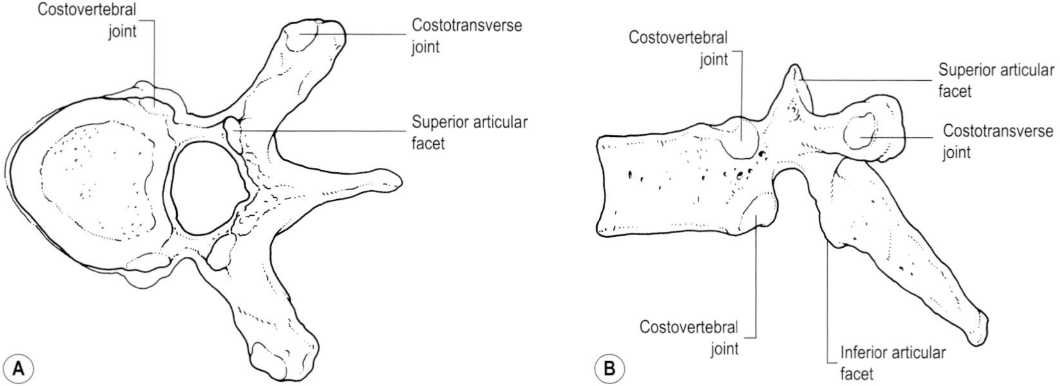

Fig. 5.31 A typical thoracic vertebra, T7. (A) Superior view. (B) Lateral view.

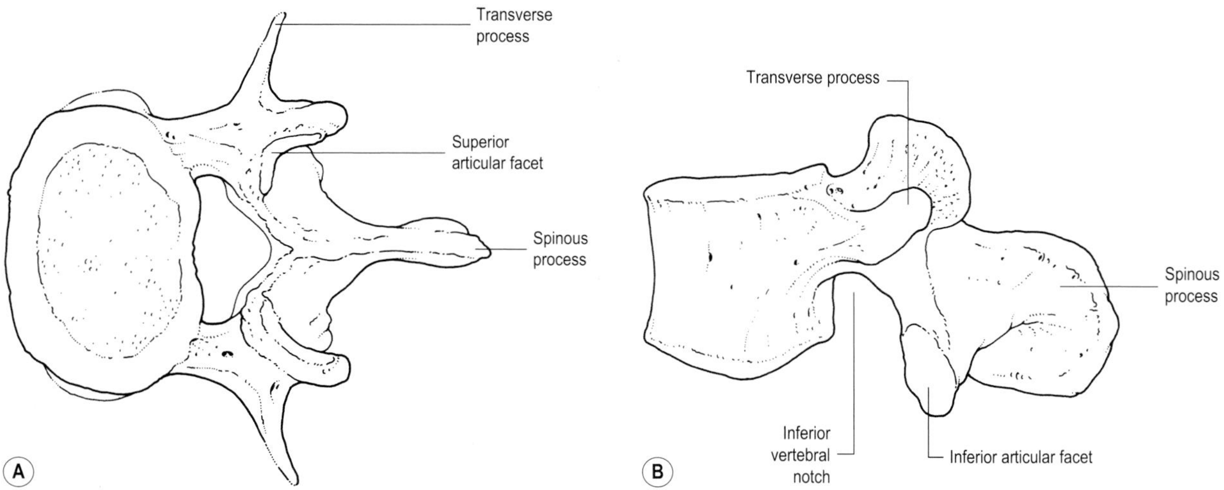

Fig. 5.32 A typical lumbar vertebra, L4. (A) Superior view. (B) Lateral view.

- Each intervertebral disc consists of:
  - peripheral annulus fibrosus, which is adherent to the thin, cartilaginous plate on the vertebral body above and below
  - nucleus pulposus, which is gelatinous fluid surrounded by the annulus fibrosus.
- Intervertebral discs constitute approximately one-quarter of the length of the spine, as well as accounting for its secondary curvatures.
- In old age the intervertebral discs atrophy, resulting in shrinkage and return of the curvature of the spine to the C-shape of the newborn.
- Movement of the spine occurs particularly at the cervicodorsal and dorsolumbar junctions, which are the two commonest sites of vertebral injury.
- The joints between atlas, axis and the skull are shown in Fig. 5.34.

Clinical Points

- The posterior part of the annulus fibrosus is relatively thin and prone to rupture owing to degeneration or injury; the nucleus pulposus protrudes posteriorly into the vertebral canal or intervertebral foramen, i.e. 'slipped disc'.
- Most posterior disc lesions pass lateral to the posterior longitudinal ligament (paracentral disc), causing compression of the transiting nerve root (Fig. 5.35). Far lateral discs may compress the exiting nerve root.
- Commonest site for 'slipped disc' is L4/5, L5/S1, or in the neck C5/6 or C6/7.

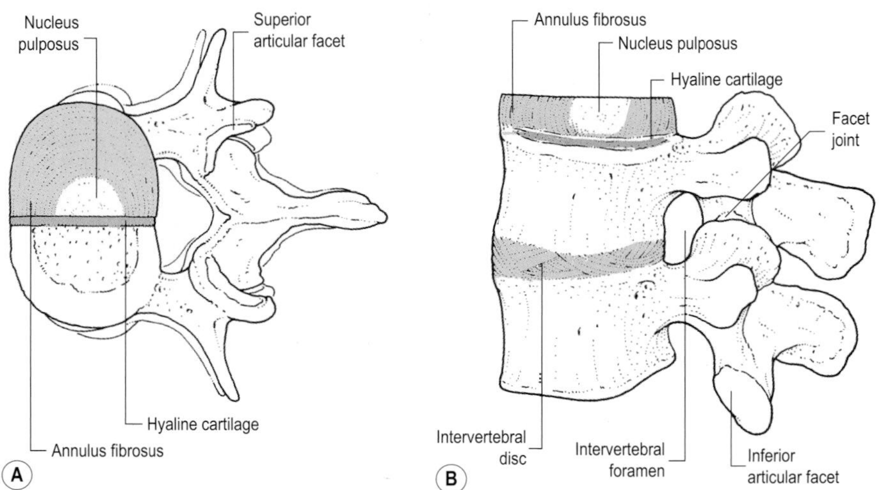

Fig. 5.33 The joints between adjacent vertebrae L3 and L4. The left half of the L2/3 disc has been cut away to show the plate of hyaline cartilage at the upper surface of L3. This has also been cut away to the left of the midline, exposing the upper surface of L3. (A) Superior view. (B) Lateral view.

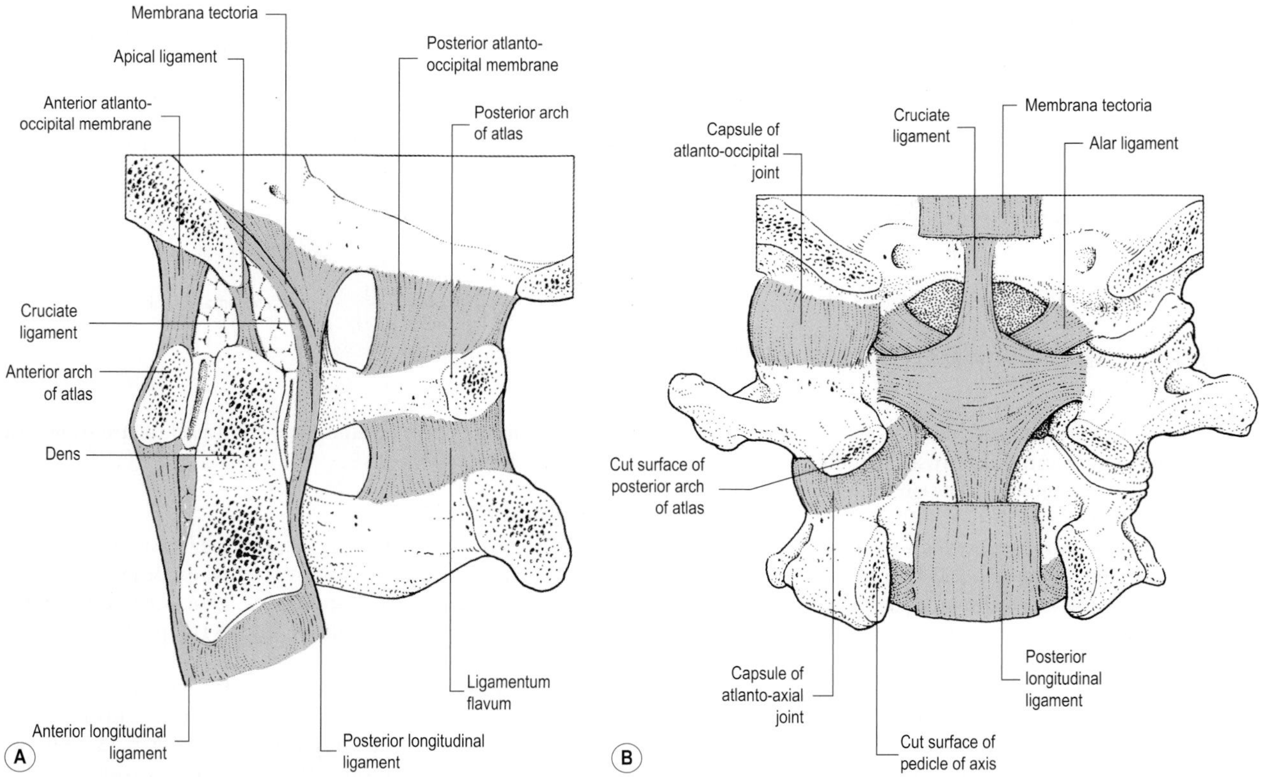

Fig. 5.34 The ligaments joining the axis, atlas and skull. (A) Midline sagittal section. (B) Posterior surface. The posterior arch of the atlas and the vertebral arch of the axis have been removed.

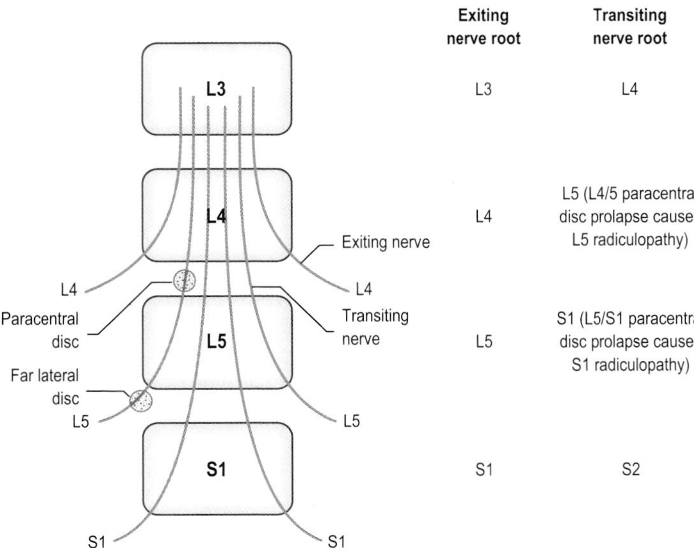

Fig. 5.35 Prolapsed intervertebral disc. Radiculopathy in relation to exiting and transiting nerve roots. Paracentral disc lesions compress the transiting nerve. Far lateral disc lesions compress the exiting nerve.

- Prolapsed L4/5 disc produces pressure on the root of L5 nerve and that of L5/S1 on S1 nerve. Pain is referred to the back of the leg and foot along the distribution of the sciatic nerves (sciatica).
- With L5 lesion there will be weakness of ankle dorsiflexion and big toe extension. There will be numbness over the lower and lateral part of the leg and medial side of the foot.
- With S1 lesion ankle jerk may be diminished or absent, there will be weakness of the evertors of the foot and there will be numbness over the lateral side of the foot.
- Direct posterior prolapse of the disc (central disc prolapse) may compress the cauda equina, giving rise to cauda equina syndrome.
- Cauda equina syndrome causes compression of the sacral outflow, saddle paraesthesia, reduced anal sphincter tone, reduced bladder coordination, painless retention and overflow, loss of anal reflex and bilateral leg symptoms. It is a surgical emergency.

OSCE SCENARIOS

OSCE Scenario 5.1

A 55-year-old female undergoes a right superficial parotidectomy for a pleomorphic adenoma of the parotid gland.

1. What is the order of structures traversing the gland from without in?
2. Name the divisions of the facial nerve within the gland.
3. How would you test the integrity of the individual branches of the facial nerve in the postoperative period to exclude intraoperative damage?
4. What is Frey's syndrome? Explain its anatomical basis.

OSCE Scenario 5.2

A 50-year-old male presents to a general surgery clinic with a lump in the right side of his neck.

1. What are the boundaries of the anterior and posterior triangles of the neck? Examination reveals that the lump is in the right posterior triangle.
2. What are the possible differential diagnoses? On further examination you suspect lymphoma and discuss the case with a haematologist. The haematologist requests an excision biopsy. The lump lies centrally in the posterior triangle.
3. What structure do you need to avoid at surgery and what is the effect of injury to this structure?

OSCE Scenario 5.3

A 40-year-old female is to undergo a subtotal thyroidectomy for a multinodular goitre.

1. Describe the gross anatomy of the thyroid gland.

2. When exposing the gland at surgery, which structures are encountered?
3. Describe the arterial blood supply of the thyroid gland.
4. Where are the nerves situated in relation to the gland and when are they in danger of damage?

OSCE Scenario 5.4

A 35-year-old female is referred to the ENT clinic after recurrent episodes of nasal congestion, nasal discharge, fever, headache, tiredness, and facial pain in the right cheek. COVID-19 swabs were negative on several occasions and the GP is seeking advice for management of possible chronic sinusitis and is concerned that the symptoms are unilateral.

1. What are the paranasal sinuses and where are they located?
2. Where do they drain into?
3. How would you go about draining the maxillary sinus surgically?
4. How can carcinoma of the maxillary sinus present?

OSCE Scenario 5.5

A 29-year-old male presented to Accident and Emergency with mandibular pain and inability to occlude the teeth following a bout of excessive laughter while watching a comic movie in the cinema. Examination of the temporomandibular joint (TMJ) revealed prominent mandibular head anteriorly.

1. What is the likely diagnosis and what other events can cause it?
2. What would you find on examination?
3. What type of joint is TMJ?
4. How would you treat the patient?

Answers in Appendix pages 440–442

Please check your eBook at https://studentconsult.inkling.com/ for more self-assessment questions. See inside cover for registration details.

6

The Nervous System

THE BRAIN

The brain is divided into the:
- forebrain
- midbrain
- hindbrain.

These are further subdivided as shown in Box 6.1.

Cerebral Hemispheres (Figs. 6.1 and 6.2)

- Frontal lobe lies in anterior cranial fossa with the frontal pole at its anterior extremity.
- Temporal lobe lies in middle cranial fossa with the temporal pole at its anterior extremity and an upturned projection on its medial surface, the uncus.
- Parietal lobe lies above temporal lobe between frontal and occipital lobes.
- Occipital lobe lies above tentorium cerebelli with the occipital pole at its posterior extremity.

BOX 6.1 Major Subdivisions and Parts of the Brain

Major subdivisions	Parts	
Forebrain	Cerebral hemisphere or telencephalon (lateral ventricle); Diencephalon containing thalamus and hypothalamus (third ventricle)	
Midbrain	Mesencephalon (cerebral aqueduct)	Brainstem
Hindbrain	Pons, medulla and cerebellum (fourth ventricle)	Brainstem

The parts of the ventricular system are shown in brackets

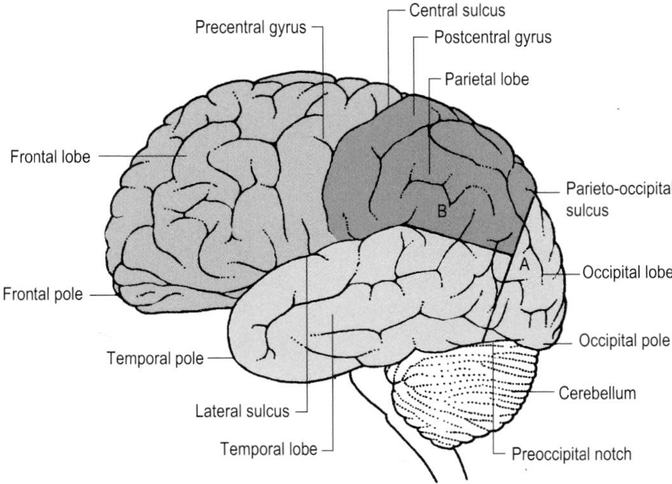

Fig. 6.1 The brain, lateral view. *Line A* indicates the posterior border of the temporal lobe and *Line B* indicates the superior border of the temporal lobe (along with the lateral sulcus).

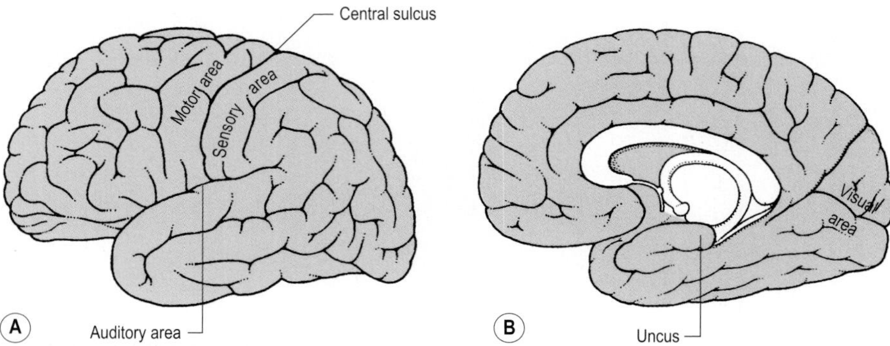

Fig. 6.2 The major areas of the cortex. (A) Lateral view. (B) Medial view.

The cerebral hemisphere:

- has a layer of grey matter on its external surface, the cerebral cortex
- has white matter internal to this, in which are the nuclei of the basal ganglia
- has a cavity in each hemisphere, i.e. the lateral ventricles.

Cerebral Cortex (Figs. 6.1 and 6.2)

- Composed of a large number of sulci (clefts) and gyri (folds).
- The large lateral sulcus on the superolateral surface separates the temporal lobe from the parietal and frontal lobes.
- The central sulcus separates the precentral gyrus (motor area) from the postcentral gyrus (sensory area).
- The parieto-occipital sulcus on the medial surface of the hemisphere separates the occipital from the parietal lobe.
- The calcarine and postcalcarine sulci lie on the medial aspect of the occipital lobe and are concerned with visual centres.
- The corpus callosum lies between the two hemispheres and links them.

Frontal Lobe

Important areas of the frontal lobe are:

- motor cortex situated in the precentral gyrus, from which fibres pass through the internal capsule to motor nuclei of the cranial and spinal nerves. Receives afferents from the thalamus and cerebellum and is concerned with voluntary movement
- Broca's area, in the posterior part of the inferior frontal gyrus of the dominant hemisphere, which controls the motor elements of speech
- frontal cortex, which comprises a considerable part of the frontal lobe. The lateral part of the frontal lobe is related to 'intellect'; the medial and orbital surfaces to affective behaviour.

Parietal Lobe

Important areas of the parietal lobe are:

- sensory cortex in the postcentral gyrus, which receives afferents from the thalamus and is concerned with all forms of somatic sensation
- parietal association cortex, the remainder of the lobe, which is concerned with recognition of somatic sensory stimuli and their integration with other forms of sensory information. It receives afferents from the thalamus.

Temporal Lobe

Important areas of the temporal lobe are:

- the auditory cortex lying on the superior temporal gyrus, which receives afferents from the medial geniculate body and is concerned with auditory stimuli
- the temporal association cortex, which surrounds the auditory cortex and is responsible for the perception of auditory stimuli and their integration with other sensory modalities
- the uncus on the medial surface of the temporal lobe, which is concerned with olfactory stimuli.

Occipital Lobe

Important areas of the occipital lobe are:

- the visual cortex, surrounding the calcarine and postcalcarine sulci, which is concerned with vision of the opposite half-field of sight
- the occipital association cortex, lying anterior to the visual cortex, which is concerned with recognition and integration of visual stimuli.

Clinical Points

- Frontal cortex: damage results in impairment of emotions and intellect.
- Motor cortex: damage results in weakness of the opposite side of the body. Lesions low down on the cortex affect the face; higher up they affect the arm; and higher

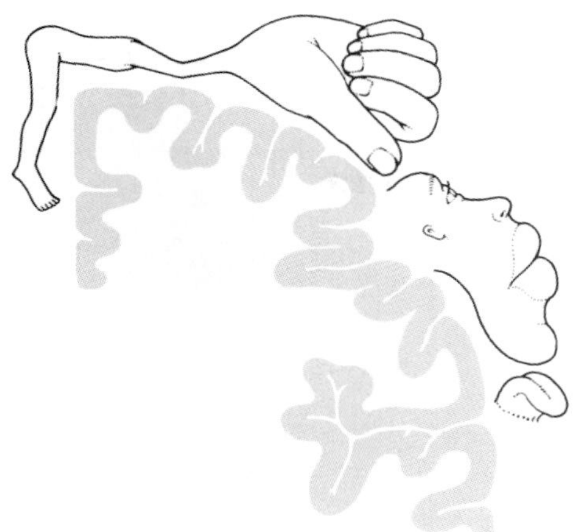

Fig. 6.3 The motor homunculus, showing proportional somatotopic representation in the precentral gyrus.

lesions affect the leg. Both precentral and postcentral gyri have somatotopic representation (Fig. 6.3).

- Sensory cortex: damage results in contralateral hemianaesthesia (same pattern as motor cortex distribution) affecting sensory modalities such as stereognosis and two-point position sense. Astereognosis is inability to recognize sensory stimuli: put an object in a patient's hand; they are aware of the object but cannot identify it.
- Temporal association cortex: damage results in auditory agnosia, i.e. inability to recognize or understand the significance of meaningful sounds.
- Occipital cortex: damage results in contralateral homonymous hemianopia.
- Lesions affecting the lower region of the sensory cortex and the auditory association cortex will cause dysphasia.

Basal Ganglia

- Consists of corpus striatum (caudate nucleus, putamen, globus pallidus), claustrum, amygdaloid nucleus and thalamus.

Midbrain

- Connects pons and cerebellum to diencephalon (thalamus and hypothalamus).
- Contains cerebral peduncles (corticobulbar and corticospinal tract), red nucleus, substantia nigra, nuclei of cranial nerves III and IV, and portion of sensory nucleus of cranial nerve V.
- Ascending fibres travel in medial and lateral lemniscus.
- Descending motor fibres pass through to reach pons and spinal cord.

Pons

- Lies between medulla and midbrain.
- Connected to cerebellum by middle cerebellar peduncle.
- Dorsal surface of lower pons forms floor of fourth ventricle.
- Contains nuclei of cranial nerves VI, VII and VIII.
- Sensory nucleus of cranial nerve V extends from midbrain through pons and medulla to upper cervical cord.
- Motor nucleus of cranial nerve V lies in pons.
- Corticospinal tracts cross in lower pons.

Medulla

- Continuous above with pons and below through the foramen magnum with the spinal cord.
- Connected to cerebellum by inferior cerebellar peduncle.
- Contains nucleus ambiguus (motor to cranial nerves IX and X).
- Contains nucleus of tractus solitarius (sensory for cranial nerves VIII, IX and X).
- Contains cranial nerve nuclei IX, X, XI and XII.
- Dorsal column nuclei cross to form the medial lemniscus.
- Sensory decussation contains some uncrossed fibres.

Cerebellum

- Largest part of hindbrain.
- Made up of two lateral cerebellar hemispheres separated by the vermis.
- Connected to brainstem by three pairs of cerebellar peduncles.
- The bulge of the lateral lobe that projects inferiorly posterolateral to the medulla is the tonsil.
- The structural organization of the cerebellum is uniform and similar to that of the cerebral hemisphere, i.e. a thin layer of cortex outside and deeper white matter containing the various cerebellar nuclei.
- Blood supply is derived from three pairs of arteries:
  - posterior inferior cerebellar branches of vertebral arteries
  - anterior inferior cerebellar branches of the basilar artery
  - superior cerebellar branches of basilar artery.

Clinical Points

- Cerebellum is concerned with balance, regulation of posture, muscle tone and muscle coordination. Cerebellar lesions give rise to symptoms and signs on the same side of the body. Cerebellar lesions may cause unsteady gait, tremor, nystagmus, dysarthria.
- In cases where there is raised intracranial pressure the cerebellar tonsil can herniate into the foramen magnum and compress the medulla oblongata, e.g. following lumbar puncture.

SPINAL CORD

- Extends from foramen magnum (continuous with medulla oblongata to lower border of first or upper border of the second lumbar vertebra.
- Approximately 45 cm long.
- Tapers inferiorly into the conus medullaris from which a prolongation of pia mater, the filum terminale, extends downwards to be attached to the coccyx (Fig. 6.4).
- Dura mater fuses with filum terminale at S2 and obliterates the subarachnoid space at this level.
- Spinal cord fills the whole of vertebral canal during the first 3 months of intrauterine life.
- Vertebral column grows more rapidly than cord, such that at birth the cord extends as far as the third lumbar vertebra; it then gradually reaches its adult level (between first and second lumbar vertebrae).
- A total of 31 pair of nerves originate from the cord:
  - eight cervical
  - twelve thoracic
  - five lumbar
  - five sacral
  - one coccygeal.
- The lumbar and sacral nerve roots below the termination of the cord form the cauda equina.

Figs 6.5 and 6.6 show the relationships of the spinal cord to the meninges and vertebral column.

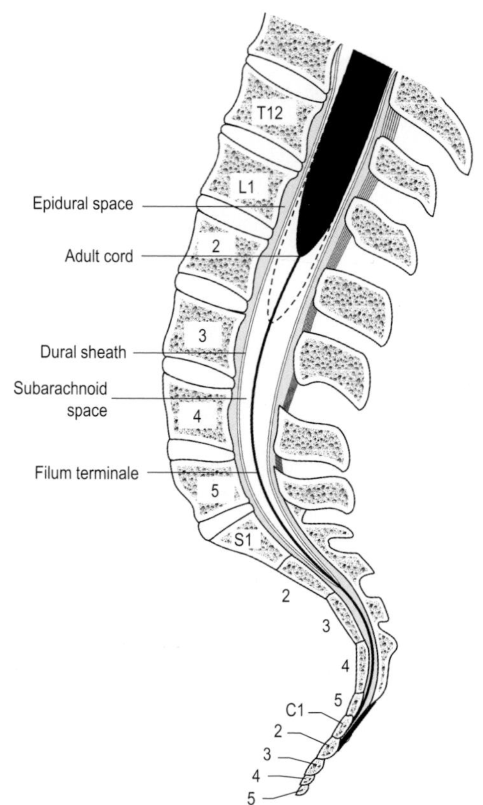

Fig. 6.4 The termination of the spinal cord in the adult showing its variations (solid black to dashed line). The figure also shows the termination of the dural sheath.

Clinical Points

- Lumbar puncture should be carried out at L3/4, L4/5 or L5/S1 interspace. The L4/5 or L5/S1 interspace should be used in children as the spinal cord ends at L3.
- As a landmark a line joining the iliac crests passes through the fourth lumbar vertebra.
- The spine should be fully flexed to increase the space between the spinous processes.
- The lumbar puncture needle passes through the following structures:
  - skin
  - supraspinous ligament
  - interspinous ligament
  - ligamentum flavum—there is a sudden 'give' as it is penetrated
  - dura mater—there is another 'give' as the needle penetrates the dura mater and enters the subarachnoid space.

Internal Structure of Spinal Cord (Fig. 6.7)

- Divided into grey and white matter.
- In transverse section the central canal is seen surrounded by the H-shaped grey matter.
- This is surrounded in turn by white matter containing the long ascending and descending tracts.
- Dorsal horn of grey matter (posterior horn) is capped by the substantia gelatinosa and contains the sensory fibres entering via the posterior nerve roots.
- Ventral horn of grey matter (anterior horn) contains motor cells giving rise to fibres of ventral roots.
- Lateral horns are found in the thoracic and upper lumbar cord; they contain the cells of origin of preganglionic sympathetic system.
- White matter is divided into dorsal, lateral and ventral columns, each containing a number of ascending and descending tracts.

The Tracts of the Spinal Cord (Fig. 6.8)

Descending Tracts

- Lateral corticospinal tract (crossed pyramidal):
  - commences in motor cortex
  - decussates in the medulla

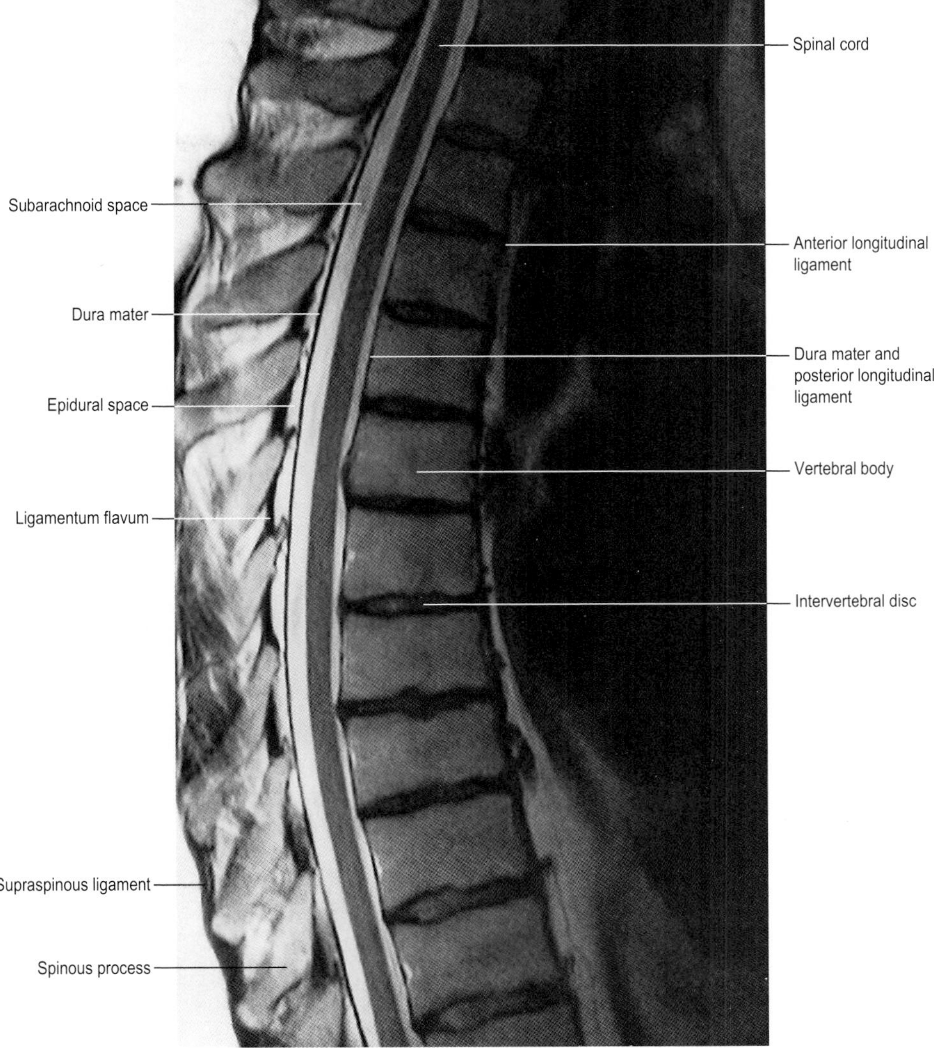

Fig. 6.5 Sagittal MRI of the thoracic spine. (From Jacob S: Atlas of Human Anatomy. Churchill Livingstone 2002, with permission.) MRI, Magnetic resonance imaging.

- descends in the pyramidal tract on the contralateral side of the cord
- at each spinal segment, fibres enter the anterior horn and synapse with motor nuclei—the tracts therefore get progressively smaller as they descend
- fibres are somatotopically arranged in the tract, fibres for the lower part of the cord laterally, and those for the upper half medially.

- Anterior corticospinal tract (direct pyramidal tract):
    - fibres do *not* cross in the decussation in the medulla
    - fibres eventually cross the midline at segmental levels and terminate close to those in the lateral corticospinal tract.

Ascending Tracts

- Lateral and anterior spinothalamic tracts:
    - conduct pain and temperature as well as some tactile sensations
    - fibres enter the posterior roots, ascend a few segments and relay in the substantia gelatinosa

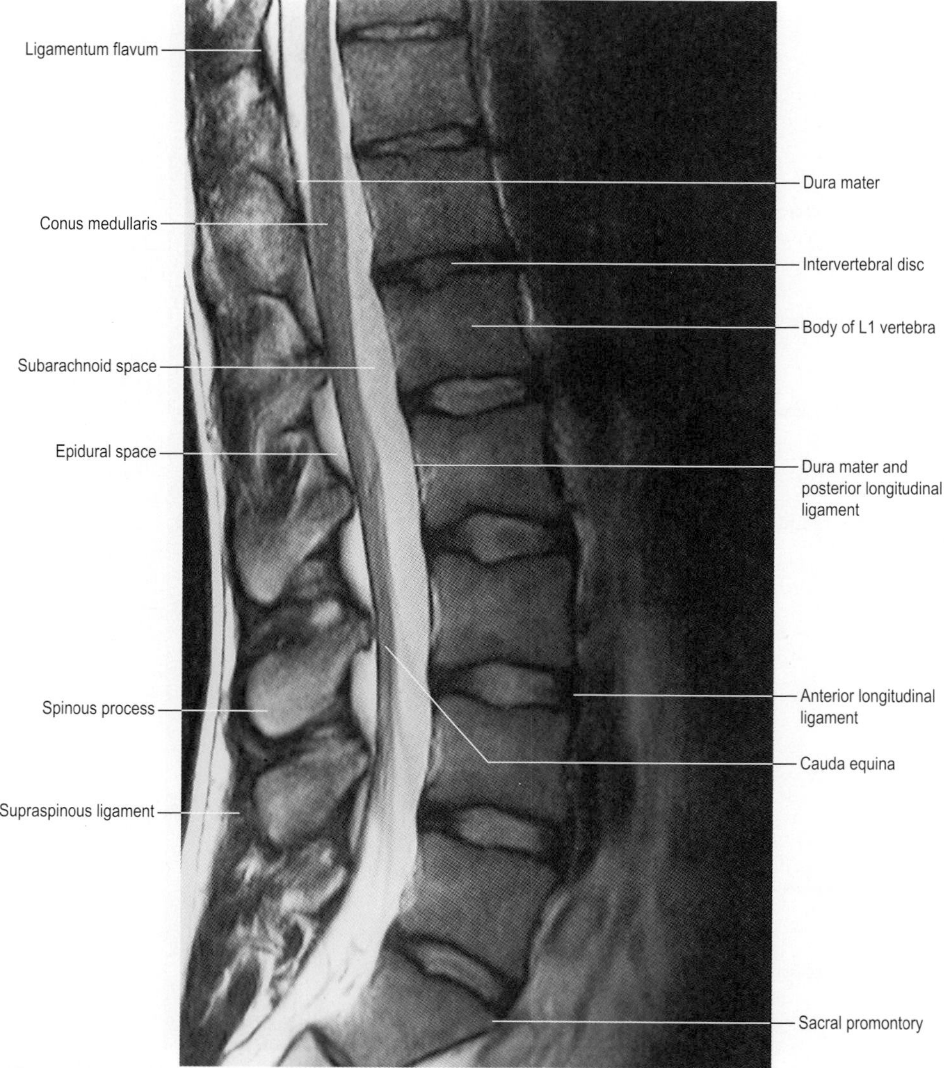

Fig. 6.6 Sagittal MRI of the lumbar spine. (From Jacob S: Atlas of Human Anatomy. Churchill Livingstone 2002, with permission.) MRI, Magnetic resonance imaging.

- they then cross to the opposite side in the ventral grey commissure close to the central canal
- they ascend in spinothalamic tracts to the thalamus, whence they are relayed to the sensory cortex
- fibres are somatotopically arranged in the lateral spinothalamic tract, those for the lower limb superficial and those for the upper limb deepest.
- Anterior and posterior spinocerebellar tracts:
  - ascend on the same side of the cord
  - enter the cerebellum through the superior and inferior cerebellar peduncles, respectively
  - concerned with the maintenance of equilibrium.
- Posterior (dorsal) columns:
  - composed of the medial fasciculus gracilis (of Goll) and the lateral fasciculus cuneatus (of Burdach)
  - contain fibres subserving fine and discriminative tactile sensation, proprioception (position sense) and vibration sense
  - as cord is ascended, fibres are added to lateral part of posterior columns—hence the fasciculus gracilis deals mostly with the lower limb and the fasciculus cuneatus with the upper limb

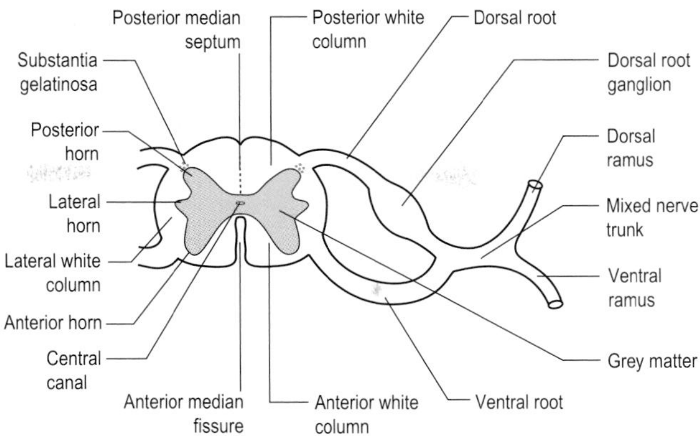

Fig. 6.7 Spinal cord in cross-section showing grey and white matter and spinal nerve roots.

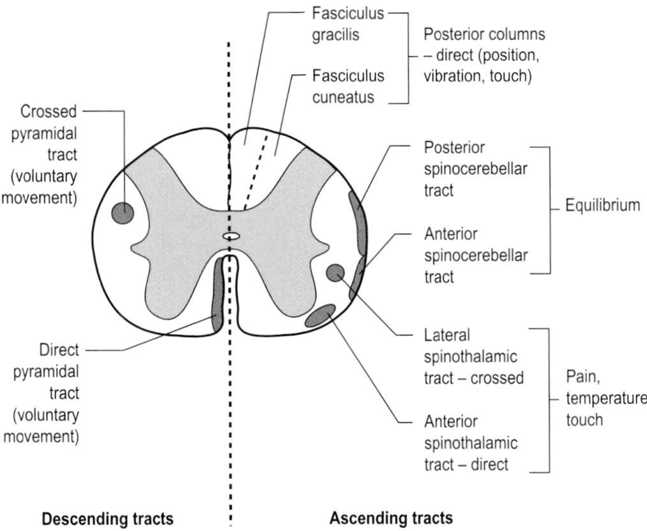

Fig. 6.8 Cross-section of the spinal cord showing important ascending and descending tracts.

- fibres in dorsal columns are uncrossed
- synapse in gracile and cuneate nuclei in medulla
- second-order fibres cross in the sensory decussation whence they synapse in the thalamus
- third-order fibres pass to the sensory cortex
- some fibres pass from medulla to cerebellum along the inferior cerebellar peduncle.

Blood Supply of the Spinal Cord

- Anterior and posterior spinal arteries from the vertebral arteries.
- Anterior spinal arteries supply the whole of the cord in front of the posterior grey columns.
- Posterior spinal arteries supply the posterior grey columns and dorsal columns on either side.
- Spinal artery reinforced at segmental level by radicular arteries, i.e. branches of the ascending cervical, cervical part of the vertebral, posterior intercostal and lumbar arteries.
- Radicular arteries may be compromised in resection of segments of the aorta in aneurysm surgery.

Clinical Points

A cross-section of the spinal cord demonstrating the representation of the various areas in the spinal tracts is shown in Fig. 6.9.

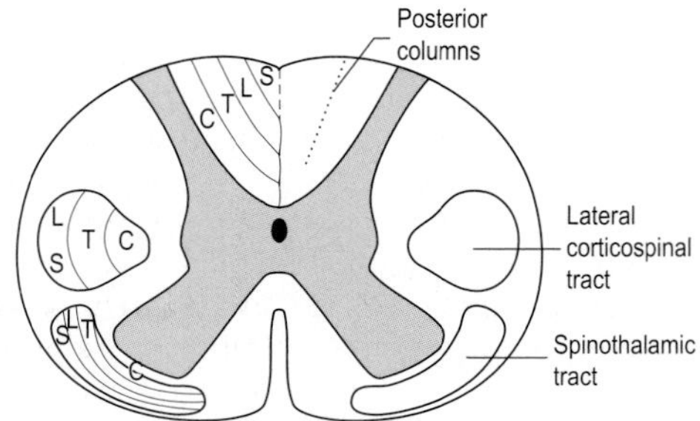

Fig. 6.9 Cross-section of the spinal cord showing the representation of the cervical (C), thoracic (T), lumbar (L) and sacral (S) areas in the various spinal tracts.

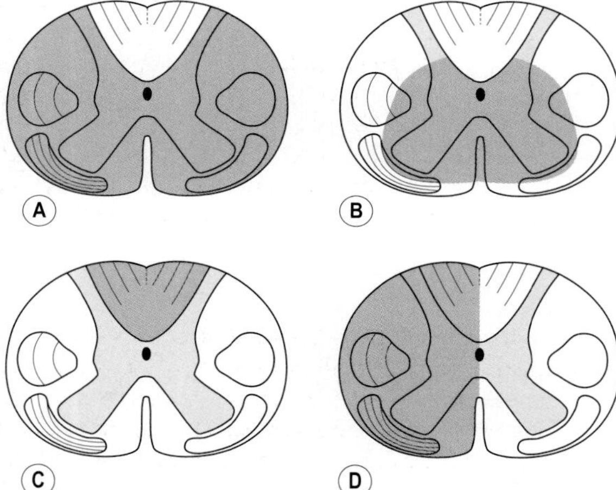

Fig. 6.10 Incomplete spinal cord injury. (A) Anterior cord syndrome. (B) Central cord syndrome. (C) Posterior cord syndrome. (D) Brown–Séquard syndrome. The dark shaded area shows the region of the cord involved.

Complete Transection of Spinal Cord

- Total loss of voluntary movement distal to level of transection; this loss is irreversible.
- Loss of all sensation from those areas which depend on ascending pathways crossing the site of injury.

Incomplete Spinal Cord Injury (Fig. 6.10)

- Anterior cord syndrome:
  - associated with flexion/rotation injuries producing anterior dislocation or compression fracture of vertebral body with bone encroaching on the vertebral canal
  - loss of power below level of lesion
  - loss of pain and temperature below the lesion
  - in addition to direct damage, the anterior spinal artery may be compressed
  - the dorsal columns remain intact so that touch and proprioception are not affected.
- Central cord syndrome:
  - occurs in syringomyelia and centrally placed tumours
  - initially involves decussating spinothalamic fibres so that pain and temperature are lost below the lesion
  - later the lateral corticospinal tract is involved, with the more centrally placed cervical tract supplying the arm being involved more than the peripheral tracts supplying the legs. Classically there is flaccid weakness of the arms, but because the distal leg and sacral motor and sensory fibres are spared, perianal sensation and some leg movement and sensation may be preserved
  - proprioception and fine touch are preserved in the dorsal columns until late.
- Posterior cord syndrome:
  - seen in hyperextension injuries with fractures of the posterior elements of the vertebra
  - loss of proprioception with profound ataxia with unsteady and faltering gait
  - usually good power and pain and temperature sensation below the lesion.
- Brown–Séquard syndrome:
  - hemisection of the cord
  - stab injury or damage to lateral mass of vertebrae
  - paralysis on affected side below lesion (pyramidal tract)
  - loss of proprioception and fine discrimination (dorsal columns) on affected side below lesion
  - loss of pain and temperature on opposite side below lesion (normal on affected side because of decussation below level of hemisection)
  - therefore the *uninjured side* has good power, but absent sensation to pinprick and temperature.
- Cauda equina syndrome:
  - compression of lumbosacral nerve roots below the conus medullaris
  - caused by bony compression or disc protrusion in the lumbosacral area
  - lower motor neuron lesion
  - bowel and bladder dysfunction together with leg numbness and weakness.

THE MENINGES

- Dura mater.
- Arachnoid mater.
- Pia mater.

Dura Mater

- Outer endosteal layer.
- Inner meningeal layer.
- Meningeal layer continuous into vertebral canal as dura covering spinal cord.
- The two layers are fused together except where they form the walls of dural venous sinuses.
- Folds of dura mater divide the cranial cavity into compartments.
- These folds are:
  - falx cerebri
  - tentorium cerebelli
  - falx cerebelli.

Falx Cerebri

- Lies between the two cerebral hemispheres.
- Attached anteriorly to crista galli.
- Attached posteriorly to tentorium cerebelli.
- Superior sagittal sinus lies in its attached superior border.
- Inferior sagittal sinus lies in its free inferior border.
- The straight sinus is seen where the falx meets the tentorium cerebelli.

Tentorium Cerebelli

- Attached anteriorly to the posterior clinoid process of sphenoid bone.
- Attachment runs posteromedially along the superior border of the petrous temporal bone where superior petrosal sinuses enclosed.
- Where latter empties into transverse sinus, attached border runs posteromedially along the lips of the groove for the transverse sinus to reach the internal occipital protuberance.
- It then continues on the opposite side of the skull to reach the other posterior clinoid process.
- Free border of tentorium is attached to anterior clinoid processes.
- Runs posterior and medially, curving round the midbrain, forming tentorial notch.
- Just behind the apex of the petrous temporal bone, the inferior layer prolongs into the middle cranial fossa as the trigeminal cave.

Falx Cerebelli

- Lies between the two lateral lobes of the cerebellum.
- Lies below the tentorium in the posterior cranial fossa.

Diaphragma Sellae

- Fold of dura forming the roof of the pituitary fossa.
- Covers the pituitary gland and has an opening through which the infundibulum passes.

Arachnoid Mater

- Separated from dura by subdural space.
- The subarachnoid space contains cerebrospinal fluid (CSF) and major blood vessels.
- Arachnoid and subarachnoid spaces extend into vertebral canal to the level of the second piece of the sacrum.
- Deep surface of the arachnoid projects into the venous sinuses to form arachnoid villi; these are most numerous along the superior sagittal sinus. Collections of arachnoid villi are known as arachnoid granulations.
- Arachnoid granulations are sites of reabsorption of CSF into superior sagittal sinus and probably other dural sinuses.

Subarachnoid Cisterns

- Subarachnoid space varies in size as arachnoid follows surface of dura and pia follows surface of brain.
- This arrangement gives rise to cisterns:
  - cerebellomedullary cistern (cisterna magna): posterior to medulla below cerebellum
  - pontine cistern: anterior to pons
  - interpeduncular cistern: between cerebral peduncles and optic chiasma—contains circle of Willis and cranial nerves III and IV.

Pia Mater

- Closely follows surface of brain.
- Dips down to sulci.
- Blood vessels enter brain in a sleeve of pia mater.
- At the choroid fissure of lateral ventricles and the roof of the third and fourth ventricles, the pia is invaginated by blood vessels to form the tela choroidea and choroid plexus.

Production and Circulation of CSF

- Produced by choroid plexus in all four ventricles.
- Flows from lateral ventricles to third ventricle to cerebral aqueduct to fourth ventricle to subarachnoid space.
- Absorbed into venous system through arachnoid granulations along dural venous sinuses.
- The interventricular foramen (of Monro) connects the lateral ventricle to third ventricle.
- The fourth ventricle has three openings on its roof which connect it to the subarachnoid space:
  - the foramen of Magendie in the midline
  - the paired foramina of Luschka laterally.
- Through these, CSF flows from the ventricular system into the subarachnoid space.
- Total volume about 100–150 mL.
- Pressure 8–10 cmH_2O.

Blood Supply to the Brain (See Fig. 5.22)

- Two vertebral arteries.
- Two internal carotid arteries.

Vertebral Arteries

- Enter cranial cavity via foramen magnum.
- Lie in subarachnoid space.
- Unite at lower border of pons to form basilar artery.

Branches

- Posterior spinal artery.
- Anterior spinal artery.
- Posterior inferior cerebellar artery.

Basilar Artery

Branches

- Anterior inferior cerebellar.
- Labyrinthine artery.
- Pontine arteries.
- Superior cerebellar arteries.
- Posterior cerebral artery (terminal branches of basilar artery) supplies visual area of occipital lobe; occlusion causes blindness in contralateral visual field.

Internal Carotid Arteries

Branches

- Posterior communicating artery.
- Anterior cerebral artery.
- Middle cerebral artery.
- Anterior choroidal artery.

Middle Cerebral Artery

- Larger of terminal branches of internal carotid artery.
- Supplies lateral surface of frontal, parietal and temporal lobes (except narrow strips supplied by anterior cerebral artery).
- Occlusion results in contralateral motor and sensory paralysis of face and arm.

Circle of Willis (Fig. 6.11)

- Formed by the two vertebral and two internal carotid arteries on the inferior surface of the brain.
- Each half of the circle is formed by:
  - anterior communicating artery
  - anterior cerebral artery
  - internal carotid artery
  - posterior communicating artery
  - posterior cerebral artery.
- Despite interconnection, there is only minimal mixing of blood passing through the arteries.
- When one artery is blocked the arterial circle may provide collateral circulation.

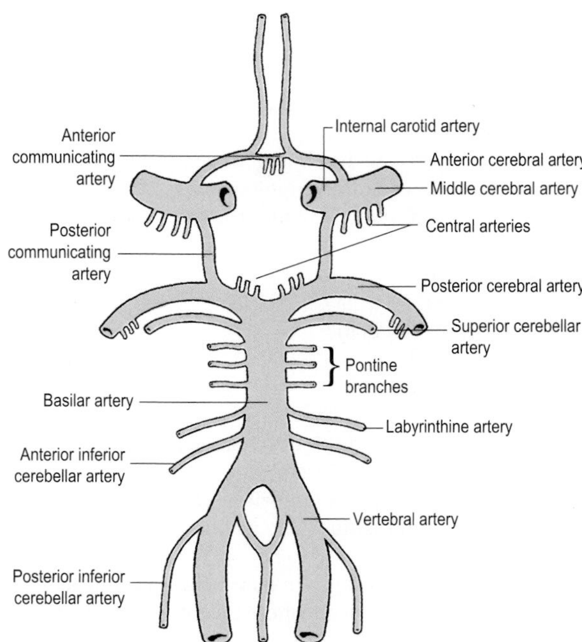

Fig. 6.11 The circle of Willis. The central arteries supply the corpus striatum, internal capsule, diencephalon and midbrain.

Venous Drainage of Brain

The veins lie alongside the arteries in the subarachnoid space. They pierce the pia mater and drain into the dural venous sinuses. The major veins are:

- superior cerebral veins
- superficial middle cerebral vein
- basal vein
- great cerebral vein.

Dural Venous Sinuses (Fig. 6.12)

- Situated within the dura mater.
- Devoid of valves.
- Drain eventually into internal jugular vein.

The cranial venous sinuses are:

- superior sagittal sinus
- inferior sagittal sinus
- straight sinus
- transverse sinus
- sigmoid sinus
- confluence of sinuses
- occipital sinus
- cavernous sinus.

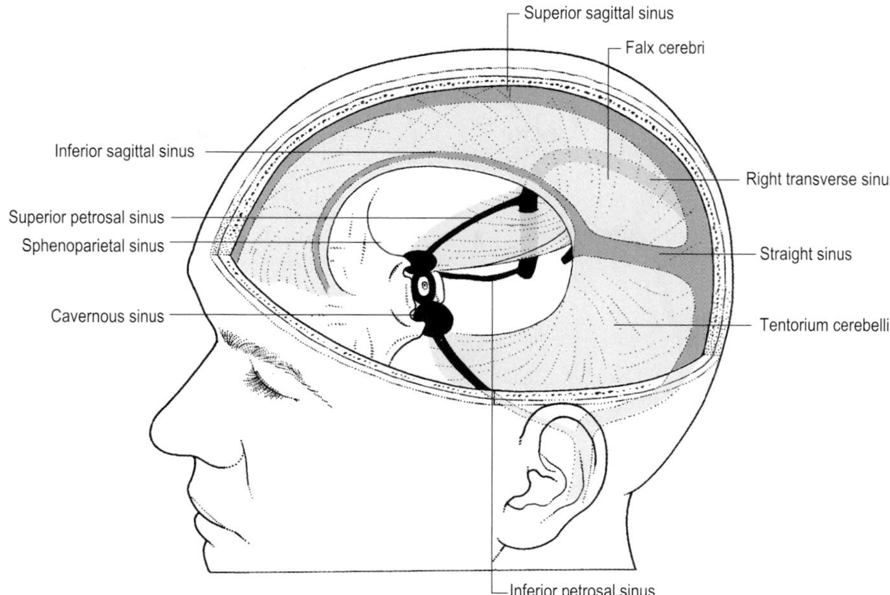

Fig. 6.12 The venous sinuses.

Superior sagittal sinus

- Commences at crista galli.
- Courses backwards along attached border of falx cerebri.
- Usually becomes continuous with right transverse sinus at the internal occipital protuberance.
- Venous lacunae lie along its course and open into the sinus.
- Sinus and lacunae are invaginated by arachnoid granulations.
- Superior cerebral veins drain into superior sagittal sinus.

Inferior sagittal sinus

- Lies along inferior border of falx cerebri.
- Receives cerebral veins from medial surface of hemispheres.
- Joins great cerebral vein to form straight sinus.

Straight sinus

- Formed by union of inferior sagittal sinus and great cerebral vein.
- Lies in attachment of falx cerebri to tentorium cerebelli.
- Usually becomes continuous with left transverse sinus near internal occipital protuberance.

Transverse sinus

- Lies in groove on inner surface of occipital bone along posterior attachment of tentorium cerebelli.
- On reaching petrous temporal bone it curves downwards into posterior cranial fossa to follow a curved course as sigmoid sinus.

Sigmoid sinus

- Passes through jugular foramen.
- Becomes continuous with internal jugular vein.

Confluence of sinuses

- Formed by the two transverse sinuses near the internal occipital protuberance.

Occipital sinus

- Small sinus extending from foramen magnum.
- Drains into confluence of sinuses.
- Lies along falx cerebelli and connects vertebral venous plexuses to transverse sinus.

Cavernous sinus (Fig. 6.13)

- One on each side.
- Situated on body of sphenoid bone.
- Extends from superior orbital fissure to apex of petrous temporal bone.
- Relations:
  - medially: pituitary gland and sphenoid sinus
  - laterally: temporal lobe of brain.
- Internal carotid artery and abducens nerve (VI) pass through it.
- On the lateral wall from above down are:
  - oculomotor nerve (III)
  - trochlear nerve (IV)
  - ophthalmic nerve (V)
  - maxillary nerve (V).
- Ophthalmic veins drain into the anterior part of sinus.

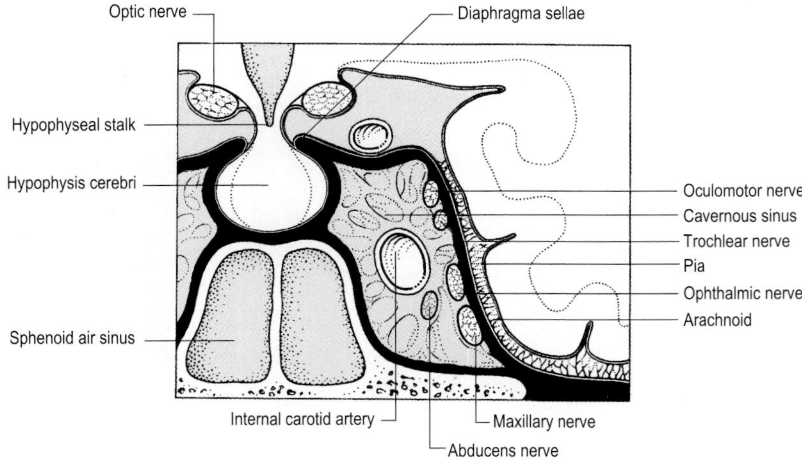

Fig. 6.13 The cavernous sinus.

- Posteriorly the sinus drains into the transverse or sigmoid sinus through superior and inferior petrosal sinuses.
- Emissary veins passing through the foramina of the middle cranial fossa connect the cavernous sinus to the pterygoid plexus and facial veins.
- The two sinuses are connected by anterior and posterior intercavernous sinuses lying in front of and behind the pituitary gland, respectively.

Clinical Points

- Cavernous sinus thrombosis may occur as a result of spread of infection from the lips and face via the anterior facial and ophthalmic veins, or from deep infections via the pterygoid venous plexus, all of which drain into the sinus.
- Blockage of the venous drainage of the orbit consequent on cavernous sinus thrombosis results in a characteristic clinical picture:
  - oedema of the conjunctiva and eyelids
  - exophthalmos with transmitted pulsations from the internal carotid artery
  - ophthalmoplegia due to pressure on the contained cranial nerves
  - ophthalmoscopy demonstrates papilloedema and retinal haemorrhages.

CRANIAL NERVES

I Olfactory Nerve

- Axons from olfactory mucosa in nasal cavity pass through the cribriform plate of the ethmoid bone to end in the olfactory bulb.
- A cuff of dura, arachnoid and pia mater surrounds each bundle of nerves.
- Synapse with mitral cells in olfactory bulb.
- Axons of mitral cells pass backwards in the olfactory tract to terminate in the cortex of the uncus.

Clinical Points

- Head injuries involving fractures in the anterior cranial fossa may sever the olfactory nerves, resulting in bilateral anosmia. In addition, fractures in the anterior cranial fossa may also cause CSF rhinorrhoea.
- Unilateral anosmia may be a sign of frontal lobe tumours.
- Olfactory cortex consists of the uncus and anterior perforated substance.
- Tumours in the region of the uncus may result in an 'uncinate fit', characterized by olfactory hallucinations associated with impairment of consciousness and involuntary chewing movements.

II Optic Nerve (Fig. 6.14)

- Commences at lamina cribrosa, where axons of ganglion cells of retina pierce sclera.
- Covered by dura, arachnoid and pia mater, it runs posteromedially in the orbit to enter the optic canal.
- Accompanied by the ophthalmic artery.
- Reaches the optic groove on the dorsum of the body of sphenoid bone.
- Fibres from medial half of retina, i.e. temporal visual field, cross over in the optic chiasma to the optic tract of the opposite side.
- Fibres from the lateral half of the retina, i.e. nasal visual field, pass backwards in the optic tract of the same side.

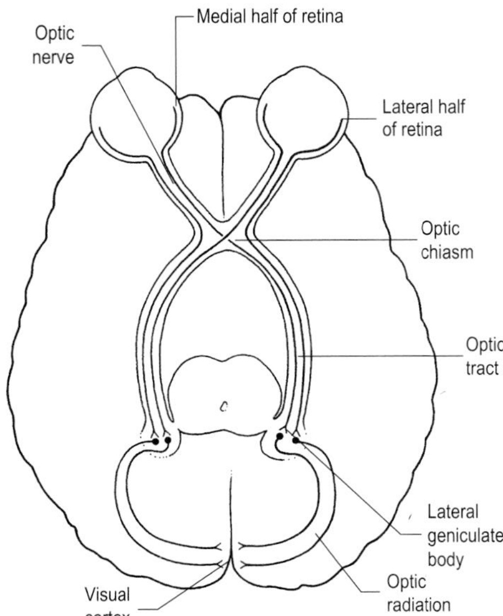

Fig. 6.14 The visual pathways.

- Optic tract passes posterolaterally from the optic chiasma.
- The majority of fibres in the optic tract end in the lateral geniculate body of thalamus.
- A small proportion of optic tract fibres bypass the lateral geniculate body, ending in the superior colliculus or pretectal nucleus. These fibres subserve pupillary, ocular and head and neck reflexes (afferent limb of light reflexes).
- From the lateral geniculate bodies, fibres of the optic radiation pass laterally and backwards to the visual cortex of the occipital lobe.
- The upper half of the retina is represented in the upper lip of the calcarine fissure, the lower half on the lower lip.

Clinical Points

- Lesions of the optic nerve result in ipsilateral blindness.
- Lesions of the optic tract and central visual pathway result in contralateral homonymous hemianopia.
- Lesions of the optic chiasma (e.g. from expanding pituitary lesions) will cause bitemporal hemianopia (loss of vision of both temporal fields).

III Oculomotor Nerve

- Two main components:
  1. Somatic motor fibres supplying:
     - superior rectus
     - inferior rectus
     - medial rectus
     - inferior oblique
     - levator palpebrae superioris.
  2. Preganglionic parasympathetic fibres supplying the sphincter of the pupil via the ciliary ganglion.
     - Somatic efferent nucleus (ocular muscles and Edinger–Westphal nucleus; parasympathetic) lie in midbrain at level of superior colliculus.
     - Oculomotor nerve emerges between cerebral peduncles.
     - Passes forwards between superior cerebellar artery and posterior cerebral artery.
     - Pierces dura to lie on lateral wall of cavernous sinus.
     - Divides into superior and inferior branch before entering into superior orbital fissure.
     - Superior division supplies superior rectus and levator palpebrae superioris.
     - Inferior division supplies medial rectus, inferior rectus and inferior oblique.
     - Parasympathetic fibres leave the branch to the inferior oblique to synapse in the ciliary ganglion (lies at the apex of the orbit just lateral to the optic nerve).
     - Postganglionic fibres pass to ciliary muscles and constrictor pupillae via the short ciliary nerves.
     - Stimulation of the nerve results in pupillary constriction and accommodation of the lens.

Clinical Points

- Complete division of the nerve results in:
  - ptosis, due to paralysis of levator palpebrae superioris
  - divergent squint, caused by unopposed action of lateral rectus and superior oblique
  - dilatation of the pupil, caused by unopposed action of dilator pupillae (supplied by sympathetic fibres in the long ciliary branches in the nasociliary nerve)
  - loss of accommodation and light reflexes, due to paralysis of ciliary muscles and constrictor pupillae
  - diplopia.
- Oculomotor nerve may be paralysed by:
  - aneurysm of posterior cerebral, superior cerebellar and posterior communicating arteries
  - raised intracranial pressure associated with herniation of uncus into tentorial notch
  - tumours in region of sella turcica.

IV Trochlear Nerve

- Smallest cranial nerve.
- Supplies superior oblique muscle.
- Nucleus lies at level of inferior colliculus.
- Fibres pass dorsally around cerebral aqueduct and decussate in superior medullary velum.

- Emerges from dorsum of pons (only cranial nerve to arise from dorsum of brainstem).
- Winds round cerebral peduncle.
- Passes forwards between superior cerebellar and posterior cerebral arteries to pierce dura.
- Runs forward on lateral wall of cavernous sinus between oculomotor and ophthalmic nerves.
- Enters orbit through superior orbital fissure lateral to tendinous ring from which recti take origin.
- Passes medially over optic nerve to enter superior oblique muscle.

Clinical Point

- Injury to trochlear nerve results in paralysis of superior oblique, resulting in diplopia when patient looks downwards and laterally. The patient complains of difficulties when walking downstairs.

V Trigeminal Nerve

The trigeminal nerve comprises three divisions:

- ophthalmic: sensory
- maxillary: sensory
- mandibular: mixed sensory and motor.

It is distributed as follows:

- sensory: to face, scalp, teeth, mouth, nasal cavity, paranasal sinuses and most of dura mater
- motor: to muscles of mastication, mylohyoid, anterior belly of digastric, tensor tympani and tensor palati
- ganglionic connections to the ciliary, sphenopalatine, otic and submandibular ganglia.

The nuclei of the trigeminal nerve lie as follows:

- Motor nucleus:
  - situated in upper part of pons near floor of fourth ventricle.
- Sensory nuclei:
  - mesencephalic nucleus (concerned with proprioception) is in the midbrain
  - the chief sensory nucleus, concerned with touch, tactile discrimination and position sense, lies in the pons
  - the nucleus of the spinal tract, concerned with pain and temperature, is in the medulla and extends caudally into the upper segments of the spinal cord.

Trigeminal Ganglion

- Lies in invaginated pocket of dura in the middle cranial fossa.
- Lies near apex of petrous temporal bone in a hollow (Meckel's cave).
- Motor root of nerve and greater superficial petrosal nerve pass deep to ganglion.
- Hippocampal gyrus of temporal lobe lies above.
- Medially lies the internal carotid artery and part of the cavernous sinus.

Ophthalmic Division

- Smallest division.
- Wholly sensory.
- Innervates skin of forehead, upper eyelid and most of nose.
- Passes forwards to enter lateral wall of cavernous sinus.
- Lies below trochlear nerve in cavernous sinus.
- Divides into three branches just before entering orbit:
  1. Frontal:
     - runs forwards beneath roof of orbit
     - divides into supratrochlear and supraorbital nerves supplying upper eyelid and scalp as far back as the lambdoid suture.
  2. Lacrimal:
     - to lacrimal gland via postganglionic parasympathetic fibres from pterygopalatine ganglion, which it reaches via the maxillary nerve
     - to the lateral part of the conjunctiva and upper eyelid.
  3. Nasociliary:
     - to ciliary ganglion
     - eyeball
     - cornea and conjunctiva of medial part of upper eyelid
     - dura of anterior cranial fossa
     - mucosa and skin of nose.

Maxillary Division

- Wholly sensory.
- Passes forwards to leave skull through foramen rotundum.
- Emerges into pterygopalatine fossa.
- Continues through inferior orbital fissure and infraorbital canal, becoming the infraorbital nerve supplying the skin of the cheek and lower eyelid.
- Branches:
  - zygomatic, giving zygomaticotemporal and zygomaticofacial branches to the skin of the temple and cheek, respectively
  - superior alveolar branches to teeth of upper jaw
  - branches from the pterygopalatine ganglion.

Pterygopalatine ganglion

- Lies in pterygopalatine fossa.
- Receives parasympathetic (secretomotor) root via the greater superficial petrosal branch of cranial nerve VII; sensory component from two pterygopalatine branches of maxillary nerve; and sympathetics from the internal carotid plexus.

- Parasympathetic efferents pass to lacrimal gland.
- Sensory and sympathetic fibres to nose, nasopharynx, palate and orbit.

Mandibular Division

- Largest division.
- Motor and sensory.
- Supplies:
  1. Sensory:
     - skin of temporal region
     - part of auricle
     - lower face
     - mucous membrane of the anterior two-thirds of the tongue and floor of the mouth.
  2. Motor:
     - muscles of mastication.
  3. Parasympathetic:
     - secretomotor to parotid gland.
- Passes forwards from trigeminal ganglion to enter foramen ovale.
- Gives off nervus spinosus to supply dura mater and nerve to medial pterygoid, from which otic ganglion is suspended.
- Divides into small anterior and large posterior trunk.
- Anterior trunk:
  - sensory branch, i.e. buccal nerve to skin of cheek and mucous membrane of cheek
  - motor to masseter, temporalis and lateral pterygoid.
- Posterior trunk:
  - auriculotemporal nerve (sensory to temple and auricle; secretomotor fibres from otic ganglion to parotid gland)
  - lingual nerve:
    - parasympathetic secretomotor fibres from the chorda tympani join the lingual nerve to supply the submandibular gland
    - terminal branches are distributed to the anterior two-third of the tongue, the floor of the mouth and the lingual surface of the gums
  - inferior alveolar nerve:
    - enters mandibular canal and supplies teeth of lower jaw
    - emerges through mental foramen, supplying skin of chin and lower lip
    - also supplies motor nerves, i.e. nerve to mylohyoid, supplying mylohyoid and anterior belly of digastric.

Otic Ganglion

- Lies immediately below foramen ovale, lying close to the medial surface of the mandibular nerve.
- Parasympathetic fibres through the lesser superficial petrosal branch of the glossopharyngeal nerve relay in the ganglion, and pass via the auriculotemporal nerve to the parotid as secretomotor supply.
- Sympathetic fibres—from plexus on middle meningeal artery—are vasoconstrictor.
- Sensory fibres via auriculotemporal nerve to parotid gland.
- Motor fibres (not present in any other cranial ganglion) pass through the ganglion from the nerve to medial pterygoid to supply tensor tympani and tensor palati.

Submandibular Ganglion

- Lies between hyoglossus and deep part of submandibular gland.
- Suspended from lower aspect of lingual nerve.
- Parasympathetic fibres from chorda tympani of facial nerve conveyed by lingual nerve carrying secretomotor fibres to sublingual and submandibular gland.
- Sympathetic fibres from superior cervical ganglion via plexus on facial artery supply vasoconstrictor fibres to sublingual and submandibular glands.
- Sensory component via lingual nerve to salivary glands and mucous membrane of floor of mouth.

Clinical Points

- Division of the whole trigeminal nerve results in unilateral anaesthesia of the face and the anterior part of the scalp, the auricle, and the mucous membranes of the nose, mouth and anterior two-thirds of tongue. Paralysis and wasting of the muscles of mastication occur on the affected side.
- Pain is frequently referred from one segment to another. A patient with a carcinoma of the tongue (lingual nerve) may complain of earache (via the auriculotemporal nerve). The classical description used to be the case of an elderly man sitting in outpatients spitting blood with a piece of cotton wool in his ear.

VI The Abducens Nerve

- Supplies lateral rectus.
- Nucleus in floor of fourth ventricle in upper part of pons.
- Fibres of facial nerve wind round nucleus to form facial colliculus.
- Emerges between medulla and pons.
- Passes forwards through pontine cistern.
- Pierces dura mater to enter cavernous sinus lying on lateral aspect of internal carotid artery.
- Enters orbit through tendinous ring at superior orbital fissure.

Clinical Points

- Has a long intracranial course and therefore frequently involved in injuries to base of skull.
- Damage gives rise to diplopia and a convergent squint.

VII Facial Nerve

- Supplies muscles of facial expression.
- Conveys parasympathetic fibres to:
  - lacrimal gland
  - glands in nasal cavity
  - submandibular salivary glands
  - sublingual salivary glands.
- Transmits taste fibres from anterior two-thirds of tongue.
- Motor nucleus in lower pons.
- Motor fibres loop round abducens nerve nucleus (facial colliculus) and emerge at cerebellopontine angle with nervus intermedius (contain sensory and parasympathetic fibres).
- Sensory fibres synapse in nucleus of tractus solitarius in the pons.
- Autonomic fibres originate in the superior salivary nucleus in the pons.
- Nervus intermedius lies lateral to motor fibres of facial nerve in between latter and vestibulocochlear nerve.
- Motor fibres of facial nerve and nervus intermedius pass through the pontine cistern and enter the internal acoustic meatus, where the two join together to form the facial nerve.
- Nerve then passes through facial canal in petrous temporal bone.
- Runs laterally over vestibule to reach medial wall of middle ear, where it bends sharply backwards over the promontory.
- This sharp bend, the genu, has the geniculate ganglion.
- Nerve passes downwards on posterior wall of middle ear to emerge through the stylomastoid foramen at the base of the skull.
- Branches given off in the petrous temporal bone are:
  - greater petrosal nerve
  - nerve to stapedius
  - chorda tympani.
- Greater petrosal nerve transmits preganglionic parasympathetic fibres to sphenopalatine ganglion, the postganglionic fibres supplying the lacrimal glands and nasal cavity glands.
- Chorda tympani carries parasympathetic fibres to submandibular and sublingual salivary glands and taste fibres from anterior two-thirds of tongue.
- After emerging from the stylomastoid foramen, the nerve enters the parotid gland and divides into the following branches:
  - temporal
  - zygomatic
  - buccal
  - mandibular
  - cervical.
- Testing of individual branches of the facial nerve is important after head and neck surgery, e.g. superficial parotidectomy. The following tests may be carried out to assess the various branches of the facial nerve:
  - to test frontalis, ask patient to raise eyebrows. Normally wrinkles are seen on the forehead. Tests temporal branch
  - to test orbicularis oculi, ask patient to close eyelids tightly against resistance. Tests temporal and zygomatic branches
  - to test levator anguli oris, ask patient to show teeth to check that the angles of the mouth move equally on both sides. Tests buccal branch
  - to test orbicularis oris, ask patient to purse lips tightly against resistance. Tests buccal and marginal mandibular branch
  - to test buccinators, ask patient to blow out the cheeks, keeping the mouth shut. Tap the cheek to see if air escapes from the closed mouth. Tests buccal branch
  - to test risorius, ask patient to smile. The angle of the mouth will not move on the side of the lesion. Tests buccal nerve
  - to test depressor anguli oris (draws the angle of the mouth downwards and laterally), ask patient to smile. The lower lip on the side of the lesion remains elevated thus distorting the smile. Tests marginal mandibular branch
  - to test platysma, ask patient to clench the teeth and simultaneously depress the angles of the mouth. Normally, longitudinal folds of skin become obvious in the neck when platysma contracts. Tests cervical branch.

Clinical Points

- Infranuclear paralysis may be caused by malignant tumours of the parotid, parotid surgery, acoustic neuroma and its surgery, and fracture of the base of the skull.
- It is important to distinguish between a supranuclear facial palsy and a nuclear or infranuclear facial palsy.
- Nuclear and infranuclear palsy affects all muscles on the same side of the face.
- Supranuclear palsy affects contralateral facial muscles but spares the frontalis and orbicularis oculi, since the part of the facial nucleus supplying these muscles receives fibres from both cerebral hemispheres, i.e. there is bilateral cortical representation. Supranuclear palsy is likely to result from cerebrovascular accidents involving the corticobulbar pathways. If a patient with a right cortical defect is asked to look up and smile, the patient will be unable to raise the left side of the mouth but the

forehead is spared, as evidenced by wrinkling caused by the action of frontalis. Also, a patient with a unilateral supranuclear lesion will be able to close the eye on that side.

VIII Vestibulocochlear (Auditory) Nerve

- Consists of two sets of fibres: cochlear and vestibular.
- The nerve emerges from the brain at the cerebellopontine angle and leaves the cranium via the internal auditory meatus with the facial nerve.
- Enters internal auditory meatus with the facial nerve.
- Cochlear fibres subserve hearing.
- Vestibular fibres subserve equilibrium.
- Cochlear:
  - cerebral processes of bipolar spiral ganglion cells of cochlea
  - pass through internal auditory meatus to reach lateral aspect of medulla (at cerebellopontine angle with cranial nerve VII)
  - terminate in dorsal and ventral cochlear nuclei.
- Vestibular:
  - to utricle, saccule and semicircular canals
  - cells originate in the vestibular ganglion
  - fibres enter the medulla just medial to the cochlear division, and terminate in the vestibular nuclei in the floor of the fourth ventricle
  - vestibular connections with cranial nerves III, IV, V and XI, and upper cervical cord via vestibulospinal tract bring eye and neck muscles under reflex vestibular control.

Clinical Points

- Temporal lobe tumours may give rise to auditory hallucinations if they encroach upon the auditory gyrus.
- Unilateral lesions of the auditory pathway do not greatly affect hearing because of the bilateral nature of the auditory projections (unless the cochlea itself is damaged).
- Lesions of the cochlear division result in deafness, which may or may not be accompanied by tinnitus.
- The differential diagnosis between middle ear and inner ear deafness (cochlear or auditory nerve lesions) may be made clinically by using a tuning fork. Air conduction with the fork being held next to the ear is normally louder than bone conduction (the fork being held on the mastoid process). If the middle ear is damaged, then the reverse will be true.

IX Glossopharyngeal Nerve

The glossopharyngeal nerve:

- has sensory fibres, including taste from the posterior third of the tongue and the oropharynx (tonsillar fossa)
- supplies stylopharyngeus
- has parasympathetic fibres supplying the parotid gland
- innervates the carotid sinus and carotid body.

The glossopharyngeal nerve has the following nuclei in the medulla:

- nucleus ambiguus: fibres to stylopharyngeus; also innervates the muscles of the pharynx, larynx and soft palate via the vagus nerve
- inferior salivatory nucleus, supplying the parotid gland
- nucleus of tractus solitarius, which receives taste fibres via the glossopharyngeal nerve
- dorsal motor nucleus of vagus (shared with vagus) for general sensation from the posterior third of the tongue and oropharynx.

The course of the glossopharyngeal nerve is as follows:

- emerges on brainstem between olive and inferior cerebellar peduncle
- passes forwards and laterally to leave skull through jugular foramen
- emerges from foramen, giving off tympanic branch (supplying middle ear), which continues as lesser superficial petrosal nerve carrying parasympathetic fibres to the otic ganglion to supply parotid gland
- in upper part of neck accompanies stylopharyngeus (which it supplies) to enter pharynx, passing between the middle and superior constrictor muscles of the pharynx
- terminal branches supply the posterior third of the tongue and oropharynx.

Clinical Points

- Complete section of the nerve results in sensory loss in the pharynx, loss of taste and common sensation over the posterior third of the tongue, and loss of salivation from the parotid gland.
- Isolated lesions of the glossopharyngeal nerve are rare.

X Vagus Nerve

- Contains sensory fibres:
  - mucosa of pharynx and larynx
  - those transmitting visceral sensation from organs in the thorax and abdomen
  - fibres carrying general sensation from dura, part of external auditory meatus, external surface of tympanic membrane; taste fibres from epiglottis.
- Contains preganglionic parasympathetic fibres to all thoracic and abdominal viscera (up to splenic flexure of colon).
- Cranial part of accessory nerve is also distributed with vagus.
- Nuclei associated with vagus in brainstem:

  - dorsal nucleus of vagus in floor of fourth ventricle in medulla; receives general visceral sensation from various organs supplied by vagus; its motor component gives rise to preganglionic parasympathetic fibres in vagus
  - nucleus of tractus solitarius, shared with facial nerve and glossopharyngeal nerve for taste fibres
  - nucleus ambiguus: origins of fibres of cranial part of accessory nerve which are distributed along with vagus.
- Emerges on brainstem in groove between olive and inferior cerebellar peduncle, below roots of glossopharyngeal nerve.
- Passes through jugular foramen.
- Bears two ganglia: in foramen (superior) and just below foramen (inferior).
- Joined by cranial part of accessory nerve.
- Branches and distribution:
  - meningeal: supplies dura of posterior cranial fossa
  - auricular: supplies medial aspect of auricle (small area), external auditory meatus and outer surface of tympanic membrane
  - pharyngeal: supplies muscles of soft palate and pharynx
  - superior laryngeal: divides into external laryngeal branch to cricothyroid, and internal laryngeal branch supplying sensation to the laryngeal pharynx and the laryngeal mucosa above the level of the vocal cord
  - recurrent laryngeal nerve
  - cardiac branches
  - pulmonary branches
  - branches to abdominal viscera.

Clinical Points

- Isolated lesions of the vagus nerve are uncommon.
- Injuries to the recurrent laryngeal nerve are discussed under the section on larynx.

XI Accessory Nerve

- Small cranial root and larger spinal root.
- Cranial part arises from the nucleus ambiguus and emerges with fibres of vagus from brainstem.
- Joins spinal root for short distance and then branches off to rejoin vagus to be distributed to muscles of soft palate, pharynx and larynx.
- Spinal root arises from upper five segments of cervical spinal cord.
- Enters skull through foramen magnum.
- Joins cranial root.
- Leaves skull through jugular foramen.
- Immediately below jugular foramen, spinal root passes backwards to supply sternocleidomastoid and trapezius.

Clinical Points

- Isolated lesions of the cranial root are rare.
- May be involved jointly with lesions of vagus, giving rise to paralysis of the laryngeal and pharyngeal muscles, resulting in dysphonia and dysphagia.
- Damage to the spinal root may occur in block dissection of the neck and operations on the posterior triangle.
- Damage in the posterior triangle will result in inability to shrug the shoulder and wasting of trapezius (loss of contour of side of neck).

XII Hypoglossal Nerve

- Supplies all extrinsic and intrinsic muscles of tongue (except palatoglossus).
- Nucleus lies in medulla in floor of fourth ventricle.
- Emerges as rootlets between pyramid and olive, which unite to form nerve.
- Leaves skull through hypoglossal canal.
- Lies initially between internal jugular vein and internal carotid artery.
- Crosses superficial to internal carotid artery and external carotid artery.
- Passes forwards deep to mylohyoid to supply muscles of the tongue.

Clinical Points

- Division of the hypoglossal nerve results in ipsilateral paralysis and wasting of the muscles of the tongue.
- On protrusion, the tongue deviates to the affected side.
- Supranuclear paralysis (owing to an upper motor neuron lesion involving the corticobulbar pathways) leads to paralysis but not atrophy of the muscles on the contralateral side.

Relationships of the nerves emerging from the brain are shown in Fig. 6.15.

PERIPHERAL NERVOUS SYSTEM

The peripheral nervous system is formed by the cranial and spinal nerves carrying somatic and autonomic nerve fibres. The cranial nerves have already been described above. The sympathetic nervous system is described later in this chapter.

Spinal Nerves and Their Distribution (Fig. 6.7)

- Each spinal nerve is formed by the union of a dorsal and ventral root.
- The ventral root contains motor fibres with cell bodies in the ventral horn of the spinal cord.
- The dorsal root contains sensory fibres with cells of origin in the dorsal root ganglion.

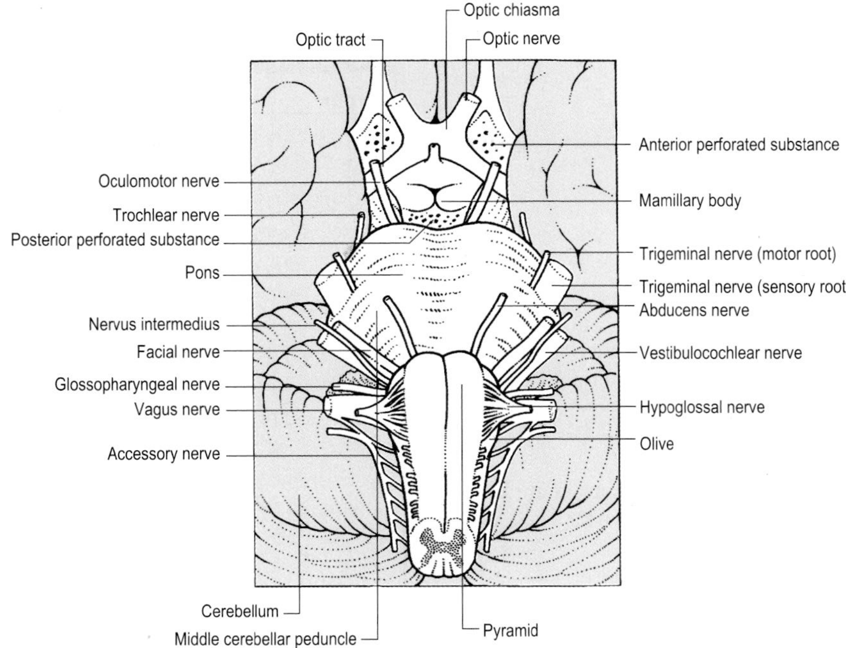

Fig. 6.15 The brainstem and cerebellum, ventral view.

- The ventral and dorsal roots lie in the vertebral canal within the dural sac.
- Ventral and dorsal roots join together to form the spinal nerve in the intervertebral foramen (mixed motor and sensory and sympathetic).
- Immediately beyond the intervertebral foramen the nerve divides into a dorsal and ventral ramus.
- The dorsal ramus passes backwards to innervate the muscles of the back and the ligaments and joints of the vertebral column. They also supply cutaneous branches to the skin of the posterior aspect of the head, trunk and gluteal region (dorsal rami of C1, L4, L5 have no cutaneous branches).
- Ventral rami in the thoracic region form the intercostal nerves.
- The lower six intercostal nerves extend onto the anterior abdominal wall to innervate the muscles and overlying skin in segmental fashion.

Spinal Nerves

There are 31 pairs of spinal nerves:

- eight cervical
- twelve thoracic
- five lumbar
- five sacral
- one coccygeal.

The first cervical nerve lies above the first cervical vertebra, but since there are eight nerves and only seven cervical vertebra, the eighth nerve lies below the seventh cervical vertebra, and from here down each nerve lies below the vertebra of the corresponding number.

- The remaining spinal nerves supply the head and neck and limbs, and are dealt with in detail in the appropriate sections.
- At cervical, lumbar and sacral levels the ventral rami form a plexus:
  - cervical plexus: C1–4
  - brachial plexus: C5–8, T1
  - lumbar plexus L1–4, with contribution from T12
  - sacral plexus S1–5, with contribution from L4, 5.

Cervical Plexus

- C1–4 ventral rami.
- Motor to:
  - prevertebral muscles
  - levator scapulae
  - scalene muscles
  - sternocleidomastoid and trapezius via accessory nerve
  - diaphragm.
- Sensory to:
  - skin of anterior and lateral neck
  - shoulder

- lower jaw
- external ear.

Brachial Plexus

- C5–8 ventral rami, T1 (part).
- Motor to muscles and joints of upper limb.
- Sensory to skin of upper limb.

Lumbar Plexus

- L1–4 ventral rami plus T12 (part).
- Supplies muscles and skin of thigh through obturator and femoral nerve.
- Small nerves from plexus innervate muscles of lower part of abdominal wall, skin of foot, lateral part of hip and external genitalia.

Sacral Plexus

- Ventral rami S1–5 and contribution of ventral rami L4–5.
- Innervate muscles and skin of lower limb, pelvic floor and perineum.

UPPER AND LOWER MOTOR NEURONS

- Upper motor neuron commences in the motor cortex.
- Groups of cells control movements rather than individual muscles.
- Upper motor neurons synapse with anterior horn cells in the spinal cord.
- Lower motor neurons are from the anterior horn cells and end in voluntary muscle.
- Peripheral nerves contain motor and sensory fibres.
- Lesions of anterior horn cells and ventral nerve roots will be entirely motor. Lesions of peripheral nerves will be mixed motor and sensory.
- Lower motor neuron is influenced by upper motor neuron and by extrapyramidal system; modifications of muscle tone and reflexes result when correct balance between these neurons is lost.
- The clinical distinction between upper and lower motor neuron lesions is shown in Box 6.2.

Dermatomes

- The skin of the trunk is supplied segmentally by the intercostal nerves. In the limbs a similar segmental supply is furnished by the cutaneous nerves. The area of skin supplied by one spinal nerve is called a dermatome. Dermatomes of the body are shown in Fig. 6.16.

Motor Root Values and Peripheral Nerve Supply of Important Muscle Groups

These are shown in Table 6.1.

BOX 6.2 Distinction Between Upper and Lower Motor Neuron Lesion

Upper	Lower
Paralysis affects movements rather than muscle	Individual or groups of muscles affected
Wasting slight	Wasting pronounced
Muscles hypertonic (clasp-knife rigidity)	Muscles hypotonic (flaccidity)
Tendon reflexes increased	Tendon reflexes absent or diminished
No trophic skin changes	Skin often cold, blue and shiny
Superficial reflexes diminished: • absent abdominal reflexes • Babinski sign present (both are corticospinal reflexes in which the afferent arc is via a small number of ascending fibres in the corticospinal tracts)	Superficial reflexes unaltered unless sensation also lost

Tendon and Abdominal Reflexes

These are shown in Table 6.2.

AUTONOMIC NERVOUS SYSTEM

- The autonomic nervous system consists of two separate parts:
  - sympathetic nervous system
  - parasympathetic nervous system.

Sympathetic Nervous System

The patterns of distribution of the sympathetic nerve fibres are shown in Fig. 6.17. The sympathetic nervous system:

- plays a major role in regulating the internal environment of the body
- is concerned with stress reactions of the body
- when stimulated, the following occur:
  - sweating
  - pupillary dilatation
  - vasoconstriction
  - bronchial dilatation
  - diminished peristalsis
  - increased heart rate.

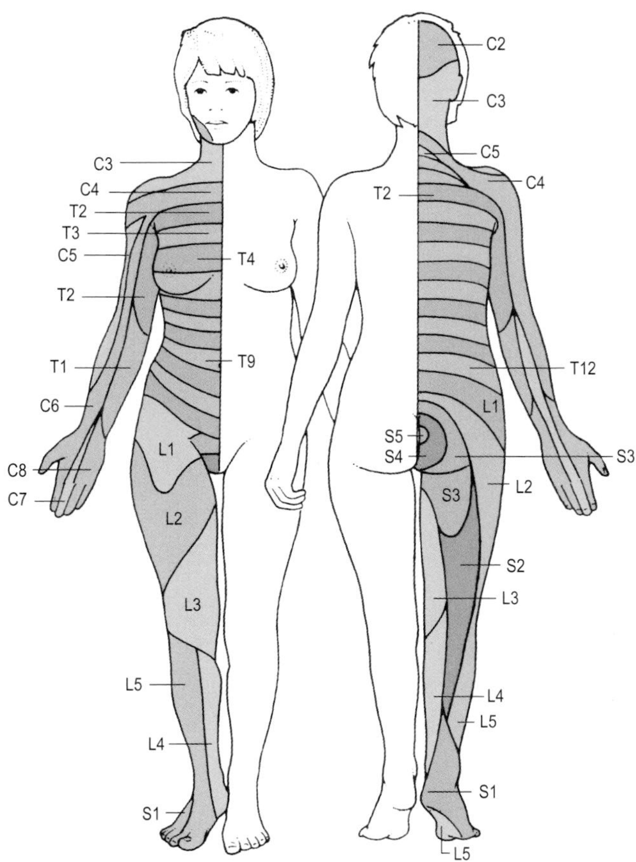

Fig. 6.16 The dermatomes of the body.

Origin of Sympathetic Outflow

- Preganglionic efferent fibres lie in the lateral horn of grey matter of T1–L2.
- The pattern of sympathetic outflow is shown in Table 6.3.

Sympathetic Trunk

- Ganglionated chain.
- Extends from base of skull to coccyx.
- Lies on either side of vertebral bodies about 2.5 cm from the midline.
- Ganglia are associated with each spinal segment except in the neck, where there are only three ganglia.

Distribution of Preganglionic and Postganglionic Fibres

- Myelinated preganglionic fibres from T1–L2 segments of the spinal cord, which leave the corresponding spinal nerves through white rami communicantes, have a number of possible destinations:
  - end by synapsing in the corresponding ganglion of the sympathetic chain
  - enter the chain and travel various distances up and down before synapsing at a ganglion
  - enter the chain and leave without synapsing as splanchnic nerves to synapse in coeliac, aortic or pelvic ganglia, associated with the corresponding autonomic plexuses in the abdomen.
- Synapses in the ganglionic neurons provide amplification and facilitate widespread reaction on stimulation.
- Unmyelinated postganglionic axons may also take one of a number of routes:
  - some leave in the grey rami communicantes, which join the spinal nerve for distribution to skin and blood vessels
  - some leave to form plexuses around arteries
  - cardiac nerves are postganglionic fibres from the cervical and upper thoracic ganglia, which innervate the thoracic viscera through the cardiac and pulmonary plexuses.

TABLE 6.1 Motor Root Values and Peripheral Nerve Supply of Important Muscle Groups

Joint Movement	Muscle	Root Value	Peripheral Nerve
Shoulder			
Abduction	Deltoid	C4, 5	Axillary
External rotation	Infraspinatus	C4, 5	Suprascapular
Adduction	Pectoralis/latissimus dorsi	C6–8	Medial and lateral pectoral
Elbow			
Flexion	Biceps	C5, 6	Musculocutaneous
Extension	Triceps	C7, 8	Radial
Pronation		C6, 7	
Supination	Biceps/	C5, 6	Musculocutaneous
	brachioradialis	C6	Radial
Wrist			
Flexion	Flexor muscles of forearm	C7, 8	Median and ulnar
Dorsiflexion	Extensor muscles of forearm	C7	Radial
Finger			
Flexion	Long finger flexors	C8	Median and ulnar
Extension	Long finger extensors	C7	Radial
Opposition of thumb or splaying of fingers	Small hand muscles	T1	Ulnar
Hips			
Flexion	Iliopsoas	L1–3	–
Extension	Glutei	L5, S1	Sciatic
Adduction	Adductors	L2, 3	Obturator
Abduction	Glutei and tensor fasciae latae	L4, 5, S1	Sciatic
Knee			
Flexion	Hamstrings	L5, S1, 2	Sciatic
Extension	Quadriceps	L3, 4	Femoral
Ankle			
Dorsiflexion	Anterior tibial	L4, 5	Sciatic (common peroneal)
Plantarflexion	Calf (gastrocnemius and soleus)	S1, 2	Sciatic (tibial)
Eversion	Peronei	L5, S1	Sciatic (common peroneal)
Inversion	Anterior tibial and posterior tibial	L4	Sciatic (common peroneal)
		L4, 5	Sciatic (tibial)
Toes			
Flexion	Flexor hallucis longus	S2, 3	Sciatic (tibial)
Extension	Extensor hallucis longus	L5, S1	Sciatic (common peroneal)

Note: All muscles on back of upper limb (triceps, wrist and finger extensors) are innervated by C7.

From Easterbrook P Basic Medical Sciences for MRCP Part 1, 2nd edn Churchill Livingstone 1999, with permission.

TABLE 6.2 Tendon and Abdominal Reflexes

Reflex	Muscle	Root Value
Knee	Quadriceps	L3, 4
Ankle	Gastrocnemius	S1
Biceps	Biceps	C5, 6
Triceps	Triceps	C7
Supinator	Brachioradialis	C6
Abdominal	Abdominal muscle	T8–12
Cremasteric	Cremaster	L1, 2
Anal	Anal sphincter	S3, 4

Head and Neck

- Superior cervical ganglion (C2–4).
- Middle cervical ganglion (C5–6).
- Inferior cervical ganglion (fused with first thoracic ganglion) to form stellate ganglion (C7, 8, T1).
- Preganglionic fibres arise from T1–2 segments of cord and relay in superior cervical ganglion.
- Supply head and neck, ciliary muscle, iris, blood vessels and sweat glands.
- Division of head and neck supply results in Horner's syndrome, i.e. miosis, ptosis, anhidrosis, on side of lesion.

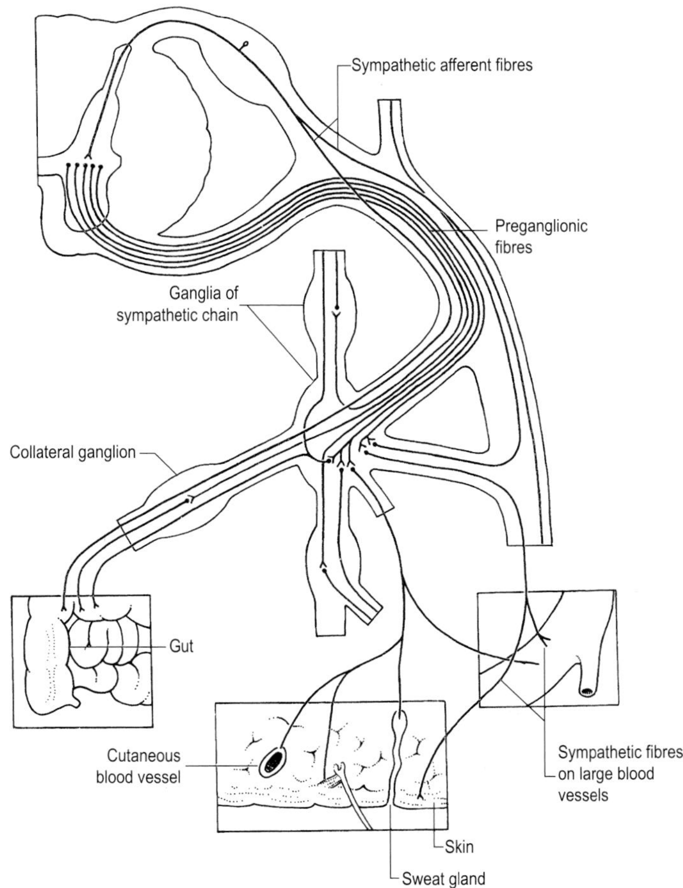

Fig. 6.17 The patterns of distribution of the sympathetic fibres.

TABLE 6.3 Sympathetic Outflow (T1–L2)

Spinal Segments	Sympathetic Innervation	Destination
T1–2	Via internal carotid and vertebral arteries	Head and neck Ciliary muscle and iris Blood vessels Sweat glands
T1–4	Via cardiac and pulmonary plexuses	Heart and bronchi
T2–7		Upper limb
T4–L2	Via coeliac, mesenteric, hypogastric and pelvic plexuses	Adrenal medulla Alimentary tract Colon and rectum Bladder and genitalia
T11–L2		Lower limb

T1–4: relay in sympathetic ganglion.
T4–L2: do not relay in sympathetic ganglion.

From Easterbrook P Basic Medical Sciences for MRCP Part 1, 2nd edn Churchill Livingstone 1999, with permission.

Upper Limb

- Preganglionic fibres arise from T2–7 segments.
- Postganglionic fibres from middle cervical and stellate ganglion are distributed to limb mainly through the brachial plexus.
- Control of palmar hyperhidrosis and vasospastic disorders can be achieved by removing second and third thoracic ganglia (the first is not removed as this would cause Horner's syndrome).

Lower Limb

- Preganglionic fibres from T12–L2 spinal segments synapse in lumbar and sacral ganglia.
- Postganglionic fibres are distributed to the limb via lumbosacral plexus.
- Lumbar sympathectomy (for plantar hyperhidrosis or vasospastic diseases) removes third and fourth lumbar ganglia and intervening chain.
- First lumbar ganglion is preserved to avoid compromising ejaculation.

Abdominal and Pelvic Viscera

- These receive sympathetic innervation via:
  - coeliac plexus
  - aortic plexus
  - hypogastric plexus.
- Coeliac plexus lies around coeliac axis.
- Continues downwards over abdominal aorta as aortic plexus.
- Hypogastric plexus lies in front of fifth lumbar vertebra as continuation of aortic plexus.
- Plexuses supply gastrointestinal tract, bladder and genitalia.
- Hypogastric and aortic plexuses may be damaged in aortic aneurysm surgery and extensive pelvic surgery, e.g. anterior resection of the rectum: ejaculation may be compromised.

Parasympathetic Nervous System

- Craniosacral outflow.
- Often antagonizes sympathetic nervous system.
- Supply limited to viscera and glands; no distribution to skin and skeletal muscle.
- The distribution of the parasympathetic nervous system may be summarized as follows:
  - oculomotor nerve supplying sphincter pupillae and ciliary muscles in the eye
  - facial nerve supplying the lacrimal, submandibular and sublingual glands as well as glands in the nasal cavity and mucosa of the palate
  - glossopharyngeal nerve supplying the parotid gland
  - vagus nerve supplying thoracic and abdominal viscera up to the left colic flexure
  - S2–4 sacral nerves supplying the pelvic viscera and descending and sigmoid colon.

There are four ganglia associated with the parasympathetic nervous system in the head and neck. These are:

- Ciliary ganglion in orbit:
  - site of synapse of preganglionic fibres accompanying oculomotor nerve
  - postganglionic fibres supply ciliary muscles and constrictor pupillae.
- The sphenopalatine ganglion in the pterygopalatine fossa:
  - site of synapse of preganglionic fibres accompanying facial nerve
  - postganglionic fibres supply lacrimal glands and glands in nasal cavity and palate.
- Submandibular ganglion attached to lingual nerve:
  - site where preganglionic fibres accompanying facial nerve and chorda tympani synapse
  - postganglionic fibres supply submandibular and sublingual glands, and glands in tongue and floor of mouth.
- Otic ganglion attached to trunk of mandibular nerve in infratemporal fossa:
  - site of synapse of preganglionic fibres accompanying the glossopharyngeal nerve
  - postganglionic fibres supply parotid gland.

OSCE SCENARIOS

OSCE Scenario 6.1

An 18-year-old male is assaulted at a party. He is struck on the left temporal region with a bottle. He briefly loses consciousness. He is taken to hospital where on examination his GCS (Glasgow Coma Scale) is 15. Four hours following admission, he suddenly deteriorates with a GCS of 8 and his left pupil dilates.

1. What is the most likely diagnosis?
2. What is the explanation for the 'lucid' interval?
3. What is the anatomical basis for the left pupillary dilatation?
4. Where would you locate the middle meningeal artery for the purpose of making a burr hole?
5. What layers of the scalp would you encounter in your incision?

OSCE Scenario 6.2

A 55-year-old male presents with low back pain, bilateral sciatica, numbness over the buttock area and weakness in the lower limbs. He has also developed difficulty in passing urine. Examination reveals reduced lower limb reflexes and loss of anal tone and sensation.

1. What is the most likely diagnosis?
2. At what level does the spinal cord end in the adult?
3. Describe the level and type of disc lesion that is likely to cause the symptoms.
4. Describe the anatomy of an intervertebral disc.
5. Explain the anatomical basis of bladder and bowel dysfunction.
6. What investigation would you carry out to confirm the diagnosis and what action would you take if the diagnosis was confirmed?

OSCE Scenario 6.3

A 55-year-old insulin-dependent diabetic develops a boil on the right upper lip. She does not seek treatment. A few days later she develops a severe headache and redness and swelling around the right orbit. A diagnosis of cavernous sinus thrombosis is made.

1. Describe the anatomy of the cavernous sinus.
2. Why does cavernous sinus thrombosis develop following an infection on the upper lip?
3. Describe the characteristic clinical picture of cavernous sinus thrombosis.

OSCE 6.4

A 75-year-old male has been referred to you by the Accident and Emergency department for a possible stroke. His main symptom is left arm and leg weakness.

1. Which hemisphere has suffered a stroke?
2. If the patient had suffered left-sided amaurosis fugax, which hemisphere would have been affected?
3. The patient is right-handed and has had dysphasia only. Which hemisphere is the most likely to have been affected and why?

OSCE 6.5

A 70-year-old non-smoking female presents with a hoarse voice. A CT angiogram is shown below (Figs. 6.5Q).

1. What is the diagnosis?
2. What are the treatment options?
3. What is the anatomical explanation for the hoarse voice?

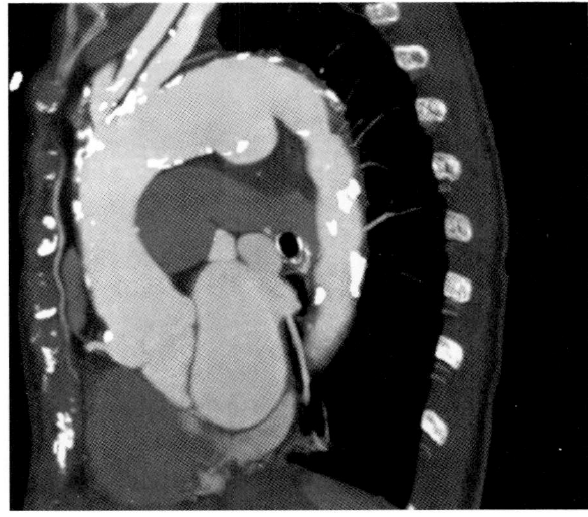

Fig. 6.5Q CT angiogram of the thoracic aorta.

Answers in Appendix pages 442–444

Please check your eBook at https://studentconsult.inkling.com/ for more self-assessment questions. See inside cover for registration details.

SECTION II

Physiology

7

General Physiology

HOMEOSTASIS

Homeostasis = maintenance of a constant internal environment.

The composition of extracellular fluid (ECF), and therefore the cellular environment, is maintained in a constant state through homeostatic mechanisms that monitor and regulate the functions of:

- circulatory system
- alimentary system
- respiratory system
- renal system.

Monitoring and regulation are co-ordinated through the nervous and endocrine systems, requiring:

- receptors
- central integration
- effectors.

Homeostatic mechanism = a regulating mechanism, triggered by an alteration in a physiological property or quantity, acting to produce a compensatory change in the opposite direction. This requires:

- Receptors: specialized to detect alterations in certain variables, e.g. osmoreceptors, chemoreceptors.
- Effectors, e.g.
  - circulatory system, carrying O_2 to cells and removing waste products of metabolism
  - alimentary system, providing nutrients
  - respiratory system, carrying out gaseous exchange
  - renal system, excluding waste products.
- Co-ordinating and integrating systems:
  - nervous
  - hormonal.

Nervous System

- Afferent fibres link receptors to co-ordinating systems in brain and spinal cord.
- Efferent fibres carry information from co-ordinating systems to effector organs.
- Somatic nervous system uses skeletal muscle as effectors for purposeful behaviour and reflex actions.
- Autonomic nervous system sends efferent fibres to glands, heart, hollow organs and blood vessels.

Hormonal System

- Endocrine glands secrete hormones to effect function of target cells.
- Actions generally slower than those of nervous system.
- Under control of nervous system via hypothalamic–pituitary axis with negative feedback.

Thermoregulation

Thermoregulation = balance between heat gain and heat loss. It is controlled by the nervous system.

Body temperature is altered by:

- small adjustments by altering skin blood flow
- large adjustments by shivering and sweating.

Heat Production

- Increased voluntary muscle effort.
- Shivering.
- Controlled via hypothalamus.

Heat Loss

- Controlled by sympathetic nervous system.
- Controlled from hypothalamus.
- Altering skin flow alters thermal conductivity.
- Sweating increases heat loss by increasing evaporation.

Regulation of Body Temperature

Temperature-sensitive receptors are found in the anterior hypothalamus:

- Activation of heat-sensitive neurons causes:
  - skin vasodilatation
  - sweating.
- Activation of cold-sensitive neurons causes:
  - inhibition of heat-sensitive neurons
  - vasoconstriction
  - shivering.

Peripheral Thermoreceptors

- Respond to warm and cold
- Connect centrally to cortex (conscious sensation and hypothalamus).

Reflex Vasoconstriction

Direct contact with a cold stimulus on a limb leads to vasoconstriction on ipsilateral and contralateral sides.

- Afferent neuron: cutaneous nerve.
- Centre: hypothalamus and spinal cord.
- Efferent neuron: sympathetic nerves.

Reflex Vasodilatation

Reflex vasodilatation occurs when radiant heat is applied to part or the whole of a body.

- Afferent neuron: cutaneous nerve.
- Centre: above C5 of the spinal cord.
- Efferent pathway: sympathetic nerves (reduced activity).

Receptors on Internal Surfaces

- Respiratory and gastrointestinal tracts possess thermoreceptors.
- Inhalation of cold air leads to shivering during inspiration.
- Hot food causes sweating and vasodilatation.

Body Temperature

The body does not have the same temperature throughout.

Core Temperature

- Temperature of thoracic, abdominal contents and brain.
- Must be kept at optimal temperature.
- Usually measured as rectal temperature.
- 0.5°C higher than mouth and axilla.
- Shows diurnal variation: higher in evening than in early morning.
- Varies during menstrual cycle: 0.5°C higher in latter half.

Peripheral Temperature

- Less than core temperature, heat being lost from surface to environment.
- Heat is lost from the body via:
  - conduction and evaporation from skin to air
  - convection from skin due to air movement; from lungs via convection of tidal air flow
  - radiation from naked skin (and to some extent between layers of clothing).

Abnormal Temperature Regulation

The core temperature is maintained between 36°C and 37.5°C. It is thought that there is a set-point temperature around which the core temperature is regulated by the hypothalamus. If the set-point temperature is raised then the hypothalamus activates mechanisms leading to increasing core temperature and vice versa.

Fever (Pyrexia)

- Fever may be caused by:
  - illness
  - exercise
  - heatstroke
  - anterior hypothalamic lesions, e.g. neoplasia, ischaemia, surgery
  - hyperthyroidism
  - malignant hyperpyrexia (abnormal muscle response to anaesthetics)
  - failure of heat-loss mechanism, e.g. dehydration.
- Set-point temperature is increased; therefore, the body feels cold as the core temperature is lower.
- As a result the hypothalamus activates responses to increase body temperature:
  - vasoconstriction
  - piloerection ('goose flesh')
  - shivering.
- Aspirin returns set-point temperature to normal and therefore patient feels hot, as core temperature is higher than set-point temperature.
- Hypothalamus then responds to increase heat loss by:
  - activating vasodilatation
  - activating sweating.

Heatstroke

- Occurs with body temperature above 41°C.
- Unacclimatized individuals undertaking exercise in hot, humid conditions.
- Symptoms:
  - nausea
  - vomiting
  - weakness
  - headache
  - skin feels hot
  - circulatory failure
  - cerebral oedema
  - hepatic failure
  - renal failure.

Hypothermia

- Core temperature (rectal) below 35°C.
- If temperature is <30°C, temperature regulatory mechanism fails completely.
- Therefore no response occurs to elevated temperature.
- Often fatal if temperature is <32°C.
- Symptoms:

- shivery and feeling cold at 32–35°C
- bradycardia, hypotension, respiratory depression, muscle stiffness, metabolic abnormalities at <32°C
- death occurs from cardiac arrhythmias, especially ventricular fibrillation.

Factors Affecting Thermoregulation

- Anaesthetics:
  - depress hypothalamic function
  - vasodilatation with increased heat loss
  - lack of shivering
  - consequent drop in body temperature.
- Exercise:
  - increases body temperature
  - hypothalamus cannot launch responses that result in loss of heat faster than its production from muscle metabolism.
- Circulatory shock:
  - reduced tissue perfusion
  - reduced cellular metabolism and heat production
  - results in decreased body temperature
  - compensatory mechanisms include vasoconstriction, piloerection and increased secretion of catecholamines
  - skin feels cold
  - exception is septic (endotoxic) shock, where there is vasodilatation and skin feels hot.
- Spinal injuries:
  - thermoregulatory mechanisms lost below level of injury
  - vasoconstriction lost; therefore, heat loss increased
  - patient unable to shiver
  - sweating in relation to hyperthermia lost below level of lesion
  - quadriplegics tend to assume temperature of environment.
- Hyperthyroidism:
  - increased basal metabolic rate (BMR)
  - increased O_2 consumption
  - patient hyperactive
  - all of above contribute to increased temperature
  - patient intolerant of heat and feels hot.
- Hypothyroidism:
  - opposite effects to hyperthyroidism
  - patient feels cold, intolerant of cold weather
  - body temperature low
- Neonates and premature babies:
  - large surface area to body weight ratio
  - inability to shiver
  - less insulating fat
  - temperature regulating mechanisms less developed
  - therefore predisposed to increased heat loss.

FLUID BALANCE AND FLUID REPLACEMENT THERAPY

Body Water

In healthy adults water constitutes approximately 60% of the body weight. Body water is partitioned into two components:

- intracellular
- extracellular.

Extracellular component may be divided further into:

- intravascular
- extravascular (interstitial).

For a 70-kg man there would be approximately:

- 25 L of intracellular water
- 19 L of extracellular water.
- Of the extracellular water:
  - 3 L is in blood plasma
  - 15 L is interstitial fluid
  - 1 L is transcellular fluid, e.g. CSF, peritoneal fluid, intraocular fluid.

Functions of the Kidney

See Chapter 11.

DIURESIS

There are two types of diuresis:

- water
- osmotic.

Water Diuresis

- Occurs when water is ingested or administered in excess of body's requirements.
- Antidiuretic hormone (ADH) secretion is suppressed.
- Collecting ducts become relatively impermeable to water and excess water is lost without solute.
- The kidney can therefore adjust to excretion of water without markedly affecting its handling of solutes.

Osmotic Diuresis

This results when more solute is presented to the tubules than they can reabsorb.

Examples of osmotic diuresis include:

- Diabetes, where the concentration of glucose in the plasma rises so that the filtered load exceeds the tubular maximum.
- The administration of mannitol, which is filtered but is a non-reabsorbable solute.
- Inhibition of tubular function, e.g. by drugs that block reabsorption of sodium chloride in one or more parts of the tubule.

WATER BALANCE

Normally body water remains constant over a 24-h period; therefore, intake and loss of water must balance exactly.

Intake comprises drinking fluids, solid food (which may contain as much as 1 L of fluid in 24 h), and the water of oxidation of metabolites (about 300 mL in 24 h). Water is lost in the following ways:

- evaporation via the respiratory system: 500 mL
- skin (insensible): 400 mL
- faeces: 100 mL
- urine (obligatory): 500 mL
- total = 1500 mL.

Urine water loss is variable. About 600 mosmol of solutes must be excreted each day in the urine. The maximal achievable urinary osmolality is about 1200 mosmol/L and therefore the obligatory volume of urine is about 500 mL per day. In practice, water intake is such that 1.5 L of urine is excreted each day.

Regulation of Total Body Water

Although the movement of certain ions and proteins between the various compartments is restricted, water is freely diffusible. Consequently the osmolality of all components is identical, being maintained within a narrow range of 285–295 mosmol/L. Control of osmolality occurs by two mechanisms:

- adjustments in secretion of ADH
- thirst-mediated water intake.

If water loss exceeds gain there is a reduction in total body water content and the osmolality of the body fluid increases. This has two effects:

- thirst, resulting in ingestion of water
- release of ADH so that water is retained by the kidneys.

Conversely, excess intake of water dilutes the body fluids, reducing osmolality. This eliminates thirst and inhibits the release of ADH, thus allowing diuresis and consequent removal of excess water.

In health, both thirst and ADH release are determined by the osmolality of plasma-perfusing nuclei in the hypothalamus. The receptors indicating thirst have an osmotic threshold of about 10 mosmol higher than that of the osmoreceptors involved in ADH release. Under normal circumstances therefore, thirst is not experienced until ADH release has ensured that ingested water is retained by the kidneys.

Other mechanisms are available for the stimulation of thirst and ADH release. These are important in conditions where circulating blood volume falls. They include:

- reduced arterial blood pressure (signals via carotid and aortic baroceptors)
- reduced central venous pressure (signals via atrial low pressure receptors)
- increased angiotensin II in the brain.

DISTURBANCES OF TOTAL BODY WATER CONTENT

Changes in total body water affect the concentration of solutes in all the body compartments.

Water Depletion

Pure water depletion is rare in clinical practice. More usually it is associated with sodium depletion. Pure water depletion usually results from decreased water intake.

Causes of water depletion include:

- Diminished oral intake:
  - exhaustion
  - inability to swallow, e.g. comatose
  - restricted intake after gastrointestinal surgery.
- Loss of fluid from the lungs.
- Hyperventilation with unhumidified air.
- Diabetes insipidus.
- Diuretic phase of acute renal failure.

Pure water deficiency is reflected biochemically by hypernatraemia. This is associated with:

- increase in plasma osmolality
- concentrated urine
- a low urine sodium concentration despite the hypernatraemia.

Clinical manifestations are usually due to the hypernatraemia, which can depress the central nervous system (CNS), leading to lethargy or coma. The sodium plasma level is usually in excess of 160 mmol/L. Treatment consists of administration of water intravenously as 5% dextrose in water.

Water Intoxication

This is more common in clinical practice. It occurs with the administration of excessively large amounts of water in patients who are unable to excrete it. It is difficult to produce water intoxication in health, the kidneys having a maximal excretory rate of about 750 mL water per hour.

Causes of water intoxication include:

- Impaired renal excretion of water, e.g.
  - renal failure with excessive intake
  - excessive administration of 5% dextrose in the postoperative period when ADH secretion is high
  - ADH-secreting tumours.
- Cardiac failure.
- Liver disease.
- Hypoalbuminaemia.

TABLE 7.1 Disturbances of Body Water

	Osmolality of Body Fluid	Compartment Affected	Clinical Manifestation
Water Excess			
Primary	Reduced	ICF ↑, ECF ↑	Water intoxication
Secondary to Na^+ ↑	Normal	ECF ↑	Oedema
Water Depletion			
Primary	Increased	ICF ↓, ECF ↓	Thirst
Secondary to Na^+ ↓	Normal	ECF ↓	Circulatory collapse

The commonest cause of water intoxication in surgical practice is excessive fluid administration in patients with compromised renal function.

Pure water excess is reflected by:

- peripheral oedema
- raised central venous pressure (CVP)
- pulmonary oedema.

Treatment depends on the degree of overhydration. If it is associated with gross pulmonary oedema and is life-threatening, dialysis or continuous veno–venous haemofiltration is indicated. With less severe causes and previous normal renal function, water restriction and the administration of a diuretic will suffice. If cardiac failure is present, digitalization may be indicated. A summary of the disturbances of body water is shown in Table 7.1.

ELECTROLYTE DISORDERS

Sodium

- Major cation in the ECF.
- 100–300 mmol Na^+ are consumed daily in a typical diet.
- Almost all this is absorbed from the gastrointestinal tract, only about 5–10 mmol daily being lost in faeces.
- Excretion of sodium is chiefly renal, the only other route in health being from the skin as sweat.
- Loss of Na^+ in sweat is extremely variable.
- Each litre of sweat contains 30–50 mmol Na^+; loss of a few litres of sweat can cause a significant loss of sodium from ECF.

Regulation of Sodium

This occurs by both:

- renal mechanisms
- extrarenal mechanisms.

Renal

- 99% of the filtered sodium is reabsorbed: 65% in the proximal tubule, 25% in the loop of Henle, and approximately 10% in the distal tubules and collecting ducts.
- Regulation of sodium balance in the kidney is determined by:
  - glomerular filtration rate (GFR)
  - renin–angiotensin mechanism
  - several prostaglandins.
- Angiotensin II has two important intrarenal effects:
  - stimulates Na^+ reabsorption in most nephron segments
  - constricts the glomerular arterioles.
- Above two factors favour Na^+ retention and restoration of ECF volume.

Extrarenal

- Renin–angiotensin mechanism via aldosterone.
- Atrial natriuretic peptide (ANP).
- Circulating angiotensin II stimulates release of aldosterone from zona glomerulosa of adrenal gland.
- Aldosterone promotes sodium reabsorption in the distal tubule and collecting ducts as well as in colonic epithelium and the ducts of salivary and sweat glands.
- ANP is released from the cardiac atria in response to stretch.
- ANP increases the excretion of Na^+:
  - by increasing GFR
  - inhibiting Na^+ reabsorption in the collecting ducts
  - reducing the secretion of renin and aldosterone.

Sodium Excess

Hypernatraemia is usually a sign of water depletion, but other causes may be apparent. These are shown in Box 7.1.

With sodium retention:

- The osmolality of ECF increases.
- This results in the release of ADH and retention of water in distal tubule.
- This increases the volume of ECF and restores osmolality to normal.
- Sodium excess presents with dependent oedema, increase in body weight and eventually pulmonary oedema.

BOX 7.1 Causes of Hypernatraemia

Sodium excess
- Excessive intravenous sodium therapy, especially postoperatively
- Conn's syndrome (primary hyperaldosteronism)
- Cushing's syndrome
- Steroid therapy
- Chronic congestive cardiac failure (CCF)
- Cirrhosis of the liver

Water depletion
- Reduced water intake, e.g. coma, confusion
- Renal, e.g. osmotic diuresis, diuretic phase of acute renal failure, post-relief of obstructive uropathy, diabetes insipidus
- Others, e.g. fever, burns, diarrhoea, fistulae

- Treatment of sodium excess is aimed at a reduction of intake together with treatment of the underlying cause, e.g. the use of spironolactone in Conn's syndrome or liver disease, or digitalization in congestive cardiac failure.
- If hypernatraemia is a reflection of water depletion then increase in water intake by intravenous administration of 5% dextrose will usually suffice.

Sodium Depletion

- Hyponatraemia may be the result of:
  - water retention
  - sodium depletion.

  The causes of sodium deficiency are shown in Box 7.2.

BOX 7.2 Causes of Sodium Deficiency

- Low intake:
  - saline-free intravenous solutions
  - reduced oral intake, e.g. coma, dysphagia
- Excessive loss via gastrointestinal tract
  - diarrhoea
  - intestinal obstruction
  - fistulae
  - paralytic ileus
- Excessive sweating, e.g. fever
- Burns
- Drainage of ascites
- Addison's disease
- Diuretics
- Inappropriate secretion of ADH:
  - bronchogenic carcinoma
  - head injury

Sodium depletion initially results in:

- decrease in osmolality of ECF
- as long as osmoregulation continues, loss of Na^+ leads to loss of water at a rate of 1 L per 150 mmol of Na^+
- water loss is shared between plasma and extravascular ECF
- consequences are more serious for the circulation than those of primary water depletion since ECF and plasma are chiefly affected by the water deficiency
- chief manifestation of depletion of body Na^+ is peripheral circulatory failure. Treatment involves:
  - hyponatraemia due to ECF depletion: usually treated with isotonic saline, as sodium loss is invariably accompanied by water loss. Infusion of normal saline requires close monitoring with checking of serum electrolytes and measurement of urinary sodium, which increases with adequate sodium repletion
  - hyponatraemia: an apparently normal or high ECF volume should be treated by water restriction. Avoidance of a diuretic is advisable since this may remove nearly as much sodium as water
  - severe hyponatraemia (<119 mEq/L) with clinical symptoms such as fits, confusion or coma, should be treated with hypertonic saline.

Potassium

Potassium is the chief intracellular cation, 98% of it being within cells. The intracellular concentration (150 mmol/L) is not critical but a two- to threefold increase or decrease in the extracellular concentration can paralyze muscle or cause cardiac arrest. Rapid loss of 5% of intracellular K^+ into the ECF would be lethal.

Factors affecting plasma potassium include:

- aldosterone: increases renal excretion by effects on distal tubule
- insulin: promotes entry of K^+ into cells
- acid–base balance: acidosis results in increased plasma K^+ due to reduced entry into cells and reduced urinary excretion. Alkalosis causes the opposite effect
- hydration: K^+ is lost from cells in dehydration and returns when the patient is rehydrated
- catabolic states, e.g. trauma, major surgery, infection: K^+ is lost from the cells.

Hyperkalaemia

Hyperkalaemia is a potentially fatal condition of insidious onset. The causes are shown in Box 7.3.

Clinically, signs may be difficult to detect and sudden cardiac arrhythmia with cardiac arrest may be the first sign. Laboratory tests will confirm high serum K^+ with acidosis. Electrocardiogram (ECG) changes include:

BOX 7.3 Causes of Hyperkalaemia

- Excess administration of potassium, especially rapidly
- Renal failure
- Haemolysis
- Crush injuries
- Tissue necrosis, e.g. burns, ischaemia
- Metabolic acidosis
- Adrenal insufficiency (Addison's disease)

- peaked T-waves
- loss of P-waves
- widening of the QRS complex.

Urgent treatment of hyperkalaemia is required. The following methods are available:

- infusion of calcium gluconate
- infusion of glucose and insulin
- ion-exchange resins, e.g. resonium
- haemodialysis.

Hypokalaemia

Potassium depletion is usually the result of abnormal losses from:

- gastrointestinal tract
- renal tract.

The causes are shown in Box 7.4.

BOX 7.4 Causes of Hypokalaemia

Inadequate intake

- Potassium-free intravenous fluids
- Reduced oral intake:
  - coma
  - dysphagia

Excessive loss

- Renal:
  - diuretics
  - renal tubular disorders
- Gastrointestinal:
  - diarrhoea
  - vomiting
  - fistulae
  - laxatives
  - villous adenoma
- Endocrine:
  - Cushing's syndrome
  - steroid therapy
  - hyperaldosteronism (primary and secondary)

The following are features of hypokalaemia:

- clinical fatigue and lethargy with eventual muscle weakness
- low serum K^+ together with alkalosis
- ECG changes include low broad T-waves in the presence of U-waves
- treatment is by correction with oral supplements, or in severe cases slow intravenous replacement with careful monitoring.

ACID–BASE BALANCE

During the course of daily metabolism, approximately 70 mEq of hydrogen ion is released into the body fluids. A large amount of carbon dioxide is produced, which combines with water to form carbonic acid (H_2CO_3). Methods to eliminate this acid are necessary, otherwise the pH of the body fluids would fall rapidly.

The following are important buffer systems in the body:

- proteins
- haemoglobin
- phosphate
- bicarbonate.

The bicarbonate system is important in that:

- CO_2 is excreted in the lungs and can be regulated by changes in ventilation
- bicarbonate excretion is also regulated in the kidney.

Carbonic Acid–Bicarbonate System

The carbonic acid–bicarbonate system ($H_2O + CO_2 \leftrightharpoons H_2\ CO_3^- \leftrightharpoons HCO_3^-$) is catalysed by carbonic anhydrase. The Henderson–Hasselbach equation is derived from this, i.e.

$$pH = pK + \log\frac{[HCO_3^-]}{[H_2CO_3]}$$

The pK for the HCO_3^-/H_2CO_3 system is 6.1. The carbonic acid is more usually expressed in terms of carbon dioxide, and the equation then becomes:

$$pH = 6.1 + \log\frac{[HCO_3^-]}{0.03 \times PCO_2}$$

where 0.03 is the solubility of CO_2 expressed in mmol/L. mmHg and PCO_2 in mmHg.

The equation makes it clear that pH depends on the ratio of $[HCO_3^-]$ to PCO_2, i.e. the buffer pair. $[HCO_3^-]$ is controlled slowly by the kidneys while CO_2 is controlled rapidly by the lungs.

If the CO_2 rises so will the bicarbonate to keep the $[HCO_3^-]/PCO_2$ ratio constant.

Similarly, if bicarbonate falls there will be a fall in PCO_2 to prevent a change in pH. If the primary change is an alteration in CO_2 it is called a respiratory acidosis or alkalosis;

if it is a primary change in [HCO_3^-] it is called a metabolic acidosis or alkalosis.

A simple way of looking at the Henderson–Hasselbach equation is:

$$pH = constant + \frac{kidney\ function}{lung\ function}$$

Basically, the regulation of pH is achieved through control of:

- excretion of H^+ and re-absorption of [HCO_3–] by the kidneys
- excretion of CO_2 by the lungs through regulation of alveolar ventilation
- buffering of H^+ by other buffering systems within the body.

Disturbances of Acid–Base Balance

- Primary respiratory disturbances cause changes in PCO_2 and produce corresponding effects on blood hydrogen ion concentration.
- Primary metabolic disturbances affect the plasma bicarbonate.
- Whether the disturbance is primarily respiratory or metabolic, some degree of compensation occurs in either numerator or denominator of the Henderson–Hasselbach equation to limit or negate the change in blood pH.
- Changes in PCO_2 from respiratory disturbances are compensated for by renal tubular handling of bicarbonate.
- The metabolic disturbances are compensated for by appropriate respiratory change.

Respiratory Acidosis

The causes are shown in Box 7.5.

- Caused by CO_2 retention due to inadequate alveolar ventilation.
- ↓pH ↑PCO_2.
- Compensation occurs by:
  - ↑HCO_3– by bicarbonate buffer system
  - ↓H^+ by kidneys.
- In acute respiratory acidosis there is little time for bicarbonate to increase as a consequence of raised arterial CO_2; therefore, bicarbonate may be normal.
- In chronic CO_2 retention, although CO_2 levels may be high, the pH is not so depressed, because kidneys compensate by retaining bicarbonate in response to increased PCO_2.

Respiratory Alkalosis

The causes are shown in Box 7.6.

- Occurs when carbon dioxide is lost via excessive pulmonary ventilation.
- ↑pH ↓PCO_2.

BOX 7.5 Causes of Respiratory Acidosis (Any Cause of Hypoventilation)

Respiratory depression
- CNS depression:
  - head injury
  - drugs, e.g. opiates, anaesthetics
  - coma
  - cerebrovascular accident (CVA)
  - encephalitis
- Neuromuscular disease:
  - myasthenia gravis
  - Guillain–Barré syndrome
- Skeletal disease:
  - kyphoscoliosis
  - ankylosing spondylitis
  - flail chest
- Artificial ventilation (uncontrolled and unmonitored)
- Impaired gaseous exchange:
  - thoracic injury, e.g. pulmonary contusions
  - obstructive airway disease (acute and chronic)
  - alveolar disease e.g. pneumonia, ARDS

BOX 7.6 Causes of Respiratory Alkalosis (Any Cause of Hyperventilation)

Stimulation of respiratory centre
- High altitude (hypoxia)
- Pneumonia
- Pulmonary oedema
- Pulmonary embolism
- Fever
- Head injury
- Metabolic acidosis (overcompensation)

Increased alveolar gas exchange
- Hyperventilation, e.g. hysteria, pain, anxiety
- Artificial ventilation (uncontrolled)

- Compensation occurs by:
  - ↓HCO_3– by bicarbonate buffer system
  - ↑H^+ by kidneys.
- Acute hyperventilation lowers the PCO_2 without concomitant changes in plasma HCO_3^-.
- In chronic hyperventilation HCO_3^- is reduced.

Metabolic Acidosis

The causes are shown in Box 7.7.

- Results from increased production of hydrogen ion from metabolic causes or from excessive bicarbonate losses, leading to a decrease in pH and a compensatory decrease in PCO_2.

BOX 7.7 Causes of Metabolic Acidosis

Excessive production of H^+
- Diabetic ketoacidosis
- Lactic acidosis secondary to hypoxia
- Septicaemia
- Starvation

Impaired excretion of H^+
- Acute renal failure
- Chronic renal failure

Excess loss of base
- Diarrhoea
- Intestinal, biliary and pancreatic fistulae

BOX 7.8 Causes of Metabolic Alkalosis

Excess loss of H^+
- Vomiting
- Nasogastric aspiration
- Gastric fistula
- Diuretic therapy (thiazide or loop)
- Cushing's syndrome
- Conn's syndrome

Excessive intake of base
- Antacids, e.g. milk–alkali syndrome

- ↓pH ↓HCO_3^-.
- Compensation occurs by:
  - ↓PCO_2 by hyperventilation
  - ↓H^+ by kidneys (unless renal failure).

Metabolic Alkalosis

Causes are shown in Box 7.8.

- Results from primary disturbance of an increase in HCO_3^- or a decrease in H^+.
- ↑pH ↑HCO_3^-.
- Compensation occurs by:
  - ↑PCO_2 by hypoventilation (limited by hypoxia)
  - ↓HCO_3^- by kidneys.

Mixed Acid–Base Disorders

- In many situations mixed disorders occur.
- Commonest example in surgical practice is a combination of a metabolic acidosis and respiratory alkalosis.
- This may occur in:
  - renal failure
  - sepsis
  - septic shock.
- As the two acid–base disorders tend to cancel one another out, the disturbance in H^+ is usually small.
- Respiratory acidosis and metabolic acidosis may occur together in:
  - adult respiratory distress syndrome (ARDS)
  - cardiac failure
  - cardiorespiratory arrest.
- Respiratory alkalosis and metabolic alkalosis in combination is rare, but may occur when over-ventilating a patient with chronic respiratory acidosis.

A summary of disturbances of acid–base balance is shown in Table 7.2.

Interpretation of Acid–Base Changes

A blood gas analyser usually prints out the variables shown below (normal values).

- temperature: 37°C
- pH: 7.35–7.45
- PCO_2: 4.6–5.8 kPa (35–44 mmHg)
- PO_2: 10–13 kPa (75–100 mmHg)
- HCO_3^- (actual): 22–28 mmol/L
- total CO_2: 24–28 mmol/L
- standard bicarbonate: 22–26 mmol/L
- base excess: −2 to +2 mmol/L
- standard base excess: −3 to +3 mmol/L
- O_2 saturation: >95%
- Hb: 11.5–15.5 g/dL.

As the patient's acid–base status varies, three factors are changing at the same time:

- pH
- PCO_2
- HCO_3^-.

TABLE 7.2 Disturbances of Acid–Base Balance

Abnormality	Primary Disturbance	pH	Base Excess	Compensatory Mechanism
Metabolic acidosis	$[HCO_3^-]$ ↓	↓	−ve	PCO_2 ↓
Respiratory acidosis	PCO_2 ↑	↓		$[HCO_3^-]$ ↑
Metabolic alkalosis	$[HCO_3^-]$ ↑	↑	+ve	PCO_2 ↑
Respiratory alkalosis	PCO_2 ↓	↑		$[HCO_3^-]$ ↓

Blood gas machines measure PO_2, pH and PCO_2 directly. Bicarbonate is calculated from the Henderson–Hasselbach equation. The standard bicarbonate is a value obtained after correction of the PCO_2 to 40 mmHg (5.3 kPa). This correction is required in order to remove any respiratory component. In other words, it indicates what the bicarbonate would be if there was no respiratory disturbance.

- The normal standard bicarbonate is 22–26 mmol/L.
- Values above this range indicate metabolic alkalosis.
- Values below this range indicate metabolic acidosis.

Interpretation of blood gas analysis should be performed systematically:

1. First the pH should be noticed; this indicates whether the patient is acidotic or alkalotic.
2. Next, the PCO_2 is noted; this will indicate the respiratory component, i.e. it will be elevated in respiratory acidosis and decreased in respiratory alkalosis.
3. Next, the standard bicarbonate or base excess is noted; both give the same information, i.e. metabolic acid–base status after correcting for the PCO_2.
4. Serum electrolytes should be checked and the anion gap calculated.

Anion gap

- Normally between 10 and 19 mmol/L.
- Reflects the concentration of those anions present in the serum but not routinely measured, e.g. phosphates, organic acids.
- For electrochemical neutrality of the ECF, the number of anions must equal the number of cations.
- Normally only Na^+, K^+, HCO_3^- and Cl^- are measured in the laboratory.
- When the normal values of these are added they do not balance, i.e. Na^+ (140) + K^+ (5)=145; and HCO_3^- (25) + Cl^- (105)=130.
- The difference, 15 mEq/L, is known as the anion gap and represents anions that are not usually measured.
- With excessive bicarbonate loss, e.g. diarrhoea, fistulae, decrease in plasma HCO_3^- is matched by an increase in serum Cl^- so that the anion gap remains around normal level.
- Metabolic acidosis resulting from an increase in production of acid is associated with an increased anion gap, e.g. lactic acidosis secondary to hypoxia, ketoacidosis of diabetes and renal failure.

FLUID BALANCE AND FLUID REPLACEMENT THERAPY

An average adult normally loses between 2.5 and 3 L of fluid in 24 h, approximately 1 L being lost from the skin and lungs (insensible losses), 100 mL in the faeces and the remainder in the urine. About 100–150 mmol of Na^+ and 50–100 mmol K^+ are lost in the urine each day. This is usually balanced by normal dietary intake.

Fluid Balance in the Uncomplicated Patient

- Requires 2.5–3 L intravenous fluid containing 150 mmol of Na^+ and 60 mmol of K^+ per day.
- A suitable fluid regimen for 24 h would therefore be as follows:
  - 500 mL 0.9% sodium chloride + 20 mmol KCl
  - 500 mL 5% dextrose
  - 500 mL 5% dextrose + 20 mmol KCl
  - 500 mL 0.9% sodium chloride
  - 500 mL 5% dextrose + 20 mmol KCl
  - 500 mL 5% dextrose.

  Each bag of fluid is given over 4 h.

Change in Fluid and Electrolyte Requirements in Response to Surgery and Trauma

Following surgery or trauma, certain physiological responses occur in the body:

- catecholamines are released
- stress stimulates the hypothalamo–pituitary–adrenal axis with an increased secretion of cortisol and aldosterone
- these hormones produce conservation of sodium and water by the kidney, resulting in a reduction of urine volume and urine sodium concentration
- if renal perfusion falls, e.g. due to haemorrhage or fluid loss into other spaces, the renin–angiotensin–aldosterone mechanism is activated
- this promotes reabsorption of sodium and water, and more potassium is lost in the urine
- ADH secretion from the posterior pituitary also leads to water conservation
- despite loss of potassium in the urine, serum K^+ does not usually fall but may even rise, due to release of potassium from tissue damage caused by trauma or surgery or administration of stored blood containing excessive potassium.

These factors must be taken into account when prescribing intravenous fluids, particularly in the first 24 h after major surgery. The regimen described above for an uncomplicated patient may not be appropriate, and an appropriate regimen for the first 24 h postoperatively is as follows:

- 500 mL 0.9% sodium chloride
- 500 mL 5% dextrose
- 500 mL 5% dextrose
- 500 mL 5% dextrose.

  Each bag of fluid is given over 6 h.

Fluid and Electrolyte Problems in Surgical Patients

The common causes of fluid and electrolyte loss in surgical patients are shown in Box 7.9.

BOX 7.9 Causes of Fluid Loss in Surgical Patients

Blood
- Trauma
- Surgery

Plasma
- Burns

Gastrointestinal
- Nasogastric aspiration
- Vomiting
- Diarrhoea
- Intraluminal:
  - intestinal obstruction
  - paralytic ileus
- Fistulae
- Stomas

Exudate in peritoneal cavity
- Peritonitis
- Acute pancreatitis (also into the retroperitoneum)
- Septicaemia

Excess insensible loss
- Fever
- Sweating
- Hyperventilation

Blood and Plasma

- Blood loss may be rapid, the loss of 1 L causing hypotension and hypovolaemic shock.
- Blood is normally replaced by blood, but initially plasma expanders such as gelatin solutions are used until cross-matched blood is available.
- Less rapid haemorrhage allows time for the loss to be replaced from the extracellular extravascular compartment.
- Greater volumes may be lost slowly before the circulation is compromised.
- Plasma lost from severe burns is replaced by plasma, the anticipated losses being replaced according to a standard formula.

Gastrointestinal Losses

- 6–10 L of electrolyte-rich fluid are secreted in the upper GI tract daily (Table 7.3).
- Most of this is reabsorbed lower down in the intestine.
- Abnormal fluid losses must be measured or estimated as accurately as possible.
- With sequestration of fluid in the bowel lumen, e.g. in ileus, only an estimate can be made, but with fistulae the amount can be measured accurately and its electrolyte content assessed.
- As a general rule, gastrointestinal fluid loss should be replaced with normal saline with the addition of potassium as necessary.
- Regular assessment of serum electrolytes will provide information regarding their requirements.

Intraperitoneal Fluid Loss

- Peritonitis and acute pancreatitis will result in loss of fluid into the peritoneal cavity.
- In pancreatitis, fluid is also lost into the retroperitoneum.
- These losses should be made good by plasma substitutes and normal saline.

Septicaemia

- Septic shock associated with peripheral vasodilatation causing relative hypovolaemia.
- Large increase in capillary permeability results in extensive loss of protein and electrolytes into the extracellular space.
- This loss combined with peripheral vasodilatation results in collapse and shock.
- Fluid replacement is with plasma expanders and normal saline.
- Exact fluid loss is difficult to estimate but should be monitored by:
  - urine output
  - blood pressure

TABLE 7.3 Normal Daily Gastrointestinal Secretion Volumes and Electrolyte Composition

Secretion	Volume (L)	Na^+ (mmol/L)	K^+ (mmol/L)	Cl^- (mmol/L)	HCO_3 (mmol/L)
Saliva	1–1.5	20–80	10–20	20–40	20–160
Gastric juice	1–2.5	40–100	5–10	120–140	0
Bile	0.5–1.5	140–200	5–10	40–60	20–60
Pancreatic juice	1–2	130	5–10	10–60	80–120
Succus entericus	2–3	140	5	variable	variable

- central venous pressure (CVP)
- pulmonary wedge pressure monitoring.

Excessive Insensible Fluid Loss

- Insensible fluid loss may be greatly increased in the ill patient.
- Pyrexia increases insensible losses by about 10% for each °C rise in temperature.
- Loss is chiefly from the lungs as expired water vapour.
- Excessive sweating causes loss of sodium-rich fluid, sweat containing about 50 mEq Na^+/L
- May be overlooked in the pyrexial patient in hot, humid ward in summer months.

COLLOID AND CRYSTALLOID SOLUTIONS

Colloids are osmotically active particles in solution.

Types

- Albumin: human albumin solution.
- Dextran: dextran 70 in 0.9% saline or 5% glucose.
- Gelatin: polygeline (Haemaccel); succinylated gelatin (Gelofusin).
- Hydroxyethyl starch: hetastarch (Hespan).
- Pentastarch (Pentaspan).

Uses

- Maintenance of plasma volume.
- Acute replacement of plasma volume deficit.
- Short-term volume expansion (gelatin, dextran).
- Medium-term volume expansion (albumin, pentastarch).
- Long-term volume expansion (hetastarch).

Albumin

- 5% and 20% human albumin solution.
- Used for replacement of plasma protein and expansion of plasma volume.
- No evidence that maintenance of plasma albumin levels, as opposed to maintenance of plasma colloid osmotic pressure with artificial plasma substitutes, is advantageous.
- 20% albumin used for replacement of plasma protein:
  - in severe hypoproteinaemia in renal or liver disease
  - after large-volume paracentesis
  - after massive liver resection.
- Some leaks through capillary membrane (in patients with capillary leak).
- Suppresses albumin synthesis.

Dextran

- Glucose polymers of different molecular weights.
- Dextran 70 formerly popular as plasma substitute.
- Interferes with cross-matching.
- Interferes with coagulation (factor VIII↓; inhibits platelet aggregation).
- Relatively high incidence of allergic reactions.

Gelatins

- Prepared by hydrolysis of bovine collagen.
- Do not affect coagulation per se.
- Low incidence of allergic reactions.
- Small average particle size; therefore, stay in intravascular space shorter period of time.
- Polygeline (Haemaccel):
  - contains K^+; also contains Ca^{2+}, which can cause coagulation if mixed with citrated blood in giving set
  - stays shorter time in circulation.
- Succinylated gelatin (Gelofusin):
  - larger molecular weight than polygeline; therefore, slightly longer effect
  - does not contain calcium.

Hydroxyethyl Starch

- Longer half-life in plasma.
- 10% solutions hyperoncotic; hence increasing plasma volume by more than volume infused.
- Hetastarch (Hespan):
  - 6% in saline has largest molecular weight of any plasma expander and therefore stays in circulation longer
  - most useful in capillary leak
  - may cause coagulopathy
  - high degree of protection from metabolism.
- Pentastarch (Pentaspan):
  - lower degree of protection from metabolism
  - shorter-lasting effect than Hetastarch.

Choice of Plasma Expanders

- Succinylated gelatin (Gelofusin) has most advantages in acute hypovolaemia:
  - short-acting
  - useful until blood becomes available
  - no calcium; therefore, does not cause coagulation if mixed with citrated blood in giving set
  - cheap.
- Hetastarch (Hespan):
  - has most advantages in chronic (continuing) hypovolaemia
  - longer-acting
  - larger molecules better retained in circulation when capillaries leaky, e.g. septic shock
  - high degree of protection from metabolism.

General Problems of Plasma Expanders

- Dilution coagulopathy.
- Allergic reactions.

TABLE 7.4 **Composition of Common Crystalloid Solutions**

mmol/L	N Saline	Hartmann's Solution	4% Dextrose/ 1/5N Saline	5% Dextrose	Sodium Bicarbonate (1.26%)
Na^+	155	131	30	0	150
K^+	0	5	0	0	0
Ca^{++}	0	2	0	0	0
Cl^-	155	111	30	0	0
HCO_3^-	0	29[a]	0	0	150
Osmolality (mosmol/L)	308	280	284	278	300

[a]In the form of lactate which is metabolized to bicarbonate in the liver.

- Interfering with cross-matching (dextran 70).
- Persistence of colloid effect dependent on molecular size and protection from metabolism.
- All artificial colloids are polydisperse, i.e. there is a range of molecular sizes.

Crystalloids

Crystalloids are salt ions in water.

Common Types

- Normal saline (0.9%).
- 4% dextrose/(1/5) normal saline.
- Glucose, e.g. 5% glucose or stronger solutions.
- Sodium bicarbonate, e.g. 1.26%, 8.4%.
- Potassium chloride.

The content of these solutions is shown in Table 7.4.

Uses

- Provision of daily requirements of water and electrolytes.
- Plasma volume should be replaced with colloids, since crystalloids are rapidly lost from plasma.
- Of a volume of crystalloid infused initially, one-third stays in intravascular compartment and two-thirds pass to ECF; therefore, risk of oedema if excessive infusion.
- Advantage that ECF deficit is replaced in shock.
- 5% glucose is used to supply intravenous water requirements, 50 g/L glucose being present to ensure an isotonic solution.
- Hartmann's solution has no practical advantages over 0.9% saline for fluid maintenance; however, may be useful if large volumes of crystalloid are exchanged (e.g. during continuous haemofiltration) to maintain acid–base balance.
- Higher concentrations of glucose are used to prevent or treat hypoglycaemia.
- Sodium bicarbonate is used to correct metabolic acidosis.
- Potassium chloride is used to supplement K^+ in crystalloid fluids. Safety rules for giving K^+ include:
  - urine output of at least 40 mL/h
  - not more than 40 mmol to be added to 1 L of fluid
  - infusion rate no faster than 40 mmol/h.

OEDEMA AND LYMPHATIC FUNCTION

Oedema is an increase in the volume of interstitial fluid above normal levels.

- A hydrostatic pressure difference across the capillary endothelium results in flow from vessel to tissue space.
- Retention of plasma proteins within the vasculature is an opposing force, i.e. the plasma oncotic pressure.
- The Starling equilibrium describes the relationship between hydrostatic pressure, oncotic pressure (colloid osmotic pressure) and fluid flow across the capillary membrane.
- The Starling equilibrium states:
  - capillary hydrostatic pressure + tissue oncotic pressure (pressure tending to drive fluid out of the capillary) = interstitial fluid pressure + plasma oncotic pressure (pressure tending to hold fluid into the capillary).

The Starling equilibrium across the capillary is shown in Fig. 7.1. Filtration is favoured at the arterial end of the capillary, while absorption is favoured at the venous end of the capillary. Any fluid not reabsorbed from the interstitium by the capillaries is returned to the circulation by the lymphatic system.

Causes of Oedema

Causes of oedema are:

- Increased capillary hydrostatic pressure:

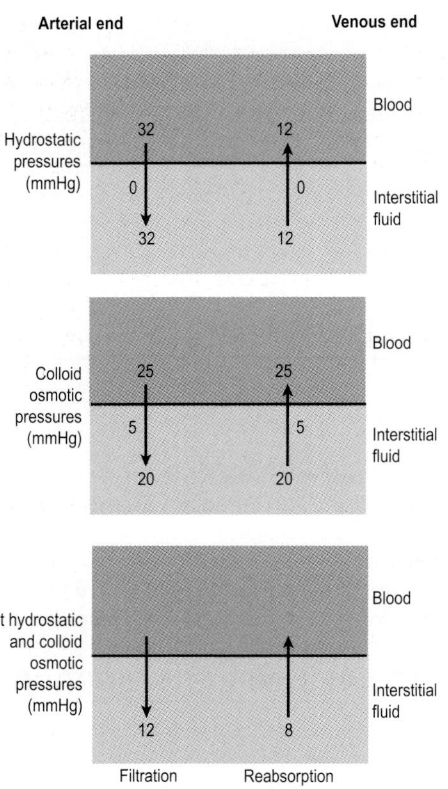

Fig. 7.1 Starling equilibrium across capillary.

- chronic right heart failure
- venous obstruction
- increased fluid volume (e.g. overtransfusion).

- Decreased plasma oncotic pressure due to hypoproteinaemia:
  - starvation
  - cirrhosis
  - nephrotic syndrome.
- Increased capillary permeability:
  - inflammatory reactions
  - allergic reactions.
- Increased tissue oncotic pressure:
  - lymphatic blockage
  - protein accumulation in burns.

Obstruction to Lymphatics

Lymphatics remove protein and excess fluid that has been filtered at the arterial end of the capillary and not reabsorbed at the venous end. If lymphatics are obstructed, then this fluid cannot return to the vascular system and accumulates behind the obstruction, causing oedema. Lymphatic obstruction may occur due to lymph node pathology as a result of:

- surgical removal, e.g. axillary clearance with mastectomy or block dissection
- metastatic tumours
- irradiation
- filariasis.

OSCE SCENARIOS

OSCE Scenario 7.1

A 64-year-old male is admitted for a right hemicolectomy and is found to have a serum sodium of 120 mmol/L.

1. What are the possible causes of hyponatraemia in this patient?
2. Describe what investigations you would carry out in order to identify the cause of the hyponatraemia.
3. How would you correct it?

OSCE Scenario 7.2

An 82-year-old male is transferred to ITU following a Hartmann's procedure for perforated diverticular disease. He has been anuric for 3 h. A number of fluid challenges have been given, achieving a BP of 120/90, pulse of 87 and a CVP of 10. ABG analysis shows a pH of 7.2 and U&Es reveal serum potassium of 7.1 mmol/L.

1. What are the possible causes of hyperkalaemia in this patient?
2. What are the ECG changes associated with hyperkalaemia?
3. What would be your possible treatment options for this patient? Explain how each works to lower the serum potassium.

OSCE Scenario 7.3

A 56-year-old male is admitted with severe dehydration and vomiting. His urea came back raised at 15 mmol/L and his creatinine level was at 215 μmol/L. A blood gas analysis shows the following abnormalities – pH 7.55, PO_2 10.9 kPa, CO_2 6.9 kPa and HCO_3 is 21.

1. What type of metabolic abnormality is this patient displaying?
2. How has it occurred?
3. The patient has a 'sucussion splash' on examination. What is the diagnosis?
4. How would you manage this condition?

OSCE Scenario 7.4

A 35-year-old female patient with weight of 70 kg underwent uncomplicated appendicectomy. As she arrives back to the ward, the nurses ask you to prescribe her intravenous fluids for the next 24 h as she is unable to eat and drink due to nausea.

1. What are the volumes of the fluid compartments of the body?
2. In general, what are the average daily fluid and electrolyte requirements?
3. What intravenous fluids would you prescribe for the next 24 h?

OSCE Scenario 7.5

A 65-year-old male patient is brought to the Accident and Emergency department with acute abdominal pain. He looks very unwell and is in obvious pain and is very confused. He is wearing a medical alert bracelet informing you he is diabetic. He has a temperature of 39°C and his blood pressure is 90/50 with a heart rate of 110. He has a rather strange smell of acetone or 'pear drop' sweets.

1. What is the diagnosis?
2. What would you expect his blood gases to show and why?
3. How would you manage this patient, explaining which electrolyte needs specific management?

Answers in Appendix pages 444–446

Please check your eBook at https://studentconsult.inkling.com/ for more self-assessment questions. See inside cover for registration details.

8

Respiratory System

INTRODUCTION

Components

The respiratory system is composed of:

- Nasal passages.
- Olfactory system.
- Conducting airways:
  - nasopharynx
  - larynx
  - trachea
  - bronchi
  - bronchioles
  - respiratory portions of the lung (alveoli).

Function

The functions of the respiratory system include:

- cleaning of inhaled air
- warming or cooling of inhaled air
- moistening of inhaled air
- respiratory gas exchange
- facilitation of olfaction and sound production.

Airway Function

The airways have three main functions:

- passage of inhaled gases
- protection against inhaled foreign material
- warming and humidification of inhaled gases.
- Passage of inhaled gases:
  - the flow of gases depends on the pressure gradient between the atmosphere and the alveoli

$$\text{Airflow}\ (V) = \frac{P_{\text{Alveoli}} - P_{\text{Atmosphere}}}{R}$$

  V: rate of airflow
  P: pressure
  R: resistance

  - the smooth muscle within the bronchi and bronchioles can influence airflow
  - bronchoconstriction, under parasympathetic control, leads to an increase in resistance (*R*) and thus a decrease in airflow
  - bronchodilatation, under sympathetic control, leads to a decrease in resistance (*R*) and thus an increase in airflow.
- Protection against inhaled foreign material:
  - inhaled air is filtered by the nasal hairs
  - any particles passing through the nose become trapped on the mucus coating the airways
  - motile cilia lining the airways transport the mucus to the pharynx, where it is swallowed
  - the epiglottis closes during swallowing, thus preventing food matter from entering the airways
  - if any food matter is inhaled, it stimulates a reflex cough that will expel the material.
- Warming and humidifying gases:
  - as inhaled air passes through the respiratory system, it is warmed and saturated with water vapour; this produces a water vapour pressure of 6.3 kPa (47 mmHg) at 37°C.

MECHANICS OF VENTILATION

Pulmonary Ventilation

- At the beginning of inspiration the intrapleural pressure is around −4 cmH_2O.
- Contraction of the respiratory muscles increases the volume of the chest; this decreases the intrapleural pressure to about −9 cmH_2O.
- The change in intrapleural pressure causes the lungs to expand, and thus generates a negative intra-alveolar pressure as the alveoli are pulled open.
- As the atmospheric pressure is higher and air flows from high to low pressure, air is inhaled (approximately 500 mL air during quiet ventilation).
- During exercise, other accessory muscles of respiration are used and can generate more negative intrapleural pressures, i.e. −30 cmH_2O. Pressures of this magnitude can lead to the inhalation of 2–3 L of air.

- Expiration is a passive process due to the elastic recoil of the chest wall.
- During exercise, contraction of internal intercostals and abdominal muscles can generate intrapleural pressures as high as +20 cmH_2O to expel air more rapidly.

Lung Pressures (Fig. 8.1)

- There are three forces acting on the lung:
  - elastic nature of the lungs: under normal conditions the lungs are stretched; this results in a force that pulls inwards on the visceral pleura
  - surfactant: lines the alveoli and exerts an inward or collapsing pressure
  - negative intrapleural pressure: opposes the above two forces. This negative pressure is created by the chest wall and diaphragm pulling the parietal pleura outwards. As the two layers of pleura are pulled in opposite directions, they generate a negative pressure.
- The pressure in the alveoli equals the atmospheric pressure as they are both in direct contact via the airways; atmospheric pressure is zero and the intrapleural pressure is between −4 and −9 cmH_2O. This produces the transmural or transpulmonary pressure; it is this that keeps the lungs distended.

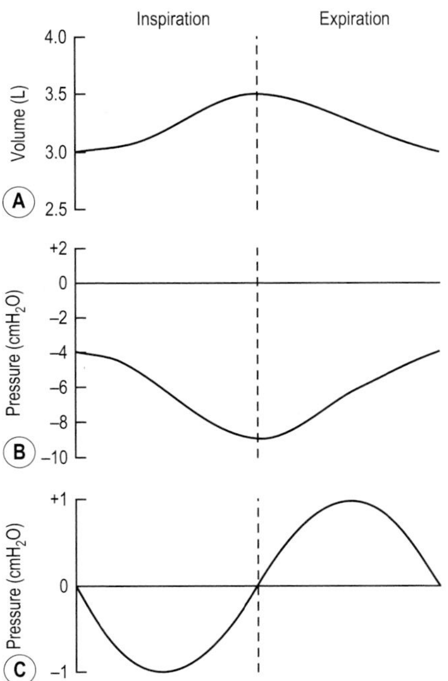

Fig. 8.1 Graphs demonstrating the relationship between (A) lung volume, (B) intrapleural, and (C) intra-alveolar pressure during normal quiet respiration. (From McGeown JG. Physiology, 2nd edn. Churchill Livingstone, Edinburgh, 2000, with permission.)

Surfactant and Surface Tension (Fig. 8.2)

- Phase 1: it takes a considerable pressure increase before there is a change in volume.
- Phase 2: expansion of the lung is proportional to the increase in pressure.
- Phase 3: maximum capacity.
- Phase 4: in the initial stage the lung volume is maintained until the pressure has fallen considerably (approximately 8 cmH_2O).
- The unequal pressure needed to maintain a given lung volume in inspiration and expiration is called hysteresis.
- Surfactant is a phospholipid-rich detergent produced by type II alveolar cells; it coats the luminal surface of alveoli and produces a force called surface tension.
- Surface tension is present at all air–fluid interfaces.
- Surface tension occurs because water molecules are attracted more to each other than they are to gas molecules. When any liquid surrounds a gas, i.e. in the alveolus, this produces an inward pressure.
- Lungs inflated with normal saline do not exhibit hysteresis; there is no air–fluid interface, so there is no surface tension; the only force opposing expansion is the elasticity of the lung parenchyma.

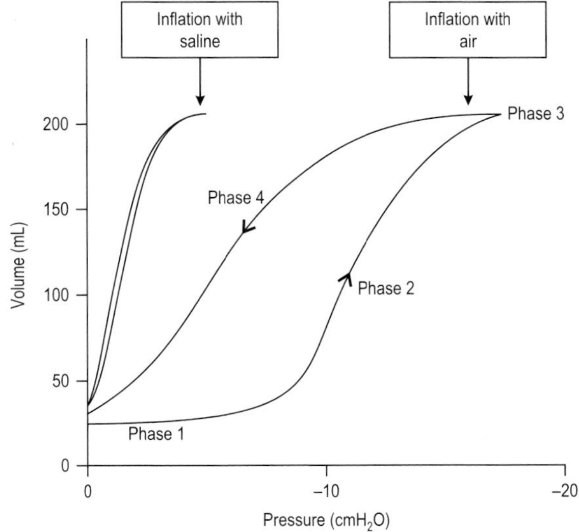

Fig. 8.2 Graph illustrating the differences in compliance between the lungs inflated with air and the lungs inflated with saline. The greater compliance in saline-filled lungs is explained by the lack of surface tension.

- In air-inflated lungs the surface tension at the air–fluid interface opposes expansion; surface tension accounts for almost two-thirds of the elastic recoil of the lungs.
- Surfactant has several other functions:
  - by lowering the surface tension, surfactant increases compliance and reduces the work of breathing
  - prevents fluid accumulating in the alveoli
  - reduces the tendency of alveoli to collapse (alveolar instability).
- Alveolar instability is related to changes in alveolar diameter and can be explained by the law of Laplace:

$$\Delta P \propto \frac{T}{r}$$

ΔP: alveolar distending pressure
T: surface tension
r: radius

- As alveoli decrease in size, the radius (r) will tend to increase (assuming surface tension [T] remains constant). If surfactant were not present, this would mean that pressure would be greater in small alveoli and lower in larger alveoli; this would result in collapse of the alveoli as air moves from the smaller to the larger alveoli.
- As the alveolar radius decreases, then the concentration of surfactant increases and thus reduces surface tension (T). Therefore, surface tension and radius increase or decrease in tandem and this results in very little change in alveolar pressure.

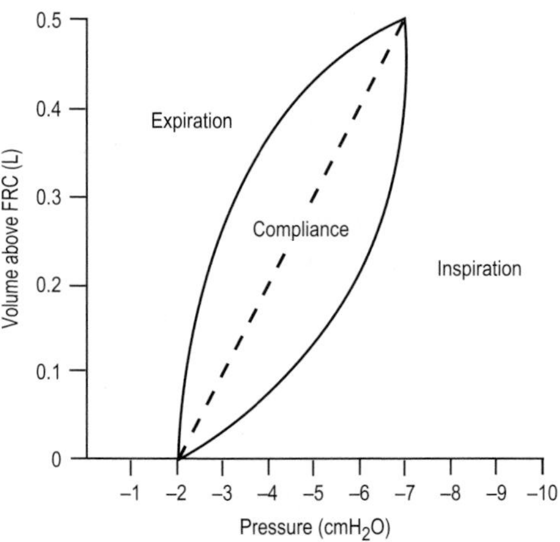

Fig. 8.3 Pressure–volume curve for a single respiratory cycle. It represents the volume change if the work of respiration was against elastic resistance only. To the right of the compliance line represents the additional pressure required to overcome airflow resistance and other resisting forces. To the left of the compliance line is the work required during passive expiration. (From Pocock G & Richards CD. Human Physiology: The Basis of Medicine, 2nd edn. Oxford University Press, Oxford, 2004, with permission.)

Compliance (Fig. 8.3)

- Compliance is the ease with which the lungs can be inflated:

$$\text{Compliance} = \frac{\Delta V}{\Delta P} = \frac{500\ \text{mL}}{5\ \text{cmH}_2\text{O}} = 100\ \text{mL/cmH}_2\text{O}$$

ΔV: change in volume
ΔP: change in pressure
↑ compliance means lungs are easy to expand.
↓ compliance means lungs resist expansion.

- Two principal factors govern compliance:
  - elasticity of the lung parenchyma
  - surface tension.
- Normal lungs have high compliance as the elastic tissue is easily stretched and surfactant reduces surface tension.
- Conditions which decrease compliance include:
  - scarring or fibrosis of lung parenchyma
  - pulmonary oedema
  - deficiency of surfactant, e.g. premature babies
  - decreased lung expansion, e.g. respiratory muscle paralysis
  - supine position
  - mechanical ventilation (due to reduced pulmonary blood flow)
  - age
  - breathing 100% O_2.
- Conditions which increase compliance include:
  - emphysema (due to destruction of elastic fibres in the lung parenchyma).

Respiratory Muscles

See Anatomy section (Chapter 1).

Work of Breathing (Fig. 8.4)

- Work of breathing is the work required to move the lung and chest wall.
- During inspiration, work consists of two components:
  - work needed to overcome the elastic forces of the chest wall and lungs
  - work needed to overcome non-elastic forces of the chest wall and lungs.

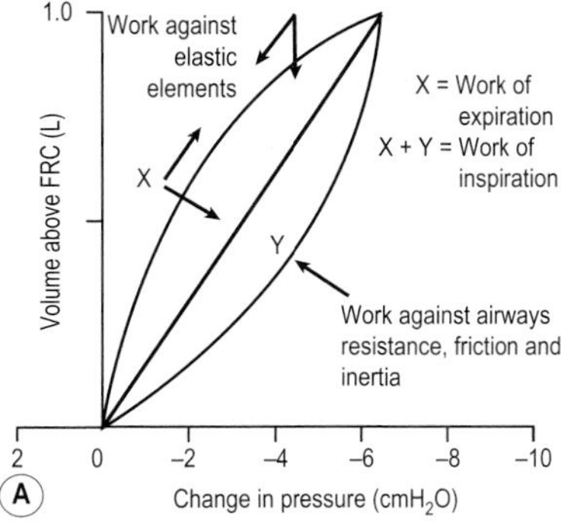

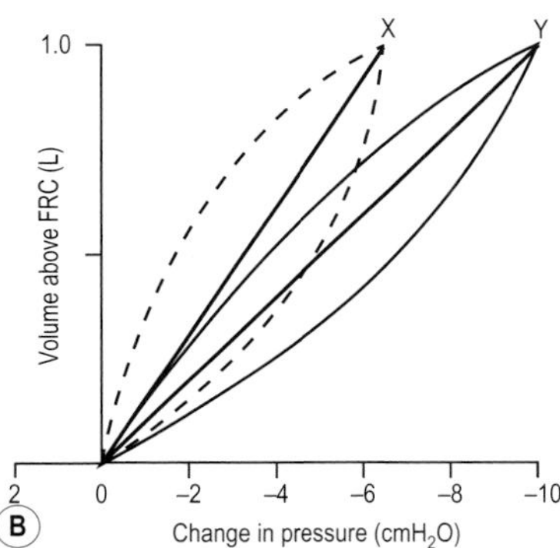

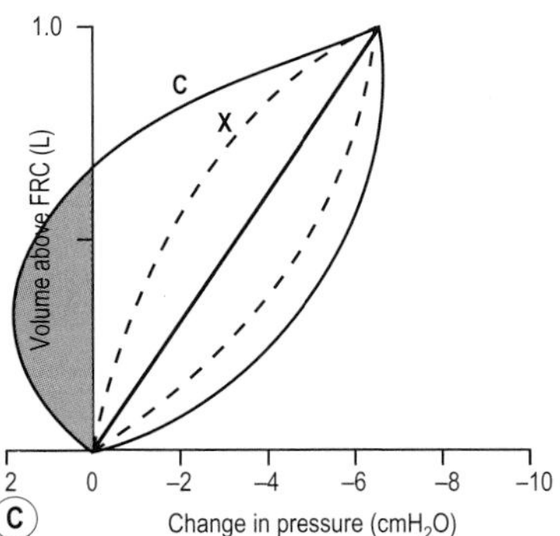

Fig. 8.4 (A) Graph demonstrating the work of respiration. The increasing volume above functional residual capacity (FRC) is plotted against the change in intrapleural pressure. The work of inspiration is greater than expiration. Energy for expiration is from the stretching of elastic lung tissue. (B) The increased pressure required to move an equal volume of air with reduced lung compliance. (C) The increased resistance to expiration and increased energy required to expire a similar volume of air in a patient with increased airways resistance. (From Pocock G & Richards CD. Human Physiology: The Basis of Medicine, 2nd edn. Oxford University Press, Oxford, 2004, with permission.)

- Non-elastic forces include:
  - airway resistance (most significant)
  - frictional forces
  - inertia of the air and tissues.
- One-third of airway resistance occurs in the upper airways – nose, pharynx and larynx. This can be greatly reduced by breathing through the mouth (e.g. during exercise).
- Two-thirds of the resistance is in the tracheobronchial tree, mainly in the medium-sized bronchi (high flow but low cross-sectional area).
- Resistance in the terminal bronchioles is very low due to the high cross-sectional area.
- Resistance falls as the volumes of the lungs increase; the elastic parenchyma pulls open bronchioles and thus resistance decreases.

Regional Variations in Ventilation (Fig. 8.5)

- In the upright position the lung is not evenly ventilated; the upper parts are not ventilated as well as the lower parts.
- There are two reasons to explain this:
  - the weight of the lungs
  - the compliance curve is sigmoid, and the upper and lower parts of the lung lie on different parts of this curve.
- Transpulmonary pressure is the difference between the intrapleural pressure and the alveolar pressure.
- During phase 1, when the lung volume is near residual volume, the compliance is low, thus it takes a large change in pressure to cause a change in volume.
- In phase 2, the compliance is at its maximum and lung volume increases linearly with an increase in pressure.
- In phase 3, the compliance falls as the lungs become fully expanded.
- The lower parts of the lungs lie on the diaphragm and are compressed, whereas the upper parts are already stretched by their own weight; therefore, inflation begins further along the pressure–volume curve.

Clinical Physiology

Pneumothorax

There are a number of types of pneumothorax:

Spontaneous (primary) pneumothorax

- Occurs in young males. The cause is unknown; there is rarely any associated respiratory disease. Occasionally the patient has Marfan's syndrome with an associated apical pleural bleb.

Spontaneous (secondary) pneumothorax

- Occurs in patients due to underlying respiratory pathology; causes include:
  - asthma
  - chronic obstructive pulmonary disease (COPD)

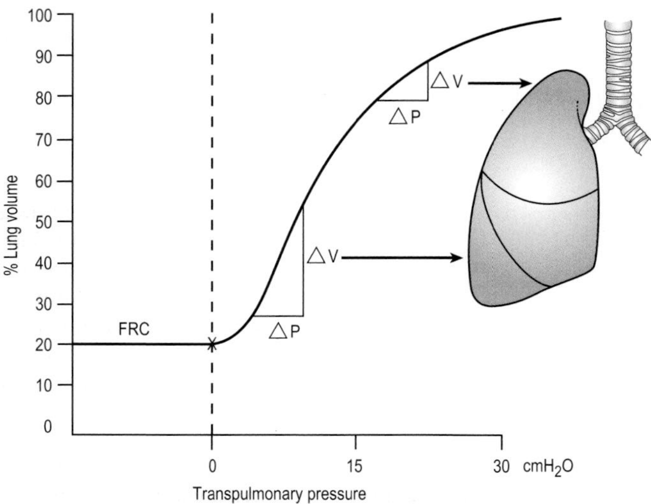

Fig. 8.5 Pressure–volume curve for lung inflation and its influence on the distribution of ventilation during inspiration from functional residual capacity (FRC).

- cancer
- lung abscess.

Traumatic (closed) pneumothorax

- Iatrogenic, e.g. mechanical ventilation or lung biopsy.
- Non-iatrogenic, e.g. stab wound or road traffic accident.

Tension pneumothorax

- A pneumothorax occurs when air enters the pleural space due to the disruption of either the visceral (ruptured pleural bleb) or parietal pleura (stab wound).
- The air entering the pleural space leads to loss of the negative intrapleural pressure and thus the lung collapses; this is the type of pneumothorax seen in spontaneous and traumatic closed pneumothoraces.
- In a tension pneumothorax the lung injury may form a valve in which air leaks into the pleural cavity during inspiration but closes during expiration; this leads to a positive intrapleural pressure (can be as high as 20 cmH_2O), and pushes mediastinal structures into the opposite side of the chest.

Open pneumothorax or 'sucking' chest wound

- In an open pneumothorax there is a defect in the chest wall, e.g. due to a gunshot wound; this allows intrathoracic pressure to equalize with atmospheric pressure. If the defect is greater than two-thirds of the diameter of the trachea then air will preferentially enter through the hole in the chest wall as this is the path of least resistance; this leads to impaired ventilation and hypoxia.

Pulmonary Assessment

Lung Volumes (Table 8.1)

- Lung volumes can be measured using a spirometer.
- The definition of each lung volume is as follows:
  - tidal volume (TV): the air taken in and exhaled during quiet breathing
  - inspiratory reserve volume (IRV): the maximum volume of air that can be inspired in excess of normal inspiration
  - expiratory reserve volume (ERV): the maximum amount of air that can be forcefully expired after normal expiration
  - functional residual capacity (FRC): the volume of gas left in the lungs after expiration during normal breathing

TABLE 8.1 Values for Respiratory Variables in a Healthy Adult Male

Lung Volume	Value (L)
Total lung volume	6.0
Vital capacity	4.8
Residual volume	1.2
Tidal volume	0.5
Functional residual capacity	2.2
Inspiratory capacity	3.8
Expiratory reserve volume	1.0

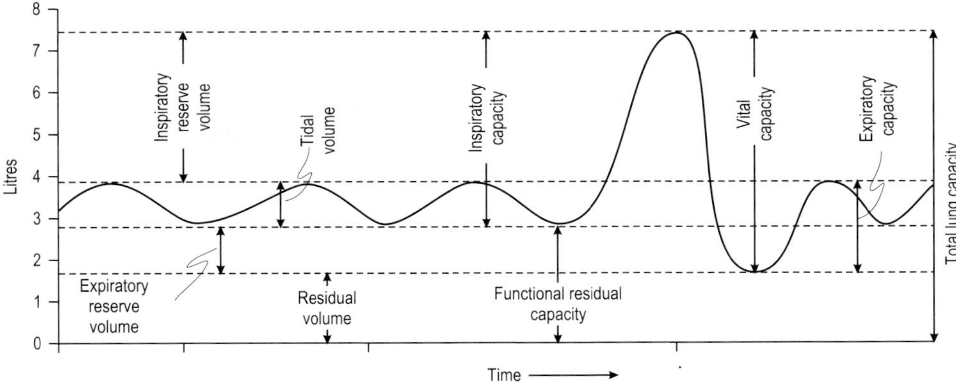

Fig. 8.6 Normal adult lung volumes.

- residual volume (RVol): the volume remaining after maximal expiration; it cannot be measured directly but can be estimated from other lung volumes:

$$RV = FRC - ERV$$

- total lung capacity (TLC): the sum of all lung volumes plus the residual volume
- vital capacity (VC): the volume of air that is expelled from maximal inspiration to maximal expiration.

- Normal spirometry traces are shown in Fig. 8.6; they may vary for size, weight and gender.
- The FRC can be determined by the helium dilution method. The subject breathes normally from a spirometer filled with a known volume of air and helium. As the subject breathes in and out the helium is diluted in the air that is left in the lungs:

$$FRC = \frac{\text{(Initial helium concentration)} \times \text{volume of spirometer}}{\text{(Final helium concentration)}}$$

- The RV can be calculated by the same method, but the subject takes a maximal expiration (i.e. only RV in the lungs) before breathing from the spirometer.

Dead Space and Alveolar Ventilation Rate

- Dead space is the volume of air which has to be ventilated, but does not actually take part in gas exchange.
- Dead space can be anatomical or physiological:
  - anatomical dead space is the volume of gas that does not mix with the air in the alveoli
  - physiological dead space is the volume of gas that may reach the alveoli but, due to a lack of perfusion, does not take part in gas exchange (this includes air in the anatomical dead space).

- The anatomical dead space can be determined using Fowler's method (Fig. 8.7). The subject breathes through a tube connected to a nitrogen analyser. The subject takes a single breath of pure oxygen, holds the breath for several seconds and then breathes out. By performing this manoeuvre the composition of air within the alveoli will differ from that within the airways (i.e. alveoli will contain nitrogen but airways higher up will have pure oxygen).
- Subject breathes out pure O_2 (from conducting airways).
- As subject starts to expire, the nitrogen content of alveolar air is measured.
- A plot of exhaled volume to nitrogen concentration is produced; the dead space is the volume at the midpoint between nitrogen first being detected and its plateau.
- Physiological dead space can be determined from the Bohr equation.
- The principles of this equation rely on two facts:
  - all of the expired CO_2 comes from the alveoli
  - dead space is atmospheric air and thus has negligible CO_2 content.
- The Bohr equation is:

$$V_D = V_E\left(1 - \frac{F_E}{F_A}\right)$$

V_D: volume of dead space
V_E: volume of expired CO_2
F_E: fraction of expired CO_2
F_A: fraction of alveolar CO_2

- F_E can be measured simply by measuring the CO_2 content of expired air.
- F_A can be measured from:
  - the last part of the expired air, which will have the same composition as alveolar air
  - arterial blood gas (more accurate).

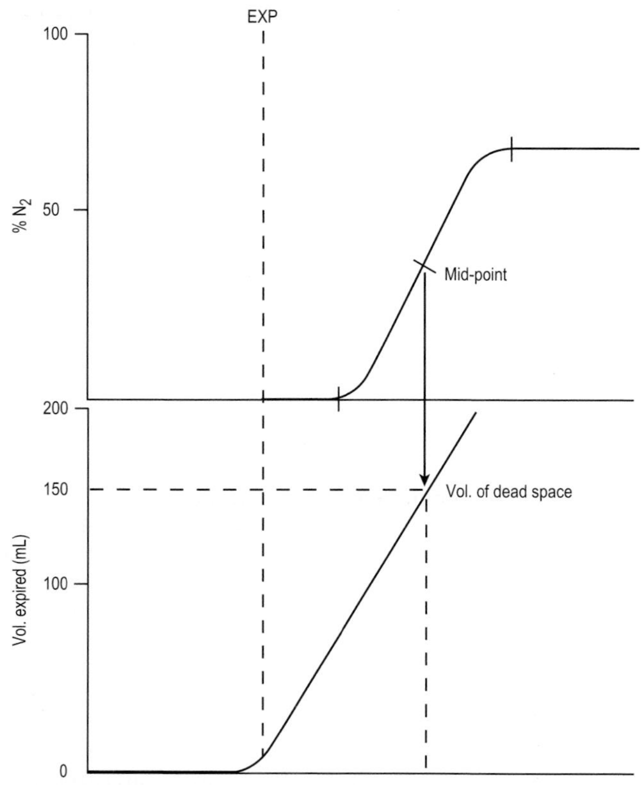

Fig. 8.7 Fowler's method for determination of the anatomical dead space.

- For a normal subject with a tidal expiration of 500 mL, expired CO_2 = 3.5% and alveolar CO_2 = 5%; the dead space:

$$V_D = 500\left(1 - \frac{3.5}{5.0}\right)$$

$$V_D = 500 \text{ mL}$$

- Factors that increase anatomical and physiological dead space are given in Table 8.2.
- Alveolar ventilation rate is the rate at which gas in the alveoli is replaced:

$$\begin{aligned}\text{Alveolar ventilation rate} &= (\text{TV} - \text{dead space}) \\ &\quad \times \text{Respiratory rate (RR)} \\ &= (500 - 150) \times 12 \\ &= 4.2 \text{ L/min}\end{aligned}$$

Peak Expiratory Flow Rate (PEFR)

- A simple bedside test of respiratory function.
- Patient is asked to take maximal inspiration and then to blow out as fast as possible into the peak flow meter.
- Values will vary for age, sex and weight, but a value of around 4–500 L/min is normal.

TABLE 8.2 Factors Increasing Anatomical and Physiological Dead Space

Anatomical Dead Space	Physiological Dead Space
Increasing size of the subject	Hypotension
Standing position	Hypoventilation
Increased lung volume	Emphysema and PE
Bronchodilatation	Positive pressure ventilation

- Values will fall dramatically in respiratory disease; PEFR is particularly useful in assessing the severity of acute asthma attacks.

Closing Capacity

- This is the volume of the lungs at which small airways at the base of the lung start to close.
- The significance of the closing capacity is that as air leaves the lungs some airways close and trap air in the

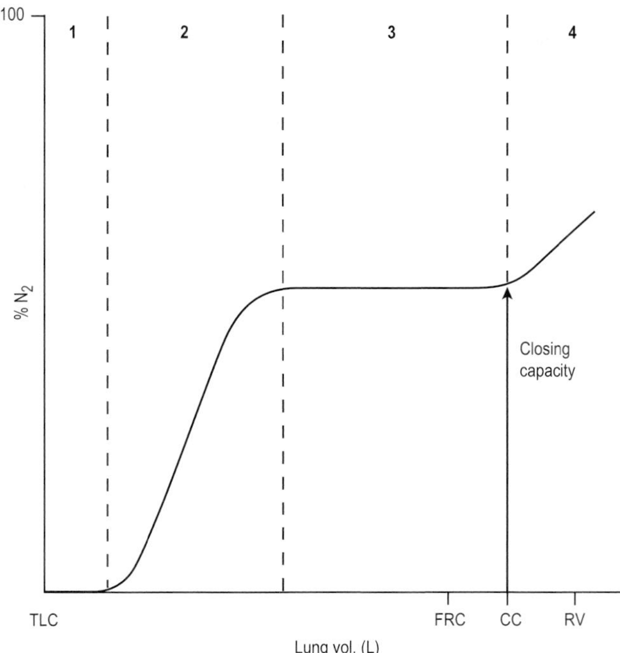

Fig. 8.8 The concentration of nitrogen following a single inspiration of 100% oxygen. The closing capacity is indicated at the point of abrupt increase in the nitrogen concentration.

alveoli; these alveoli cannot play a full part in respiratory gas exchange.

- Closing capacity can be measured by the following technique:
  - the subject breathes out to residual volume and then takes a maximal inspiration of 100% O_2
  - the subject then takes a full expiration through a nitrogen meter
  - the plot of nitrogen concentration to lung volume gives a characteristic plot with four phases (Fig. 8.8):
    - phase 1: pure dead space is exhaled and is therefore 100% O_2
    - phase 2: mixture of dead space and alveolar gas (nitrogen concentration from alveoli increases concentration)
    - phase 3: pure alveolar gas (plateau phase)
    - phase 4: abrupt increase in nitrogen concentration as airways at the base of the lung close. Expired air at this point is from the apex, which has received less O_2, and thus the nitrogen is less dilute.
- Closing capacity is normally 10% of the vital capacity.
- Factors affecting the closing capacity include:
  - age: increases with age
  - posture: in a supine position in a 40-year-old subject, the closing capacity is equal to the FRC
  - anaesthesia: decrease in lung volumes results in closing capacity exceeding FRC, even in the youngest patients.

Flow–Volume and Volume–Time Curves

- Spirometry values should always be assessed with flow–volume and volume–time curves. Diseases of the lung produce characteristically shaped curves.
- Flow–volume curves (Fig. 8.9).
- Volume–time curves (Fig. 8.10).

Diffusion Capacity

- Diffusion capacity (D_LCO) or transfer factor (T_LCO) is a test that reflects both the diffusion capacity of the alveolar membrane and also the pulmonary vasculature.
- It can be measured by inhaling very small concentrations of carbon monoxide and measuring the increase in arterial CO.
- D_LCO is reduced with:
  - ↑ in diffusion distance, i.e. pulmonary oedema
  - loss of alveolar area, i.e. emphysema.

PULMONARY BLOOD FLOW

Structure of the Lung

See Anatomy section (Chapter 1).

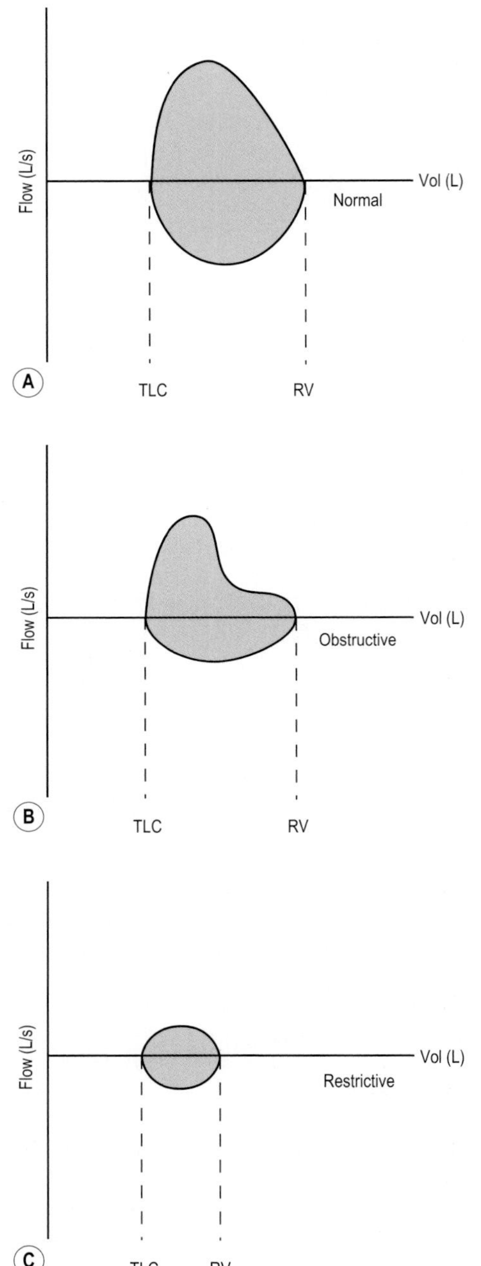

Fig. 8.9 (A) A normal flow–volume curve. (B) An obstructive defect with characteristic concave shape during expiration. (C) The relatively unaffected shape but significantly decreased volume seen in restrictive lung disease.

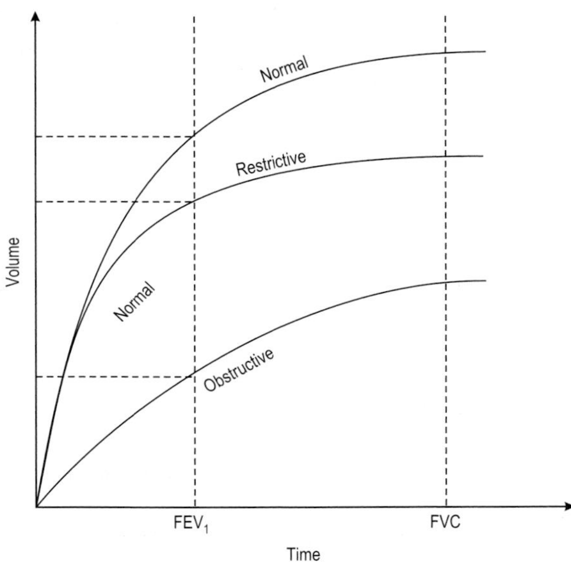

Fig. 8.10 FEV_1/FVC ratios. Normal = 4 L/5 L = 80%. Obstructive FEV_1/FVC = 1.2/3 = 40%. Restrictive FEV_1/FVC = 2.9/3.2 = 93%. FEV_1, Forced Expiratory Volume in the first second; FVC, Forced Vital Capacity.

Regulation of Pulmonary Blood Flow

- Pulmonary arterioles do not appear to play an important role in the regulation of pulmonary blood flow, but the calibre of small alveolar vessels is altered by the PO_2 and PCO_2.
- Hypoxia (↓PO_2) or hypercapnia (↑PCO_2) result in constriction of vessels and thus divert blood to areas that are better oxygenated; this is termed hypoxic pulmonary vasoconstriction (HPV).
- This is a local response and differs from other vascular beds in that the opposite response is usually seen (i.e. hypoxia causes vasodilatation).

Regional Variations in Pulmonary Blood Flow

- Perfusion pressure and resistance determine flow.
- Pressure in the pulmonary artery is low in comparison with the systemic circulation: 25/8 mmHg compared with 120/80 mmHg.
- Blood flow in the lung is determined by three pressures:
  - hydrostatic pressure in the pulmonary arteries (PA)
  - pressure in the pulmonary veins (PV)
  - pressure of air in the alveoli.
- With these forces in mind the blood flow to the lung can be divided into three zones:
  - zone 1: this is at the apex of the lung; the alveolar pressure is similar to the PA pressure; smaller vessels will be compressed and resistance will be high. Blood flow is low in this zone

  - zone 2: pressure in the PA is higher than the alveolar pressure; blood flow is better in this zone, increasing towards zone 3
  - zone 3: PA pressure greatly exceeds the alveolar pressure and thus vessels are fully open. Blood flow is very good.
- The variations in regional blood flow are abolished on lying down.

Cardiac Output and Pulmonary Vascular Resistance

- During exercise the CO to the lungs increases but the pressure within the PA changes relatively little; this is due to two mechanisms which decrease resistance when CO increases:
  - distension of vessels already open
  - recruitment of additional vessels (at rest many capillaries are closed).
- The response to the increase in CO is passive.

Ventilation and Perfusion

- Ventilation and perfusion (V/Q) varies throughout the lung, depending on the height above or below the origin of the PA.
- The V/Q ratio expresses this variation:
  - in alveoli that are ventilated but not perfused V/Q = infinity
  - in alveoli that are perfused but not ventilated V/Q = 0
  - at the apex V/Q = 3, thus indicating that the alveoli are ventilated better than they are perfused
  - at the base V/Q = 0.6, thus indicating that the alveoli are perfused better than they are ventilated
  - the ideal V/Q = 1 and is found approximately two-thirds of the way up the chest
  - the average V/Q ratio, assuming an alveolar ventilation rate of 4.2 L/min, and a cardiac output of 5 L/min, would be 0.84.

Clinical Physiology

Pulmonary Embolus

- A pulmonary embolus results from a thrombus breaking off from a thrombus formed in the large leg/pelvic veins; this clot then lodges in the pulmonary arteries.
- A pulmonary embolus can also occur with fat, amniotic fluid, air or tumour fragments; these are all very rare.
- The effect of the embolus will depend on its size: clinical presentation varies from complete obstruction and sudden death, to the insidious development of hypoxia due to numerous small emboli.
- The physiological changes associated with a pulmonary embolus include:
  - increased pulmonary vascular resistance
  - pulmonary hypertension
  - increased right ventricle (RV) afterload (leading to RV dilatation and dysfunction)
  - reduced left ventricle output
  - impaired gas exchange, due to shunting of blood through non-perfused segments of lung
  - decreased lung compliance, due to bleeding and loss of surfactant over the area affected by the embolus.

Pleural Effusion

- This refers to the abnormal presence of fluid within the pleural cavity.
- The physiological consequences are similar to those of pneumothorax, i.e. hypoxia occurs as lung tissue is compressed by the fluid and prevents normal gas exchange.
- The fluid can be classified as a transudate or an exudate:
  - an exudate has a high protein content (>30 g/L) and is usually due to infection or cancer
  - a transudate has a low protein content (<30 g/L) and most commonly is due to left ventricular failure.

Pulmonary Oedema

- Pulmonary oedema is the abnormal accumulation of fluid in the lung parenchyma.
- Starling's law states that hydrostatic forces push fluid out of the circulation and osmotic forces draw fluid back.
- Normally the balance of hydrostatic and osmotic forces leads to 20–30 mL of excess fluid in the lung interstitium; this is transported back to the circulation as lymph.
- Pulmonary oedema occurs in stages:
  - interstitial oedema: this has little effect on respiration, but will eventually overwhelm lymphatic recirculation and lead to alveolar oedema
  - alveolar oedema: as alveolar oedema develops, the alveoli fill with fluid; this increases surface tension and causes the alveoli to shrink
  - airway oedema: as fluid accumulation continues then fluid will begin to fill the airways; this presents as blood-tinged frothy sputum.
- The physiological effects of pulmonary oedema include:
  - decreased lung compliance due to the reduction in surface tension and alveolar shrinkage
  - increased airway resistance: this can occur due to the reduction in lung volume and fluid filling the airways. Resistance is also due to reflex bronchoconstriction.
- Alveolar oedema leads to a ventilation–perfusion mismatch as alveoli filled with fluid are still perfused but not ventilated.
- Pulmonary vascular resistance increases due to hypoxic vasoconstriction and external compression from interstitial oedema.

- There are numerous causes of pulmonary oedema; these include:
  - raised pulmonary hydrostatic pressure, the commonest cause, occurs with left ventricular failure – left atrial pressure rises and this is transmitted into the pulmonary circulation, resulting in increased pulmonary capillary pressure, and thus capillary hydrostatic pressure. This type of pulmonary oedema can also be seen with fluid or transfusion overload
  - increased pulmonary capillary permeability: this can occur with endotoxic shock, irritant gases and adult respiratory distress syndrome (ARDS)
  - blocked lymphatic drainage: this can occur in the face of normal pulmonary hydrostatic pressures and normal capillary permeability. The commonest cause is obstruction of lymphatics due to tumour cells. The normal 20–30 mL of interstitial fluid normally removed by lymphatics accumulates and leads to pulmonary oedema – it is called lymphangitis carcinomatosa
  - high altitude: the exact cause is unclear, but is likely to be due to hypoxic vasoconstriction leading to elevated pulmonary artery pressure and thus an increase in the hydrostatic pressure
  - neurogenic: frequently seen in severe head injury patients, it is thought to occur due to overactivity of the sympathetic nervous system.

Adult Respiratory Distress Syndrome

- ARDS is the pulmonary component of the systemic inflammatory response syndrome (SIRS).
- It can be caused by direct (contusion, near drowning, aspiration, smoke inhalation) or indirect (trauma, sepsis, pancreatitis) insults.
- Criteria for its diagnosis include:
  - known cause
  - acute onset of symptoms
  - hypoxia refractory to O_2
  - new, bilateral 'fluffy' infiltrates on chest X-ray
  - no evidence of cardiac failure (pulmonary artery wedge pressure <18 mmHg).
- ARDS develops in two phases:
  1. acute exudative: the insult (direct or indirect) leads to neutrophil activation and the release of inflammatory mediators such as tumour necrosis factor (TNF), platelet activating factor (PAF), interleukin (IL)-1 and IL-6; there is also the release of proteases and toxic oxygen radicals that damage the lung parenchyma. This lung damage leads to increased capillary permeability and allows protein-rich exudates to fill the alveoli and form hyaline membranes. There is thrombosis in alveolar capillaries and haemorrhage into the alveoli. This leads to alveolar collapse and decreased surfactant production, leading to decreased lung compliance
  2. late organization: there is regeneration of type II pneumocytes; the hyaline membranes organize with pulmonary fibrosis, leading to interstitial fibrosis and obliteration of alveolar spaces and alveolar microvasculature.

Gas Diffusion and Exchange

Gas Diffusion

- Three factors affect the diffusion of gases, both in the lungs and in the peripheral tissues:
  - pressure gradient: gas flows from an area of high pressure to an area of low pressure. This is usually referred to as the partial pressure
  - diffusion coefficient: a measure of the ease with which a gas can diffuse. It is determined by its solubility in water and its molecular weight
  - tissue factors: the tissue at the site of diffusion should have a large surface area and a short diffusion distance. The surface area of the lungs is about 70 m^2 and the diffusion distance is 0.2 μm.
- The diffusion distance for oxygen consists of:
  - pulmonary surfactant
  - alveolar epithelium
  - alveolar epithelium basement membrane (BM; often fused with capillary BM)
  - pulmonary capillary endothelium.

Gas Exchange (Table 8.3)

- The exchange of gases in both peripheral tissues and alveoli relies on partial pressure gradients. In alveoli the gradient is between alveolar gas and pulmonary blood gas, while in the periphery the gradient is between capillary blood and metabolically active tissues.
- Room air: mixture of nitrogen and oxygen, water vapour (variable) and a tiny amount of carbon dioxide.
- Humidified air: inspired air becomes fully saturated with water; the partial pressure of water vapour is 6.3 kPa; the addition of water vapour leads to a decrease in the partial pressures of all other gases.
- Alveolar air: differs from room air due to the addition of water vapour and the constant removal of oxygen and carbon dioxide i.e. oxygen levels are lower and carbon dioxide levels are higher in comparison to room air.

Gas Transport (Fig. 8.11)

- Systemic venous blood is pumped into the pulmonary artery from the right ventricle. PO_2 is 5.3 kPa and PCO_2 is 6 kPa. Alveolar PO_2 is 13.7 kPa and the PCO_2 is 5.3 kPa.
- Following the principle of gases flowing from areas of high partial pressure to low partial pressure, oxygen will

TABLE 8.3 Standard Values for Respiratory Gases

Gas	Room Air (kPa)	Humidified Air (kPa)	Alveolar Air (kPa)
N_2	79.79	74.83	75.6
O_2	21.17	19.87	13.7
CO_2	0.04	0.04	5.3
H_2O	0	6.3	6.3
Total	101	101	101

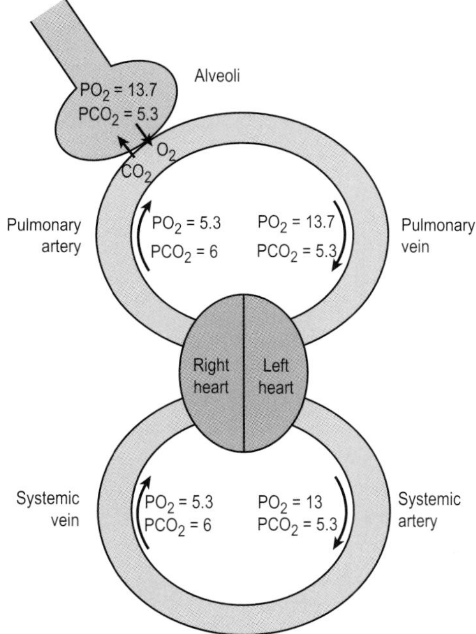

Fig. 8.11 The gas exchange between the lungs and tissues.

diffuse into the blood and carbon dioxide will diffuse into the alveoli.

- Oxygenated blood is returned to the heart via the pulmonary veins and then to the left ventricle.
- PO_2 of systemic blood is slightly lower than pulmonary venous blood, due to the addition of deoxygenated blood from bronchial veins (13.7 kPa → 13 kPa).
- The deoxygenated blood from bronchial veins is referred to as 'shunting'; it describes the passage of blood through the lungs without coming into contact with ventilated alveoli. Other causes of shunt include:
  - pneumonia (due to consolidation of lung parenchyma)
  - atrial septal defect
  - ventricular septal defect
  - patent ductus arteriosus.

Oxygen transport

- Haemoglobin:
  - consists of four peptide chains; two α and two β. Each peptide has a haem group which consists of a protoporphyrin ring surrounding a ferrous iron molecule (Fe^{2+})
  - each haemoglobin (Hb) molecule can carry four oxygen molecules
  - normal Hb values for a male and female are 15 g/dL and 13 g/dL, respectively. Each gram of Hb can carry 1.34 mL of O_2; therefore, O_2-carrying capacity varies between 20 and 17.5 mL per 100 mL blood
  - the vast majority of O_2 is transported via Hb; only a negligible amount is dissolved, approximately 0.225 per kPa of O_2.
- Oxygen dissociation curve (Fig. 8.12):
  - the oxygen dissociation curve illustrates the relationship between the partial pressure of O_2 and the concentration of O_2 in the blood
  - the characteristic shape of the curve reflects the increasing ability of Hb to take up O_2 following the binding of the first molecule
  - the curve reaches a plateau at a PO_2 of around 15–16 kPa
  - a number of factors will alter the position of the curve. A right shift decreases oxygen affinity and thus oxygen will be released at a higher partial pressure. A left shift increases oxygen affinity
  - a right shift is caused by:
    - ↑temperature
    - ↑2,3-diphosphoglycerate (2,3-DPG)
    - ↑H^+
  - the right shift of the dissociation curve is called the Bohr effect; the factors causing a right shift would be present in active tissues; the Bohr effect represents a mechanism to increase oxygen extraction
  - anaemia does not affect the dissociation curve. The shape and position are the same; to see the effect of anaemia you would need to plot partial pressure against oxygen content.

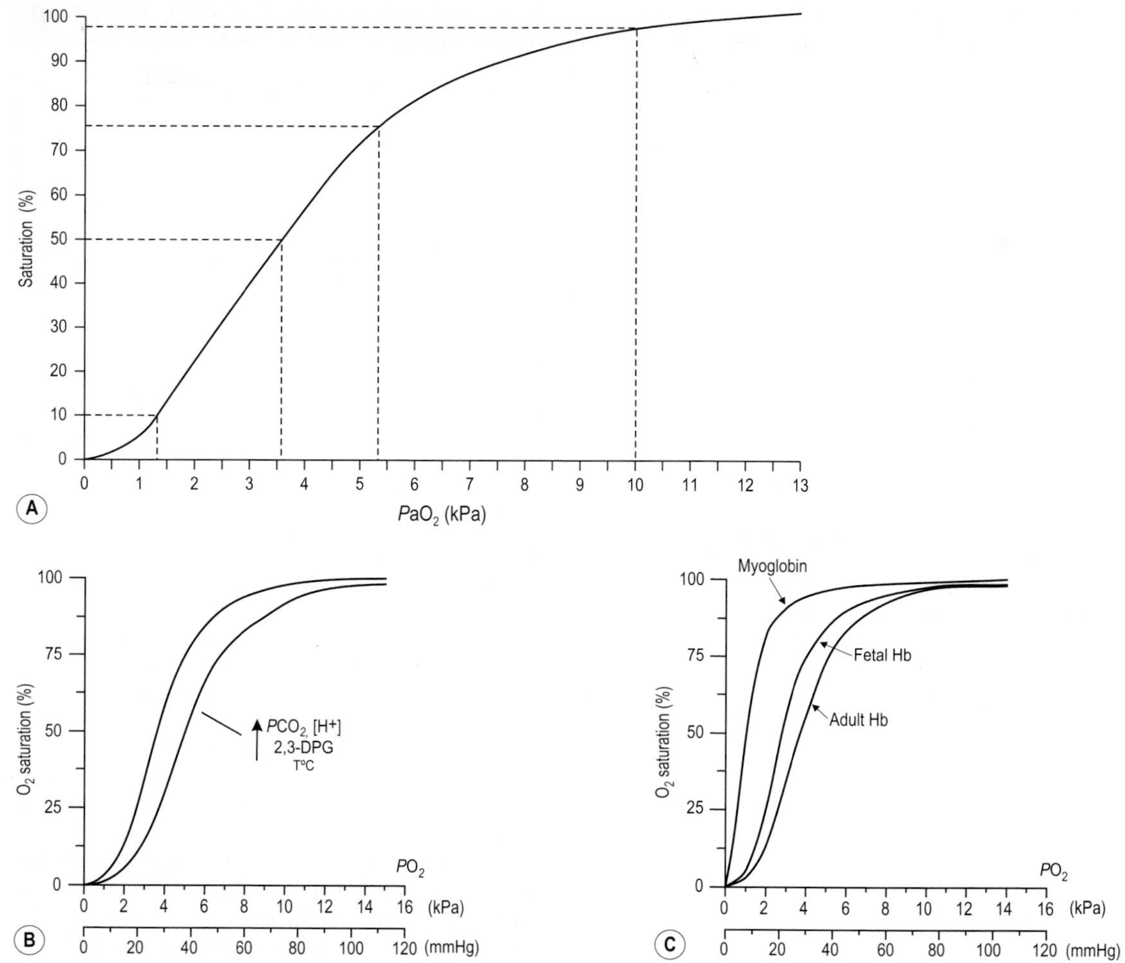

Fig. 8.12 (A) Oxyhaemoglobin dissociation curve. (B) Factors that shift the oxyhaemoglobin curve to the right and increase O_2 dissociation. (C) Different O_2 affinities for fetal haemoglobin and myoglobin in comparison with the O_2 dissociation curve for adult Hb.

- Fetal haemoglobin and myoglobin:
  - fetal haemoglobin (HbF) has different globin chains to adult Hb (two α and two γ); the change in globin chain results in a greater affinity for O_2 and allows the fetus to extract blood from the maternal circulation
  - the curve for HbF is to the left of adult Hb, reflecting the increased affinity for O_2
  - the curve for myoglobin lies further to the left; it acts as an oxygen storage molecule and only releases O_2 when the partial pressure has fallen considerably
  - the function of myoglobin is to provide additional O_2 in muscles during periods of anaerobic respiration (i.e. during sustained contractions when blood vessels are compressed).

Carbon dioxide transport

- Carbon dioxide is transported in three main ways:
  - carbamino groups: these are formed between CO_2 and proteins or peptides. Most of these reactions are with the globin portions of haemoglobin, accounting for 20–30% of transported CO_2
  - dissolved CO_2 accounts for about 10% of the transported CO_2
  - HCO_3^- accounts for about 60–70% of the transported CO_2. The CO_2 diffuses into the red blood cells and reacts with water to form carbonic acid (a reaction catalysed by the enzyme carbonic anhydrase). The carbonic acid dissociates into H^+ and HCO_3^-; the H^+ binds to haemoglobin and the HCO_3^- diffuses

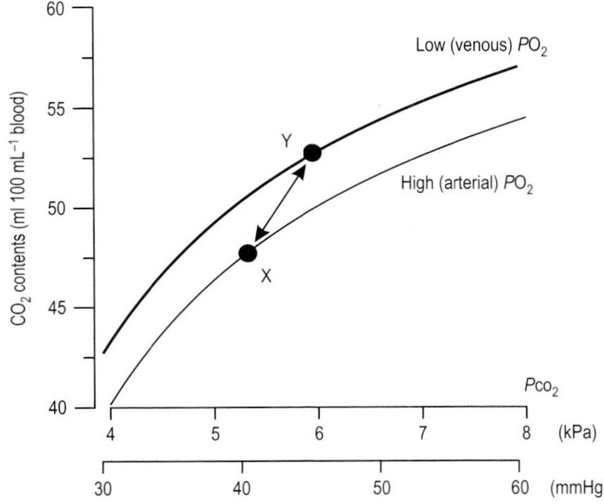

Fig. 8.13 The CO_2 dissociation curve – Haldane effect. X indicates CO_2 content in systemic arterial blood (↑O_2) and Y indicates CO_2 content in venous blood (↓O_2).

out of the cell into the plasma. To maintain cellular balance Cl^- diffuses into the red cell (chloride shift). This process is reversed in the alveoli, producing CO_2 in preparation for expiration.

- The CO_2 dissociation curve is for total CO_2 and not one form; there are several differences between it and the oxygen dissociation curve (Fig. 8.13):
  - the solubility of CO_2 is greater than oxygen
  - the normal range of CO_2 is much smaller: 5.3–6 kPa compared with 5.3–13.3 kPa for oxygen
  - blood cannot be saturated with CO_2, therefore the graph has no plateau phase.
- The CO_2 dissociation curve is influenced by the partial pressure of O_2. Essentially the amount of carbon dioxide carried increases as the oxygen level falls; this effect is called the Haldane effect.
- The significance of the Haldane effect is that as arterial blood (PCO_2 5.3 kPa) passes through the capillary network (PCO_2 6 kPa), the dissociation curve moves upwards and allows the increased uptake of CO_2.

Regulation of Respiration

The body maintains the amount of PO_2 and PCO_2 at appropriate levels through an interaction between neurological and chemical control mechanisms.

Neurological Regulation

- There are a number of areas in the brain that exert differing degrees of control on respiration. These areas include:
  - medulla oblongata
  - pons
  - cerebral cortex
  - limbic system and hypothalamus.
- Medulla oblongata: there are two groups of cells within the respiratory centre in the medulla:
  - the inspiratory neurons: these demonstrate rhythmical firing of action potentials with intervening periods of inactivity. These action potentials stimulate the diaphragm and external intercostals to contract, and thus initiate inspiration. Expiration occurs during the intervening pauses of inactivity
  - the expiratory neurons: these neurons are usually inactive during normal quiet respiration; however, during periods of exercise or increased respiration they fire action potentials during the inactive period of the inspiratory neurons to stimulate the internal intercostals and abdominal muscles to contract, and thus aid expiration.
- Pons: there are two areas within the pons; they are not essential for respiration, but can influence the pattern of breathing:
  - apneustic centre: this is located in the lower pons; it tends to prolong inspiration and results in short expiratory efforts
  - pneumotaxic centre: this is located in the upper pons; it tends to inhibit the inspiratory neurons and shortens inspiration.
- Cerebral cortex: this can override the neurons within the medulla and increase ventilation (hyperventilate) or hold the breath.
- Limbic system and hypothalamus: in extreme states of emotion, such as fear or anger, these areas may influence the respiratory pattern.

Chemical Regulation

- The rhythmical firing of neurons in the medulla is regulated by the input of a number of chemoreceptors, which monitor changes in chemical factors and then signal the medulla to increase or decrease the respiratory rate to normalize the detected chemical change.
- These chemoreceptors monitor changes in the following:
  - arterial PCO_2
  - arterial pH
  - arterial PO_2.
- These chemoreceptors can be further subdivided into:
  - central chemoreceptors
  - peripheral chemoreceptors.
- Central chemoreceptors:
  - situated in the CNS, close to the respiratory centre in the medulla
  - particularly sensitive to changes in the arterial PCO_2

- CO_2 diffuses from the blood into the brain and reacts with water to produce H^+ and causes the pH to fall, thus directly stimulating the chemoreceptors
- any elevation in CO_2 leads to a central acidosis that stimulates the chemoreceptors and leads to an increased respiratory rate in order to blow off the excess CO_2. The opposite effect is seen with low levels of CO_2
- central chemoreceptors are the main determinant of respiration, as the level of CO_2 is the most important stimulus to respiration.

- Peripheral chemoreceptors:
  - located in the carotid bodies, close to the bifurcation of the common carotid and in the aortic bodies, which lie along the aortic arch
  - less important than the central chemoreceptors
  - they respond to changes in arterial pH and to low levels of PO_2; the response to pH is of secondary importance to respiratory control but does allow compensation for acid–base disturbances
  - for instance, a fall in arterial pH due to a metabolic acidosis will stimulate respiration and thus will lower the level of CO_2 and favour an increase in pH back towards normal. The opposite effect is seen with an alkalosis
  - the response to low O_2 only comes into effect when levels are abnormally low, i.e. PO_2 8 kPa or less
  - these receptors can become important in severe longstanding lung disease with persistently elevated levels of CO_2. Patients may become accustomed and lose the controlling influence of CO_2. They therefore rely on the low level of O_2 to stimulate respiration. This is called hypoxic drive.
- There are several other factors which may influence respiration:
  - Hering–Breuer reflex: this reflex prevents over-inflation of the lungs. Stretch receptors in the lung send inhibitory signals via the vagus. Only significant at high tidal volumes (>1.5 L)
  - 'J' receptors: these receptors lie in the alveoli in close association with the capillaries. Their function is unclear but injection of chemicals into the pulmonary circulation triggers these receptors and causes a marked inhibition of inspiration
  - irritant receptors: lie in the epithelia lining the airways; they respond to noxious gases and cause bronchospasm and inhibition of inspiration
  - vasomotor centre: low blood pressure detected by baroreceptors results in an increase in the ventilatory rate. An increase in blood pressure has the opposite effect.

Hypoxia and Respiratory Failure

Hypoxia and Hypoxaemia

- Hypoxia: a deficiency of oxygen in the tissues.
- Hypoxaemia: reduction in the concentration of oxygen in the arterial blood.
- There are four types of hypoxia:
  1. Hypoxic hypoxia: results from a low arterial PO_2; examples include:
     - high altitude
     - pulmonary embolism
     - hypoventilation
     - lung fibrosis
     - pulmonary oedema.
  2. Anaemic hypoxia: a decrease in the amount of haemoglobin and thus a decrease in oxygen content of arterial blood; examples include:
     - haemorrhage
     - decreased red cell production
     - increased red cell destruction
     - carbon monoxide poisoning.
  3. Stagnant hypoxia: due to low blood flow; examples include:
     - vasoconstriction
     - decreased cardiac output: due to the low blood flow there is increased extraction of oxygen from the blood; this leads to very low venous oxygen and produces peripheral cyanosis.
  4. Histotoxic hypoxia: poisoning of the enzymes involved in cellular respiration. Oxygen is available but cannot be utilized; the main example is cyanide poisoning.
- There are five main causes of hypoxaemia:
  1. Hypoventilation, accompanied by $\uparrow PaCO_2$; oxygen therapy can improve the hypoxaemia; common causes of hypoventilation include:
     - central depression of respiratory drive, e.g. drugs
     - trauma, i.e. cervical cord injury
       - neuromuscular disorders, e.g. myasthenia gravis
       - chest wall deformity.
  2. Impaired diffusion: $PaCO_2$ is usually normal due to its increased solubility; oxygen therapy can also improve the hypoxaemia. Causes of impaired diffusion include:
     - asbestosis
     - sarcoidosis
     - ARDS.
  3. Shunt (see Gas Transport section): $PaCO_2$ is usually normal, but unlike other causes of hypoxaemia the administration of oxygen will not raise the PaO_2; this

is characteristic of hypoxaemia due to shunt, and occurs because of the differences between the dissociation curves for O_2 and CO_2.

4. Ventilation and perfusion inequality: (see Ventilation and Perfusion section), usually seen in chronic lung disease, i.e. chronic obstructive airways disease (COAD). It means that ventilation and blood flow are mismatched. Oxygen therapy can improve the hypoxaemia.
5. Reduction in inspired oxygen tension.

Respiratory Failure

- Respiratory failure is present if PaO_2 is <8 kPa; this can be further divided into types I and II based on the level of carbon dioxide:
  1. Type I: $PaCO_2$ is <6 kPa; it is referred to as hypoxaemic respiratory failure. It is due to ventilation–perfusion mismatching. $PaCO_2$ is normal or low as the increased ventilatory rate in remaining alveoli can compensate for increases in CO_2. Compensation cannot occur for O_2, as the dissociation curve is sigmoid and will reach a plateau:
     - causes of type I respiratory failure include:
       - pneumothorax
       - pneumonia
       - contusion
       - pulmonary embolism
       - ARDS.
  2. Type II: $PaCO_2$ is >6 kPa; it is referred to as ventilatory failure and is due to inadequate movement of air. The relative state of hypoventilation causes the PaO_2 to fall and the $PaCO_2$ to rise:
     - causes of type II respiratory failure include:
       - COPD
       - neuromuscular disorders
       - airway obstruction
       - central respiratory depression
       - chest wall deformity.

Clinical Physiology

Response to Hypoxia

Acute

- PaO_2 is a relatively weak stimulus to respiration; the respiratory rate does not alter significantly until PaO_2 falls to 8 kPa.
- The carotid bodies are responsible for detecting this change and initiating the physiological changes – they respond to the decrease in PaO_2 by increasing the rate and depth of respiration (minute volume); this leads to a decrease in $PaCO_2$ and reduced respiratory drive from the central chemoreceptors.
- In these situations respiration is stimulated by hypoxia rather than the level of CO_2; this is called hypoxic drive.
- The carotid bodies also elicit cardiovascular changes in response to hypoxia:
  - increased heart rate
  - increased cardiac output
  - vasoconstriction in the skin and splanchnic circulation.

Chronic

There are several physiological changes that occur with chronic hypoxia; these include:

- ↑ minute volume: although this causes a respiratory alkalosis by decreasing $PaCO_2$, there is renal compensation by the excretion of excess bicarbonate.
- ↑ number of red cells and haemoglobin: this is stimulated by erythropoietin, released by the kidney in response to hypoxia. In addition there is increased 2,3-DPG by red cells; this shifts the oxygen dissociation curve to the right and increases the ease of oxygen release.
- ↑ cardiac output: this produces increased blood flow to organs and thus increased oxygen delivery.
- ↑ vascularity of organs: the diameter of capillaries increases and they become more tortuous; this aids in the delivery of oxygen to the tissues.

Oxygen Therapy and Mechanical Ventilation

Oxygen Therapy

Oxygen therapy can be via variable or fixed performance masks:

- Variable performance masks, i.e. Hudson mask or nasal cannula, do not deliver a constant concentration of oxygen and are dependent on the patient's peak inspiratory flow rate (PIFR). As PIFR ↑ then more air will be entrained and will decrease oxygen concentration.
- Fixed performance masks, i.e. Venturi masks, deliver a constant oxygen concentration, irrelevant of the patient's PIFR. The mask entrains air at a fixed rate and thus oxygen dilution does not occur. Different colours signify different oxygen flow rates.

Mechanical Ventilation

Indications

These can be divided into:

- Inadequate ventilation:
  - apnoea
  - respiratory rate >35
  - $PaCO_2$ > 8 kPa.
- Inadequate oxygenation: PaO_2 <8 kPa with 60% FiO_2.
- Surgical indications:
  - head injury
  - chest injury
  - facial trauma
  - high spinal injury.

Intermittent positive pressure ventilation (IPPV)

- The basis for mechanical ventilation is called intermittent positive pressure ventilation (IPPV); the principle of IPPV is the same as normal ventilation in the fact that air flows down a pressure gradient. However, during normal ventilation air flows from atmospheric pressure to negative intra-alveolar pressure; in IPPV the driving pressure is positive to zero (as opposed to zero to negative). Expiration remains a passive event.
- Following the decision to commence mechanical ventilation, the settings and mode of ventilation must be selected.
- An example of initial ventilator settings may be:
  - $FiO_2 = 0.5$
  - tidal volume = 10–12 mL/kg
  - respiratory rate = 10–12 per min
  - inspiration:expiration (I:E) ratio = 1 : 2
  - limit airway pressure = 40 cmH_2O
  - positive end expiratory pressure (PEEP) = 2.5–10 cmH_2O.
- Modes of ventilation include:
  - controlled mandatory ventilation (CMV): the patient makes no respiratory effort and the ventilator delivers a set volume
  - synchronized intermittent mandatory ventilation (SIMV): the patient requires less sedation and paralysis; the patient receives a combination of ventilator breaths and breaths initiated by the patient; the ventilator co-ordinates the breaths so that they do not occur together
  - pressure controlled ventilation (PCV): in CMV and SIMV modes the ventilator will deliver a given volume of air irrelevant of the pressure required to do so. Controlling the pressure reduces the risk of barotrauma to the lung
  - pressure support ventilation (PSV): this mode of ventilation can be used with SIMV and PCV. It allows the patient to wean from the ventilator by triggering each breath. The ventilator simply delivers a preset pressure to assist the patient; this pressure can be gradually reduced, allowing the patient to do increasing amounts of work.
- Another important concept in mechanical ventilation is the recruitment of collapsed alveoli by using positive pressure throughout the respiratory cycle. This has the effect of allowing oxygenation to occur throughout the respiratory cycle and also increases FRC, which places the lung on the efficient part of the compliance curve. Examples of this include:
  - PEEP: used during mechanical ventilation
  - continuous positive airways pressure (CPAP): used during spontaneous breathing by a tight-fitting face-mask
  - reversal of I:E ratio: normally the ratio is 1 : 2, which allows time for passive expiration; increasing the inspiratory time and allowing less time for expiration (i.e. 1 : 1, 2 : 1 or 3 : 1) will leave progressively more air in the alveoli and thus prevent their collapse; this is called auto-PEEP.

Complications

The complications of mechanical ventilation include:

- ventilator-induced injury
- volutrauma
- barotrauma
- hypotension and decreased cardiac output: decreased venous return due to positive intrathoracic pressure
- respiratory muscle atrophy
- nosocomial infections
- technical complications, e.g. disconnection
- increase in intracranial pressure (ICP) due to the increase in intrathoracic pressure.

OSCE SCENARIOS

OSCE Scenario 8.1

A 59-year-old male with severe acute gallstone pancreatitis has been on the ward for 5 days. He is complaining of acute shortness of breath with a respiratory rate of 32 and an SpO_2 of 88% despite oxygen by facemask. The junior doctor has obtained arterial blood gases, the results of which are shown below:

pH 7.25
PaO_2 7.7 kPa
$PaCO_2$ 7 kPa
Base excess −9 mmol/L
HCO_3^- 18 mmol/L

1. What are the possible differential diagnoses for the shortness of breath?
2. How is respiratory failure classified?
3. What is adult respiratory distress syndrome (ARDS)?
4. How is ARDS diagnosed?
5. How is ARDS managed?

OSCE Scenario 8.2

A 52-year-old male, seven days post-right total knee replacement, has become acutely short of breath. He has severe chest pain on inspiration.

1. What is the differential diagnosis?
2. What changes on ECG would support a diagnosis of pulmonary embolism (PE)?
3. What is the treatment for PE?
4. Describe the physiological changes that lead to hypoxia and hypotension which occur in PE.

OSCE Scenario 8.3

A 19-year-old male is involved in a fight. He has been stabbed in the left side of the chest. He is brought into A&E very pale and struggling to breathe.

1. What possible chest injury could he have?
2. What would be the examination findings in each?
3. How would you manage this patient?

OSCE 8.4

A 56-year-old male has recently had major knee surgery and you are called to the ward as he has difficulty breathing. He also has pleuritic chest pain. You suspect a pulmonary embolism (PE).

1. What other signs may be associated with a PE?
2. What would you expect to see on arterial blood gases and why would you see these changes?
3. How would you investigate and treat this patient?

OSCE 8.5

A 26-year-old male has been shot in the chest with a shotgun and has a sizeable chest injury. He is very short of breath. Bubbles are coming from the wound.

1. What type of chest injury is this and how would you treat it?
2. He has hypoxia and hypoxaemia – which type of hypoxia and hypoxaemia does he have?
3. What other types of chest injury can you describe?

Answers in Appendix pages 446–449

Please check your eBook at https://studentconsult.inkling.com/ for more self-assessment questions. See inside cover for registration details.

9

Cardiovascular System

CARDIAC MUSCLE

- Myocytes surrounded by cell membrane, in which there are voltage-operated ion channels.
- Myocytes contain myofibrils, which are made up of sarcomeres.
- Sarcomeres consist of actin (thin) and myosin (thick) filaments, which are responsible for contraction.
- Actin filaments are associated with troponin and tropomysin, which regulate the process of contraction.
- Actin and myosin filaments slide over each other to shorten the sarcomere. Shortening of several sarcomeres is the mechanism by which the myocyte contracts.
- In the absence of calcium the troponin/tropomysin complex inhibits cross-bridging between actin and myosin filaments.
- When calcium binds to troponin, formation of cross-bridging occurs between the filaments. The filaments then slide over one another to cause contraction.
- ATP is required to detach myosin and actin so that the procedure can be repeated.
- Functionally, heart must act as a syncytium, i.e. a single cell formed from a number of fused cells. Therefore, when one part of the heart depolarizes, a wave of depolarization passes through the entire cardiac muscle.
- Myocytes contain large numbers of mitochondria, generating energy via aerobic metabolism.
- Myocyte function depends on optimal concentrations of Ca^{2+}, Na^+ and K^+.
- Myocytes have two systems of intracellular membranes:
    - T-tubules
    - sarcoplasmic reticulum.

Cardiac Action Potential (Fig. 9.1)

- The action potential is the electrical signal that travels throughout the cardiac muscle to initiate contraction.
- Cardiac action potentials have different characteristics in different regions of the heart: one for the Purkinje fibres and ventricular muscle, one for atrial muscle and one for the sinoatrial (SA) and atrioventricular (AV) nodes.
- A typical action potential is divided into four phases:

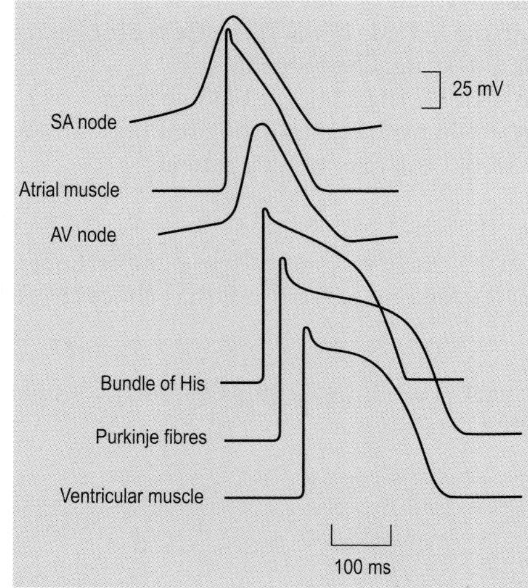

Fig. 9.1 Shape, duration and sequence of cardiac action potentials; note also the delays caused by the anatomical sequence of depolarization and by the relative conduction velocities down the conducting system. (From Hoffman BF & Cranefield PF. Electrophysiology of the Heart. McGraw-Hill, New York, 1960.)

Phase 0

Initial rapid depolarization, rapid increase in sodium permeability.

Phase 1

Rapid repolarization, rapid decrease in sodium permeability, small increase in potassium permeability.

Phase 2

Slow repolarization – plateau effect due to inward movement of calcium. Plateau lasts about 200 ms.

Phase 3

Rapid repolarization – increase in potassium permeability and inactivation of slow inward Ca^{2+} channels.

Phase 4

The resting membrane potential of the ventricular muscle is about −90 mV. The SA node and conducting system do not have a resting membrane potential – they are constantly depolarizing.

Excitation/Contraction Coupling

- Mechanism by which the cardiac action potential causes the myofibrils to contract.
- Arrival of the action potential allows Ca^{2+} to move from the sarcoplasmic reticulum into the cytoplasm.
- Ca^{2+} binds to troponin C, eventually activating the actin–myosin complex, resulting in contraction.
- The plateau phase, the result of further calcium influx, prolongs and enhances contraction.
- The cardiac action potential is very long (200–300 ms). After the contraction there is a refractory period when no further action potentials can be initiated and therefore no contraction occurs. The long action potential and refractory periods ensure contraction and relaxation of the heart, allowing the chambers to fill during relaxation and empty during contraction.
- Intracellular Ca^{2+} is the most important factor controlling myocardial contractility:
  - increased intracellular Ca^{2+} increases force of myocardial contraction
  - decreased intracellular Ca^{2+} decreases the force of myocardial contraction.

Generation and Conduction of Cardiac Impulse

- Cardiac tissue has two types of cell:
  - cells that initiate and conduct impulses, i.e. SA, AV nodes
  - cells that conduct and contract; muscle mass of the heart.
- SA node is situated in the right atrium near the entrance of the superior vena cava (SVC).
- SA node is the pacemaker dictating the rate of beating of the heart because it has the highest frequency of firing.
- From SA node, action potentials are conducted from one atrial cell to another, ensuring that both atria contract simultaneously.
- AV node is located in the atrioventricular fibrous ring on the right side of the atrial septum. It is the only electrical pathway through the fibrous ring.
- AV node is activated by atrial electrical activity, which results in activation of Purkinje cells.
- Conduction through the AV node is slow, delaying transmission from atria to ventricles, ensuring that atrial contraction is finished before ventricular contraction begins.
- From the AV node, action potentials travel in the bundle of His down the ventricular septum and along the right and left bundle branches to enter the Purkinje system of fibres.
- Conduction is rapid in the Purkinje cells and the action potential is rapidly transmitted to myocytes at the apex of the heart.
- Myocytes at the apex of the ventricle are excited and the action potential spreads upwards towards the fibrous ring.
- Cells of the SA node, AV node, Purkinje system have the ability to depolarize themselves at regular intervals (self-excitation).
- These cells also have a long refractory period. Therefore the cells with the highest frequency of firing will control the heart rate.
- A denervated heart (e.g. transplanted heart) will continue to beat. The rate can increase via circulating adrenaline but atropine does not have any effect (vagal denervation) on the heart rate.
- Failure of the SA node results in cells with the next highest firing frequency, i.e. AV node, taking over pacemaker function.
- Vagal stimulation (parasympathetic) slows the heart by action on the SA node. Stimulation of the sympathetic innervation and sympathomimetic hormones act to increase the heart rate.

Generation of Cardiac Output

- All cardiac muscle has intrinsic capacity for rhythmic excitation.
- Cardiac tissue spontaneously depolarizes until an action potential occurs and contraction is initiated. This is independent of other influences.
- Various fibres have different rates of depolarization, but since they form a functional syncytium with specialized conducting tissue, depolarization spreads from cell to cell leading to co-ordinated contraction.
- This rhythmic activity produces alternate contraction/relaxation, i.e. systole/diastole.

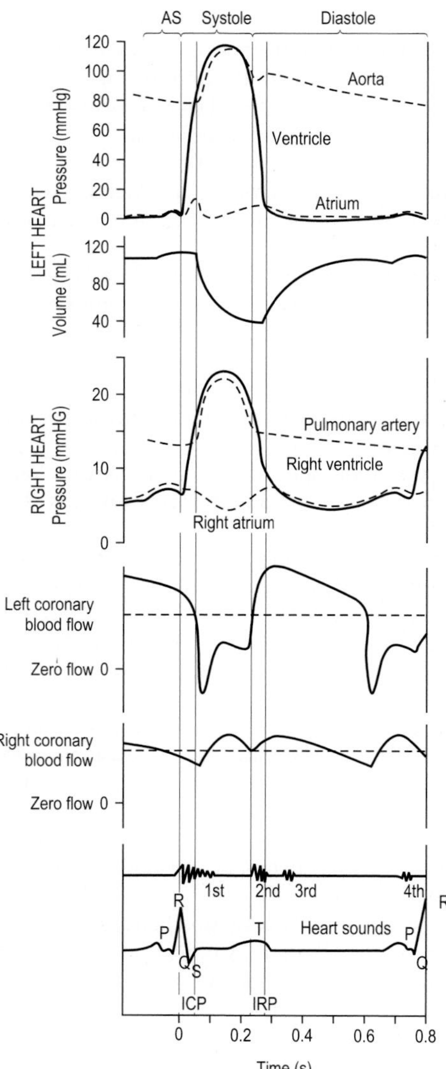

Fig. 9.2 The cardiac cycle. ICP, Isometric contraction period, IRP, isometric relaxation period, AS, atrial systole.

Phases of the Cardiac Cycle (Fig. 9.2)

- Systole:
  - contraction (I): mitral and tricuspid valves close
  - ejection (IIa, b): aortic and pulmonary valves open.
- Diastole:
  - relaxation (III): aortic and pulmonary valves close
  - filling (IVa, b, c): mitral and tricuspid valves open.

Phase IVc

- Atrial systole.
- SA node depolarizes.
- Atrial muscle contracts.
- Blood flows through AV valves to ventricles, completing the last 15% of ventricular filling.

Phase I

- Isovolumetric contraction of ventricles.
- AV valves close.
- Aortic and pulmonary valves close.
- Volume of blood in heart remains constant as pressure rapidly increases (isovolumetric contraction).

Phase IIa

- Ejection.
- Pressure in ventricles exceeds that in aorta and pulmonary artery; valves open.
- Blood ejected in aorta and pulmonary artery.

Phase IIb

- Ejection.
- Aortic and pulmonary pressures equalize with ventricles.

Phase III

- Diastolic relaxation.
- Isovolumetric relaxation.
- Ventricular pressure falls.
- Aortic and pulmonary valves close.

Phase IVa

- Filling phase of diastole.
- AV valves reopen.
- Passive ventricular filling.
- Rapid filling of ventricles.
- Low atrial pressures due to 'suction' effect results in rapid filling.

Phase IVb

- Decline in rate of filling as atrial volume increases.
- Finally, active atrial contraction begins again, i.e. phase IVc.
- During phase III the ventricle ejects about 60% of its volume, i.e. the ejection fraction.

$$\text{Ejection fraction} = \frac{\text{Stroke volume (SV)}}{\text{Left ventricular end diastolic volume (LVEDV)}}$$

- During phase IVc the ventricles are topped up by 15% at rest, but more at higher heart rates.
- Failure of atrial contraction therefore at higher heart rates, e.g. fast atrial fibrillation (AF); exercise may be life-threatening.

Intracardiac Pressures

Normal values for aortic and intra-cardiac pressures are shown in Fig. 9.3.

Heart Sounds

First Heart Sound

- Due to closure of AV valves.
- Best heard at apex.
- Louder in mitral stenosis, hyperdynamic circulation, tachycardia.

Second Heart Sound

- Due to closure of aortic and pulmonary valves.
- Physiological splitting may occur (A_2–P_2 intervals). This is due to prolongation of ventricular ejection periods during inspiration resulting from increased stroke volume secondary to increased venous return.

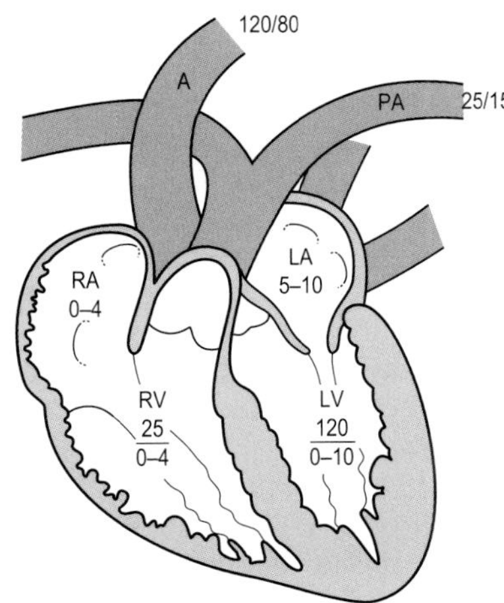

Fig. 9.3 Normal values for intracardiac, aortic and pulmonary artery pressure (mmHg as measured by cardiac catheterization). A = aorta, PA = pulmonary artery, RA = right atrium, LA = left atrium, RV = right ventricle, LV = left ventricle.

Third Heart Sound

- Due to rapid ventricular filling.
- Best heard in children.

Fourth Heart Sound

- Due to ventricular distension (stiff ventricle) caused by forceful atrial contraction.
- Indicates ventricular hypertrophy or heart failure.

Venous Pulse (Fig. 9.4)

a-Wave

- Atrial systole.
- Absent in atrial fibrillation (AF).
- Cannon waves in complete heart block.
- Giant waves in pulmonary hypertension, tricuspid and pulmonary stenosis.

c-Wave

- Bulging of tricuspid valve leaflets in right atrium during isovolumetric contraction.
- Synchronous with pulse wave in carotid artery.

v-Wave

- Rise in right atrial pressure before tricuspid valve opens.

x-Descent

- Due to tricuspid valve moving down during ventricular systole.

y-Descent

- Tricuspid valve opens.
- Right atrial pressure falls as blood flows to right ventricle.

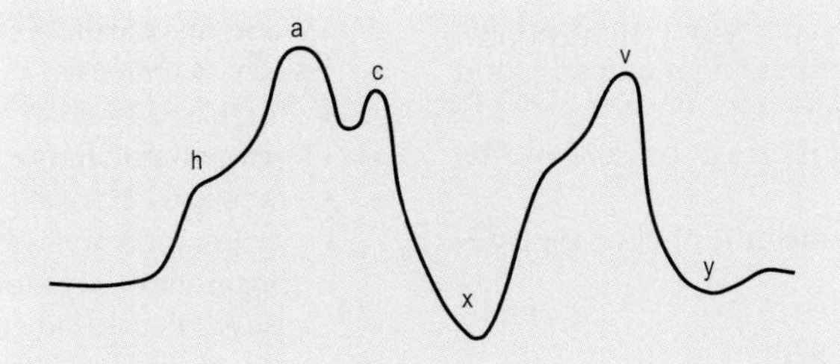

Fig. 9.4 Venous pulses: 'a'-wave: atrial systole, not seen in atrial fibrillation, increased in tricuspid or pulmonary stenosis; heart block causes variable 'a'-waves and even 'cannon' waves. 'c'-wave: leaflets of the tricuspid valve bulge into the right atrium during isovolumetric contraction. 'v'-wave: right atrium is rapidly filled while tricuspid valve is closed. 'x'-descent: atrium relaxes and tricuspid valve moves down. 'y'-descent: tricuspid valve opens, and blood flows from right atrium to right ventricle.

Coronary Circulation

See also Chapter 1 – Blood Supply of Heart.

- Coronary blood flow is about 250 mL/min at rest.
- Rises to 1 L/min on exercise.
- Coronary flow is reduced during systole (especially during isovolumetric contraction) due to compression of the intramyocardial arteries.
- Coronary flow therefore occurs mainly during diastole.
- Conditions resulting in low diastolic BP or increased intramyocardial tension during diastole (e.g. an increased end diastolic pressure) may compromise coronary blood flow.
- Subendocardial muscle, where the tension is highest, is particularly vulnerable.
- Diastolic time is important. At fast rates, inadequate myocardial perfusion occurs.
- Normally, autoregulation of coronary blood flow occurs by changes in diameter in the coronary vessels; the diameter is controlled by vessel tone and wall pressure exerted by the myocardial muscle.
- The tone of vessels is determined by local metabolites, adenosine, K^+ and lack of oxygen.

Cardiac Output (CO)

- Cardiac output is the volume of blood ejected by the heart in 1 min.

  CO = stroke volume (SV) × heart rate (HR),
  i.e. 70 mL (SV) × 70 bpm (HR) = 5 L/min (approximately)

- May increase three- to fourfold in strenuous exercise.
- Cardiac index (CI) is the CO per square metre of body surface area (BSA), i.e. 3.2 L (average).

Regulation of Cardiac Output

Regulation of the vascular system ensures that:

- Each organ receives its minimum required blood flow.
- Redistribution of blood flow occurs where appropriate.
- The heart is not overtaxed by providing maximal blood flow to organs that do not require it.
- The heart has the capacity to increase or decrease its output according to demand.
- Each organ has its own mechanism for achieving adequate blood flow.

Starling's Law of the Heart (Fig. 9.5)

- Starling's law: the energy of contraction of a cardiac muscle fibre is a function of the initial length of the muscle fibre.
- The greater the stretch of the ventricle in diastole, the greater the stroke volume.

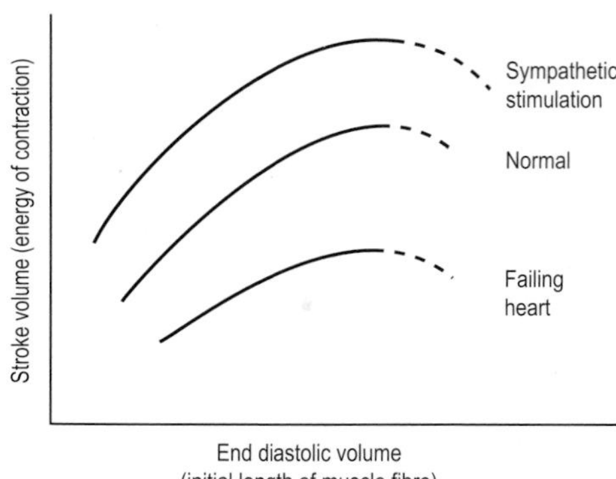

Fig. 9.5 Starling's law of the heart. In humans the initial fibre length cannot be measured, so end diastolic volume is used instead.

- The more blood in the heart, i.e. the higher the end-diastolic volume, the more sarcomeres are stretched.
- Up to a point, increasing the venous return increases the force that the heart muscle can exert.
- Beyond the critical point, further increase in the amount of blood decreases the force that the heart muscle can exert.

Factors Modifying Cardiac Output

- Heart rate:
  - intrinsic rhythmicity
  - extrinsic factors:
    - sympathetic increases rate and force
    - parasympathetic reduces rate.
- Stroke volume:
  - contractility
  - preload
  - afterload.

1 Contractility

- The force of myocardial contraction determines the CO, SV and myocardial O_2 demand.
- Causes of increased contractility include:
  - increased preload
  - sympathetic nerve stimulation
  - increased extracellular calcium
  - drugs: inotropes, digoxin
  - hormones: catecholamines, thyroxine, glucagons.
- Causes of decreased contractility:
  - reduced filling (Starling's law)
  - hypoxia
  - hypercapnia
  - acidosis
  - ischaemia and cardiac disease
  - parasympathetic stimulation

- electrolyte imbalance: Ca^{2+}, K^+
- drugs: beta-blockers, antiarrhythmic drugs, anaesthetics.
- Contractility measured by:
  - stroke volume and CO
  - ejection fraction on echocardiography.

2 Preload

- Dependent on:
  - venous return
  - atrial systole (fibrillation)
  - myocardial distensibility.
- Measured by:
  - central venous pressure (CVP)
  - pulmonary artery occlusion pressure (PAOP).

3 Afterload

Afterload is the tension in the ventricular wall during ventricular ejection.

- Increased by:
  - raised aortic pressure
  - aortic valve resistance (aortic stenosis)
  - ventricular cavity size; increased ventricular volume; requires greater tension to contract (Laplace's law)
  - raised systemic vascular resistance (SVR), e.g. shock
  - increased afterload increases cardiac work and therefore oxygen consumption.
- Decreased by:
  - vasodilator drugs: at constant preload and contractility, SV is inversely related to afterload, i.e. decrease in the peripheral resistance with a vasodilator increases SV
  - vasodilator metabolites in septic shock.

Measurement of Cardiac Output

Cardiac output may be measured by the following methods:

- Fick method.
- Thermodilution.
- Dye dilution.
- Doppler ultrasound.

The direct Fick method is rarely used in clinical practice, but most methods are based on this principle. The thermodilution method and Doppler ultrasound are more likely to be used in clinical practice.

Fick Method

- Fick principle states that the amount of substance taken up by an organ per unit time is equal to the blood flow multiplied by the difference in concentration of that substance between arterial and mixed venous blood.
- O_2 consumption by whole body is measured for about 15 min. During this time, blood samples are taken from a systemic artery and pulmonary artery (mixed venous) blood:

$$\text{CO} = \frac{\text{Oxygen consumption rate by body (mL/min)}}{\text{Arterial } O_2 - \text{mixed venous } O_2}$$

$$\text{i.e. } \frac{250 \text{ mL } O_2\text{/min}}{190 \text{ mL } O_2\text{/L blood} - 140 \text{ mL } O_2\text{/L blood}}$$

$$\text{CO} = 5 \text{ L/min}$$

Thermodilution

This is the most commonly used technique in the intensive treatment unit (ITU).

- A bolus of ice-cold 5% dextrose is rapidly injected into the right atrium via the proximal lumen of a pulmonary artery catheter.
- The dextrose mixes with blood and causes a fall in temperature, which is recorded by a thermistor at the catheter tip in the distal pulmonary artery.
- Computerized integration of the temperature curves allows derivation of the CO.
- When CO is known it is possible to calculate SVR, pulmonary vascular resistance (PVR) and ventricular stroke work.

Dye Dilution

- Uses the same principle as the thermodilution technique but a dye is used rather than ice-cold dextrose.

Doppler Ultrasound

- A Doppler probe is placed in the suprasternal notch.
- Changing frequency of ultrasound waves caused by reflection from blood moving through the ascending aorta is detected.
- From analysis of the velocity waveform and aortic diameter, the stroke volume can be estimated and hence CO measured.

Blood Pressure

- BP = CO × SVR.
- Systolic pressure = maximum pressure recorded during systole (100–200 mmHg).
- Diastolic pressure = minimum pressure recorded during diastole (60–80 mmHg).
- Pulse pressure = systolic pressure minus diastolic pressure (40 mmHg).
- Mean arterial pressure = diastolic pressure plus ⅓ of the pulse pressure (70 mmHg).

Control of Blood Pressure (General Systemic Blood Pressure)

- Regulation of CO and SVR controls BP.
- Baroceptors of the autonomic nervous system (aortic arch and carotid) and higher centres of midbrain exert effects on BP.
- Baroceptors are stretched by increased BP; this leads to reflex reduction in vasoconstriction and venoconstriction, and reduction in heart rate, with consequent fall in SVR, CO and BP.
- When BP falls baroceptors are less stretched; vasoconstriction, venoconstriction and heart rate increase and BP rises in reflex.
- Autonomic neuropathy may render these reflexes ineffective.
- Renin–angiotensin mechanism also controls BP.

Factors Determining Arterial Blood Pressure

- Systolic pressure increases when there is an increase in:
  - stroke volume
  - ejection velocity (without an increase in stroke volume)
  - diastolic pressure of the preceding pulse
  - arterial rigidity (arteriosclerosis).
- Diastolic pressure increases when there is an increase in:
  - total peripheral resistance
  - arterial compliance (distensibility)
  - heart rate.

Control of Local Blood Pressure and Blood Flow

The overall determinant of flow is CO, but each organ has its own superimposed regulatory mechanisms. Regulation of blood flow is mainly achieved by alteration to the diameter of vessels, which is influenced by the smooth muscle of the vessel walls.

Tone in smooth muscle is affected by:

- neural activity, e.g. sympathetic, parasympathetic
- hormones, e.g. adrenaline, noradrenaline, vasopressin, angiotensin
- local control – autoregulation: hypoxia, adenosine, nitric oxide, CO_2, H^+, K^+, prostaglandins.

Peripheral Resistance (Systemic Vascular Resistance; SVR)

- Resistance to flow of blood through arterioles.
- By constricting and dilating, arterioles control the blood flow to capillaries according to local needs.

$$SVR = \frac{\text{Mean arterial pressure} - \text{mean right atrial pressure}}{\text{Cardiac output}}$$

- Repeated measurements of SVR in the critically ill patient are useful in monitoring the effects of fluid and inotropic therapy.

Monitoring the Circulation

- There is no one single monitoring measure which will define the problem.
- A series of measurements and monitoring systems over a period of time is required.

Methods used include:

- ECG
- blood pressure
- central venous pressure
- pulmonary wedge pressure (pulmonary artery occlusion pressure)
- pulse oximetry
- cardiac output
- urine output
- echocardiography
- echo Doppler.

ECG

The events recorded in a standard ECG recording are shown in Fig. 9.6. The ECG gives information on:

- heart rate
- rhythm (regular or irregular)
- disorders of conduction or excitation
- size and muscle mass of the heart
- damage, e.g. ischaemia or infarction, to different parts of the heart
- electrolyte disturbances, e.g. K^+, Ca^{2+}
- pericardium, e.g. inflammation or effusion.

Blood Pressure

- Monitored by manual sphygmomanometry, automatic dynamap, or best by intra-arterial catheter, usually in the radial artery.
- In the critically ill there should be continuous observation of the pressure trace.
- The rate of pressure increase (up-slope) of the pressure trace is proportional to myocardial contractility.
- The area under the wave-form is proportional to stroke volume.

Central Venous Pressure

- Gives a good indication of preload in patients with normal heart.
- Useful guide to fluid replacement in hypovolaemic patients, e.g. dehydration, haemorrhage.
- Cannula inserted via internal jugular vein; tip should be in right atrium.

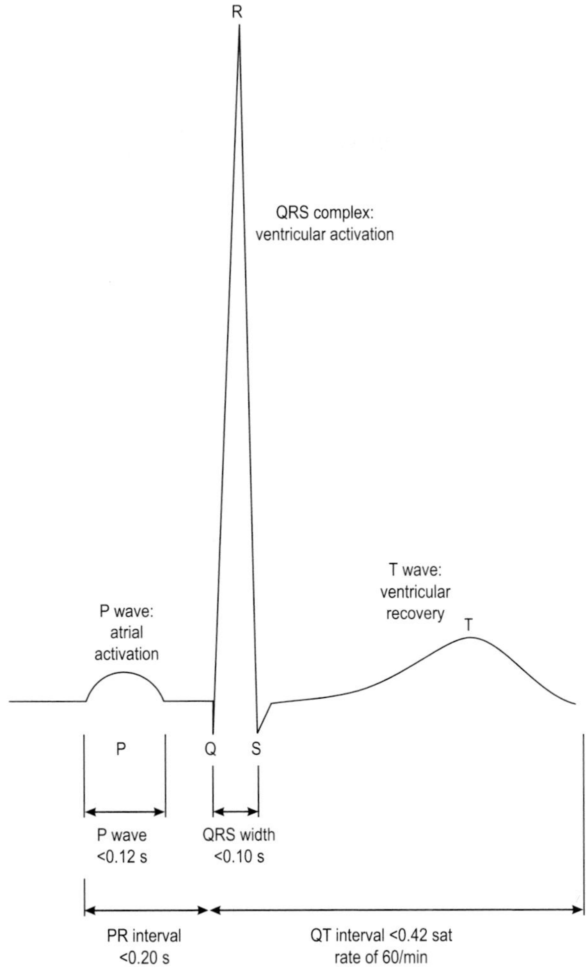

Fig. 9.6 Standard ECG recording during the timing of various events in the cardiac cycle.

- A correctly positioned catheter should give a normal venous pressure wave form (i.e. a, c, v waves).
- Measurement should be made after 'zeroing' the transducer to the level of the right atrium.
- Isolated readings are of little use due to:
  - individual variations in the condition of the heart
  - some patients can compensate with a remarkable degree of vasoconstriction in the presence of hypovolaemia, such that CVP may become transiently elevated.
- Normal CVP ranges 5–12 mmHg.
- Low CVP indicates hypovolaemia.
- High CVP usually indicates fluid overload.
- If there is disparity between function of the right and left ventricles (e.g. right ventricular infarction, pulmonary embolism [PE], left ventricular disease), the filling pressure of the right heart, i.e. CVP, may not reflect the filling pressure of the left heart. Therefore CVP will not be accurate and pulmonary capillary wedge pressure measurement is required.

Pulmonary Capillary Wedge Pressure (Pulmonary Artery Occlusion Pressure; PAOP)

- PAOP reflects left atrial pressure as the resistance in the pulmonary veins is low.
- A flotation balloon catheter is passed through the right heart into the pulmonary artery.
- Inflation of the balloon excludes flow from the right side of the heart, allowing a fluid bridge to complete the connection to the left atrium.
- The pressure at the catheter tip equates to that in the left atrium.
- The balloon is deflated between readings to avoid pulmonary infarction.
- The normal pulmonary artery occlusion pressure (PAO) is 6–12 mmHg. It should be kept below 15 mmHg to minimize the risk of pulmonary oedema.
- The major advantage of the catheter is that it can be used to measure CO.

Pulse Oximetry

- Measures the arterial oxygen saturation (SaO_2).
- It relies on the measurement of the different absorption of oxyhaemoglobin and deoxyhaemoglobin at different wavelengths.
- The instrument pulses infrared light at wavelengths of 660–940 nm.
- The pulsation component of absorption is measured and the constant background component not due to arterial blood, i.e. absorption by skin, venous blood and fat, is subtracted.
- Because oxygenated and deoxygenated Hb absorb differing amounts at the two wavelengths, pulse oximetry is able to calculate a percentage of saturated Hb from the ratio of the two.
- The problems with pulse oximetry include:
  - delay: calculations are made from a number of pulses and there is a 20 s delay between actual and displayed values
  - irregular pulse: atrial fibrillation
  - venous pulsation (tricuspid incompetence)
  - hypotension
  - vasoconstriction
  - abnormal Hb (carboxy-), and methaemoglobin
  - bilirubin

- methylene blue dye
- other factors: electrical interference (diathermy), flickering lights, patient movement, shivering, nail varnish (coloured or not).

Cardiac Output

- Useful as *part* of overall assessment of circulation.
- Once CO is known it is possible to derive values for SVR, the amount of work the heart is performing, oxygen delivery and oxygen consumption.
- Specific pharmacological therapy can then be given to optimize the circulation.

Urine Output

- Directly related to renal perfusion.
- Good indicator of overall fluid balance.

Echocardiography

- Transthoracic echocardiography allows non-invasive real-time imaging at the bedside.
- Provides information on cardiac structure, function and haemodynamics.

Echo Doppler

- Measures blood flow in the aorta via an oesophageal probe.
- Gives indication of contractility and CO.
- Contraindicated with oesophageal pathology, e.g. stricture and varices.

Cardiovascular Support

- Ventilate.
- Infusion.
- Pump.

Ventilate

- Improves oxygenation and gas exchange.
- Controls acidosis (by CO_2 control).
- Reduces oxygen demand by respiratory muscle.

Infusion

- Ensure adequate filling pressure.
- Fluid challenge with monitoring, e.g. CVP, PAOP.

Pump

- Maintain blood pressure.
- Monitor CO.
- Ensure organ blood flow.
- If SVR low, use vasopressor to improve perfusion pressure.

Pharmacological Support

- Inotropes: increase force of ventricular contraction, usually β-effect.
- Vasopressor: constricts blood vessels, α-effect.
- Vasodilator: dilates blood vessels.
- Chronotrope: increased heart rate, β-effect.

Adrenaline

- Both α- and β-effects.
- Inotrope, vasopressor, chronotrope.
- β_2-effect at low doses causes vasodilatation in skeletal muscle, lowering SVR.
- α-vasoconstrictor effect at higher doses increases SVR and myocardial oxygen demands, with adverse effect on cardiac output.

Noradrenaline

- α-effect.
- Vasopressor.
- Indicated in septic shock when hypotension due to peripheral vasodilatation persists despite adequate volume replacement.

Isoprenaline

- Exclusively β-effect.
- Inotrope, chronotrope.
- Vasodilatation in skeletal muscle; therefore reduces SVR.
- Tachycardia limits clinical use.
- Used to increase rate in heart block while awaiting pacing.

Dopamine

- Low dose dilates renal, cerebral, coronary and splanchnic vessels, via D_1 and D_2 receptors and β_1 receptors, resulting in increased cardiac contractility and heart rate.
- High dose stimulates α-receptors, causing vasoconstriction.

Dobutamine

- β_1 and β_2.
- Inotrope, vasodilator.
- β_1 effect increases heart rate and force of contraction.
- Mild β_2 effect causes vasodilatation.
- First choice inotrope in cardiogenic shock due to left ventricular dysfunction.
- Dobutamine and low-dose dopamine in conjunction used in cardiogenic shock to increase BP via increased cardiac contractility and urinary output (UO; via increased renal perfusion).

Dopexamine

- β_2 and D receptors.
- Inotrope, chronotrope.
- Peripheral vasodilatation, increased splanchnic blood flow and increased renal perfusion (increased UO).

Vasodilators

- Nitrates: venodilators reducing preload.
- Nitroprusside: chiefly arterial vasodilator with short half-life given by infusion.
- Hydralazine: arterial vasodilator reduces afterload.

Phosphodiesterase Inhibitors

- Decrease the rate of breakdown of cAMP by phosphodiesterase III.
- Inotropic and vasodilator effect. Little chronotropic effect.
- Increased myocardial contractility (increased CO) with reduced PAOP and SVR.
- No significant rise in heart rate or myocardial oxygen consumption.

OSCE SCENARIOS

OSCE Scenario 9.1

An 80-year-old male is 5 days post-repair of abdominal aortic aneurysm. He has suddenly developed a tachycardia and become hypotensive. His ECG shows atrial fibrillation with a rate of 140.

1. What are the causes of atrial fibrillation?
2. What are the physiological mechanisms which explain the hypotension seen in fast atrial fibrillation?
3. How would you diagnose atrial fibrillation?
4. Describe your initial management of the patient.

OSCE Scenario 9.2

An 89-year-old male is 8 days post-laparotomy for repair of a perforated duodenal ulcer. He has developed a severe postoperative chest infection and is pyrexial and hypotensive.

1. Describe your initial management of this patient.
2. Why does sepsis lead to hypotension?
3. Which inotrope is commonly used in sepsis and what is its mode of action?
4. What is Starling's law of the heart and how do inotropes affect it?

OSCE Scenario 9.3

A 58-year-old male is admitted with severe interscapular back pain. He is hypertensive with a BP of 200/140. A CT angiogram shows a type B aortic dissection.

1. What is the difference between a type A and B dissection?
2. How is a type A dissection managed?
3. How is an uncomplicated type B dissection managed?

OSCE Scenario 9.4

A 72-year-old male patient underwent elective open abdominal aortic aneurysm repair. An infra-renal aortic cross clamp was required.

1. What are the physiological and cardiovascular changes that result from aortic cross clamping?
2. What techniques would the anaesthetists use to reduce these effects?
3. What are the physiological and cardiovascular changes that result from releasing aortic cross clamp?
4. What techniques would the anaesthetists use to reduce these effects?

OSCE Scenario 9.5

A 75-year-old female patient underwent difficult open anterior resection. She has past medical history of hypertension, ischaemic heart disease and transient ischaemic attack (TIA). The procedure was complicated with significant blood loss that necessitated intraoperative blood transfusion. Postoperatively, she was admitted to the high-dependency unit as she required vasopressors support.

1. What methods can be utilised to monitor the cardiovascular system?
2. What is the best indicator to assess adequate fluid balance?
3. How does the pulse oximetry work?
4. What are the problems and pitfalls that can occur when reading pulse oximetry?
5. What is a vasopressor? Give some examples used in common clinical practice.

Answers in Appendix pages 449–451

Please check your eBook at https://studentconsult.inkling.com/ for more self-assessment questions. See inside cover for registration details.

10

Gastrointestinal System

FUNCTIONS

The functions of the various components of the gastrointestinal (GI) system are:

- Oral cavity: teeth crush and tear food; the tongue forms a food bolus in preparation for swallowing; saliva secretion initiates carbohydrate digestion.
- Pharynx and oesophagus: conveys food from the oral cavity to the stomach.
- Stomach: stores food; mechanically and chemically digests food; regulates the passage of chyme into the duodenum; secretes intrinsic factor.
- Small bowel: food passes from the stomach into the small intestine; this is where the majority of food digestion and absorption occurs.
- Large bowel: water is removed from undigested food, which is then stored in the rectum in preparation to be excreted; vitamin K and some B vitamins are produced by resident bacterial flora.
- Liver: an important site for carbohydrate, protein and lipid metabolism; involved in the synthesis of several plasma proteins and clotting factors; the primary site for detoxification and elimination of body waste and toxins.
- Gall bladder: stores and concentrates bile.
- Pancreas: has both exocrine and endocrine functions, secreting the majority of digestive enzymes.

Nervous and Hormonal Regulation Within the GI Tract

Nervous Regulation

The nervous system of the GI tract consists of:

- Intrinsic or enteric system.
- Extrinsic system:
  - sympathetic
  - parasympathetic.
- The intrinsic nervous system is found in the wall of the GI tract and forms two well-defined plexuses:
  - myenteric or Auerbach's plexus: this lies between the circular and longitudinal muscle layers; it is mainly involved in motor function
  - submucosal or Meissner's plexus: this lies within the submucosa; it is mainly sensory.
- The enteric nervous system responds to numerous gut transmitters such as cholecystokinin, substance P, vasoactive intestinal peptide (VIP) and somatostatin; it is responsible for the majority of gut secretion and motility.
- The enteric nervous system also receives input from the autonomic (extrinsic) nervous system:
  - Sympathetic: fibres terminate in the submucosal and myenteric plexuses; stimulation of the sympathetic system leads to:
    - blood vessels: vasoconstriction
    - glandular tissue: inhibits secretion
    - sphincters: contraction
    - circular muscle of bowel: inhibits (↓ motility).
  - Parasympathetic: fibres terminate in the myenteric plexus only; stimulation of the parasympathetic system leads to:
    - glandular tissue: increases secretion
    - sphincters: relaxation
    - circular muscle of bowel: stimulates (↑ motility).

Hormones and Neurotransmitters

- Play an important role in regulating GI motility and secretion; these include:
  - gastrin
  - secretin
  - cholecystokinin (CCK)
  - pancreatic polypeptide
  - gastric inhibitory polypeptide (GIP)
  - motilin
  - enteroglucagons
  - neurotensin.
- These hormones and neurotransmitters will be discussed individually in the relevant sections.

Oral Cavity, Pharynx and Oesophagus

Chewing

- Food is ingested through the mouth and is divided between two regions:
  - vestibule: space between the teeth, lips and cheeks
  - oral cavity: inner area bound by the teeth.
- Chewing or mastication has a number of functions:
  - teeth are able to cut, grind and tear food, allowing it to be swallowed more easily
  - mixes food with saliva and mucus; this lubricates it in preparation for swallowing, and starts carbohydrate digestion with salivary amylase.

Saliva

- Saliva is secreted by a number of glands:
  - parotid: watery secretion lacking mucus; accounts for around 25% of saliva secretion; also contains salivary amylase and IgA
  - submandibular: produces a more viscous saliva (a mixed serous and mucosal saliva); accounts for approximately 70% of saliva secretion
  - sublingual: contains mucoproteins; accounts for only 5% of saliva secretion.
- Numerous saliva glands are present over the tongue and palate.
- Saliva has a number of functions:
  - lubrication to help swallowing: mucus
  - speech
  - taste
  - antibacterial action: lysozyme and IgA
  - starch digestion: amylase.
- Formation of saliva within the salivary glands is a two-stage process:

1. Isotonic fluid of similar composition to the extracellular fluid (ECF) is secreted by the acinar component of the salivary gland.
2. The isotonic fluid is modified as it moves along the duct; Na^+ and Cl^- is removed and K^+ and HCO_3^- are added by means of ATP transport proteins.

- During low rates of secretion the saliva is dilute as there is plenty of time for ductal modification.
- During high rates of secretion the Na^+, HCO_3^- and Cl^- content increases and is thus more concentrated.
- Control of the secretion of saliva is via the autonomic nervous system; this reflex is stimulated by the salivary nuclei in the medulla; secretion of saliva is stimulated by:
  - stimulation of mechanoreceptors and chemoreceptors in the mouth
  - higher centres in the CNS, i.e. smelling or thinking about food.
- Parasympathetic impulses via cranial nerves VII and IX stimulate saliva secretion; sympathetic impulses lead to vasoconstriction and a decrease in saliva secretion.

Swallowing

Swallowing can be divided into a number of phases:

- Oral phase: voluntary; a food bolus is pushed against the roof of the mouth by the tongue; this forces the food into the oropharynx and then into the pharynx.
- Pharyngeal phase: involuntary; the superior constrictor raises the soft palate (preventing food entering the nasopharynx). In addition it initiates a wave of contraction (peristalsis) that pushes the food through the upper oesophageal sphincter. At this stage respiration is inhibited so as to prevent food entering the respiratory system.
- Oesophageal phase: the wave of contraction, which was initiated by the superior constrictor in the pharynx, continues into the oesophagus. This wave of contraction propels the food into the stomach. If the food fails to enter the stomach then the resulting distension initiates a secondary peristaltic wave.

Oesophageal Sphincter

- The oesophageal sphincter is an area of high pressure (15–25 mmHg) in the region 2 cm above and 2 cm below the diaphragm; it is a physiological sphincter as there are no anatomical differences to identify it as the sphincter.
- The oesophageal sphincter acts to prevent gastric juices refluxing from the stomach into the oesophagus.
- In addition to the physiological sphincter there are a number of other factors that assist in preventing reflux:
  - the right crus of the diaphragm compresses the oesophagus as it passes through the oesophageal hiatus
  - the acute angle at which the oesophagus enters the stomach acts as a valve
  - mucosal folds in the lower oesophagus act as a valve
  - closure of the sphincter is under vagal control; however, the hormone gastrin causes the sphincter to contract (secretin, CCK and glucagon cause it to relax).

STOMACH

Gastric Mucosa

- The gastric mucosa contains a variety of secretory cells; the mucosa is divided into:
  - columnar epithelium: secretes a protective mucus layer
  - gastric glands: intersperse the mucosa; they contain a variety of secretory cells.

- These secretory cells include:
  - mucus cells: secrete mucus and are situated at the opening of the gastric gland
  - peptic or chief cells: found at the base of the gastric glands and secrete pepsinogen
  - parietal or oxyntic cells: secrete hydrochloric acid and intrinsic factor
  - neuroendocrine cells: secrete a number of peptides that regulate GI motility and secretion, i.e. gastrin.
- The predominant cell type in the gastric glands varies throughout the various regions of the stomach:
  - fundus and body: peptic and parietal cells predominate
  - antrum and pylorus: parietal cells are less common; mucus and neuroendocrine (secreting gastrin) cells predominate
  - cardia: gastric glands are composed almost completely of mucus cells.

Gastric Secretion

Gastric Acid (Fig. 10.1)

- The stomach secretes approximately 2–3 L/day; it contains:
  - hydrochloric acid
  - pepsinogen
  - mucus
  - intrinsic factor
  - salt and water.
- Stomach acid has a pH of around 1–3; it plays a number of roles:
  - tissue breakdown
  - converts pepsinogen to the active pepsin
  - forms soluble salts with calcium and iron; this aids their absorption
  - acts as an immune defence mechanism by killing micro-organisms.
- Gastric acid is secreted by the parietal cells; when activated, deep clefts form in the apical membrane; these canaliculi allow the acid to be secreted into the stomach.
- Chloride and hydrogen ions are pumped from the parietal cells; this process is energy dependent.
- H^+ ions are pumped from the cell by the H^+/K^+ ATPase system.
- Cl^- ions are pumped from the cell by two routes: one is a chloride channel, the other is a Cl^-/K^+ co-transport system (K^+ is thus cycled into the cell via the H^+/K^+ ATPase system and out via the Cl^-/K^+ system).
- H^+ ions are produced by oxidative processes; this also produces a hydroxyl ion; in a reaction catalysed by carbonic anhydrase this results in the formation of HCO_3^-, which is then exchanged for Cl^- on the basolateral surface of the cell.
- The secretion of HCO_3^- is a protective mechanism that prevents the gastric acid from damaging the mucosa; it is referred to as the 'alkaline tide'; the production of HCO_3^- can be influenced by prostaglandins.

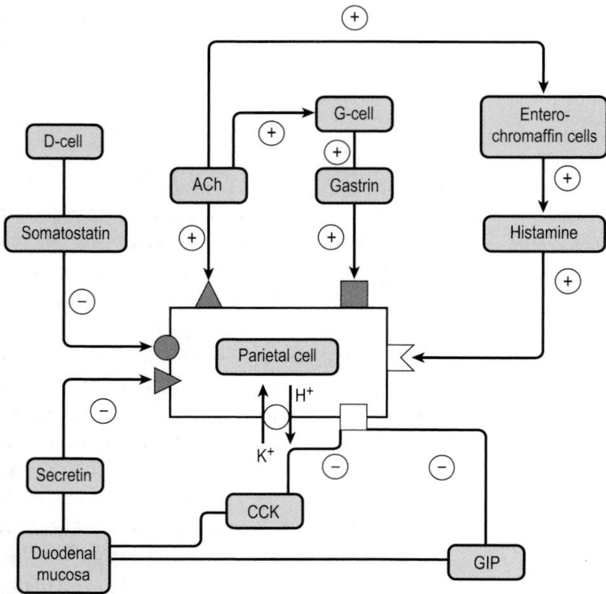

Fig. 10.1 Regulation of acid secretion by the parietal cell. (From McGeown JG. Physiology, 2nd edn. Churchill Livingstone, Edinburgh, 2002, with permission.)

Pepsinogen Secretion

- The peptic cells produce pepsinogen, a proteolytic enzyme that hydrolyses peptide bonds in proteins.
- The enzyme is secreted into the gastric glands in an inactive form (pepsinogen); exposure to the acid environment in the stomach activates the enzyme (pepsin).

Mucus Secretion

- Mucus is secreted from cells at the neck of the gastric glands; the secreted mucus forms a layer (mucosal barrier) over the gastric epithelium and prevents the gastric acid and secreted pepsins from digesting the stomach lining.
- The mucus is alkaline; this helps to neutralize gastric acid.
- Additional factors which protect the stomach from digestion include:
  - tight epithelial junctions prevent acid reaching deeper tissues
  - prostaglandin E secretion has a protective role by increasing the thickness of the mucus layer, stimulating HCO_3^- production and increasing blood flow in the mucosa (bringing nutrients to any damaged areas).

Intrinsic Factor Secretion

- Secreted from parietal cells; the stimulus for excretion is the same as for acid secretion.
- Intrinsic factor (IF) binds to vitamin B_{12}; it is then absorbed in complex with the IF via specialized receptors in the ileum (see below).

Regulation of Gastric Secretion

- Divided into three phases:
  - cephalic
  - gastric
  - intestinal.
- Cephalic phase: sight, smell and even the anticipation of food lead to impulses from the appetite centre in the hypothalamus to the stomach; it contributes to almost 30% of gastric secretions. This descending input is parasympathetic and runs in the vagus; vagal activity stimulates gastric secretion in a number of ways:
  - direct stimulation of the gastric glands via acetylcholine release
  - release of gastrin from the neuroendocrine cells (G-cells) in the antrum; gastrin stimulates acid and pepsin secretion
  - release of histamine from mast cells; this stimulates parietal cells via H_2 receptors, which leads to acid production (gastrin also stimulates histamine release).
- Gastric phase: food entering the stomach stimulates the gastric phase; this is the primary stimulus to secretion and accounts for around 60% of gastric secretion. Distension of the stomach and the chemical composition of food lead to acetylcholine release from the vagus.
- Intestinal phase: only accounts for 5% of gastric secretion; the stimulation is the presence of food in the duodenum; this results in the release of gastrin from G-cells in the duodenal mucosa.
- There are a number of other influences on gastric secretion:
  - the secretion of gastrin is inhibited when the pH falls to around 2–3
  - somatostatin secreted from neuroendocrine cells (D-cells) inhibits gastrin secretion
  - secretin from the duodenal mucosa is released in response to acid in the duodenum; it inhibits gastrin release
  - fatty food in the duodenum leads to the release of CCK and GIP; both inhibit gastrin secretion.
- The action of hormones released in the duodenum is referred to as the enterogastric reflex.

Gastric Motility

- The main functions of the stomach are storage and mixing and propulsion of food into the intestine; the storage area consists of the fundus and body, whereas the mixing and propulsion area is the antrum and pylorus.

Storage

- The stomach has a resting volume of around 50 mL and an intragastric pressure of 5–6 mmHg; however, it is able to accommodate significantly greater volumes with little change in pressure (approximately 1 L). As the stomach is distended, parasympathetic input from the vagus inhibits muscle contraction.

Mixing and Propulsion

- The stomach has three muscle layers: longitudinal, circular and oblique.
- Contractions in the stomach are more intense in the more muscular pyloric area in comparison with the gentle contractions in the storage area of the fundus.
- Peristaltic waves push food or chyme towards the pylorus; as pressure increases the pyloric sphincter will open and a small amount of food is allowed through to the duodenum.
- Parasympathetic impulses tend to increase motility whereas sympathetic impulses decrease motility.
- The amount of food allowed in to the duodenum is carefully regulated by a number of factors:
  - gastric volume: $\uparrow$volume then more rapid emptying
  - fatty food: CCK and GIP are released by the small intestine in response to fatty foods; they increase contractility of the pyloric sphincter

- proteins: proteins and amino acids stimulate gastrin release; gastrin increases contractility of the pyloric sphincter
- acid: acid entering the duodenum results in a vagally mediated delay in gastric emptying and also leads to secretin release. Secretin inhibits antral contractions and increases contractility in the pyloric sphincter. Secretin also stimulates HCO_3^- release from the pancreas to neutralize the acid
- hypertonic chyme: delays gastric emptying.

Clinical Physiology

Vomiting

- The reflex action of ejecting the contents of the stomach through the mouth.
- Prior to vomiting, autonomic symptoms such as salivation, pallor, sweating and dizziness often occur.
- The events which occur during vomiting are:
  - respiration is inhibited
  - the larynx closes and the soft palate rises
  - the stomach and pyloric sphincter relax and the duodenum contracts, propelling intestinal contents into the stomach
  - the diaphragm and abdominal wall contracts → intragastric pressure rises
  - the gastro-oesophageal sphincter relaxes and the pylorus closes
  - stomach contents expelled through the mouth.
- The vomiting reflex is co-ordinated by the vomiting centre in the medulla; stimulation of the vomiting centre leads to motor impulses passing along cranial nerves V, VII, IX and XII, and to the intercostals and abdominal muscles and diaphragm.
- Causes of vomiting include:
  - stimulation of the posterior oropharynx
  - excessive distension of the stomach or duodenum
  - stimulation of the labyrinth, e.g. motion sickness
  - severe pain
  - raised intracranial pressure
  - stimulation of the chemoreceptor trigger zone by noxious chemicals
  - bacterial irritation of the upper GI tract.

Treatment of Peptic Ulceration

- The treatment of peptic ulcer disease can be divided into medical and surgical.

Medical treatment

- The choices for medical treatment are:
  - reduce acid secretion
  - mucosal protection
  - antacids (pH increasers).
- There are three groups of drugs used in the reduction of acid secretion:
  - histamine (H_2-receptor) antagonists, e.g. cimetidine and ranitidine: these drugs act by blocking H_2-receptors on parietal cells. Although these cells also possess gastrin and muscarinic receptors, both gastrin and acetylcholine mainly stimulate acid production indirectly by stimulating histamine release. The blocking of H-receptors prevents the intracellular increase in cAMP, and thus acid production
  - muscarinic antagonists, i.e. pirenzepine: this is only of historical value, as this drug is no longer in clinical use. Pirenzepine was a selective M_1-receptor antagonist that was selective for the muscarinic receptors on parietal cells but did not produce the unwanted symptoms of blurred vision, dry mouth, etc.
  - proton pump inhibitors (PPIs), e.g. omeprazole: this group of drugs acts directly on the proton pump (H^+/K^+ ATPase). It is inactive at neutral pH but is activated by the acidic conditions in the stomach; it then irreversibly binds to sulfydryl groups on the proton pump.
- The mucosal protectants aim to support the mucus layer that normally protects the gastric mucosa; there are three types:
  - sucralfate: formed from sulphated sucrose and aluminium hydroxide, it polymerizes at $pH < 4$ to form a sticky layer that adheres to the base of the ulcer
  - bismuth chelate: acts in a similar manner to sucralfate; in addition it has been shown to eradicate *Helicobacter pylori*
  - misoprostol: a synthetic analogue of prostaglandin E_2. This prostaglandin is thought to protect gastric mucosa by stimulating the secretion of mucus and bicarbonate, and increasing the mucosal blood flow.
- Antacids are a very simple treatment for peptic ulcers, and simply consist of alkaline substances that increase the pH within the stomach; examples include:
  - sodium bicarbonate
  - magnesium hydroxide and magnesium trisilicate
  - aluminium hydroxide.

Surgical treatment

- With the advent of PPIs surgical treatment has become much less common. Indications include:
  - chronic unhealed ulcer
  - failure to heal after more than two courses of treatment
  - possible malignancy
  - complications, i.e. bleeding, perforation.
- The options for surgical treatment include (Fig. 10.2):
  - Bilroth I partial gastrectomy
  - Bilroth II partial gastrectomy
  - truncal vagotomy and gastrojejunostomy

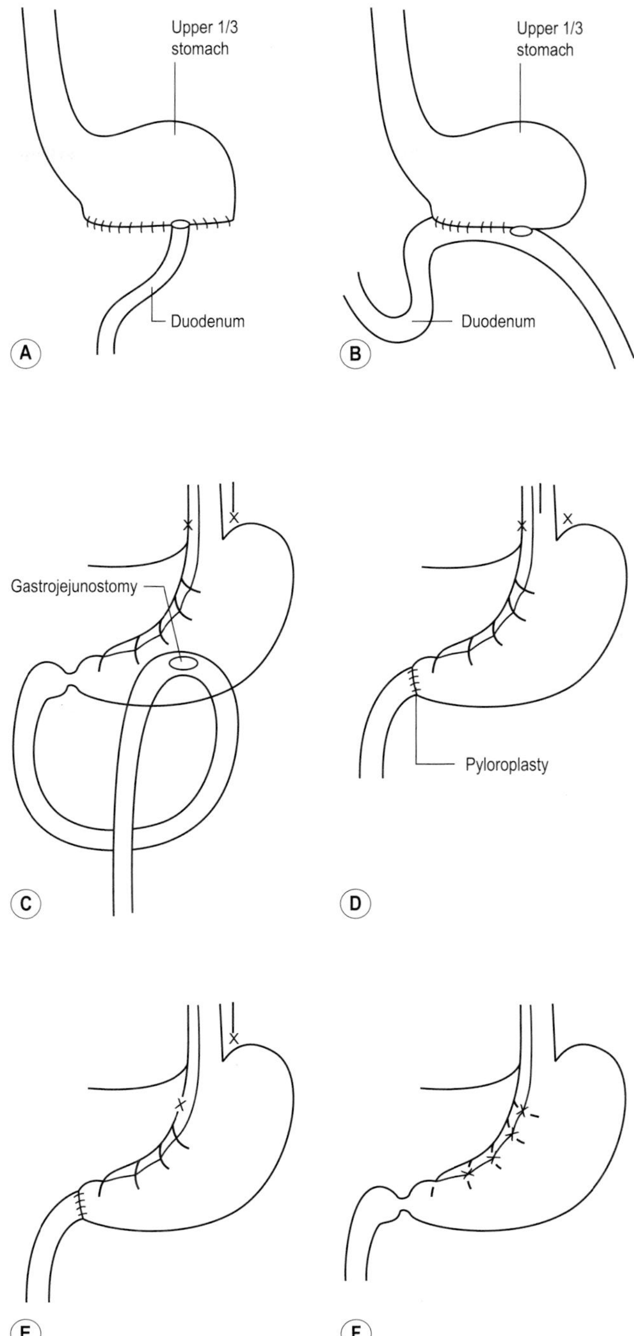

Fig. 10.2 Surgical options for peptic ulceration. (A) Bilroth I. (B) Bilroth II or Polya. (C) Truncal vagotomy and gastrojejunostomy. (D) Truncal vagotomy and pyloroplasty. (E) Selective vagotomy and pyloroplasty. (F) Highly selective vagotomy (no drainage procedure needed). (From McGeown JG. Physiology, 2nd edn. Churchill Livingstone, Edinburgh, 2002, with permission.)

  - truncal vagotomy and pyloroplasty
  - selective vagotomy and pyloroplasty
  - highly selective vagotomy (no drainage procedure needed).
- The surgical treatment of peptic ulcers is associated with a number of complications. These can be divided into post-gastrectomy syndromes and those that occur post-vagotomy.

Post-gastrectomy syndromes

- Malnutrition: occurs due to small capacity stomach, rapid gastric emptying and rapid intestinal transit.
- Deficiency:
  - iron deficiency, as it is in the wrong ionic state for absorption
  - vitamin B_{12} deficiency, due to a lack of intrinsic factor.
- Dumping syndromes: these can be early or late. Early dumping occurs 30–45 min after eating and is due to rapid gastric emptying of a hyperosmolar meal into the small bowel; this results in fluid moving into the small bowel by osmosis (third space loss) and results in dizziness, weakness and palpitations. Late dumping is due to rapid swings in insulin secretion in response to the glucose load in the small bowel; this leads to rebound hypoglycaemia.
- Diarrhoea: due to early gastric emptying and passage of hyperosmolar chyme attracting fluid into the bowel.
- Bilious vomiting: the loss of the pylorus allows reflux of duodenal contents; this leads to bilious vomiting. The refluxed bile can also lead to gastritis and further ulcer development.
- Infection: there is a decreased ability to destroy bacteria, particularly tuberculosis.
- Carcinoma: the duodenal reflux increases the risk of developing gastric cancer in the gastric remnant.

Effects of vagotomy

- Reduced gastric acid secretion.
- Delayed gastric emptying.
- Failure of the pylorus to relax prior to gastric peristaltic wave.
- Reduced pancreatic exocrine secretions.
- Diarrhoea secondary to loss of vagal control of the small bowel.
- Increased risk of large bowel cancer due to excessive bile salts reaching the colon.

SMALL INTESTINE

Small Intestine Mucosa

- The primary function of the small bowel is the absorption of nutrients; a number of characteristics make it particularly suited to this role:
  - large surface area
  - circular folds called plicae circulares, which cause the chyme to spiral round, and thus increase the time for absorption to take place
  - the circular folds are covered with villi—finger-like projections approximately 1 mm high; each of these villi is further covered with microvilli ('brush-border'). These serve to further increase the surface area.
- Interspersed among the villi are the crypts of Lieberkuhn. These are analogous to the gastric glands and contain a number of different cell types:
  - undifferentiated cells that constantly replace enterocytes
  - D-cells: produce somatostatin
  - S-cells: produce secretin
  - N-cells: produce neurotensin
  - Enterochromaffin cells: produce 5-hydroxytryptamine.
- The 'brush-border' secretes a number of enzymes involved in digestion:
  - disaccharidases: maltase, sucrase
  - peptidases
  - phosphatases
  - enteropeptidase or enterokinase (activates pancreatic trypsinogen)
  - lactase (under 4 years).
- The duodenum contains Brunner's glands, which secrete mucus rich in bicarbonate (they are not present in the jejunum or ileum).

Absorption (Table 10.1)

- The small intestine secretes 2–3 L/day of isotonic fluid; Cl^- is transported to the bowel lumen and Na^+ and water follow. In addition, the bowel secretes a number of hormones (see above) and enzymes (see Pancreas section).
- The absorption of nutrients in the small bowel can be divided into:
  - carbohydrates
  - fats
  - proteins
  - fluids and electrolytes
  - vitamins
  - iron
  - calcium.

Carbohydrates (Fig. 10.3)

Glucose and galactose are absorbed via a Na^+-dependent process in which a Na^+/K^+ ATPase pumps out Na^+. The glucose/galactose are then absorbed with the Na^+ via a cotransport protein. A Na^+-independent process absorbs fructose.

Fats (Fig. 10.4)

The absorption of fats is a complex multistage process:

TABLE 10.1 Summary of the Absorption and Secretion of Fluid Within the GI Tract

	Absorbed	Secreted/ Ingested
Mouth	Nothing	2–3 L fluid ingested 1.5 L saliva secreted
Stomach	Lipid-soluble compounds, e.g. alcohol	2–3 L gastric juices secreted
Gallbladder	Absorbs water and concentrates bile	500 mL bile secreted
Pancreas	Nothing	1.5 L pancreatic juices secreted
Small bowel	8–9 L fluid absorbed	1.5 L intestinal secretions
Large bowel	1 L of fluid absorbed	100 mL excreted in faeces

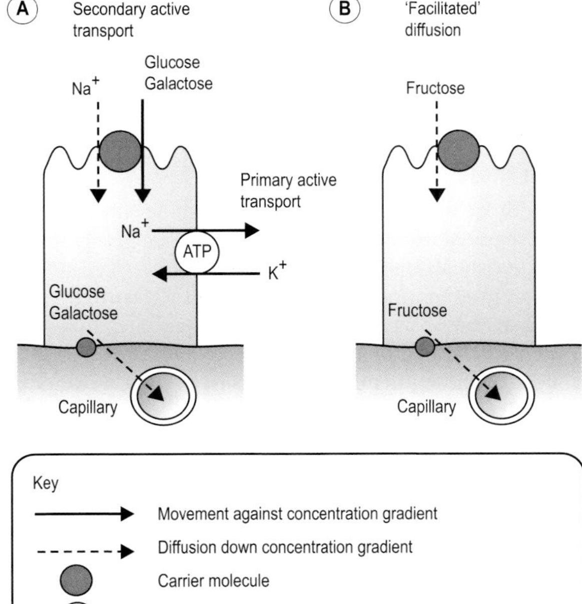

Fig. 10.3 Carbohydrate absorption mechanism. (A) Glucose and galactose are absorbed by an active transport mechanism using Na^+ as a cotransport. (B) Fructose absorption is passive, but utilizes a carrier molecule. (From McGeown JG. Physiology, 2nd edn. Churchill Livingstone, Edinburgh, 2002, with permission.)

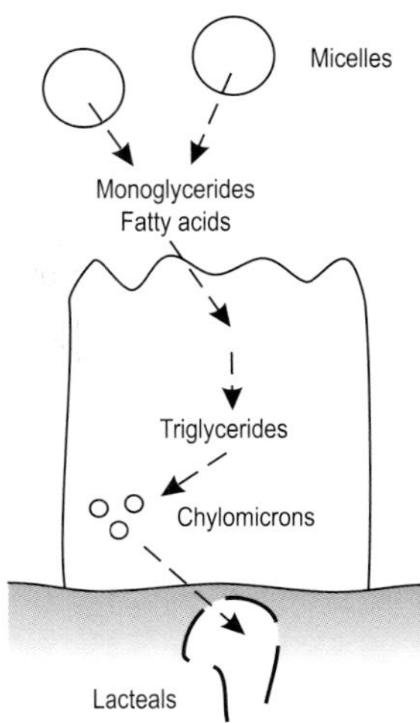

Fig. 10.4 Lipids are absorbed by diffusion as monoglycerides and fatty acids. Inside the cell they are reconstituted to triglycerides, packaged as chylomicrons, and then enter the lymphatic channels (lacteals). (From McGeown JG. Physiology, 2nd edn. Churchill Livingstone, Edinburgh, 2002, with permission.)

- fats form globules in the stomach
- globules are coated with bile salts in the duodenum
- the bile salts disperse these globules into smaller droplets; this increases the surface area exposed to pancreatic enzymes
- fatty droplets are broken down by pancreatic lipases to monoglycerides and free fatty acids (FFA)
- the monoglycerides and FFAs combine with bile salts to form micelles
- micelles have a hydrophilic outer layer and are able to diffuse into the enterocytes; the bile salt stays in the bowel lumen
- in the enterocytes, the smooth endoplasmic reticulum reforms triglycerides from the absorbed monoglycerides and FFAs
- the reformed triglycerides are formed into particles of fat called chylomicrons, which are released from the basal layer of the enterocyte to diffuse into the lacteals within the villi; from here they enter the lymphatic circulation and then into the venous circulation.

Protein (Fig. 10.5)

- Proteins are broken down into amino acids by the proteolytic enzymes released from the stomach (pepsin) and pancreas (see below).
- A Na^+-dependent cotransport mechanism absorbs amino acids.

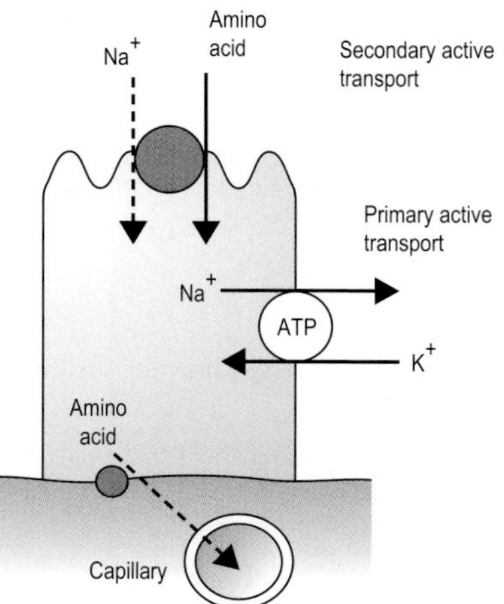

Fig. 10.5 Amino acids are absorbed using a Na^+ cotransport system. (From McGeown JG. Physiology, 2nd edn. Churchill Livingstone, Edinburgh, 2002, with permission.)

- There are four transporters:
  - neutral amino acids
  - basic amino acids
  - acidic amino acids
  - proline and hydroxyproline.
- The majority of amino acids are absorbed in the upper small intestine; any that enter the large bowel are metabolized by the resident bacterial flora.

Fluids and Electrolytes

- Approximately 2–3 L of fluid is ingested each day; another 8–9 L is secreted into the GI tract, but only 100–200 mL is excreted in the faeces.
- Na^+ absorption is coupled with the absorption of glucose and amino acids; active absorption is stimulated by aldosterone.
- K^+ is absorbed along a concentration gradient (caused by water absorption); a small amount is secreted in mucus.
- Anions such as Cl^- are generally absorbed by electrochemical gradients created by Na^+ absorption.
- The absorption of water is a result of the osmotic gradient established by the absorption of nutrients and electrolytes.

Vitamins

- Vitamins are divided into fat-soluble and water-soluble; this classification refers to the method of absorption.
- Fat-soluble vitamins (A, D, E and K) are absorbed within the micelles created during fat absorption.
- Water-soluble vitamins (C and B) are absorbed by more specific mechanisms:
  - vitamin C is absorbed by a Na^+-dependent mechanism in the jejunum
  - vitamin B_{12} is absorbed in the ileum after intrinsic factor (secreted in the stomach) binds to its specific receptor. The IF–vitamin B_{12} complex is then taken up into the cell
  - the remaining B vitamins diffuse freely across the enterocyte cell membrane.

Iron

- Iron is absorbed in the duodenum and jejunum in the ferrous (Fe^{2+}) and not the ferric (Fe^{3+}) form; gastric acid is responsible for converting iron to the ferrous form. Absorption is then via the transport protein transferrin. This binds iron and links to a membrane-bound receptor, and is then taken into the cell via endocytosis; it is then transferred to the plasma and binds to plasma transferrin.

Calcium

- Absorption is dependent on a calcium-binding protein in intestinal cells; these receptors can be increased by vitamin D, and thus the rate of calcium absorption can be increased when plasma levels fall.

Small Intestinal Motility

- There are three types of movement in the small bowel:
  - segmentation (feeding)
  - peristalsis (feeding)
  - migrating motility complex (MMC) (fasting).
- Segmentation is a movement that facilitates mixing of chyme; the circular muscle layer contracts and relaxes in adjacent segments; this results in circular movements of the chyme.
- Peristalsis is a propulsion movement that is triggered by distension. The longitudinal muscle contracts; midway through contraction of the longitudinal muscle the circular muscle also contracts. This pattern of contraction is repeated and moves food through the bowel.
- Peristaltic contractions eventually reach the ileocaecal valve and cause it to relax, thus allowing food to enter the large bowel.
- Peristaltic contractions last a few seconds and only propel the food a few centimetres; the MMC leads to contraction along the full length of the small bowel and lasts several hours. Their purpose is to push any remaining food debris into the colon. The stimulation for the MMC is not fully understood, but may involve the hormone motilin.

- The movements of segmentation and peristalsis are intrinsic and result from the basal electrical rhythm in the intestine. It can be influenced by extrinsic nervous input:
  - parasympathetic: increases rate of contraction
  - sympathetic: decreases rate of contraction.
- In addition to the autonomic input, there are several reflexes which also influence intestinal contractility:
  - ileogastric reflex: distension of the ileum decreases gastric motility
  - gastroileal reflex: increase in gastric secretion or contractility increases ileal motility.

Clinical Physiology

Physiological Effects of Duodenal Resection

Removal of the duodenum (duodenectomy) leads to a range of physiological abnormalities, including:

- Ulceration of small bowel: the duodenum is able to withstand gastric acid better than small bowel; this is due to HCO_3^- secreted from the Brunner's glands and from the pancreas—allowing the neutralization of gastric acid within the chyme. Following duodenal resection, surgical reconstruction of bowel continuity often involves small bowel; the rerouted gastric acid causes peptic ulceration in the small bowel.
- Malabsorption: Fe^{2+}, Ca^{2+} and PO_4^- malabsorption and impaired fat emulsification.
- Dumping: loss of control over gastric emptying leads to uncontrolled passage of chyme into the small bowel, resulting in dumping.

Physiological Effects of Terminal Ileal Resection

Removal of the terminal ileum (ilectomy) leads to a range of physiological abnormalities, including:

- Bile salt reabsorption: the terminal ileum is the site of bile salt absorption; loss of this mechanism leads to:
  - bile salts in the colon; this alters the bacterial flora and stool consistency, and can lead to an increased risk of colonic malignancy
  - due to the loss of enterohepatic circulation, there is a decrease in bile salt pool; this predisposes to cholesterol gallstones.
- Vitamin B_{12} deficiency: receptor-mediated reabsorption in conjunction with intrinsic factor occurs in the terminal ileum; resection of the ileum will result in deficiency of B_{12} and cause a macrocytic anaemia and degeneration of the spinal cord if not corrected.
- Water reabsorption: the ileum plays an important role in the absorption of water from bowel contents (especially in the elderly); this leads to diarrhoea and an increase in stool frequency.

PANCREAS

Exocrine Secretions

Fluid Component

- The pancreas secretes approximately 1.5 L of fluid per day; it contains a variety of enzymes and is rich in bicarbonate.
- The epithelial cells that line the ducts form the fluid component of pancreatic juice; HCO_3^- is transported into the lumen in exchange for Cl^- and directly via a luminal channel. Sodium and potassium are exchanged for H^+ formed by the reaction catalysed by carbonic anhydrase. Na^+ follows HCO_3^- to maintain electrochemical neutrality and water follows by the osmotic gradient created by the movement of Na^+ and HCO_3^-.

Enzyme Component

- The enzymes secreted by the pancreas can be divided into:
  - proteolytic
  - amylase
  - lipolytic.

Proteolytic enzymes

- These enzymes are secreted in an inactive form, called zymogen granules, from pancreatic acinar cells. The key event in the activation of these enzymes is activation of trypsinogen to trypsin. Activation of trypsinogen is by an enzyme secreted by the duodenum (enterokinase) and the alkaline environment.
- Trypsin then activates the other enzymes:
  - chymotrypsinogen: chymotrypsin (cleaves peptide bonds)
  - proelastase: elastase (cleaves peptide bonds)
  - trypsinogen: trypsin (cleaves peptide bonds)
  - procarboxypeptidase: carboxypeptidase (cleaves peptides at the C-terminus).

Amylase

- Responsible for the majority of starch digestion; it splits α-1,4-glycosidic bonds; the brush-border enzymes of the small bowel digest the resulting oligosaccharides.

Lipolytic enzymes

- As with proteolytic enzymes, the lipolytic enzymes are excreted in an inactive form; they are all activated by trypsin. These enzymes include:
  - lipase: cleaves triglycerides to FFAs and glycerol
  - co-lipase: helps bind lipase to the lipids
  - phospholipase A_2: cleaves FFAs from phospholipids
  - cholesterol esterase.

Regulation of Exocrine Secretions

- As with gastric secretion, regulation of pancreatic juice secretion is divided into three phases:
  - cephalic: vagal
  - gastric: vagal
  - intestinal: CCK and secretin.

Cephalic

- During the cephalic phase the sight, smell and taste of food cause vagal (parasympathetic) stimulation and the release of acetylcholine (ACh) and VIP. These activate the acinar and ductal cells as well as increasing blood flow via vasodilatation. A small stimulus also comes from gastrin released from the gastric antrum cells.

Gastric

- Accounts for a relatively small stimulus to secretion; gastrin secretion and distension (vagal gastropancreatic reflex) stimulate pancreatic secretion.

Intestinal

- Accounts for 60–70% of the stimulus for pancreatic secretions; two main hormones are responsible for stimulating pancreatic secretions:
  - cholecystokinin (CCK): release of a fluid rich in enzymes from acinar cells
  - secretin: release of a bicarbonate-rich fluid.
- Factors that promote secretion of these hormones (from the duodenal mucosa) include:
  - lipids (CCK)
  - peptides and amino acids (CCK)
  - acid (secretin).

Endocrine Secretions

See Chapter 12.

Clinical Physiology

Physiological Effects of Pancreatic Resection

Removal of the pancreas (pancreatectomy) leads to a range of physiological abnormalities, including:

- Malnutrition: inadequate digestion of protein and lipids due to the loss of proteolytic and lipolytic enzymes. The inadequate breakdown of protein leads to progressive weight loss and inadequate fat digestion; this leads to fatty stools and flatus (due to bacterial overgrowth). The absorption of fat-soluble vitamins (A, D, E and K) is reduced, and leads to progressive deficiencies.
- Malabsorption: loss of alkaline pancreatic secretions leads to failure to neutralize gastric chyme and leads to Fe^{2+}, Ca^{2+} and PO_4^- malabsorption; this eventually leads to anaemia and osteoporosis.
- Diabetes mellitus: loss of the pancreas leads to an absolute deficiency of insulin.

LIVER AND GALL BLADDER

Liver

Bile Production (Fig. 10.6)

- Hepatocytes secrete fluid into the canaliculi; this fluid is very similar to plasma with reference to its ion composition; however, it also contains:
  - bile acids: cholic acid and chendeoxycholic acid
  - bile salts: formed by linking the amino acids glycine and taurine to bile acids. Bile salts have a hydrophobic and hydrophilic region (amphipathic); this enables them to form an emulsion of lipids in the intestinal fluid. The emulsion produces a large surface area for pancreatic enzymes to act upon; in addition bile salts form smaller collections of FFAs and monoglycerides (micelles) to facilitate absorption into enterocytes. The bile salts are not absorbed during this process, and remain in the bowel lumen until the distal ileum, where they are absorbed (see below)
  - bile pigments: these are produced by the breakdown of the haem unit of haemoglobin; it gives bile its green/yellow colour. The destruction of ageing red blood cells (RBCs) takes place in the spleen; in this process bilirubin is released into the circulation; it is poorly soluble and is transported to the liver bound to albumin. The bilirubin is conjugated to glucuronic acid in the hepatocytes, producing a water-soluble compound that is excreted in bile. In the intestine bacteria convert these pigments to:
    - urobilinogen: some is reabsorbed in the intestine and secreted back into the bile or excreted in the urine
    - stercobilin and urobilin: give faeces brown colour
  - cholesterol
  - lecithin
  - mucus.
- There are two factors that govern bile secretion; one is dependent on bile acid recirculation (enterohepatic circulation), and the other is independent of this:
  - enterohepatic circulation: >90% of secreted bile acids are reabsorbed from the intestine (distal ileum) and returned to the liver via the portal vein; the remaining 5–10% of bile acids are altered by bacterial flora and become insoluble, and are thus excreted. The rate at which bile acids are returned to the liver will influence the rate at which they are secreted into the canaliculi
  - the remaining components of bile (water, Na^+, HCO_3^-) are secreted into the canaliculi independently of bile acid recirculation. HCO_3^- and Na^+ are both actively pumped into the lumen; water follows due to the resulting osmotic gradient. Secretion of the bicarbonate-rich fluid is stimulated by secretin, gastrin and glucagon.
- Regulation of secretion: CCK stimulates the contraction of the gall bladder and the release of bile into the duodenum.

Metabolic Functions

The liver is responsible for the handling of dietary carbohydrate, protein and lipids.

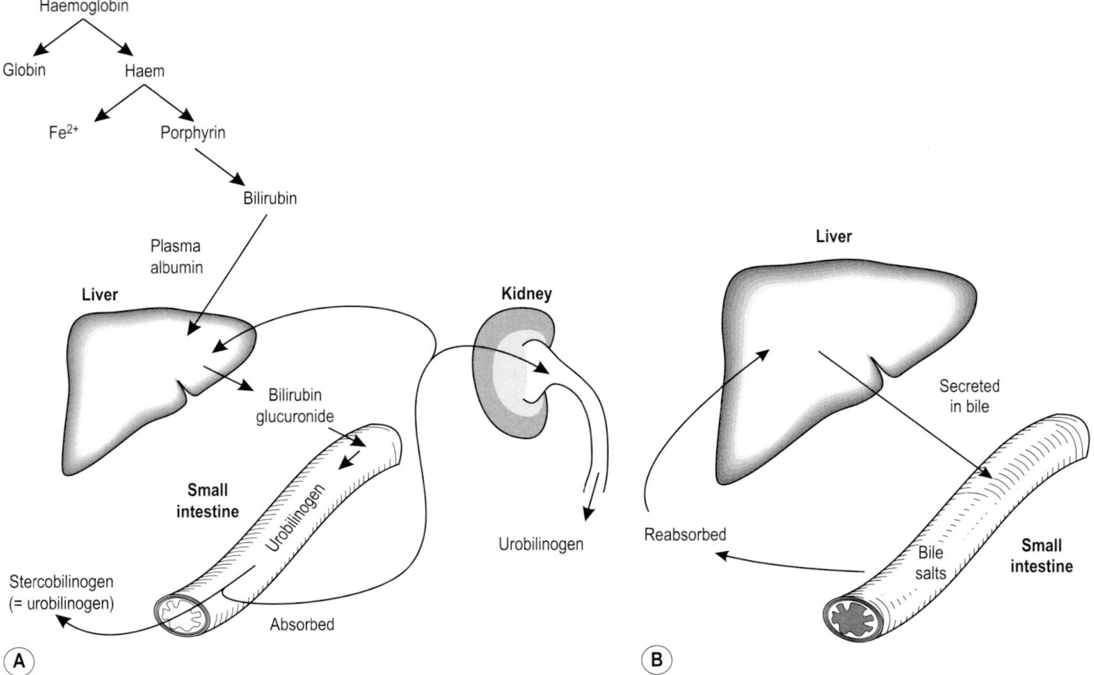

Fig. 10.6 (A) Summary of bile pigment metabolism. (B) Enterohepatic circulation of bile salts.

Carbohydrate metabolism

- Following a meal the digested components are delivered to the liver via the portal vein; the absorbed glucose is then converted to glycogen (the principal form of stored carbohydrate; glycogenesis). At times of low blood glucose or high energy demand the glycogen within the liver is converted back to glucose (glycogenolysis).

Protein metabolism

- The liver has a number of roles related to protein metabolism:
    - able to produce glucose from amino acids and other non-carbohydrate substances (gluconeogenesis); this becomes particularly important in times of prolonged exercise and depletion of glycogen stores during starvation
    - involved with synthesis of many of the plasma proteins, such as albumin and clotting factors
    - also handles the degradation products of amino acid metabolism. Use of amino acids throughout the body results in the production of ammonia, which is converted to urea.

Lipid metabolism

- The liver is involved with several facets of lipid metabolism:
    - glucose is converted to FFAs; this is then transported to adipose tissue. It is then combined with glycerol and stored as triglycerides. During starvation these stores are released, providing fatty acids (provides energy as ATP for gluconeogenesis) and glycerol (acts as a non-carbohydrate substrate for gluconeogenesis)
    - synthesizes lipoproteins and cholesterol.

Protein Synthesis

- As mentioned above, the liver synthesizes all the plasma proteins (other than immunoglobulins), all the non-essential amino acids and many of the clotting factors.

Vitamin D Activation

- Activation of vitamin D is a two-stage hydroxylation process. The liver performs the first hydroxylation to give 25-hydroxycholecalciferol, and the kidney performs the second to give 1,25-hydroxycholecalciferol.

Detoxification

- The liver detoxifies a number of substances:
    - peptide hormones: insulin, Anti-Diuretic Hormone (ADH), growth hormone
    - steroid hormones: testosterone, oestrogen, adrenal cortex hormones
    - catecholamines
    - drugs
    - toxins.

- The detoxification process involves two stages:
  - stage 1: increase in the water solubility of the substrate (i.e. the cytochrome p450 system)
  - stage 2: reduction in biological activity and toxic activity.

Vitamin and Mineral Storage

- The liver stores a number of substances; in addition to glycogen and fats, it also stores:
  - iron
  - copper
  - vitamin A, D, E, K and B_{12}.

Phagocytosis

- Kupffer cells in the hepatic sinusoids remove bacteria, debris and old RBCs.

Haemopoiesis

- In the embryo the liver is involved in haemopoiesis; in adults it only plays a role in disease states such as chronic haemolysis (extramedullary haemopoiesis).

Clinical Physiology

Jaundice

- Defined as the yellow pigmentation of the skin and eyes as a result of excess bilirubin in the circulation; this usually becomes clinically detectable at plasma levels >40 μmol/L (normal range is <22 μmol/L).
- Jaundice can be classified in three ways:
  - prehepatic (haemolytic)
  - hepatic (parenchymal)
  - post-hepatic (cholestatic).
- This classification refers to the site of the obstruction or abnormality affecting normal bilirubin metabolism.
- The following is a summary of bilirubin metabolism:
  - RBCs are broken down in the spleen and release bilirubin, a breakdown product of the porphyrin ring of haemoglobin; at this stage bilirubin is unconjugated
  - unconjugated bilirubin is not water-soluble and binds to albumin; it is in this form that it is transported to the liver
  - in the liver the bilirubin is conjugated to glucuronide; conjugated bilirubin is water-soluble
  - bilirubin is then stored in the gall bladder and excreted in the bile
  - once the bilirubin enters the bowel, intestinal bacteria convert it to urobilinogen. The urobilinogen may be absorbed and recirculated back into the bile; some is excreted in the urine, the remaining urobilinogen that is not absorbed is excreted in the faeces; it gives the faeces their brown colour. The urobilinogen that is excreted in the faeces is further altered by bacterial flora and is referred to as stercobilinogen.

Prehepatic jaundice

- This is caused by disorders that result in excessive destruction of RBCs (haemolysis); the liver is overwhelmed by the bilirubin that is being produced and is unable to conjugate it. The jaundice is thus referred to as being an unconjugated hyperbilirubinaemia. This finding is highly suggestive of a prehepatic cause for the jaundice. Other laboratory findings associated with prehepatic jaundice include:
  - no bilirubin in the urine (unconjugated bilirubin is not water-soluble)
  - ↑urobilinogen in the urine (as a result of more bilirubin being broken down in the intestine)
  - reticulocytosis: in response to the need to replace destroyed blood cells
  - anaemia
  - ↑lactate dehydrogenase (LDH)
  - ↓haptoglobin: protein that binds free haemoglobin and transfers it to the liver.
- Common causes of prehepatic jaundice include:
  - inherited:
    - red cell membrane defects, e.g. hereditary spherocytosis
    - haemoglobin abnormalities, e.g. sickle cell disease
    - metabolic defects, e.g. G6PD deficiency
  - acquired:
    - immune, e.g. transfusion reactions
    - mechanical, e.g. heart valves
    - acquired membrane defects, e.g. paroxysmal nocturnal haemoglobinuria (PNH)
    - infections
    - drugs
    - burns.
- In addition to the haemolytic causes of prehepatic jaundice, there are a group of disorders known as congenital hyperbilirubinaemias; these include:
  - unconjugated hyperbilirubinaemia:
    - Gilbert's syndrome: due to an abnormality in bilirubin uptake
    - Crigler–Najjar syndrome: due to the absence of glucuronyl-transferase
  - conjugated hyperbilirubinaemia:
    - Dubin–Johnson and Rotor's syndrome: defects in the handling of bilirubin.

Hepatocellular jaundice

- This is caused by a variety of conditions that interfere with hepatocyte function. There is usually an element of cholestasis as hepatocytes swell and obstruct the flow of bile. The hyperbilirubinaemia is a combination of conjugated and unconjugated, reflecting the impaired

hepatocyte function and partial obstruction. Laboratory tests demonstrate the following:
- liver enzymes, i.e. ↑ aspartate amino transferase (AST) and ↑ alanine amino transferase (ALT); this reflects liver damage and thus release of these enzymes from hepatocytes
- ↑alkaline phosphatase: reflects the partial cholestasis
- abnormal clotting tests reflect the impaired hepatocyte function.

- Causes of hepatocellular jaundice include:
  - viruses, e.g. hepatitis A, B, C and E; Epstein–Barr virus (EBV)
  - autoimmune disorders, e.g. chronic hepatitis
  - drugs, e.g. paracetamol overdose
  - cirrhosis
  - liver tumours and metastasis.

Cholestatic jaundice

- This is due to obstruction of the biliary system and can be further divided into intrahepatic or extrahepatic obstruction:
  - intrahepatic cholestasis is similar to hepatocellular jaundice, as the obstruction is usually due to hepatocyte swelling; causes include:
    - hepatitis
    - drugs
    - cirrhosis
    - primary biliary cirrhosis
  - extrahepatic cholestasis occurs due to obstruction of the large bile ducts distal to the canaliculi; causes include:
    - gallstones
    - biliary stricture
    - carcinoma: head of pancreas, ampulla, bile duct (cholangiocarcinoma), malignant lymph nodes at the porta hepatis
    - pancreatitis
    - sclerosing cholangitis.
- Laboratory tests demonstrate the following:
  - bilirubin in the urine (characteristic dark colouration); this occurs as the bilirubin is conjugated and thus water-soluble
  - no urobilinogen in the urine; due to the obstruction, no bilirubin enters the bowel to be converted to urobilinogen
  - ↑canalicular enzymes: alkaline phosphatase and γ-Glutamyl Transferase (GT)
  - ↑liver enzymes ALT and AST; not as significant as seen in hepatocellular causes, but biliary backpressure inevitably leads to mild hepatocyte damage.

Gall Bladder

- The gall bladder stores bile; the bile from the liver is diverted into the gall bladder due to the high tone in the sphincter of Oddi. The bile is then concentrated by the absorption of Na^+, HCO_3^-, Cl^- and water.
- The bile is released into the duodenum when the gall bladder contracts; the major stimulus is the release of CCK from the duodenum in response to fats and acid. A small amount of gall bladder contraction is mediated by the vagus when a fatty meal enters the stomach.
- CCK also stimulates pancreatic secretions and reduces the tone within the sphincter of Oddi.

Clinical Physiology

Physiological Effects of Cholecystectomy

- The removal of the gall bladder (cholecystectomy) is usually well tolerated, but does have several physiological consequences that may lead to symptoms:
  - the loss of the concentrating action of the gall bladder can lead to increased flow of bile, leading to reflux and biliary gastritis
  - the formation of micelles during fat absorption is disturbed, and can lead to fat intolerance and malabsorption; this can produce abdominal pain and diarrhoea.

Water Absorption

- The colon is the last site for water reabsorption; it absorbs up to 1 L of water per day. Na^+ is transported from the lumen under the influence of aldosterone; water follows along the osmotic gradient.
- Failure of fluid absorption in the colon leads to diarrhoea (see below).

Colonic Flora

- The colon has a huge population of both aerobic and anaerobic bacteria; these perform a number of roles:
  - fermentation of indigestible carbohydrate: produces fatty acids that the colonic mucosa is able to use as an energy source and a variety of gases, such as carbon dioxide and methane; these are released as flatus
  - degradation of bilirubin to urobilin, urobilinogen and stercobilin
  - synthesis of vitamins K, B_{12}, thiamine and riboflavin.

Large Intestinal Motility

- Food traverses the small intestine in approximately 5 h; colonic movements are considerably slower, taking up to 20 h or more before defecation.
- The colon has a number of movements:
  - mixing or retrograde peristalsis: the circular muscle contracts and narrows the lumen, the longitudinal muscle is incomplete in the colon and forms bands called taenia coli. Contraction of the taenia

coli appears to cause faecal matter to roll, and thus increase its exposure for absorption (occurs predominantly in the right colon)
    - peristalsis and mass movements: these are more common in the transverse and distal colon, and move faecal matter towards the anus. More prolonged contractions of the colon (mass movements) serve to empty the colon, and invariably produce the desire to defecate as faeces are pushed into the rectum and anus. Mass movements are initiated by distension of the stomach and duodenum (gastrocolic and duodenocolic reflexes).
- Vagal stimulation increases colonic motility and sympathetic stimulation decreases it.
- The colon is able to influence gastric motility by releasing enteroglucagon (also released from the distal ileum). This hormone is released in response to glucose and fat in the ileum and colon, and inhibits gastric and small bowel motility.

Defecation

- Mass movements lead to distension of the rectum as faeces are pushed along; this leads to the sensation of needing to defecate.
- The control of defecation (continence) is by sympathetic and parasympathetic input, but is also under somatic control. The nervous input supplies two sphincters:
    - internal sphincter: smooth muscle under involuntary control; sympathetic impulses lead to contraction of the sphincter and para-sympathetic impulses lead to relaxation
    - external sphincter: composed of skeletal muscle and allows voluntary control of defecation.
- The reflex arc that initiates defecation is (Fig. 10.7):
    - rectal distension: when faecal material enters the rectum and causes distension, impulses from stretch receptors in the rectum travel via parasympathetic fibres (S2, 3, 4) in the sacral nerves
    - conscious awareness: as a result of rectal distension there is activation of ascending sensory pathways that allow differentiation of solid faecal matter and flatus. Impulses also travel along the pudendal nerve; this results in contraction of the external sphincter
    - parasympathetic impulse: leads to an increase in the tone of the colon and relaxation of the internal sphincter
    - not convenient to defecate: voluntary contraction of the external sphincter; the urge to defecate often subsides at this point. If the distension on the rectum is due to solid faecal matter then descending impulses reinforce contraction of the external sphincter to maintain continence

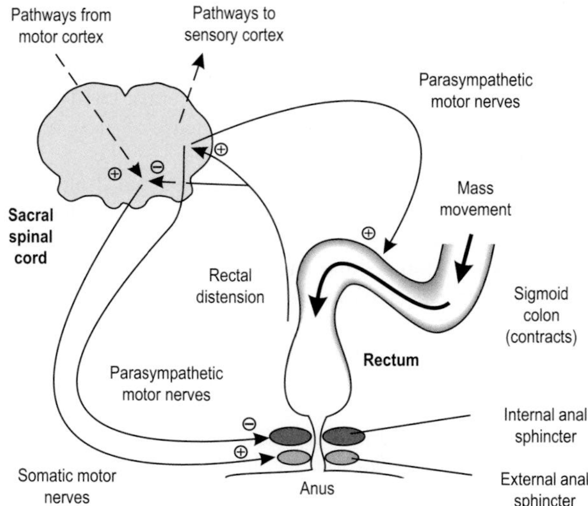

Fig. 10.7 Summary of the defecation reflex.

    - convenient to defecate: the external sphincter relaxes, allowing faeces through the anus; this is often aided by the contraction of abdominal muscles.

Clinical Physiology

Diarrhoea

- Defined as more frequent evacuation or the passage of liquid/soft faeces.
- The pathophysiological mechanisms responsible for the diarrhoea can be classified as follows.

Osmotic

- Fluid enters the bowel if there are large amounts of hypertonic substances in the lumen, e.g. purgatives, malabsorption leading to high glucose levels. The diarrhoea reduces if the patient stops eating.

Secretory

- There is active secretion and decreased absorption of fluids from the lumen. Causes include:
    - enterotoxins, e.g. cholera
    - hormones, e.g. VIP from a VIPoma
    - bile: following ileal resection
    - fats: following ileal resection
    - laxatives.
- In secretory diarrhoea stopping food has no effect.

Inflammatory

- Diarrhoea occurs due to mucosal damage and thus reduced absorption, i.e. infective diarrhoea or inflammatory bowel disease.

Abnormal motility

- Causes include diabetic neuropathy, post-vagotomy syndrome, carcinoid, thyrotoxicosis, irritable bowel syndrome (IBS) and bowel resection.

Constipation (Box 10.1)

- Defined as the infrequent or difficult passage of abnormally hard/firm faeces.
- Causes are often divided into medical and surgical.

NUTRITION

Requirements

- The energy requirements of a normal adult are around 2000–2500 kcal/day.
- Carbohydrates, proteins and fats supply this energy.
- In addition, the body needs vitamins, minerals and trace elements; deficiency can result in ill health.
- Carbohydrates: present in numerous foods, provide a rapidly used energy source, but are also converted to glycogen in the liver, and if ingested in excess quantities will be converted to fat and laid down in adipose tissue. Carbohydrates provide 4.1 kcal/g of energy.
- Protein: broken down to amino acids which then form hormones, enzymes, etc. Of the 20 different amino acids, 12 can be synthesized in the liver, but 8 are referred to as essential amino acids as they cannot be synthesized (isoleucine, leucine, lysine, methionine, phenylalanine, threonine, tryptophan, valine). Proteins provide 5.3 kcal/g of energy.
- Fats: can be saturated (found in meats, fish and dairy products) or unsaturated (vegetable); three fatty acids are referred to as essential as the body is unable to synthesize them (linolenic, linoleic and arachidonic acid). Fats have numerous roles throughout the body:
  - support of other tissues, e.g. fat around kidneys
  - stores fat-soluble vitamins
  - forms part of the nerve sheaths
  - forms part of cell membranes
  - provides 9.3 kcal/g of energy.
- Minerals: include sodium, potassium, calcium, phosphorus, iron and iodine. They are involved in numerous cellular processes (Box 10.2).
- Vitamins: required in small amounts but deficiency can lead to a variety of clinical conditions (Box 10.3). Divided into fat-soluble (A, D, E and K) and water-soluble (C and B).
- Trace elements: include zinc, copper, manganese, chromium, cobalt, selenium and molybdenum.

Regulation

- Regulation of eating and food intake is under the control of two centres in the hypothalamus:
  - hunger or feeding centre: lateral hypothalamus
  - satiety centre: ventromedial hypothalamus.

BOX 10.1 Summary of the medical and surgical causes of constipation

Medical	Surgical
Diet	Anal fissure
Lifestyle	Carcinoma of the rectum/anus
IBS	Carcinoma of the colon
↑Ca^{2+}	Foreign body
Hypothyroidism	Pelvic masses
Drugs, i.e. opiates, tricyclic antidepressants	Post-operative immobility Hirschsprung's disease (rare in adults)

BOX 10.2 Summary of the Roles of Minerals in Physiological Processes

Mineral	Role
Sodium	Main extracellular ion, and is involved in fluid regulation, muscle contraction and nerve conduction
Potassium	Main intracellular ion, and is involved in many cellular processes
Calcium	Mineralization of bone, muscle contraction and blood clotting
Magnesium	Necessary for muscle and nerve function, also needed for normal parathyroid hormone secretion
Iron	Formation of haem and oxidation of carbohydrates
Iodine	Synthesis of thyroid hormones
Selenium	Part of the enzyme glutathione peroxidase and also responsible for converting thyroxine to tri-iodothyronine in liver microsomes
Zinc	Involved in numerous metabolic pathways as a cofactor for enzymes, and vital for the synthesis of RNA and DNA
Phosphorus	Forms complexes with calcium to form bone and is essential in energy-requiring processes as part of ATP
Chromium	Facilitates the action of insulin
Copper	Required for synthesis of haemoglobin and is a component of coenzymes in the electron transport chain

BOX 10.3 Summary of the Various Disorders Caused by Vitamin Deficiencies

Vitamin	Deficiency Syndrome
Vitamin A	Night blindness, epithelial atrophy and infections
Vitamin D	Rickets (child) and osteomalacia (adults)
Vitamin E	Haemolytic anaemia
Vitamin K	Clotting disorders
Vitamin B_1	Beriberi
Vitamin B_2	Dermatitis and light sensitivity
Vitamin B_3	Pellagra
Vitamin B_6	Convulsions, anaemia, vomiting and skin lesions
Pantothenic acid	Neuropathy
Biotin	Muscle pains and skin lesions
Vitamin B_{12}	Pernicious anaemia
Folic acid	Anaemia
Vitamin C	Scurvy

- After a meal when the blood glucose is high and the stomach is distended the satiety centre is stimulated, and this inhibits feeding. When blood glucose falls the activity within the satiety centre decreases and allows impulses from the hunger centre to predominate.
- Lesions in the hunger centre lead to a lack of food intake (aphagia).
- Lesions in the satiety centre lead to increased food intake (hyperphagia).

OSCE SCENARIOS

OSCE Scenario 10.1

A 40-year-old male presents with recurrent attacks of right upper quadrant pain exacerbated by fatty food. His only significant past medical history is a right hemicolectomy five years previously for acute regional ileitis (Crohn's disease). Investigations reveal normal liver function tests but FBC reveals anaemia with a raised Mean Corpuscular Volume (MCV). Abdominal ultrasound scan demonstrates gallstones.

1. Explain the pathophysiology underlying the development of gallstones in this patient.
2. What is the cause of the patient's anaemia?
3. What would be the effects of failing to treat the anaemia?
4. How would you treat the anaemia?

OSCE Scenario 10.2

A 32-year-old female is admitted with jaundice and right upper quadrant pain. Liver function tests reveal a bilirubin of 112 µmol/L, a markedly raised alkaline phosphatase and gamma GT. Liver enzymes are normal.

1. What is jaundice?
2. At what level of bilirubin is jaundice clinically apparent?
3. Classify the types of jaundice.
4. What is the most likely cause in this case?
5. Describe the different types of gallstone.
6. List the complications of gallstones.

OSCE Scenario 10.3

A 63-year-old male is admitted with central abdominal pain radiating through to his back. He is hypotensive with a BP of 90/60 mmHg and tachycardic. The results of blood investigations are shown below:

WBC 19×10^9/L
Glucose 8 mmol/L
AST 390 U/L
LDH 500 U/L
Amylase 2235 U/L

1. The raised amylase suggests acute pancreatitis. What are the common causes of acute pancreatitis?
2. What is the patient's initial Ranson score?
3. What are the criteria measured at 48 h for the Ranson score?
4. What pancreas-related complications can occur with acute pancreatitis?

OSCE Scenario 10.4

A 50-year-old male patient presented to Accident and Emergency with epigastric pain after starting a course of NSAIDs 2 weeks ago for a flare up of arthritis. His pain was getting worse over the last 24 h. Abdominal examination revealed peritonism with guarding. His HR is 130/min, temperature 38.5°C and BP 130/70. You suspect perforated peptic ulcer.

1. What is the volume of daily gastric secretion? And what is its content?
2. What are the classes of medications that are used to treat peptic ulcers and what are their mechanisms of action?
3. The patient undErgoes emergency laparotomy, and a large friable perforated duodenal ulcer is found that could not be closed with a patch. The surgeon decides to perform distal gastrectomy with Roux-en-Y gastrojejunostomy. What are the potential complications of gastrectomy?
4. Why does dumping syndrome develop?

OSCE Scenario 10.5

A 65-year-old female patient with background of smoking and hypertension presents with chronic postprandial pain (sitophobia), weight loss and loose stools. She is found to be cachexic due to food fear and admission is for urgent investigations and addressing nutritional problems with total parenteral nutrition (TPN).

1. A CT abdomen is arranged (Fig. 10.5Q). What is the main finding on this CT scan? What is the diagnosis?
2. What are the pros and cons of enteral and parenteral feeding?
3. How would you treat this condition?

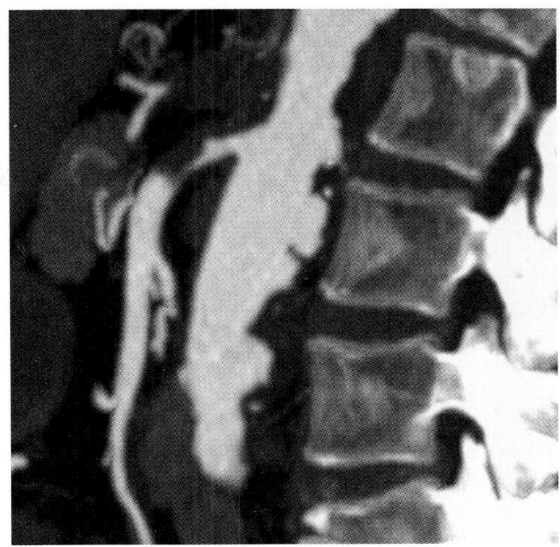

Fig. 10.5Q CT angiogram of abdominal aorta.

4. Five days after her admission, the patient is found to have low levels of K, Mg and PO_4. What is this condition called? And why does it develop?

Answers in Appendix pages 451–454

Please check your eBook at https://studentconsult.inkling.com/ for more self-assessment questions. See inside cover for registration details.

11

Urinary System

COMPONENTS

The urinary system is composed of:

- kidneys
- ureters
- bladder
- urethra.

Functions

The functions of the urinary system include:

- maintenance of electrolyte balance
- maintenance of fluid balance
- maintenance of acid–base balance
- storage and excretion of urine
- hormone production: renin, erythropoietin, 1,25-dihydrocholecalciferol.

Structure

- See Chapter 2 for further anatomical detail of the kidneys, ureter, bladder and urethra.
- Macroscopically the kidney can be divided into:
  - outer region: cortex
  - inner region: medulla, pelvis.
- Medulla is divided into several pyramids that project into the pelvis.
- The renal pyramids divide the renal pelvis into two to three areas known as the major calyces.
- The functioning portion of the kidney is the nephron; each nephron consists of a glomerulus; this consists of a collection of capillaries that are connected to afferent (a = arrive) and efferent (e = exit) arterioles.
- Each glomerulus is surrounded by epithelium, which forms Bowman's space.
- The glomerulus is the site of plasma filtration.
- From Bowman's space the filtrate passes in turn through the proximal convoluted tubules, loop of Henle, distal convoluted tubule and the collecting duct. The resulting urine passes through the papilla in the renal pyramids into the renal pelvis.

RENAL BLOOD SUPPLY

Renal Circulation

- Renal artery enters the hilum → branches to form interlobar arteries, which ascend between the pyramids → interlobar arteries branch to form arcuate arteries → arcuate arteries branch to form interlobular arteries → afferent arteries arise from the interlobular arteries.
- Afferent arterioles give rise to glomerular capillaries within Bowman's capsule → leave the glomerulus as the efferent arterioles.
- Efferent arterioles have two distinct courses:
  - supply of capillaries to the renal tubules → peritubular capillaries
  - descending vessels called the vasa recta; these provide the blood supply to the medulla; the ascending vasa recta drain into the arcuate veins → interlobar vein → renal vein.

Regulation of Renal Blood Flow

- Total renal blood flow (RBF) is approximately 1.25 L/min or 25% of the cardiac output.
- Renal blood flow is maintained by intrinsic mechanisms; it shows very little variation over a range of arterial pressures; this is termed autoregulation.
- Autoregulation fails at systolic blood pressures <80 mmHg.
- The mechanisms underlying autoregulation of renal blood flow can be divided into:
  - myogenic: ↑ in pressure due to ↑ in flow causes distension of the vessels; this elicits smooth muscle contraction and thus ↑ vascular resistance and thus ↓ blood flow
  - metabolic: metabolites from active renal tissue induce vasodilatation.
- Renal blood flow can also be influenced by:
  - humoral factors
  - prostaglandins (vasodilatation)
  - nitric oxide (vasodilatation)
  - adrenaline (vasoconstriction)

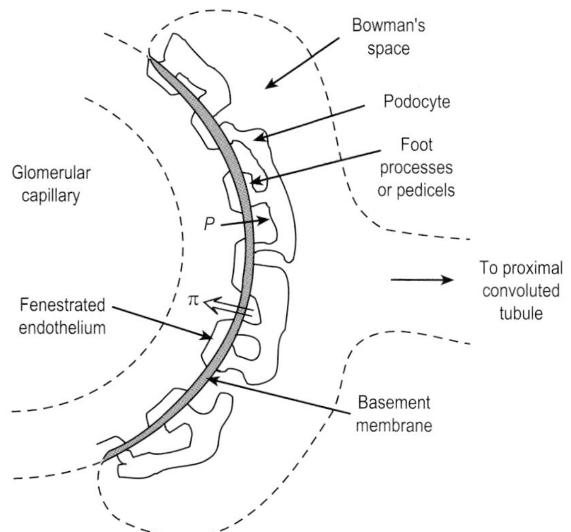

Fig. 11.1 Microscopic structure of the glomerulus. P = hydrostatic pressure, π = osmotic pressure. (From McGeown JG. Physiology, 2nd edn. Churchill Livingstone, Edinburgh, 2002, with permission.)

- noradrenaline (vasoconstriction)
- angiotensin I (vasoconstriction)
- angiotensin II (vasoconstriction).
- Renal nerves:
  - sympathetic (vasoconstriction)
  - parasympathetic (vasodilatation).

Glomerulus (Fig. 11.1)

Microscopic Structure

- The endothelium and the epithelium of Bowman's capsule have several features which allow them to perform the role of filtration:
  - the capillary endothelium is perforated by small pores; it is referred to as a fenestrated capillary; it permits the free passage of water and electrolytes
  - negative charge of glycoproteins in the basement membrane results in greater permeability to positively or neutrally charged molecules than negatively charged molecules
  - the epithelium of Bowman's capsule contains specialized cells called podocytes. These cells do not form a continuous layer, and instead they are spread over the basement membrane and pass out processes known as pedicels or 'foot processes'. This leaves gaps, which allow filtration to occur.
- In addition, the numerous glomeruli throughout the kidney produce a large surface area to allow filtration.
- The fenestrated nature of the endothelium and the gaps between podocyte processes produce low resistance to fluid movement.

Glomerular Filtration

- The glomerulus is the initial site of urine formation.
- As a result of the factors mentioned above, the kidneys show a high rate of filtration: 120 mL/min.
- The forces governing filtration are identical to filtration forces in peripheral capillaries:
  - hydrostatic pressure
  - osmotic pressure.
- Hydrostatic pressure is higher than in normal capillaries; approximately 50 mmHg; this is generated by the high resistance to outflow caused by the efferent arteriole. Pressure within Bowman's capsule is approximately 10 mmHg; this leaves a hydrostatic pressure of 40 mmHg.
- Plasma proteins generate osmotic pressure; they are not filtered and therefore produce an opposing absorption pressure to the hydrostatic pressure. Osmotic pressure is about 25 mmHg; therefore, the net filtration pressure is around 15 mmHg.
- As filtration proceeds, the remaining plasma proteins exert a greater osmotic pressure until it equals that of the filtration pressure and thus no further removal of fluid occurs.
- The fluid that is filtered by the glomerulus is identical to plasma, apart from the lack of plasma proteins and blood cells; it is often referred to as an ultrafiltrate.
- The osmolality of the ultrafiltrate is around 300 mosmol/L.

Proximal Convoluted Tubule

- The proximal convoluted tubule absorbs 70% of the filtered sodium; chloride follows by electrostatic attraction; water follows the absorption of NaCl as a result of the osmotic gradient.
- The volume of the ultrafiltrate is decreased but as the NaCl solution is isosmotic with the plasma, the osmolality of the filtrate reaching the loop of Henle is unchanged.
- The transport of Na^+ is an energy dependent process; it relies on an ATP-dependent pump.
- The proximal tubular cells are particularly vulnerable to ischaemic damage as a result of the energy requirements.

Loop of Henle

- The descending loop of Henle is permeable to NaCl and water. Due to the high osmolality of the surrounding medulla, water is removed from the ultrafiltrate and NaCl is added as ions move down the concentration gradient between the medulla and the ultrafiltrate.

- The ultrafiltrate in the descending loop of Henle is concentrated by the passive addition of NaCl from the medulla and the reduction in volume due to the absorption of water.
- The ascending loop of Henle is responsible for the active reabsorption of Na^+ (which again leads to passive Cl^- absorption). However, this region is impermeable to water; the transport of NaCl leads to a decrease in the osmolality of the ultrafiltrate but an increase in the osmolality of the surrounding medullary parenchyma.
- The osmolality of the ultrafiltrate entering the loop of Henle is approximately 300 mosmol/L. As fluid is removed and ions added in the descending loop, the osmolality increases to around 1200 mosmol/L at the bottom. As the fluid enters the ascending limb, ions are removed but water remains, as this area is impermeable to water. The osmolality is decreased as ions are removed; the concentration of the ultrafiltrate entering the convoluted tubule is about 100 mosmol/L.

Countercurrent Multiplier Mechanism (Fig. 11.2)

- The changes in osmolality of the ultrafiltrate as it moves through the loop of Henle produce very high ion concentration within the medulla, providing the necessary osmotic pressure for water reabsorption from the collecting ducts.
- The mechanism by which the high medullary osmolality is produced is called the countercurrent multiplier mechanism.
- The explanation for countercurrent exchange lies in its 'U' shape and repeated cycles of ion pumping and fluid movement. This allows fluid to be concentrated several times (osmolality changes from around 300–1200 mosmol/L, which equates to a fourfold increase in concentration); this is significantly greater than could be achieved with a parallel system.
- The 'U' shape of the loop of Henle allows solute to be continuously recycled in order to generate the high medullary osmolality.
- The other facet of the countercurrent mechanism is the fact that the vasa recta (medullary blood supply) is arranged in a similar 'U' shape; this allows the continuous recycling of solute and prevents the removal of solute and resulting decrease in medullary osmolality.

Distal Convoluted Tubule and Collecting Ducts

- The distal convoluted tubule and the collecting ducts have two important functions:
  - water reabsorption
  - Na^+ reabsorption.
- The ultrafiltrate that enters the distal tubule has a low osmolality and thus water is reabsorbed. Further

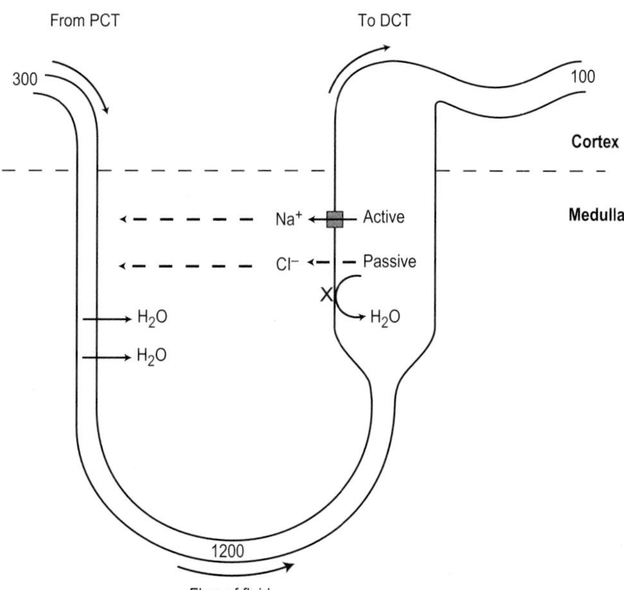

Fig. 11.2 The osmolality of the fluid entering the descending loop of Henle is approximately 300 mosmol/L. The descending loop is permeable to Na^+ and Cl^- and H_2O, thus there is osmotic removal of H_2O and an increase in the osmolality due to the influx of Na^+ and Cl^-. In the ascending limb there is an active pumping of Na^+ (Cl^- following passively), but this region is impermeable to water and thus the fluid becomes more dilute.

fluid absorption occurs in the collecting ducts as they descend through the medulla.

- The absorption of water in the distal tubule and collecting ducts leads to a decrease in the volume of urine and an increase in its concentration; therefore, under normal circumstances concentrated urine of low volume is excreted.
- The distal tubule and collecting duct also function to reabsorb the remaining Na^+. This process is energy dependent and requires ATP. A proportion of the Na^+ absorption is under the control of the hormone aldosterone (see later).

REGULATION OF NA^+ AND WATER REABSORPTION

- Three hormones are involved in the control of the extracellular fluid (ECF) volume via their actions on Na^+ and water absorption; these hormones are:
  - antidiuretic hormone (ADH or vasopressin)
  - renin–angiotensin–aldosterone (RAS) system
  - atrial natriuretic hormone.

Antidiuretic Hormone

- Produced in the supraoptic nucleus in the hypothalamus; it is then released from the posterior pituitary.
- Stimulation of ADH release is via osmoreceptors in the hypothalamus; they detect increases in the osmolality of the ECF and stimulate drinking.
- Other factors that stimulate ADH secretion include:
  - ↓ circulating blood volume
  - ↓ arterial pressure
  - angiotensin II.
- The actions of ADH include:
  - ↑ water permeability of the distal tubule and collecting ducts
  - ↑ arterial blood pressure by vasoconstriction.
- The secretion of ADH leads to the production of concentrated low-volume urine.
- Inhibition (i.e. alcohol), absence (cranial diabetes insipidus) or failure to respond to ADH (nephrogenic diabetes insipidus) leads to the production of urine with a low osmolality and a high volume.

Renin–Angiotensin–Aldosterone System (RAS)

- The RAS system is a complex interaction of hormones that influences the ECF volume and also interacts with the vascular system and affects blood pressure.
- The juxtaglomerular apparatus in the kidney is a key mechanism in monitoring changes in the ECF and renal circulation; it is composed of the juxtaglomerular cells of the afferent arteriole and the macula densa cells in the distal tubule that lie in close association.
- Juxtaglomerular cells are specialized smooth muscle cells that lie in the wall of the afferent arteriole and secrete the hormone renin.
- Renin catalyses the reactions in the RAS system; release from the juxtaglomerular cells is stimulated by:
  - decrease in afferent arteriole pressure
  - reduction in Na^+, detected by the macula densa which monitors the Na^+ load in the distal tubule
  - stimulation by renal sympathetic nerves.
- Renin stimulates the conversion of the plasma protein angiotensinogen to angiotensin I; this is then converted to angiotensin II in the lungs by the enzyme angiotensin converting enzyme (ACE).
- Angiotensin II has a number of actions:
  - stimulates arterial vasoconstriction
  - stimulates the release of ADH
  - stimulates drinking
  - stimulates the release of aldosterone.
- Aldosterone is released from the adrenal cortex and stimulates the reabsorption of Na^+ and water from the distal tubule and collecting ducts (see Chapter 12 for more details).

Atrial Natriuretic Peptide (ANP)

- Released by the heart in response to an increase in the ECF—stimulation is via atrial stretch.
- The actions of ANP are:
  - increases glomerular filtration
  - inhibits reabsorption of Na^+.
- The actions of ANP lead to increased excretion of both Na^+ and water.

Ion and Nutrient Reabsorption

Potassium

- Active reabsorption of K^+ occurs in the proximal tubule and the ascending loop of Henle in conjunction with Na^+ and Cl^- transport. By the time it reaches the distal tubule, approximately 90% of the filtered K^+ has been reabsorbed.
- The amount of K^+ present in the urine is regulated by aldosterone.
- Aldosterone stimulates the secretion of K^+ into the distal tubule and thus into the urine.

Calcium and Phosphate

- Calcium and phosphate are actively absorbed in the proximal tubule and ascending loop of Henle; any remaining is absorbed in the distal tubule and collecting duct. Only 1% of the filtered calcium is excreted.
- Absorption in the distal tubule and collecting ducts is controlled by parathormone (PTH) (see Chapter 12).
- PTH stimulates calcium reabsorption and phosphate excretion.

Hydrogen and Bicarbonate (Fig. 11.3)

- The regulation of H^+ and HCO_3^- is essential in maintaining adequate acid–base balance and a normal pH.
- The majority of the filtered bicarbonate is reabsorbed in the proximal tubule and the loop of Henle.
- Intercalated cells in the distal tubule differ from proximal tubular cells in that they actively secrete ions, namely H^+, rather than actively absorb them.
- H^+ and HCO_3^- are generated in the intercalated cells by the dissociation of carbonic acid (formed from CO_2 and H_2O and catalysed by carbonic anhydrase).
- H^+ is then transported in the distal tubular lumen and the HCO_3^- passively diffuses into the peritubular bloodstream, thus maintaining electrical neutrality.
- H^+ secretion drives the reaction with HCO_3^-; this forms carbonic acid, which in turn dissociates to H_2O and CO_2; the CO_2 diffuses into the tubular cell and begins the reaction between CO_2 and H_2O to produce H^+ and HCO_3^-.
- These reactions are able to react to changes in acid–base balance in several ways:
  - with a metabolic alkalosis there will be an increase in the filtered HCO_3^-, thus the HCO_3^- will swamp the secreted H^+ and will be excreted
  - with a metabolic acidosis the amount of HCO_3^- reabsorbed can be increased; this occurs when the secreted H^+ reacts with other buffers in the urine, and leaves HCO_3^- to diffuse into the bloodstream.

Glucose and Amino Acids

- Glucose is filtered by the glomerulus and has an identical concentration to plasma.
- As the concentration of glucose in the ultrafiltrate and plasma are identical, it cannot be reabsorbed along a concentration gradient; it therefore requires an energy-dependent process. The transport of glucose utilizes the gradient of Na^+ between the ultrafiltrate and the plasma; Na^+ and glucose bind to a carrier protein and the movement of Na^+ along the concentration gradient draws the glucose with it. The glucose leaves the cell by a separate cell membrane transport protein.
- The same mechanism is responsible for the absorption of amino acids.
- The process occurs in the proximal tubule, and under normal circumstances leads to the absence of glucose or amino acids in the urine.
- The uptake mechanism of glucose can be saturated; in these instances the excess glucose will be lost in the urine (glycosuria); the renal threshold for glucose absorption is around 11 mmol/L. Glycosuria is one of the main symptoms in diabetes mellitus.

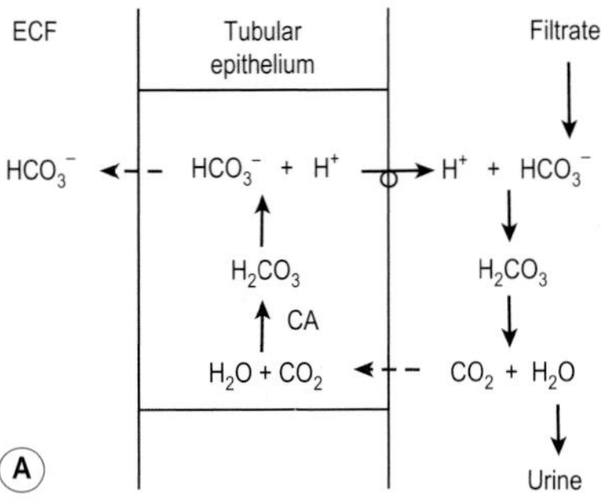

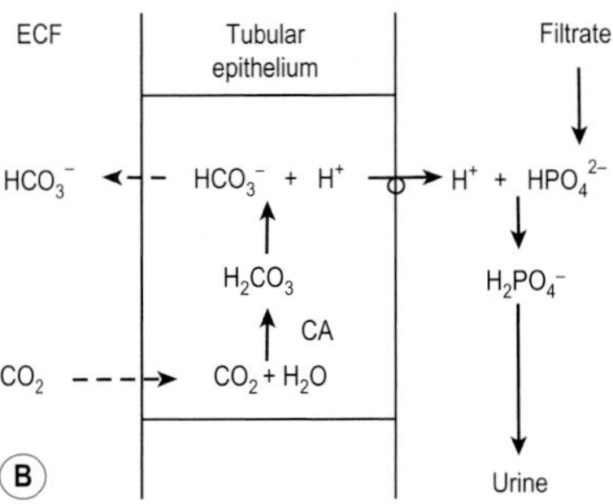

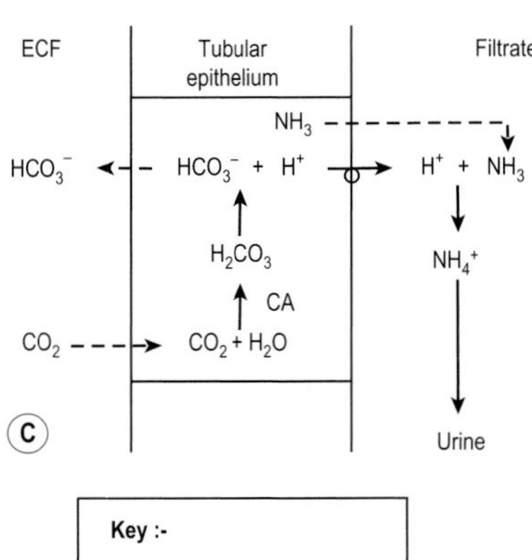

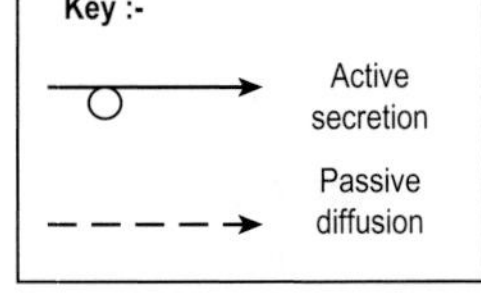

Fig. 11.3 Mechanisms for regulation of the pH of extracellular fluid. Tubular secretion of H^+ leads to reabsorption of filtered HCO_3^- (A). Secreted H^+ can also protonate filtered phosphates (B) or ammonia (C) and is then excreted. (From McGeown JG. Physiology, 2nd edn. Churchill Livingstone, Edinburgh, 2002, with permission.)

Urea

- Urea is a waste product formed in the liver during protein metabolism. It is not actively absorbed, but as water is drawn out the concentration of urea in the tubules rises and therefore there is a small amount of passive reabsorption as urea moves down the concentration gradient.

Glomerular Filtration Rate (GFR) and Renal Plasma Flow

- The concept of clearance can be used to calculate both GFR and renal plasma flow.
- Clearance is a quantitative measure of the rate of removal of a waste product from the blood by the kidneys; it is calculated from its urinary concentration, multiplied by the volume per unit time and divided by the plasma co ncentration:

$$\text{Clearance} = \frac{UV}{P}$$

U: urine concentration
V: urine volume
P: plasma concentration

Measuring GFR

- There are a number of mechanisms that can be used to calculate GFR:
  1. Inulin clearance: inulin is used as it closely obeys the following criteria needed of a substance to measure GFR:
     - must be filtered by the glomerulus
     - must not be reabsorbed
     - must not be secreted
     - must not be metabolized
     - this technique is the 'gold standard' for measuring GFR; however, it is not widely used in clinical practice.
  2. Creatinine clearance: used in clinical practice as creatinine occurs naturally; production is relatively constant but a small amount is secreted by the tubules; this can be significant at low GFR.
  3. EDTA: has similar kinetics to inulin; it can be radioactively labelled and GFR determined from subsequent blood tests.
  4. Dynamic renography: an estimate of GFR can be made from DTPA and MAG3 scans.
  5. Cockroft–Gault equation: this equation can be used to estimate creatinine clearance, and thus GFR:

$$\text{Clearance} = \frac{1.23\ (♂)\ \text{or}\ 1.04\ (♀) \times (140 - \text{age}) \times (\text{weight [kg]})}{\text{Serum creatinine } (\mu\text{mol/L})}$$

Measuring Renal Plasma Flow

- Measurement of renal plasma flow requires that a substance be completely removed from the plasma in a single pass through the kidney.
- Para-aminohippuric acid (PAH) is used for this test and is injected into the bloodstream; clearance is then calculated using UV/P.
- Renal plasma flow is around 650 mL/min.

Micturition

- Urine is formed at the rate of 1 mL/kg/h.
- Urine is transported from the renal pelvis to the bladder by the ureters by waves of peristaltic contraction.
- Urine is then stored in the bladder.
- The pressure within the bladder (intravesical pressure) is around 3 cmH_2O. The bladder will fill to a volume of about 200–300 mL of urine before the desire to urinate is felt. Before this point there is little change in intravesical pressure. As the volume increases, the intravesical pressure rises steeply and the desire to urinate increases; at this point the volume is around 400–450 mL.
- These changes in volume are sensed by stretch receptors that send impulses to the spinal cord via the pelvic nerves.
- The nervous control of bladder function is from both parasympathetic and sympathetic systems (Fig. 11.4):

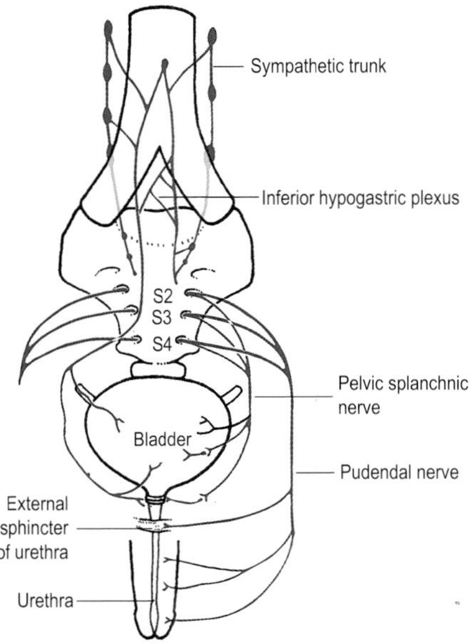

Fig. 11.4 Innervation of the bladder and urethra.

- parasympathetic: these run in the sacral outflow (S2–3) and innervate the bladder (detrusor muscle) and internal sphincter. Parasympathetic fibres also run in the pudendal nerve and control the external sphincter. They stimulate micturition by ↑ detrusor contraction and ↓ contraction of the internal sphincter
- sympathetic: these run in the hypogastric plexus; they act to inhibit micturition by ↓ detrusor contraction and ↑ contraction of the internal sphincter.

- Therefore, parasympathetic input initiates micturition and sympathetic input inhibits it.
- Once micturition is initiated, the sympathetic impulses are inhibited by impulses from the brainstem and parasympathetic impulses lead to bladder contraction and relaxation of the internal sphincter.
- Voluntary contraction of the abdominal muscles aids bladder emptying.
- In the first few years of life micturition is a reflex occurrence with no voluntary control; however, later in life it becomes a voluntary response; descending impulses inhibit parasympathetic fibres and also stimulate somatic impulses along the pudendal nerve, which allow contraction of the external sphincter.

Clinical Physiology

Bladder Function and Spinal Injury

- A normal bladder has the following innervation:
  - L1–2: sympathetic outflow (see above)
  - S2–4: parasympathetic (see above)
  - efferent sensory fibres enter the spinal cord at L1–2 and S2–4.
- Following spinal injury there are three common bladder abnormalities; these are:
  - atonic bladder
  - automatic reflex bladder
  - autonomous bladder.
- Atonic bladder: occurs during the initial phase of spinal shock and may last several weeks; the following abnormalities are seen:
  - bladder wall muscle is relaxed
  - sphincter vesicae is contracted
  - sphincter urethrae is relaxed
  - bladder becomes distended and eventually empties by overflow. If the level of the spinal injury is above L1–2 then the patient is unaware of the bladder distension; if the injury is below L1–2 then the patient is aware of the distended bladder.
- Automatic reflex bladder: this is seen once the spinal shock has subsided in patients with a spinal injury above the parasympathetic outflow (S2–4). The bladder empties reflexively every 3–4 h rather than by simple distension and overflow.
- Autonomous bladder: occurs if the sacral area of the spinal cord is damaged. The bladder is flaccid and its capacity greatly increases; the bladder fills to capacity and then overflows. Partial emptying can be performed by compression of the lower abdomen; however, backpressure leading to vesicoureteric reflux and hydronephrosis is unavoidable, and leads to frequent infections and eventually chronic renal failure.

Hormone Production

Renin

- Produced by the juxtaglomerular apparatus in the kidney.
- The action of renin is to cleave angiotensin I from angiotensinogen.
- The release of renin is stimulated by:
  - reduction in renal perfusion
  - stimulation of the sympathetic nervous system
  - catecholamine release
  - hyponatraemia.

Erythropoietin

- Majority is secreted in the kidney, although small amounts are made in the spleen and liver.
- It acts by accelerating differentiation of marrow stem cells into erythrocytes.
- There are numerous stimuli that increase the rate of erythrocyte production:
  - haemorrhage
  - respiratory disease
  - high altitude
  - vasoconstriction
  - ↑levels of red blood cells degradation products.
- In general these causes result in low tissue PO_2; this is the main stimulus for erythropoietin secretion.

1α-Hydroxylase

- 1α-hydroxylase is secreted by the kidney in response to ↓Ca^{2+}; it converts 25-hydroxycholecalciferol to 1,25-dihydroxycholecalciferol.
- 1,25-dihydroxycholecalciferol promotes Ca^{2+} reabsorption and decreases urinary loss (see Chapter 12 for further details on calcium homeostasis).

OSCE SCENARIOS

OSCE Scenario 11.1

A 70-year-old male is two days post-repair of a ruptured abdominal aortic aneurysm. Urine output has been poor, the last 4 h having been 20 mL, 10 mL, 5 mL and 5 mL per hour, respectively. The patient has been haemodynamically unstable.

1. How would you define oliguria?
   A specimen of urine is sent for examination and reveals the following results:
   Specific gravity >1020
   Urine osmolality >500 mosmol/L
   Urine sodium <20 mmol/L
   Fractional sodium excretion <1
2. What is the likely cause of the oliguria?
3. What action would you take based on these results?
   Appropriate measures fail to produce a diuresis. Serum creatinine is now 350 mmol/L and urine analysis reveals the following:
   Specific gravity <1010
   Urine osmolality 290 mosmol/L
   Urine sodium >40 mosmol/L
   Fractional sodium excretion >2
4. What is now the cause of the patient's renal dysfunction?
5. What techniques are available for renal replacement therapy in this patient?
6. What are the absolute indications for renal replacement therapy?
7. Which mode of renal replacement therapy will be the most appropriate in this patient?

OSCE Scenario 11.2

A 19-year-old male is admitted to A&E having been stabbed in the abdomen. On examination he is pale, sweating, with a tachycardia of 120 and a systolic blood pressure of 80 mmHg.

1. What are the grades of haemorrhagic shock?
2. What is renal blood flow autoregulation and how is it affected by shock?
3. Describe the hormonal response to shock with specific reference to ADH, aldosterone and the renin–angiotensin system.

OSCE Scenario 11.3

A 75-year-old male with a known lung malignancy is admitted in an acute confusional state. He is found to have a sodium level of 117 mmol/L. He is not dehydrated and has no signs of sepsis.

1. What possible explanation is there for the electrolyte abnormality?
2. What other tests would help confirm it?
3. Which type of lung cancer most commonly causes it?
4. How would you treat it?

OSCE Scenario 11.4

A 40-year-old male who was a restrained driver in a motor vehicle crash was found to be paraplegic at the level of T10. After primary and secondary survey, he was admitted to the high-dependency unit and abdominal examination revealed a palpable bladder.

1. What is the normal innervation to the urinary bladder?
2. What are the three bladder abnormalities that can occur following spinal injury?
3. Describe the bladder function following the initial phase of spinal injury.

OSCE Scenario 11.5

A 70-year-old man is admitted to the emergency surgical unit with suprapubic pain and inability to pass urine for 12 h. He reported recent history of hesitancy, weak stream and nocturia. Abdominal examination revealed a palpable distended bladder. His creatinine is found to be 220 µmol/L and GFR of 32 mL/min/1.73 m^2, while his baseline test 2 months ago showed Cr of 87 µmol/L and GFR of 60 ml/min/1.73 m^2.

1. What volume in the bladder normally triggers the urge to urinate?
2. What is the differential diagnosis?
3. What is the likely cause of his renal function deterioration?
4. The patient was found to have been recently commenced on tamsulosin by his GP. How does tamsulosin work?

Answers in Appendix pages 454-456

Please check your eBook at https://studentconsult.inkling.com/ for more self-assessment questions. See inside cover for registration details.

12

Endocrine System

INTRODUCTION

- The function of the endocrine system is the secretion of hormones into the circulation and their regulation of cellular responses by binding to target cells and initiating a particular response.
- Hormones can be divided into:
  - steroids: derived from cholesterol
  - peptides
  - altered amino acids, e.g. thyroid hormones are composed of two tyrosine residues.
- The secretion of hormones can be stimulated by:
  - level of a substance, e.g. glucose and insulin secretion
  - stimulation by another hormone, e.g. TSH stimulates the thyroid gland to secrete thyroid hormones
  - nervous control, e.g. catecholamines during the 'fight or flight' response.
- Hormones interact with receptors to exert their effects; there are three main types:

1. Receptors on the cell surface: usually protein or peptide hormones, they initiate conformational changes in the receptor that lead to the production of second messengers, which in turn modify the cell's response.
2. Cytoplasmic receptors: steroid hormones interact with receptors in the cytoplasm (or nucleus). The receptor–hormone complex then enters the nucleus and binds to a specific area of DNA and stimulates translation of a protein product.
3. Nuclear receptors: thyroid hormone receptors are found in the nucleus of cells; thyroid hormone enters the cell in conjunction with the receptor and enters the nucleus to exert its effect.

PITUITARY AND HYPOTHALAMIC FUNCTION

- The hypothalamus lies in the forebrain in the floor of the third ventricle; it is linked to the thalamus above and the pituitary below via the hypophyseal stalk.
- The pituitary is divided into anterior and posterior.
  - anterior pituitary (adenohypophysis): derived from an outpouching of tissue from the oral cavity (ectoderm); it is linked to the hypothalamus via the hypophyseal portal system
  - posterior pituitary (neurohypophysis): derived from a downgrowth of neural tissue; it is continuous with the hypothalamus. Nuclei (paraventricular and supraoptic) lie within the hypothalamus and send axons into the posterior pituitary. These axons are specialized and release hormones into the bloodstream.

Control of Pituitary Function

Anterior Pituitary

- Regulation of hormone secretion from the anterior pituitary is by hormones secreted along the hypophyseal tract from the hypothalamus.
- These releasing or inhibiting hormones act on secretory endocrine cells in the anterior pituitary.
- Release of the hormone from the target organ is regulated by feedback inhibition, either by the releasing/inhibiting hormone or by the hormone released from the target organ.

Posterior Pituitary

- The posterior pituitary stores two hormones, which are produced by two nuclei in the hypothalamus.
- These two hormones are transported to the ends of the axons that connect the hypothalamus and the posterior pituitary; they are released into the circulation following an appropriate stimulus.

Anterior Pituitary Hormones

Adrenocorticotrophic hormone (ACTH)

- Secreted in response to corticotrophin-releasing hormone (CRH) from the hypothalamus.
- Stimulates the release of glucocorticoids from the adrenal cortex; also stimulates the release of β-endorphin and precursors of melanocyte-releasing hormone (MSH).

Thyroid-stimulating hormone (TSH)
- Secreted in response to thyrotrophin-releasing hormone (TRH).
- Stimulates thyroid secretion.

Follicle-stimulating hormone (FSH) and luteinizing hormone (LH)
- Secreted in response to gonadotrophin-releasing hormone (GnRH).
- Lead to stimulation of the male and female gonads.

Prolactin
- Secretion is controlled by the inhibitory action of dopamine. Factors that decrease dopamine lead to the release of prolactin.

Growth hormone (GH)
- Secretion is stimulated by growth-hormone-releasing hormone (GHRH) and inhibited by growth-hormone-inhibiting hormone (GHIH or somatostatin).

Posterior Pituitary Hormones

Oxytocin
- Produced by cells in the paraventricular nucleus in the hypothalamus.
- Secretion is stimulated by sensory stimuli activating mechanoreceptors in the breast during suckling.
- Also stimulates the ejection of milk and uterine contractions.

Antidiuretic hormone
- Produced by cells in the supraoptic nucleus in the hypothalamus.
- Release is stimulated by sensory input into osmoreceptors and cardiac stretch receptors (see section on fluid balance in Chapter 7).

Clinical Physiology

Pituitary Disorders

Increased hormone secretion

The clinical conditions seen as a result of excess hormone secretion include:
- ↑ ACTH: Cushing's disease (see below).
- ↑ Prolactin: hyperprolactinaemia occurs with pituitary tumours (prolactinoma). Patients present with galactorrhoea, amenorrhoea, impotence, headaches and visual field defects. The effects on reproductive function are via its inhibitory effect on GnRH production.
- TSH: TSH-secreting pituitary tumours can cause hyperthyroidism but they are exceedingly rare.
- GH: abnormal release of GH results in two disorders, depending on the age at which it presents:
  - ↑ in childhood results in gigantism (see below)
  - ↑ in adult life results in acromegaly (see below).
- ↑ADH: elevated ADH leads to the syndrome of inappropriate antidiuretic hormone (SIADH). The condition is diagnosed by ↓ Na^+, ↓ plasma osmolarity, ↑ urine osmolarity, and urinary Na^+ >30 mmol/L. Causes include:
  - tumours, e.g. lung, pancreas, lymphomas
  - TB
  - lung abscess
  - CNS lesions, e.g. meningitis, abscess, head injury
  - metabolic, e.g. alcohol withdrawal
  - drugs, e.g. carbamazepine.

Decreased hormone secretion

- Deficiency of pituitary hormones can be isolated or involve all hormones (panhypopituitarism).
- The effects of individual deficiency include:
  - ↓ ACTH: results in Addison's disease (see below)
  - ↓ TSH: results in hypothyroidism (see below)
  - ↓ FSH and LH: leads to a failure in sexual function and hypogonadism
  - ↓ GH: leads to dwarfism (see below)
  - ↓ ADH: results in diabetes insipidus (cranial), also nephrogenic diabetes insipidus – this occurs due to failure at the cell receptor level in the kidney. A deficiency of ADH leads to an inability to concentrate urine and the passage of litres of urine (polyuria).
- The causes of pituitary deficiency include:
  - rare congenital deficiency, e.g. Kallman syndrome: FSH and LH deficiency
  - infection: meningitis and encephalitis
  - pituitary apoplexy: bleeding into a pituitary tumour
  - Sheehan's syndrome: infarction following post-partum haemorrhage
  - cerebral tumours
  - radiation
  - trauma, i.e. frontal skull
  - sarcoidosis.

THYROID FUNCTION

Anatomy

- See Chapter 5.
- Microscopically, the thyroid is composed of follicles; these consist of an outer layer of cuboidal epithelium and are filled with colloid.
- The follicles are responsible for the production, storage and secretion of thyroid hormone.
- Between follicles lie the parafollicular cells; these secrete calcitonin (see Calcium and Phosphate Regulation section).

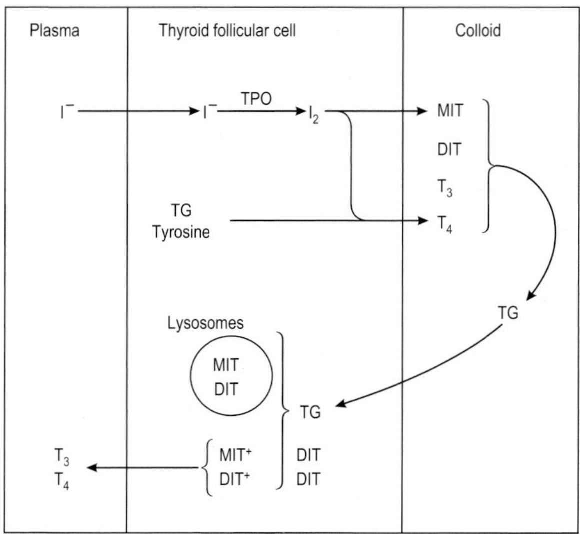

Fig. 12.1 Production of T_3 and T_4 in the thyroid gland (I^- = iodide, I_2 = iodine, TPO = thyroid peroxidase, TG = thyroglobulin, MIT = monoiodotyrosine, DIT = diiodotyrosine).

Synthesis of Thyroid Hormone (Fig. 12.1)

- Steps in the synthesis of thyroid hormones include:
  - active pumping of iodide ions in from the extracellular space to the follicular epithelium
  - iodide ions enter the colloid and are converted to iodine
  - iodine is combined with tyrosine.
- Two forms are produced: monoiodotyrosine (1 MT) and diiodotyrosine (2 DT); these then combine to form the two thyroid hormones:
  - triiodothyronine (T_3): MT + DT
  - thyroxine (T_4): × 2 DT.
- More T_4 is produced but T_3 is more biologically active.
- Thyroid hormones are stored in the colloid of the follicle and released into the circulation as needed (the thyroglobulin is detached).

Clinical Physiology

Antithyroid Drugs

The drugs used in the treatment of hyperthyroidism include:

- Thionamides, e.g. carbimazole and propylthiouracil: this group of drugs competitively inhibits the peroxidase-catalysed reaction (iodide is converted to iodine). They also block the coupling of the iodotyrosine. Propylthiouracil also inhibits the peripheral deiodination of T_4.
- Anion inhibitors, e.g. perchlorate: competitively inhibits the uptake of iodine; discontinued as it can cause aplastic anaemia.
- Iodide, e.g. Lugol's solution: iodide is thought to work by blocking the binding of iodine with tyrosine residues, inhibiting hormone release. It is also thought to decrease the size and vascularity of the thyroid gland.

Secretion and Transport of Thyroid Hormone

- Hypothalamus releases thyrotrophin-releasing hormone (TRH). TRH is transported to the endocrine cells of the anterior pituitary along the hypophyseal tract; this stimulates the release of thyroid-stimulating hormone (TSH).
- TSH stimulates thyroid hormone production and secretion.
- T_3 and T_4 have a negative feedback effect on TRH and TSH.
- Cold stress stimulates thyroid hormone secretion.
- The majority of thyroid hormone in the circulation is bound to thyroid-binding globulin (TBG); however, only the free portion is biologically active.

Effects of Thyroid Hormone

- T_3 and T_4 cross the cell membrane via diffusion; most of the T_4 is converted to T_3 in the cell.
- Thyroid hormone then bonds to receptors and initiates increased DNA transcription and protein production.
- The effects of thyroid hormone include:
  - metabolic:
    - ↑ basal metabolic rate: leading to ↑ O_2 consumption and ↑ heat production
    - ↑ absorption of glucose, glycolysis and gluconeogenesis
    - ↑ catabolism of fatty acids
    - ↓ cholesterol production
    - ↑ synthesis and catabolism of protein
  - cardiac:
    - ↑ heart rate
    - ↓ in peripheral vascular resistance (indirect, due to increased metabolic rate in tissues)
    - ↑ in cardiac output and pulse
    - ↑ β-receptor production; facilitates activation and increases the response
    - promotes erythropoiesis
  - respiratory:
    - ↑ ventilatory rate
  - gastrointestinal:
    - ↑ motility and secretion
  - CNS:
    - ↑ CNS activity and alertness
    - normal neuronal function

- growth and development:
  - necessary for normal myelination and axonal development
  - stimulation of skeletal growth
  - promotes bone mineralization.

Clinical Physiology

Thyroid Disorders

Hyperthyroidism

- Hyperthyroidism = 'overactive' thyroid.
- The causes of hyperthyroidism include:
  - primary hyperthyroidism: this includes intrinsic thyroid diseases:
    - Graves' disease: commonest cause, due to autoimmune IgG antibodies that bind to the TSH receptors and stimulate thyroid hormone production
    - solitary toxic adenoma/nodule (Plummer's disease)
    - toxic multinodular goitre
    - acute phase of thyroiditis – occurs in the early phase of cell injury and is due to the release of large amounts of stored thyroid hormone
    - drugs, e.g. amiodarone.
  - secondary hyperthyroidism: this includes causes of hyperthyroidism extrinsic to the thyroid gland:
    - pituitary/hypothalamic tumour secreting TSH/TRH; very rare
    - metastatic thyroid carcinoma: if well differentiated, may produce enough thyroid hormone to produce symptoms of hyperthyroidism
    - choriocarcinoma: this tumour usually produces HCG; however, it can also produce a substance similar to TSH
    - ovarian teratoma: a particular specialized type of teratoma – called struma ovarii – is composed of mature thyroid tissue. This may overfunction and lead to hyperthyroidism.

The clinical features of hyperthyroidism are shown in Fig. 12.2.

Hypothyroidism

- Hypothyroidism = 'underactive' thyroid.
- The causes of hypothyroidism include:
  - primary hypothyroidism: this includes diseases that directly affect the thyroid gland; these include:
    - autoimmune (atrophic): arises due to microsomal antibodies that lead to destruction and atrophy of the thyroid gland
    - Hashimoto's thyroiditis: an autoimmune inflammation of the thyroid gland; microsomal autoantibodies are also present. The condition is associated with atrophy and regeneration of the thyroid gland; this leads to goitre formation
    - iodine deficiency
    - genetic defects: inherited defects in the enzymes involved in the synthesis of thyroid hormones, e.g. Pendred's syndrome
    - iatrogenic, e.g. post-thyroidectomy and -irradiation
    - drugs, e.g. lithium
    - neoplasia: infiltration and destruction of the gland secondary to a malignant neoplasm.
  - secondary hypothyroidism: occurs due to pituitary or hypothalamic disease:
    - hypopituitarism
    - isolated TSH deficiency.

The clinical features of hypothyroidism are shown in Fig. 12.3.

Sick euthyroid syndrome

- Acute illness from any cause can result in a number of abnormalities in the markers of thyroid function without actually affecting thyroid function, i.e. the patient is euthyroid. These changes include:
  - ↓ binding proteins
  - ↓ affinity of binding proteins
  - ↓ peripheral conversion of T_4 to T_3
  - ↓ TSH.
- These patients will thus have low T_4/T_3 levels, but levels of TSH are also low.

CALCIUM AND PHOSPHATE REGULATION

Calcium

- Calcium is absorbed via the gut and is mainly excreted in the urine.
- Calcium is stored in three 'pools':
  - bone: 99% of total body calcium. Osteoclasts break down bone to release Ca^{2+} (structural bone calcium) and phosphate into the circulation; osteocytes are also able to transfer Ca^{2+} into the circulation, but do not affect the bone structure (exchangeable bone calcium)
  - intracellular: Ca^{2+} is an important mediator of intracellular signals
  - extracellular: normal levels are between 2.2 and 2.6 mmol/L. Approximately 50% is protein-bound, only the free fraction is biologically active. The extracellular pool is in constant flux with bone, Ca^{2+} absorbed from the gastrointestinal tract, and excreted in the urine.
- Calcium is important in a number of cellular processes:
  - excitability of nerve and muscle: calcium level affects the permeability of the Na^+ channel; a low calcium level will lead to increased permeability and increased Na^+ influx, and will thus depolarize the

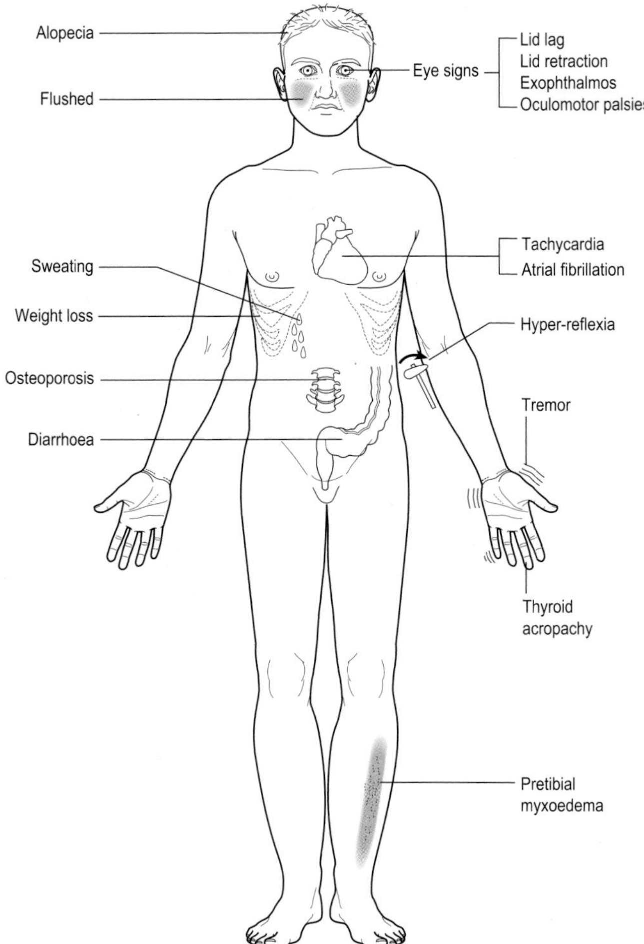

Fig. 12.2 Features of hyperthyroidism.

cell towards threshold. If the Ca^{2+} level rises then Na^{+} permeability decreases, and the threshold will rise, thus decreasing nerve and muscle activity

- muscle contraction: excitation–contraction coupling in muscle (see Chapter 13) requires an influx of calcium
- secretion processes: the products secreted from various glands is often triggered by an influx of Ca^{2+} into the cell
- clotting: Ca^{2+} is an essential blood-clotting factor; it acts as a cofactor for several of the clotting factors (see Chapter 20).

Regulation of Calcium Balance

- The regulation of calcium is by two hormones (parathormone [PTH] and calcitonin) and vitamin D.

Parathormone

- PTH is an 84-amino-acid polypeptide released from the parathyroid glands; these are found on the posterior surface of the thyroid lobes.
- A fall in extracellular fluid (ECF) Ca^{2+} stimulates the release of PTH. It increases Ca^{2+} in several ways:
  - stimulates Ca^{2+} release from bone; the initial rapid phase of Ca^{2+} release is due to osteocytes mobilizing the exchangeable bone calcium. Longer-term release of PTH will stimulate osteoclasts to release Ca^{2+} from the structural bone pool
  - increases the rate of Ca^{2+} uptake from the renal tubules, therefore reducing urinary loss
  - stimulates urinary phosphate excretion
  - stimulates the rate at which vitamin D is converted to the biologically active 1,25 form in the kidney.

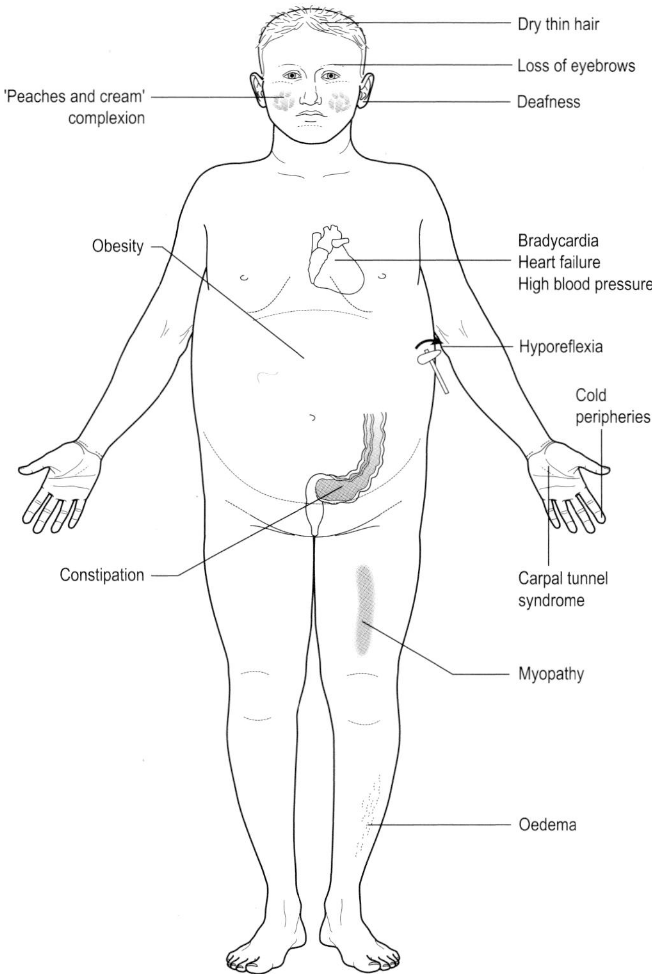

Fig. 12.3 Features of hypothyroidism.

Vitamin D

- Vitamin D is a fat-soluble vitamin, derived from two sources:
  - diet: vitamin D_2
  - skin: UV radiation converts cholesterol to vitamin D_3.
- Vitamin D (cholecalciferol) is converted to 1,25-dihydrocholecalciferol in two stages:
  - converted to 25-hydroxycholecalciferol in the liver
  - converted to 1,25-dihydroxycholecalciferol (the most active form) in the kidney.
- PTH and low phosphate levels stimulate the conversion steps for vitamin D.
- Vitamin D increases plasma Ca^{2+} by a number of mechanisms:
  - increases the rate of Ca^{2+} and phosphate uptake from the gut
  - increases renal tubular absorption of Ca^{2+} and phosphate
  - stimulates osteoclastic bone resorption
  - promotes mineralization of osteoid.

Calcitonin

- Calcitonin is a 32-amino-acid polypeptide; it is secreted by parafollicular C-cells within the thyroid gland.
- It acts to reduce the rate of Ca^{2+} release into the ECF by:
  - decreasing Ca^{2+} and phosphate reabsorption from the renal tubules
  - stimulating osteoblasts to mineralize bone and thus take Ca^{2+} from the circulation.

- The action of calcitonin is thought to be significant in periods of hypercalcaemia, but plays little role in the everyday regulation of Ca^{2+}.

Regulation of Phosphate Balance

- The regulation of phosphate levels occurs in tandem with Ca^{2+} regulation.
- PTH reduces phosphate levels (decreases renal tubular absorption and thus increases urinary loss).
- 1,25-dihydroxycholecalciferol increases phosphate levels (increases renal tubular absorption).
- ↓phosphate stimulates the renal activation of vitamin D to the 1,25 form.

Clinical Physiology

Disorders of Calcium and Phosphate Balance

Hypoparathyroidism

- Hypoparathyroidism is a rare cause of hypocalcaemia.
- Causes include:
  - congenital, e.g. DiGeorge syndrome
  - autoimmune
  - iatrogenic: following total thyroidectomy or parathyroidectomy
  - hypomagnesaemia: low magnesium levels prevent the release of PTH.

Hyperparathyroidism

- Hyperparathyroidism is a common cause of hypercalcaemia. There are several different types:
  - primary hyperparathyroidism. Causes include:
    - single adenoma (>80%)
    - multiple adenomas (<5%)
    - parathyroid hyperplasia (<10%)
    - parathyroid carcinoma (rare; <2%)
  - secondary hyperparathyroidism: with prolonged ↓ Ca^{2+} the parathyroid glands hypertrophy. In these instances, e.g. renal failure, the calcium level will be low or normal, but the PTH level will be elevated.
  - tertiary hyperparathyroidism: if secondary hyperparathyroidism develops and the cause of the ↓ Ca^{2+} is not treated, then tertiary hyperparathyroidism develops – in this case the glands produce PTH autonomously and the levels of both Ca^{2+} and PTH are elevated.
  - ectopic PTH: this condition is very rare; it occurs when tumours, e.g. squamous cell lung cancer, produce PTH-related peptide. This is a 141-amino-acid protein that is similar to PTH and is thus able to stimulate bone resorption and calcium release.

Vitamin D deficiency

- A lack of vitamin D leads to inadequate mineralization of bone; in adults this leads to osteomalacia, in children it leads to rickets.
- Causes of vitamin D deficiency include:
  - dietary insufficiency: particularly common in vegans
  - lack of sunlight: common in elderly patients and Asian women
  - malabsorption: particularly after gastric surgery, coeliac disease and disorders of bile salt production
  - renal disease: leads to inadequate conversion to the active form 1,25-dihydroxycholecalciferol
  - hepatic failure
  - Vitamin-D-resistant rickets: a familial condition with hypophosphataemia, phosphaturia and rickets.

Hypocalcaemia

- Hypocalcaemia results in symptoms related to neuromuscular irritability, e.g. paraesthesia, numbness, cramps and tetany. Neuropsychiatric disturbances may also occur, e.g. anxiety and psychosis.
- Specific signs include Chovstek's sign and Trousseau's sign.
- ECG may show a prolonged QT interval.
- Causes include:
  - hypoalbuminaemia
  - hypomagnesaemia
  - hypophosphataemia
  - hypoparathyroidism
  - acute pancreatitis
  - rhabdomyolysis
  - sepsis
  - massive transfusion (due to citrate binding)
  - post-thyroid surgery
  - vitamin D deficiency
  - osteoblastic metastases
  - hypoventilation with respiratory alkalosis and reduction in ionized plasma calcium
  - drugs, e.g. diuretics, aminoglycosides, bisphosphonates, calcitonin.

Hypercalcaemia

- Hypercalcaemia is more common than hypocalcaemia.
- Symptoms can be remembered by the rhyme, 'stones, bones, abdominal groans and psychiatric overtones', i.e. renal stones, bone pain, abdominal pain (due to peptic ulceration in some cases) and depression.
- ECG may show a reduced QT interval.
- Causes include:
  - excess PTH – primary and tertiary hyperparathyroidism, ectopic PTH secretion
  - excess vitamin D
  - sarcoidosis
  - milk–alkali syndrome (excess calcium intake)
  - drugs, e.g. thiazide diuretics
  - malignancy.
- solid tumour with lytic bony metastases, e.g. carcinoma of the breast, carcinoma of the bronchus

- solid tumour with humoral mediation, e.g. inappropriate PTH secretion with carcinoma of the bronchus, carcinoma of the kidney
- multiple myeloma
  - hyperthyroidism
  - Addison's disease
  - prolonged immobilization
  - Paget's disease of bone
  - familial hypocalciuric hypercalcaemia.

Hypophosphataemia

- Hypophosphataemia results in:
  - confusion
  - convulsions
  - muscle weakness: acute hypophosphataemia can lead to significant diaphragmatic weakness and delay weaning from a ventilator in patients in the intensive treatment unit
  - left shift of oxyhaemoglobin curve: this results in decreased oxygen delivery to tissues and is due to the reduction in 2,3-DPG.
- Causes include:
  - hyperparathyroidism: PTH reduces renal tubule absorption
  - vitamin D deficiency: vitamin D stimulates gut and tubular absorption of phosphate
  - total parenteral nutrition (TPN): refeeding with carbohydrate after fasting can result in hypophosphataemia
  - diabetic ketoacidosis
  - alcohol withdrawal
  - acute liver failure
  - paracetamol overdose: phosphaturia.

Hyperphosphataemia

- Hyperphosphataemia is usually asymptomatic and no treatment is required.
- Causes include:
  - chronic renal failure: causes itching, hyperparathyroidism and deposition of calcium in the joints and around vessels
  - tumour lysis: occurs following radio- or chemotherapy
  - myeloma.

ADRENAL FUNCTION

- The adrenal glands are located at the upper poles of both kidneys (see Chapter 2).
- They consist of an outer cortex and an inner medulla.
- The cortex secretes steroid-based hormones and is subdivided into three sections:
  - zona glomerulosa: mineralocorticoids
  - zona fasciculata: glucocorticoids
  - zona reticularis: sex hormones.
- The medulla is part of the sympathetic nervous system; it contains chromaffin cells; these are specialized sympathetic post-ganglionic neurons.
- Nerve fibres from the splanchnic nerves innervate the medulla; these release acetylcholine, which stimulates hormone release.
- The chromaffin cells release a variety of hormones when stimulated to do so; they are stored in granules and exit the cells into the circulation via exocytosis.
- The adrenal medulla produces:
  - epinephrine (adrenaline)
  - norepinephrine (noradrenaline)
  - dopamine
  - β-hydroxylase (enzyme involved in catecholamine synthesis)
  - ATP
  - opioid peptides (metenkephalin and leuenkephalin).

Cortex

Synthesis and Excretion

- Cholesterol is converted to pregnenolone in mitochondria; this provides the basic structure for the formation of all other steroid hormones.
- Conversion products of pregnenolone are shown in Fig. 12.4.
- Adrenal steroids are broken down by the liver and excreted via the kidneys and in faeces.

Actions of the Adrenal Cortex Hormones

Aldosterone

- Aldosterone is a mineralocorticoid.
- Mineralocorticoids function to regulate ECF volume by altering the rate of Na^+ reabsorption.
- Glucocorticoids have a mild mineralocorticoid action.
- Aldosterone secretion is stimulated by a number of factors:
  - renin–angiotensin system: a reduction in the ECF volume, blood pressure or Na^+ concentration in plasma (detected by the juxtaglomerular apparatus) will lead to an increase in the secretion of renin from the juxtaglomerular cells; this leads to the production of angiotensin II, which stimulates the release of aldosterone
  - ↑ K^+ in plasma
  - ACTH (does not play a role in the normal regulation of aldosterone release).
- The actions of aldosterone include:
  - stimulation of the reabsorption of Na^+ from the distal convoluted tubule in the kidney
  - secretion of K^+ into the distal convoluted tubule
  - secretion of H^+ into the distal convoluted tubule.

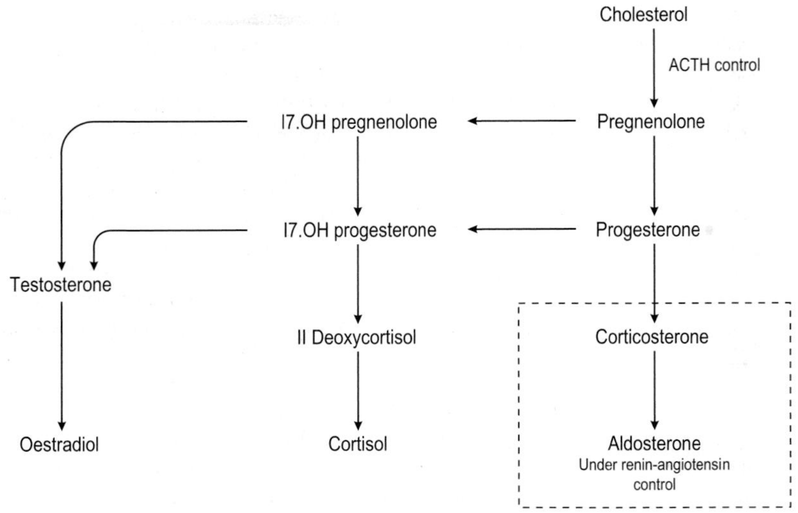

Fig. 12.4 Scheme for the production of adrenal cortical hormones.

Cortisol

- The zona fasciculata releases several glucocorticoid hormones: cortisol or hydrocortisone (the main glucocorticoid), corticosterone and cortisone.
- Cortisol is bound to a specific binding protein called transcortin (75%); approximately 15% is bound to albumin and only 10% is active or free.
- Cortisol secretion is stimulated by a number of factors:
  - ACTH: released from the anterior pituitary (promoted by CRH released from the hypothalamus); it binds to receptors in the adrenal glands and stimulates the release of cortisol. Cortisol levels then inhibit CRH and ACTH release (negative feedback)
  - circadian rhythm: cortisol levels are higher first thing in the morning (7–8 am) and fall to a lower level in the middle of the night (1–2 am)
  - stress
  - trauma
  - burns
  - infection
  - exercise
  - hypoglycaemia.
- The actions of cortisol include:
  - metabolic effects: the metabolic effects of cortisol generally oppose those of insulin; they include:
    - breakdown of protein to amino acids
    - amino acids are then converted to glucose (gluconeogenesis)
    - storage of glucose as glycogen
    - lipolysis: mobilizes free fatty acids and glycerol; these are then converted to glucose in the liver
  - cardiovascular effects: cortisol is necessary for vasopressors, e.g. epinephrine, to increase vascular tone. In the absence of cortisol, blood vessels become unresponsive to the effects of catecholamines
  - CNS: cortisol produces euphoria
  - anti-inflammatory effects: the glucocorticoids have profound anti-inflammatory actions, which include:
    - ↓ immunocompetent cells and macrophages
    - stimulate synthesis of lipocortin in leukocytes. This protein inhibits phospholipase A2 and thus prevents formation of inflammatory mediators such as prostaglandins, leukotrienes and platelet activating factor (PAF)
  - immunosuppressive effects: the immunosuppressive effects of the glucocorticoids include:
    - ↓ T-cell number and function
    - ↓ B-cell clonal expansion
    - ↓ basophils and eosinophils
    - inhibit complement
  - mineralocorticoid: the glucocorticoid hormones have very mild mineralocorticoid activity
  - permissive effects: this relates to the normal function of other hormones in the face of normal cortisol levels; they include:
    - vascular reactivity to catecholamines
    - activity of aldosterone on renal tubules
    - activity of ADH on the collecting ducts
    - gluconeogenesis
    - increases the effect of T_3 in maintaining body temperature
    - facilitates the action of growth hormone.

Androgens

- The zona reticularis produces sex steroids: androgens in men, and oestrogen and progesterone in women; the amount is insignificant in comparison with the amount produced by the testes/ovaries.
- Secretion is stimulated by ACTH released from the hypothalamus.

Medulla

- The adrenal medulla acts as an extension of the sympathetic nervous system. It contains chromaffin cells that resemble the post-ganglionic cells in the sympathetic nervous system. They do not possess axons but are similar in the fact that they release a number of neurotransmitters from intracellular vesicles once stimulated.
- The main hormones secreted by the adrenal medulla are epinephrine (adrenaline) and norepinephrine (noradrenaline); they are synthesized from the amino acid tyrosine
- Epinephrine and norepinephrine released from the adrenal medulla bind to α-receptors (mainly norepinephrine) and β-receptors (mainly epinephrine). Binding to these receptors leads to the production of second messengers such as cAMP; these second messengers lead to further intracellular reactions that ultimately alter cell function.
- The adrenal hormones are rapidly inactivated once released, by the enzymes catechol-O-methyl-transferase and monoamine oxidase, present in the liver and kidney.

The effects of epinephrine and norepinephrine are shown in Box 12.1.

BOX 12.1 Efficacy of Norepinephrine (Noradrenaline) and Epinephrine (Adrenaline) in Various Physiological Processes

Norepinephrine > Epinephrine	Epinephrine > Norepinephrine
↑gluconeogenesis (α_1)	↑glycogenolysis (β_2)
↓insulin secretion (α_2)	↑lipolysis (β_3)
Vasoconstriction: ↑BP (α_1)	↑insulin secretion (β_2)
↑tone in GI sphincters (α_1)	↑glucagon secretion (β_2)
Bronchoconstriction (α_1)	↑K^+ uptake by muscle (β_2)
	↑heart rate (β_1)
	arteriolar tone in skeletal muscle (β_2)
	↑cardiac contractility (β_1)
	bronchodilatation (β_2)

Clinical Physiology

Disorders of Adrenal Function

Addison's disease

- Addison's disease is caused by destruction of the adrenal cortex; this produces a reduction in mineralocorticoid, glucocorticoid and sex-hormone production.
- The causes of Addison's disease include:
  - primary hypoadrenalism: caused by destruction of the adrenal cortex; causes include:
    - autoimmune (>80%)
    - TB (20%)
    - haemorrhage, e.g. Waterhouse–Friderichsen syndrome in meningococcal septicaemia
    - malignant infiltration
    - drugs
  - secondary hypoadrenalism: due to pituitary disease and the resulting decrease in ACTH secretion; production of mineralocorticoids is not affected as stimulation is via angiotensin II; sex hormone secretion is also independent of pituitary function.
- The clinical features of Addison's disease are shown in Fig. 12.5.
- The clinical features of Addison's disease are mainly due to the deficiencies in mineralocorticoid and glucocorticoid:
  - mineralocorticoid deficiency: there is increased urinary Na^+ loss leading to dehydration, ↓ Na^+, ↓ blood pressure, K^+ retention leading to hyperkalaemia, and H^+ retention leading to metabolic acidosis
  - glucocorticoid deficiency: this leads to nonspecific symptoms such as weight loss, anorexia and lethargy. Hypoglycaemia may occur during fasting, and there is reduced resistance to trauma and infection.

Hyperaldosteronism

- Excess secretion of aldosterone may be primary or secondary.
- Primary hyperaldosteronism:
  - a very rare cause of ↑ blood pressure (<1%); it is caused by adrenal adenomas in 60–70% (Conn's syndrome) and bilateral hyperplasia in 20–30%.
- Secondary hyperaldosteronism:
  - results from excess secretion of renin, this stimulates angiotensin II and thus aldosterone; causes include:
    - renal artery stenosis
    - congestive cardiac failure
    - cirrhosis.

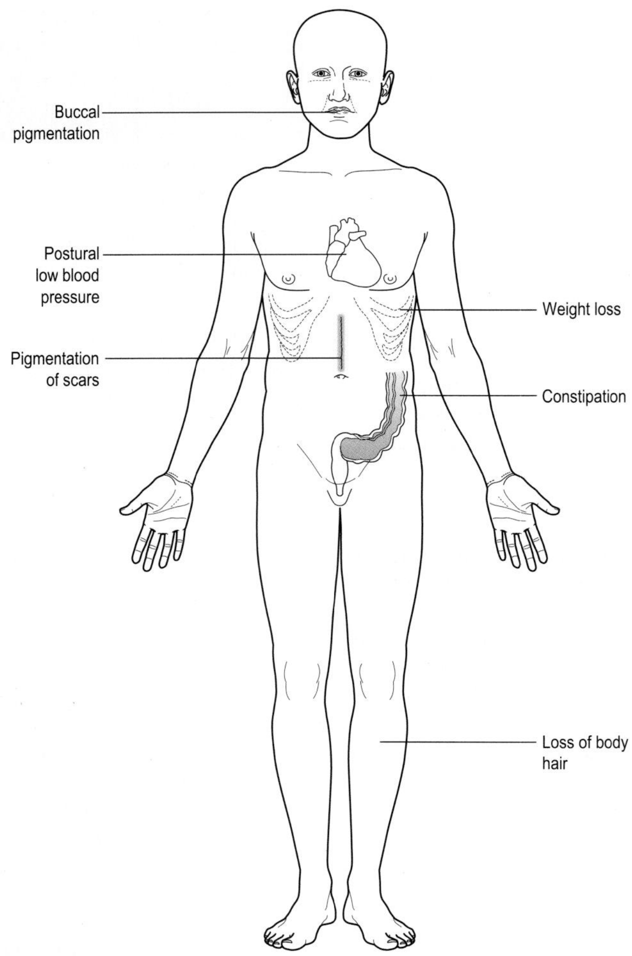

Fig. 12.5 Features of Addison's disease.

- The effects of excess aldosterone secretion include:
  - Na^+ and water retention, leading to ↑ blood pressure
  - renal K^+ loss, leading to hypokalaemia
  - renal H^+ loss, leading to metabolic alkalosis.

Cushing's disease/syndrome

- Cushing's disease/syndrome is due to excess glucocorticoid; this can occur in several situations:
  - ACTH-dependent: there is increased ACTH, which stimulates glucocorticoid secretion. The ACTH may be from the pituitary (Cushing's disease) or by ectopic secretion from a tumour
  - ACTH independent: this is caused by an excess of glucocorticoid with suppression of ACTH; this can result from:
    - adrenal adenoma
    - adrenal carcinoma
    - glucocorticoid administration.
- The clinical features of Cushing's syndrome are shown in Fig. 12.6.
- The main effects of raised glucocorticoids include:
  - hyperglycaemia
  - muscle wasting due to protein breakdown
  - osteoporosis
  - striae (stretch marks)
  - weight gain, partly due to a stimulation of appetite but also due to abnormal fat deposition in the face (moon face) and back (buffalo hump)
  - ↑ blood pressure, due to fluid retention from the mineralocorticoid activity of cortisol
  - hirsutism and acne, due to the androgenic properties of cortisol.

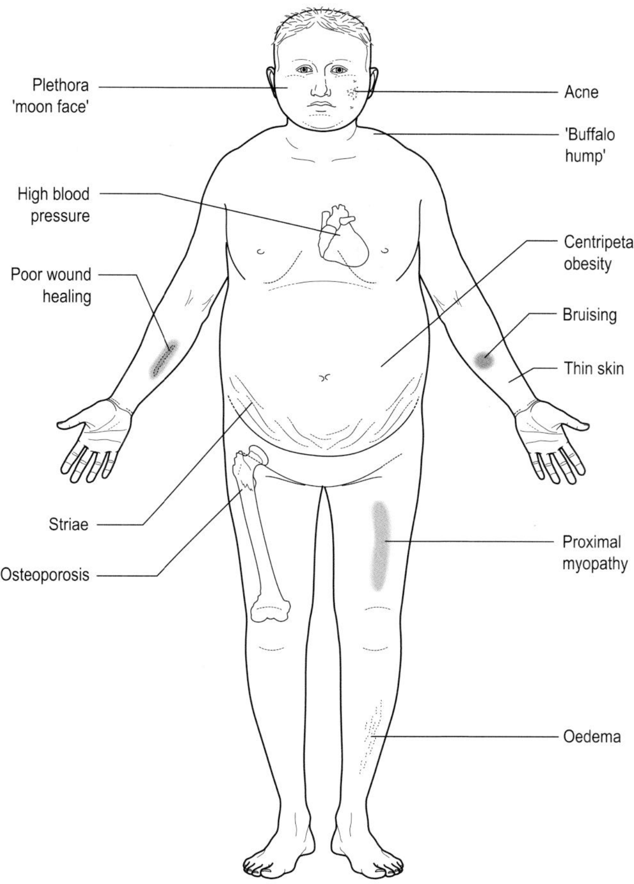

Fig. 12.6 Features of Cushing's syndrome.

Adrenogenital syndrome

- Also known as congenital adrenal hyperplasia (CAH), it results from genetic deficiencies in the enzymes in the synthesis of cortisol. The commonest defect affects the enzyme 21-hydroxylase.
- The lack of this enzyme leads to a decrease in cortisol secretion and as a result increases in ACTH secretion; this has the effect of driving the unused cortisol precursors into the androgenic hormone synthetic pathways.
- The clinical effects depend on the sex of the affected individual:
  - male: there is rapid growth in childhood and early sexual development (precocious puberty); due to early fusion of the epiphysis, these patients are often shorter than average
  - female: there is masculinization of the external genitalia with hypertrophy of the clitoris, a male body shape and hair distribution.

Phaeochromocytoma

- A rare condition characterized by oversecretion of catecholamines (epinephrine and norepinephrine) from the adrenal medulla.
- A tumour of the chromaffin cells causes the condition: 10% are malignant, 10% are multiple and 10% arise outside of the adrenal medulla ('rule of 10 s').
- The effects of the increased circulating catecholamines include:
  - palpitations and arrhythmias
  - tremors
  - sweating and flushing
  - ↑ blood pressure (episodic)
  - hyperglycaemia (episodic).

Growth Hormone

- Human growth hormone (hGH) is the main form of growth hormone; it is a large protein composed of 191 amino acids.

- Secretion is stimulated by growth hormone releasing hormone (GHRH) released by the hypothalamus and inhibited by somatostatin.
- GH is released in a pulsatile manner and demonstrates a circadian rhythm, with elevation in secretion during periods of deep sleep.
- Hypoglycaemia is a potent stimulator of GH secretion; it stimulates GHRH release and inhibits somatostatin secretion.
- A number of other stimuli promote GH secretion:
  - anxiety
  - pain
  - hypothermia
  - haemorrhage
  - trauma
  - fever
  - exercise.
- The effects of GH can be divided into those predominating in childhood and adolescence, and those that predominate in adulthood:
  - childhood and adolescence: GH stimulates skeletal growth by stimulating mitosis in the cartilage cells in the epiphyseal plates at the ends of the long bones; this process is aided by insulin-like growth factors (IGFs) that encourage matrix secretion from cartilage cells
  - adulthood: after fusion of the epiphyseal plates, GH no longer has any influence on skeletal growth; however, it still has an important role in a number of metabolic functions:
    - ↑glycogenolysis
    - ↓glucose uptake by cells
    - promotes amino acid uptake into cells
    - promotes protein synthesis
    - ↑lipolysis and release of free fatty acids (FFAs)
    - ↓LDL cholesterol.

Clinical Physiology

Disorders of Growth Hormone Secretion

Gigantism

- Caused by growth hormone hypersecretion prior to epiphyseal fusion; there is increased growth, particularly of the limbs – this results in the condition of gigantism.

Acromegaly

- In this condition there is also hypersecretion of growth hormone, but it occurs in adult life after epiphyseal fusion.
- Hypersecretion of growth hormone in adult life is called acromegaly, and results from a pituitary tumour.
- The symptoms and signs of acromegaly can be divided into those produced by the tumour and those produced by the growth hormone excess (see Fig. 12.7).

ENDOCRINE FUNCTION OF THE PANCREAS

- The exocrine role of the pancreas has been discussed in Chapter 10.
- Exocrine secretions are produced in the pancreatic acini and then discharged into the ductal system; the endocrine secretions are produced in the islets of Langerhans.
- The islets of Langerhans are highly vascular and are innervated by the sympathetic and parasympathetic nervous system.
- Three main hormones produced in the islet of Langerhans play a role in the regulation of plasma glucose levels:
  - insulin (secreted by β-cells)
  - glucagon (secreted by α-cells)
  - somatostatin (secreted by δ-cells).

Insulin

- Insulin is a small peptide consisting of 91 amino acids; it is derived from the precursor proinsulin.
- Proinsulin undergoes cleavage to form insulin.
- Insulin is stored within granules in β-cells and is secreted into the circulation by exocytosis.
- Insulin has a short half-life in the circulation (5–10 min); it is rapidly broken down by the liver and kidney.
- A number of factors are able to influence the secretion of insulin; the level of glucose is the most potent stimulus.
- Increased glucose stimulates insulin release from the β-cells; this decreases glucose concentration in the plasma and acts as a negative feedback.
- Other regulators of insulin secretion include:
  - fatty acids (+)
  - ketone bodies (+)
  - parasympathetic stimulation (+)
  - amino acids, i.e. arginine, leucine (+)
  - gastrin, cholecystokinin (CCK), secretin, gastric inhibitory polypeptide (GIP) (+)
  - prostaglandins (+)
  - drugs, e.g. sulfonylureas (+)
  - sympathetic stimulation (−)
  - dopamine (−)
  - serotonin (−)
  - somatostatin (−).
- Insulin is an anabolic hormone; it has a variety of actions, which can be divided into:
  - carbohydrate metabolism
  - protein metabolism
  - lipid metabolism.

Carbohydrate Metabolism

- Promotes glucose uptake, except in brain cells; these are freely permeable to glucose.

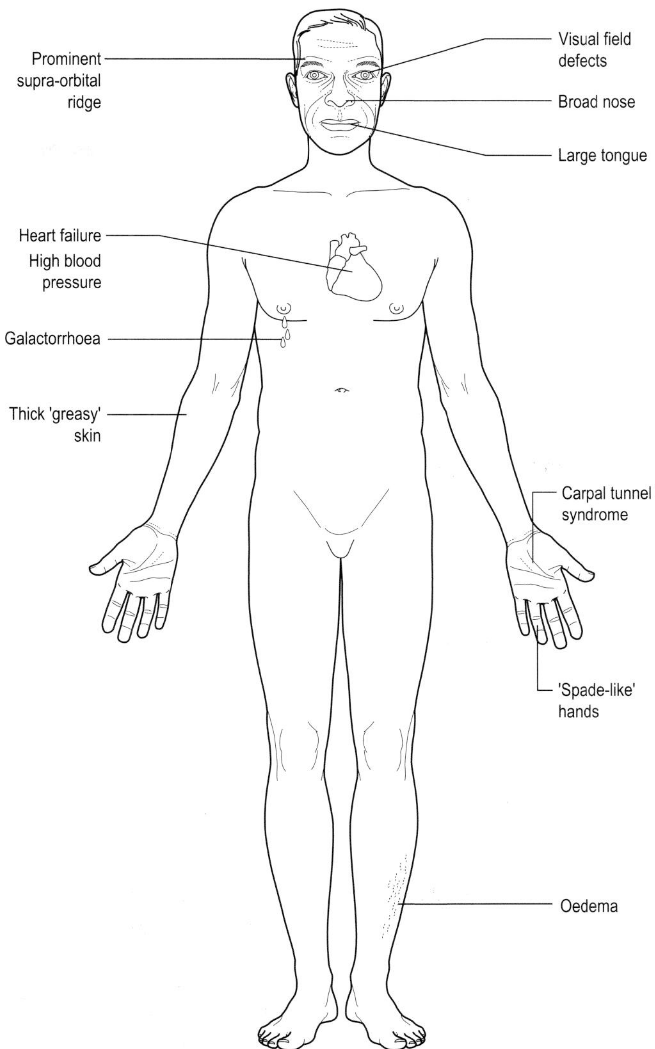

Fig. 12.7 Features of acromegaly.

- Promotes glycogen storage via ↑ glycogenesis and ↓ glycogenolysis; this allows glucose storage in the post-prandial period. Liver glycogen is converted to glucose and is able to maintain plasma glucose levels. Muscle glycogen acts as an energy store. Muscle lacks the phosphatase enzyme necessary to release free glucose and thus muscle glycogen can only be used in the muscle cells for glycolysis.
- Stimulates the use of glucose (glycolysis).

Protein Metabolism

- Stimulates amino acid uptake.
- Stimulates protein synthesis.
- Inhibits protein degradation.
- Inhibits amino acid conversion to glucose.

Lipid Metabolism

- Inhibits lipolysis by lipase.
- Stimulates lipogenesis.

Glucagon

- Glucagon is a catabolic hormone. It is a 29-amino-acid polypeptide and is released from the α-cells of the pancreas; like insulin it has a short half-life in the circulation (approximately 5 min).

- The actions of glucagons can be divided into those affecting carbohydrate metabolism and those affecting lipid metabolism.

Carbohydrate Metabolism

- ↑ Glycogenolysis.
- ↑ Gluconeogenesis.
- Glucose sparing by preferential oxidation of fatty acids; this produces ketones, i.e. acetone, acetoacetate, β-hydroxybutyrate.

Lipid Metabolism

- Stimulates lipase activity to increase plasma FFAs and glycerol.

Somatostatin

- Somatostatin is released by δ-cells in the pancreas.
- Secretion is stimulated by:
  - ↑ plasma glucose
  - ↑ plasma amino acids
  - ↑ plasma glycerol.
- The effects of somatostatin include:
  - inhibits the release of insulin and glucagons
  - ↓ gastrointestinal motility, secretion and absorption.

Effects of Other Hormones on Glucose Regulation

Glucocorticoids

- Released in response to hypoglycaemia, the effects include:
  - anti-insulin: inhibit glucose uptake
  - promote lipolysis: FFAs and glycerol are used in preference to glucose
  - promote gluconeogenesis
  - promote glycogen production.

Growth Hormone

- Released in times of fasting, the effects include:
  - anti-insulin: inhibits glucose uptake
  - promotes lipolysis
  - stimulates glycogenolysis.

Thyroid Hormone

- The role of thyroid hormone is complex: at low concentrations it is anabolic and reduces plasma glucose; at high concentrations it is catabolic and induces hyperglycaemia.
- The effects of thyroid hormone include:
  - ↑glycogenolysis
  - ↑gluconeogenesis
  - ↑absorption of glucose from the gastrointestinal tract
  - ↑uptake of glucose into cells
  - enhances the rate of insulin-dependent glycogenesis.

Catecholamines

- Release of catecholamines is stimulated when the plasma glucose falls below 4 mmol/L; their effects include:
  - ↑glycogenolysis
  - enhanced glycogen secretion
  - inhibited insulin secretion
  - lipolysis (FFAs and glycerol metabolized in preference to glucose).

Clinical Physiology

Disorders of the endocrine pancreas

Diabetes Mellitus

- Diabetes mellitus encompasses a number of conditions in which there is either a lack of insulin or a relative resistance to its effects.

The causes of diabetes mellitus include:

- Primary:
  - type I insulin-dependent diabetes mellitus (IDDM)
  - type II non-insulin-dependent diabetes mellitus (NIDDM).
- Secondary:
  - pancreatic disease:
    - pancreatitis
    - pancreatic cancer
    - pancreatectomy
    - cystic fibrosis
  - antagonists to insulin:
    - acromegaly (GH)
    - Cushing's syndrome (glucocorticoids)
    - hyperthyroidism (thyroid hormone)
    - phaeochromocytoma (catecholamines)
    - glucagonoma (glucagon)
  - drugs, e.g. corticosteroids, thiazide diuretics
  - liver disease
  - genetic syndromes, e.g. Down's syndrome, Friedreich's ataxia
  - insulin receptor abnormalities, e.g. congenital lipodystrophy
- Diabetes mellitus has a number of complications, these can be divided into:

  Acute

- Hypoglycaemia: very common complication of insulin therapy in patients with diabetes; symptoms usually develop when blood glucose falls <3 mmol/L. Symptoms include sweating, tremor and palpitations (adrenergic symptoms); in patients with long-standing disease these warning signs may not be present.
- Diabetic ketoacidosis (DKA): occurs when the body produces ketones in an uncontrolled manner. Glucose is not taken up into cells and is lost in the urine, producing an osmotic diuresis. The abnormal glucose handling

is associated with increased lipolysis, which leads to increased circulating levels of fatty acids; these are converted to acetyl-CoA and then to ketones. The ketones lead to a severe metabolic acidosis and dehydration due to nausea and vomiting.

- Hyperglycaemic hyperosmolar non-ketotic coma (HONK): occurs in the absence of ketosis; it is typically seen in patients with NIDDM. The patients present with severe dehydration and a decreased level of consciousness with a very high plasma glucose level.
- Lactic acidosis: occurs in patients on biguanide therapy; it rarely occurs nowadays as long as the dosage is not exceeded and is not used in patients where it can accumulate, i.e. renal or hepatic failure.

Chronic

- Macrovascular
  - Diabetes mellitus is a risk factor in the development of atherosclerosis. This tends to be widespread and more severe as it tends to affect vessels distally (thus making bypass surgery technically harder).
  - Disorders caused by atherosclerosis are all increased in diabetics, i.e. ischaemic heart disease (IHD), stroke, myocardial infarction (MI) and peripheral vascular disease.
- Microvascular
  - Small blood vessels are predominantly affected; this has its greatest effect at three sites:
    - eye: diabetic retinopathy
    - kidney: diabetic nephropathy
    - nerves: diabetic neuropathy.

Pancreatic Endocrine Tumours

Tumours can arise in the endocrine cells of the pancreas. When these are 'functioning' and secrete excess hormone they can lead to clinical syndromes; examples include:

- Insulinoma: 75% of endocrine tumours; they are derived from β-cells; the classic presentation is with 'Whipple's triad' – hypoglycaemic symptoms during fasting, a reduced blood sugar during these periods, and relief with intravenous glucose; 10% are malignant.
- Gastrinoma (Zollinger–Ellison syndrome): arise from pancreatic G-cells; malignant in >50% of cases; the excess gastrin leads to gastric hypersecretion, diarrhoea and widespread peptic ulceration.
- VIPomas: associated with excess secretion of VIP (vasoactive intestinal peptide); they lead to severe watery diarrhoea, ↓ K^+, and achlorhydria (absence of HCl in the stomach).
- Glucagonoma: a rare cause of secondary diabetes mellitus; other symptoms include anaemia, weight loss and a characteristic rash called necrolytic migratory erythema; the tumour arises from the α-cells; 75% are malignant.
- Somatostatinoma: a very rare tumour derived from the δ-cells of the pancreas; they cause diabetes mellitus, cholelithiasis and steatorrhoea.

Hormonal Response to Trauma/Surgery

- The body responds to a variety of noxious stimuli such as pain, infection, trauma and surgery.
- This response aims to limit the injuring process and allow the body to heal; this involves a variety of hormonal changes that alter the metabolism of carbohydrates, proteins and fats, and also involves stimulating the immune and clotting systems.
- There are four systems involved in the body's response to injury:
  1. Sympathetic nervous system: this response is the initial phase of a response to injury and occurs at the time of injury. It prepares the body for action, i.e. 'fight or flight'; the release of epinephrine and norepinephrine has a number of effects:
     - blood is redistributed to non-essential organs, thus supplying more to the heart, skeletal muscle and brain
     - ↑ glucose: provides energy
     - ↑ lipolysis: provides energy
     - ↑ ketone production: provides energy
     - inhibition of non-essential visceral functions, e.g. bowel peristalsis.
  2. Acute phase system: the acute phase response refers to the cytokine and inflammatory mediator production that occurs following tissue injury; this has local and systemic effects:
     - local effects: this involves the rapid influx of inflammatory cells such as neutrophils and macrophages (see below) into the wound; these release a variety of cytokines such as IL-1, 2, 6, TNF-α, and interferons and inflammatory mediators such as the prostaglandins, histamine, serotonin, etc. These mediators aim to limit tissue injury by producing vasodilatation, increased vascular permeability, attraction and migration of neutrophils, fibroblasts and endothelial cells, and stimulation of the clotting system and complement cascade
     - systemic effects: the cytokine cascade associated with local injury is usually limited to the area of injury; however, if the insult is severe, it may lead to cytokines spilling into the circulation; this produces systemic effects such as:
       - tachypnoea
       - fever
       - tachycardia
       - increased vascular permeability (↓ blood pressure)

- vasodilatation (↓ blood pressure)
- immune cell activation
- increased leukocyte adhesion
- effects on glucose metabolism (see below).

3. Endocrine response: a variety of hormones are involved in the response to tissue injury; these are shown in Box 12.2.
4. Vascular endothelium: the endothelium should be considered as an organ in its own right. The response to trauma has both local and systemic effects:
   - increased adhesion molecule expression: this action attracts cells such as neutrophils to destroy bacteria and digest foreign bodies; however, enzymes released and production of free radicals can lead to additional tissue damage
   - nitric oxide (NO): produces vasodilatation; this may lead to hypotension. NO also increases the number of antigen-presenting cells
   - endothelins: these oppose the action of NO and produce vasoconstriction
   - platelet-activating factor (PAF): released in response to cytokines such as IL-1 and TNF-α. The main effect is to stimulate platelet aggregation and produce vasoconstriction
   - prostaglandins: reduce platelet aggregation and cause vasodilatation.

- The changes associated with trauma and surgery lead to wide-ranging local and systemic changes and production of numerous cytokines and humoral mediators; together they produce a number of clinical changes:
- hypovolaemia: this type of fluid loss is referred to as 'third space' loss; the vasodilatation and increased vascular permeability lead to fluid being sequestered in the interstitial space
- renal changes: following injury there is reduced excretion of free water and sodium; this continues for about 24 h and is due to the release of aldosterone and ADH
- fever: injury (even in the absence of infection) is associated with a rise in temperature; this is due to changes in the thermoregulatory set point in the hypothalamus by IL-1
- haematological changes: there is a leukocytosis; albumin levels fall due to decreased production and loss into injured tissue. The coagulation system is activated. This is primarily to reduce bleeding after the injury; however, it leads to a state of hypercoagulability and an increased risk of deep vein thrombosis (DVT)
- electrolyte and acid–base changes: the electrolyte changes include ↓Na^+ (due to dilution from retained water), ↑K^+ (as a result of cell death and tissue injury), metabolic alkalosis (the absorption of Na^+ stimulated by aldosterone leads to K^+ and H^+ excretion) and metabolic acidosis (this occurs with more severe injuries with hypotension, poor perfusion and consequent anaerobic metabolism).

BOX 12.2 Summary of the Action of Various Hormones in the Body's Response to Trauma

Hormone	Action
ACTH	Stimulates glucocorticoid release and potentiates the actions of catecholamines on the heart
Glucocorticoids	Protein → glucose, glucose → glycogen. Inhibits insulin and stimulates gluconeogenesis, decreases vascular permeability, potentiates catecholamine-induced vasoconstriction, anti-inflammatory (suppresses prostaglandin synthesis), immunosuppressant (inhibits secretion of IL-2)
Aldosterone	Stimulates reabsorption of Na^+ (water follows by osmosis; this leads to a reduced urine volume) and secretion of K^+
ADH	Increased water absorption from the collecting ducts, vasoconstriction (particularly splanchnic), and stimulates glycogenolysis and gluconeogenesis
Insulin	Low in the ebb phase (due to ↓ β-cell sensitivity to glucose levels; glucagon inhibits its secretion and cortisol reduces its peripheral action), levels increase in the flow phase but hyperglycaemia remains due to continued resistance
Glucagon	Stimulates glycogenolysis, gluconeogenesis, ketogenesis, and lipolysis
Thyroxine	See Sick euthyroid syndrome section
Serotonin	Causes vasoconstriction, bronchoconstriction, ↑ heart rate and contractility, and stimulates platelet aggregation
Histamine	Causes vasodilatation and ↑ vascular permeability
Growth hormone	Stimulates protein synthesis, lipolysis and glycogenolysis

- Metabolic changes: the altered metabolism seen after trauma or surgery can be divided into two phases: the ebb phase and the flow phase:
- the ebb phase is the initial response to injury and is a phase of reduced energy expenditure and metabolic rate that lasts for approximately 24 h
- the flow phase follows: this is a catabolic phase with increased metabolic rate, hyperglycaemia, negative nitrogen balance and increased O_2 consumption. The flow phase has significant effects on the metabolism of carbohydrates, lipids and proteins:
  - carbohydrates: hyperglycaemia is seen post-injury due to mobilization of liver glycogen; this is stimulated by catecholamines and glucocorticoids (insulin resistance prevents cell uptake). After 24 h the glycogen is exhausted and the hyperglycaemia is maintained by gluconeogenesis
  - lipids: lipolysis is stimulated by catecholamines, the sympathetic nervous system, cortisol and growth hormone. They provide the primary source of energy for all tissues (leaving the brain and blood cells to utilize glucose)
  - proteins: the demand for amino acids is met by skeletal muscle breakdown; the greater the insult, the greater the breakdown and nitrogen loss. The amino acids are used in gluconeogenesis and synthesis of acute phase proteins.
- Respiratory changes: there is increased respiratory drive that leads to a respiratory alkalosis (due to ↓ $PaCO_2$); in addition, the systemic effects of the cytokine release and immune cell activation can lead to ARDS and severe hypoxia. The metabolic alkalosis created by H^+ excretion affects the oxygen dissociation curve, making it harder for O_2 to dissociate into tissues – thus exacerbating hypoxia.
- Cardiac changes: the cardiac output increases dramatically following injury.
- Immune system changes: there are a variety of defects in the immune system that occur following trauma:
  - cell-mediated immunity
  - antigen presentation
  - neutrophil function
  - opsonization of bacteria.

OSCE SCENARIOS

OSCE Scenario 12.1

A 32-year-old female is admitted with suspected acute appendicitis. She is sweating, agitated, confused and complaining of palpitations. Her symptoms do not fit with a straightforward diagnosis of acute appendicitis. Examination reveals a temperature of 40°C and a tachycardia of 140 with an irregular pulse. You check her thyroid function, which reveals an elevated T_3 and T_4 with suppressed TSH.

1. What is the most likely diagnosis?
2. What may precipitate the condition?
3. How is the condition managed?

OSCE Scenario 12.2

A 40-year-old male presents to his GP with intermittent headaches, palpitations, sweating, anxiety and intermittent chest pains. Examination reveals a blood pressure of 180/110 mmHg.

1. What endocrine condition do you need to consider? Explain the condition.
2. How could you confirm the diagnosis?
3. What measures would you take to prepare the patient for surgery?

OSCE Scenario 12.3

A 64-year-old female is admitted for major gastrointestinal surgery. She is taking 5 mg Prednisolone and has been doing so for six months.

1. What are the risks of failing to replace steroids pre-operatively?
2. How would you manage her steroid administration prior to major surgery?
3. How long after stopping steroids would a patient not require pre-operative replacement?

OSCE Scenario 12.4

A 46-year-old female has undergone a total thyroidectomy – you are called to the ward as the patient is suffering from severe cramps and numb peripheries.

1. What are Chovstek's and Trousseau's signs?
2. What is causing the above symptoms and why? What would you expect to see on an ECG and how would you treat it?
3. Why has the hypocalcaemia happened and what will be the long-term treatment?

OSCE Scenario 12.5

A 45-year-old male attends a GP surgery with some strange symptoms – he describes episodes of sweating, palpitations, being confused and forgetting things, and also abdominal pain and diarrhoea. A friend thought it might be diabetes and measures his blood sugar during an episode and found it to be 3 mmol/L.

1. What is the diagnosis and what is the classic triad associated with this condition?
2. What cells does the disorder arise from?
3. What percentages are benign or malignant?
4. What syndrome are they associated with?

Answers in Appendix pages 457–458

Please check your eBook at https://studentconsult.inkling.com/ for more self-assessment questions. See inside cover for registration details.

13

Nervous and Locomotor Systems

INTRODUCTION

Components

- The nervous system is composed of two components:
  - central
  - peripheral: sensory and motor.
- The nervous system can also be divided into somatic and autonomic:
  - somatic: supplies the skin and muscles
  - autonomic: supplies glands, sphincters and smooth muscles within blood vessels, etc.
- The central nervous system (CNS) is composed of the brain and spinal cord; it is composed of numerous specialized cells called neurons.
- The neurons are supported by neuroglia (or glial cells); these are cells that have a variety of ancillary functions including:
  - astrocytes: form the 'blood–brain barrier'
  - microglia: perform a phagocytic role in the CNS
  - oligodendroglia: produce myelin.
- The CNS is organized into two distinct areas:
  - grey matter: contains the neuronal cell bodies
  - white matter: contains the axon of the neurons.
- The peripheral nervous system consists of the cranial and spinal nerves and the autonomic nervous system and their associated ganglia. They link the CNS with sensory receptors (e.g. pain receptors) and effectors (i.e. muscles).

Functions

- The functions of the nervous system include:
  - the interpretation of sensory input such as touch, temperature, proprioception and pain
  - interpretation of electrical impulses from the special senses leading to our ability to taste, smell, hear and see
  - the initiation and co-ordination of movement and muscle contraction
  - higher functions such as thought, memory and the ability to learn.

CENTRAL NERVOUS SYSTEM

Cerebral Blood Flow (Fig. 13.1)

- Blood flow to the brain is via the internal carotid and the vertebral arteries; they anastomose to form a circle of arteries that supply the brain: the circle of Willis.
- The control of cerebral blood flow is maintained within very close limits. The brain is particularly sensitive to ischaemia, with loss of consciousness occurring within 5 s of the interruption of cerebral circulation, and irreversible damage within 2–3 min.
- The brain receives approximately 10–15% of the cardiac output.
- Cerebral blood flow is controlled by three mechanisms:
  - autoregulation: myogenic or metabolic
  - neural
  - local.

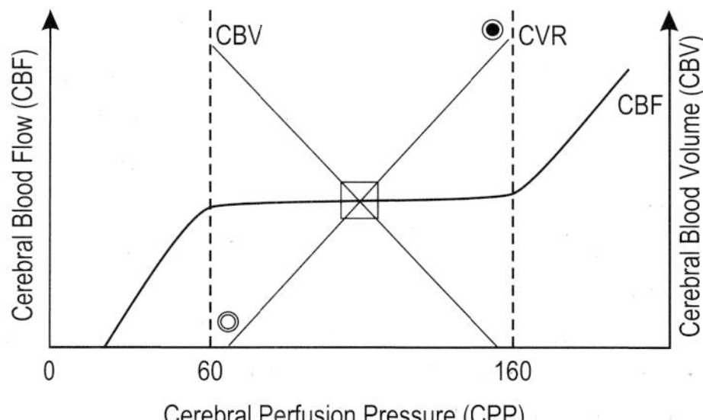

Fig. 13.1 Graph illustrating control of cerebral blood flow (CBF). The range of autoregulation is at a CPP of 60–160 mmHg. Flow is maintained by changes in the cerebrovascular resistance (CVR) with increasing vasoconstriction at high CPP and vasodilatation at low CPP. The effect of CVR can also be seen to affect cerebral blood volume (CBV): vasodilatation increasing CBV and vasoconstriction decreasing it. (From McGeown JG. Physiology, 2nd edn. Churchill Livingstone, Edinburgh, 2002, with permission.)

Autoregulation

Myogenic

- The brain will maintain a remarkably similar cerebral blood flow over a wide range of blood pressures: this is known as autoregulation.
- Myogenic autoregulation occurs when the cerebral blood vessels constrict or dilate to maintain adequate cerebral perfusion.
- When the blood pressure rises, the vessels constrict, thus decreasing flow; when the blood pressure falls, the cerebral vessels dilate in order to increase flow.
- Autoregulation has a limit to which it can compensate. At a cerebral perfusion pressure (CPP; see below) of around 50 mmHg, the dilatation of cerebral vessels will fail to maintain flow, and at a CPP of 150–160 mmHg, the cerebral vessels will begin to fail to regulate flow – indeed, at this point, they become abnormally permeable, causing cerebral oedema.
- These same mechanisms are responsible for maintaining cerebral flow in patients with head injuries.
- In patients with severe head injuries the amount of perfusion the brain is receiving is dependent upon the intracranial pressure resisting flow within the cranial cavity:

$$\text{Cerebral perfusion pressure (CPP)} \\ = \text{mean arterial pressure (MAP)} \\ - \text{intracranial pressure (ICP)}$$

- When CPP falls below 50 mmHg then cerebral ischaemia results; when it falls below 30 mmHg then death occurs.
- These changes occurring during cerebral autoregulation can be seen in Fig. 13.1:
  - autoregulation occurs over the range 50–150 mmHg
  - to maintain flow over this range you can see from the graph that CVR (cerebral vascular resistance) falls as CPP falls; this reflects the vasodilatation of cerebral vessels
  - as the CPP rises then CVR increases; this reflects the vasoconstriction of cerebral vessels
  - as the CVR varies so does the CBV (cerebral blood volume); as vessels vasodilate the CBV rises, and as CVR increases the CBV decreases.
- Myogenic autoregulation can be impaired by a number of factors, such as:
  - hypoxia
  - ischaemia
  - trauma
  - cerebral haemorrhage
  - tumour
  - infection.

Metabolic

- The activity of certain areas of the brain will differ depending on the task being performed; as a consequence, these areas will require additional blood flow.
- The increased activity results in a decrease in PaO_2 and increase in $PaCO_2$ and H^+, the changes resulting in local vasodilatation of cerebral blood vessels and thus increased perfusion.

Neural Control of Cerebral Blood Flow

- The cerebral circulation does receive some sympathetic vasoconstrictor and parasympathetic vasodilator innervation, but their effect is very weak and their precise role, if any, is unclear.

Local Control of Cerebral Blood Flow

- Cerebral blood flow is sensitive to changes in the arterial PaO_2 and $PaCO_2$.
- Increases in $PaCO_2$ are associated with an increase in CBF due to marked cerebral vasodilatation; however, just as hypercapnia results in vasodilatation, then a fall in $PaCO_2$ (hypocapnia) results in cerebral vasoconstriction.
- The effect that CO_2 has on cerebral blood flow is particularly important in head injury patients; maintaining a low–normal CO_2 prevents increases in ICP due to cerebral vasodilatation. Equally it must be remembered that overzealous ventilation to low CO_2 levels can be equally detrimental due to vasoconstriction and consequent cerebral ischaemia.
- The effect of changes in PaO_2 is not as marked; hypoxia has a significant effect only when it falls below 8 kPa. Below this level then CBF may increase dramatically.
- Increases in PaO_2 can cause mild cerebral vasoconstriction; indeed hyperbaric oxygen therapy can reduce CBF by 20–30%.
- These normal responses to PaO_2 and $PaCO_2$ can be affected by a number of factors, such as:
  - head injury
  - cerebral haemorrhage
  - shock
  - hypoxia.

Cerebrospinal Fluid

- Cerebrospinal fluid (CSF) lies in the subarachnoid space; the total volume is 130–150 mL (40 mL in the cerebral ventricles and 100 mL around the spinal cord).
- The rate of production of CSF is approximately 500 mL/day.
- The normal CSF pressure is approximately 0.5–1 kPa; obstruction to the flow of CSF leads to an increase in this pressure, i.e. hydrocephalus.
- CSF is produced by the choroid plexus in the lateral, third and fourth ventricles.

- CSF flows from the lateral ventricles to the third ventricle via the interventricular foramina; it then flows to the fourth ventricle via the cerebral aqueduct. From the fourth ventricle CSF flows into the subarachnoid space via the foramen of Luschka (lateral) and the foramen of Magendie (midline).
- The CSF circulates around the subarachnoid space and is reabsorbed back into the circulation via the arachnoid villi; these drain into the venous sinuses.
- The arachnoid villi may become blocked by blood following a subarachnoid haemorrhage and prevent reabsorption of CSF; this results in hydrocephalus.
- A small amount of CSF is also absorbed by spinal villi in the lumbar region.
- CSF has two main functions:
  - hydraulic 'cushion': serves to protect the brain from violent movements of the head
  - provides a stable ionic environment for cerebral function.

Blood–Brain Barrier (Fig. 13.2)

- Lipid-soluble molecules are able to pass freely from the blood into the interstitial space of the brain; however, ions are unable to pass freely into the brain. This enables

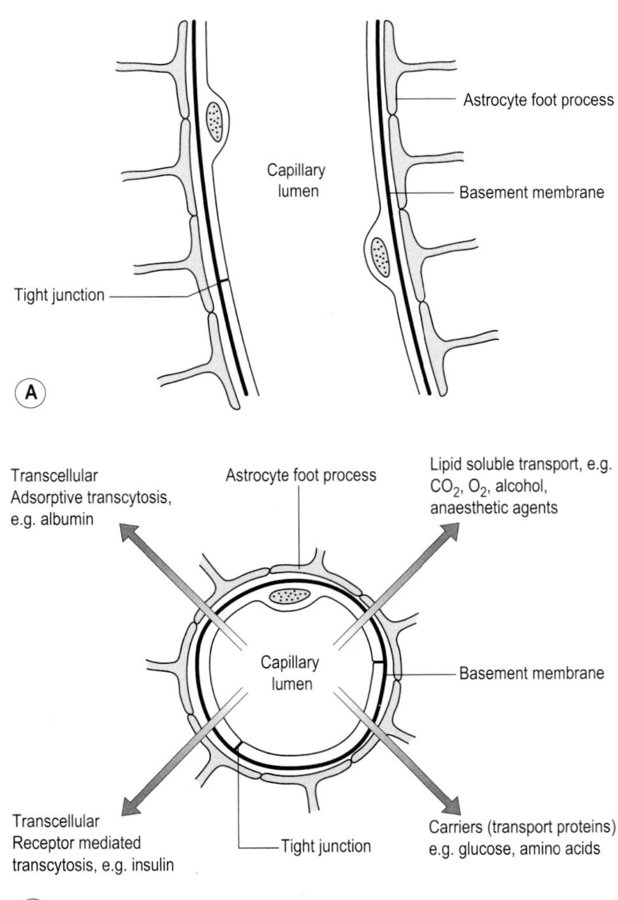

Fig. 13.2 The blood–brain barrier. (A) Longitudinal section through a capillary in the brain. The capillaries have tight cell-to-cell junctions and the astrocytes project foot processes to cover the capillary basement membrane. (B) Transverse section through a capillary in the brain, showing methods of transport across the blood–brain barrier.

the brain to maintain the ionic environment within very tight limits, thus allowing the optimal environment for neuronal communication.

- The blood–brain barrier also prevents the release of neurotransmitters from neurons into the peripheral circulation.
- The blood–brain barrier is formed by the structure of the capillaries. Rather than the freely permeable fenestrated capillaries found in other tissues, the cerebral capillaries have very tight cell-to-cell junctions in the endothelium. In addition, the end-feet of astrocytes cover the basement membrane.
- Specific functions provided by the blood–brain barrier are:
  - tight junctions restrict penetration of water-soluble substances
  - lipid-soluble molecules such as CO_2, O_2, hormones, anaesthetics and alcohol (that's why we get drunk!) can pass freely across the barrier via the lipid membranes of the capillary endothelium
  - the endothelium contains transport proteins (carriers) for nutrients such as sugars and amino acids
  - certain proteins, e.g. insulin and albumin, may be transported by endocytosis and transcytosis
  - an 'efflux pump' extrudes unwanted lipid soluble molecules back into the blood.
- The blood–brain barrier is not continuous and in some areas consists of fenestrated capillaries. These areas lie in the midline and include:
  - third and fourth ventricles: allow drugs and noxious chemicals to trigger the chemoreceptor area in the floor of the fourth ventricle; this in turn triggers the vomiting centre. In addition angiotensin II passes to the vasomotor centre in this region to increase sympathetic outflow and causes vasoconstriction of peripheral vessels
  - posterior lobe of pituitary: allows the release of oxytocin and antidiuretic hormone (ADH) into the circulation
  - hypothalamus: this allows the release of releasing or inhibitory hormones into the portal–hypophyseal tract.

BRAINSTEM DEATH

- The brainstem provides the capacity for consciousness.
- The cerebral hemispheres provide the content of consciousness.
- Brainstem death is a condition in which the heart and lungs function, but there is no cerebral activity.
- It is legally regarded as being equivalent to the more traditional mode of death, i.e. cessation of respiratory and cardiac activity.
- The diagnosis of brainstem death is important for several reasons:
  - withdrawal of treatment
  - assessment for suitability for organ donation.
- The diagnosis of brainstem death must first satisfy several preconditions and exclusions before the appropriate tests can be performed.

Preconditions for the Diagnosis of Brainstem Death

- There are four preconditions:
  - the patient must be in a coma
  - there must be a known cause for the patient's coma
  - this cause must be known to be irreversible
  - the patient must be dependent on a ventilator.

Exclusion Criteria for the Diagnosis of Brainstem Death

- There are a number of exclusion criteria:
  - no residual drug effects from narcotics, hypnotics, tranquillizers, muscle relaxants, alcohol and illicit drugs
  - core body temperature must be >35°C
  - no circulatory, metabolic or endocrine abnormality disturbance that may contribute to the coma.

Brainstem Death Tests

- The UK brainstem death criteria tests seven areas. All must be absent for the diagnosis to be made.
- The tests include:
  1. No pupillary response to light, direct or consensual: this reflex involves cranial nerves II and III.
  2. Absent corneal reflex – normally would result in blinking; this reflex involves cranial nerves V and VII.
  3. No motor response in the cranial nerve distribution to stimuli in any somatic area, e.g. supraorbital or nailbed pressure leading to a grimace.
  4. No gag reflex: back of the throat is stimulated with a catheter; this reflex tests cranial nerves IX and X.
  5. No cough reflex: no response to bronchial stimulation with a suction catheter; this reflex tests cranial nerves IX and X.
  6. No vestibulo-ocular reflex: head is flexed to 30° and 50 mL of ice-cold water is injected over 1 min into each external auditory meatus; there should be no eye movements; this reflex tests cranial nerves III, VI and VIII.
  7. Apnoea test: the patient is preoxygenated with 100% O_2 for 10 min; $PaCO_2$ is allowed to rise to 5 kPa (before testing); the patient is disconnected from the ventilator and O_2 is insufflated at 6 L/min; $PaCO_2$ is allowed to rise to 6.5 kPa; there should be **NO** respiratory effort.

- There are several other caveats to the brainstem death tests:
    - performed on two occasions
    - performed by two doctors
    - one must be a consultant
    - must be competent in the field, e.g. ITU or neurology
    - must have >5 years' experience
    - must not be part of the transplant team.
- The time of death is legally defined as the time at which the first set of brainstem tests were performed.

SPACE-OCCUPYING LESIONS AND RAISED INTRACRANIAL PRESSURE

- Space-occupying lesions (SOLs) result from a variety of causes, and may be focal or diffuse.
- Focal SOLs include:
    - tumour
    - aneurysm
    - blood or haematoma
    - granuloma
    - tuberculoma
    - cyst
    - abscess.
- Diffuse SOLs result from either vasodilatation or oedema.
- The consequences of intracranial SOLs include:
    - raised intracranial pressure
    - intracranial shift and herniation
    - hydrocephalus.

Raised Intracranial Pressure (ICP) (Fig. 13.3)

- The skull is a rigid container in which brain, CSF and blood are the only contents; it therefore follows that $ICP = V_{CSF} + V_{Brain} + V_{Blood}$.
- This formula is the basis for the Monro–Kellie hypothesis, which states that the ICP will increase if the volume of one component is increased; the increase in ICP can only be compensated for by a decrease in one or both of the other components.
- Normal ICP in the supine position is 0–10 mmHg.
- The removal of blood and CSF can accommodate a SOL of approximately 100–150 mL; after this compensatory point the ICP will increase rapidly.
- Raised ICP has a number of consequences:
    - hydrocephalus: an increase in ICP may result in the interruption of CSF flow; this is most commonly seen with posterior fossa lesions leading to compression of the cerebral aqueduct and fourth ventricle
    - cerebral ischaemia: remember that CPP=MAP − ICP. Any rise in ICP will eventually exceed autoregulation and lead to cerebral ischaemia

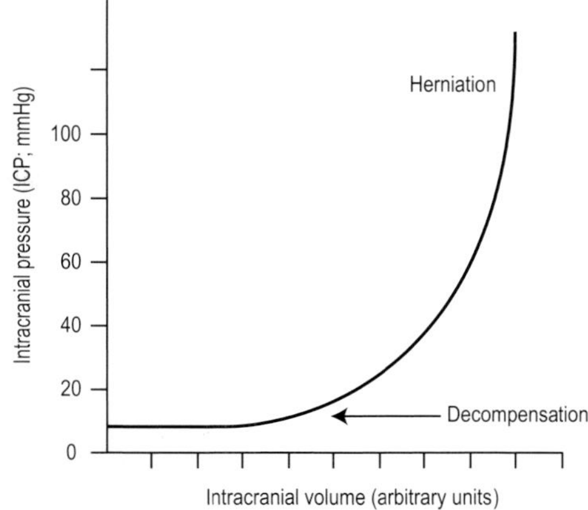

Fig. 13.3 Pressure–volume curve for intracranial pressure (ICP). The compensatory properties of the intracranial contents follow a pressure–volume exponential curve. Increased volume of any of the three components (i.e. brain, CSF, blood) can be accommodated up to a certain point without any change in intracranial pressure. Once a critical volume is reached, decompensation occurs, i.e. blood and CSF have been pushed from the cranial cavity and ICP increases exponentially to the point of herniation.

    - brain shift and herniation: as ICP increases the risk of herniation increases; this occurs at specific sites (Fig. 13.4):
        - transtentorial: the lesion lies within one hemisphere; leads to herniation of the medial part of the temporal lobe over the tentorium cerebelli
        - tonsillar: caused by a lesion in the posterior fossa; the lowest part of the cerebellum pushes down into the foramen magnum and compresses the medulla
        - subfalcial: caused by a lesion in one hemisphere; leads to the herniation of the cingulate gyrus under the falx cerebri
        - diencephalic: generalized brain swelling; leads to the midbrain herniating through the tentorium; this is termed coning
    - systemic effects: the systemic effects of raised ICP are thought to occur due to autonomic imbalance, hypothalamic overactivity (due to compression) and ischaemia of the vasomotor area; the effects include:
        - Cushing's response: ↓ respiratory rate, bradycardia and hypertension
        - neurogenic pulmonary oedema
        - Cushing's ulcers
        - preterminal events include bilateral pupil constriction followed by dilation, tachycardia, ↓ respiratory rate, and hypotension.

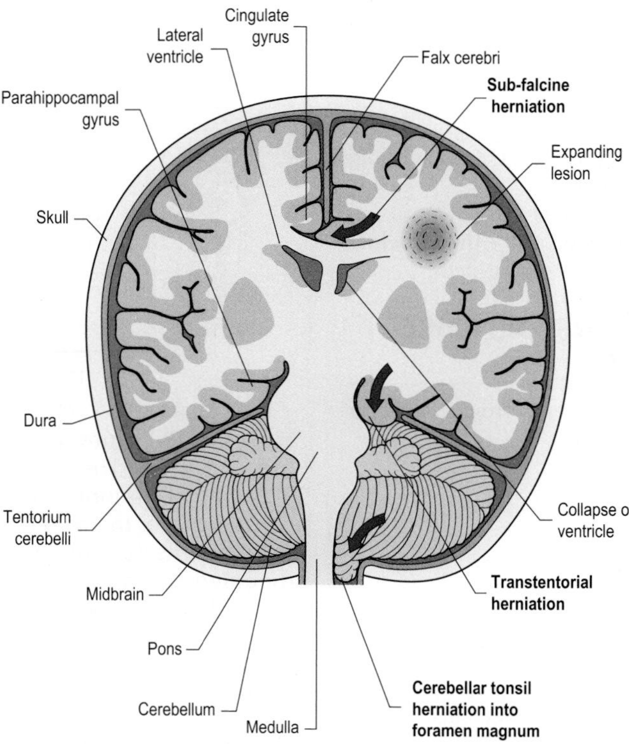

Fig. 13.4 Diagram illustrating the possible consequences of an expanding lesion, i.e. haematoma, on one side of the brain. Diencephalic herniation is caused by generalized brain swelling.

- The clinical manifestations of raised ICP include:
  - headache
  - nausea and vomiting
  - papilloedema
  - decreased conscious level.
- The clinical manifestations of cerebral herniation include:
  - oculomotor nerve compression: ipsilateral pupil dilation (transtentorial)
  - cerebral peduncles: contralateral hemiparesis (transtentorial)
  - posterior cerebral artery: cortical blindness (transtentorial)
  - cerebral aqueduct: hydrocephalus (transtentorial)
  - compression of cardio/respiratory centres in the medulla: death (tonsillar)
  - reticular activating system: coma (all types)
  - anterior cerebral artery: infarction (subfalcial)
  - distortion of the midbrain and tearing of vessels: death (all types).

Post-Operative Confusion

- One of the commonest complications occurring in elderly patients.
- The symptoms can include:
  - clouding of consciousness
  - restlessness
  - abnormalities of perception
  - incoherent speech
  - agitation
  - violence
  - pulling out lines, catheters, drains, etc.
- There are numerous factors that predispose to or cause post-operative confusion; these include:
  - dehydration
  - electrolyte abnormalities
  - hypoxia
  - infection
  - drugs
  - uraemia
  - hypoglycaemia
  - pre-existing psychiatric disorder or dementia
  - alcohol and drug withdrawal (particularly in young patients)
  - urinary retention
  - pain and anxiety
  - cerebrovascular accident (CVA)

- head injury (especially in trauma patients)
- sleep deprivation
- ITU syndrome: pain, fear and sleep deprivation can lead to visual and auditory hallucinations and inability to differentiate reality from fantasy.

- Post-operative confusion is an important complication with many serious underlying causes; a full management plan must be formulated and the cause sought. Appropriate management should include:
  - history and examination
  - FBC, U&E, LFT, glucose, ABG
  - ECG
  - sepsis screen: blood cultures, chest X-ray, sputum, midstream urine, wound swab.
- If a specific cause is found then this must be corrected, e.g. hypoxia, urinary retention; however, non-specific treatment may include:
  - eliminate drugs likely to cause or increase the confusional state
  - presence of nursing staff in a well-lit environment
  - low-dose sedation, e.g. haloperidol
  - physical restraint – only if patient at risk of harming self or others.

PERIPHERAL NERVOUS SYSTEM (PNS)

Conduction and Transmission

Action Potentials (Fig. 13.5)

- Action potentials are the method by which nerves send information; they are electrical signals and are described as 'all-or-nothing'.
- Axons have a resting membrane potential with respect to the extracellular environment; this is approximately −70 mV.
- As stimuli attempt to activate an action potential the membrane potential is decreased towards a 'threshold'; stimuli below this threshold will not result in an action potential and are described as subthreshold. If the stimulus is large enough to decrease the membrane potential above the threshold then this will result in an action potential.
- The action potential, once initiated, begins with a rapid depolarization and a reversal of the membrane potential to around 50 mV; this occurs in a few tenths of a millisecond.
- Following depolarization is repolarization: this is where the cell returns to the normal resting membrane potential; the repolarization may initially be more negative than the resting potential – hyperpolarization.
- During the action potential the cell has an 'absolute' refractory period in which no further action potential can be generated. During repolarization then a 'relative' refractory period exists; an action potential can be stimulated but will need a stimulus of greater magnitude than the initial stimulus.
- Action potentials self-propagate: once the cell is stimulated, the signal will propagate along all cells.
- The intra- and extracellular concentrations of Na^+ and K^+ differ:
  - Na^+ concentration is greater extracellularly and thus tends to diffuse into the cell, both along this concentration gradient and due to the negative membrane potential
  - K^+ has a greater concentration intracellularly and thus tends to diffuse out of the cell.
- The change in permeability of the cell to Na^+ and K^+ during an action potential is due to conformational changes in voltage-controlled ion channels by the initial stimulus depolarizing the cell membrane.

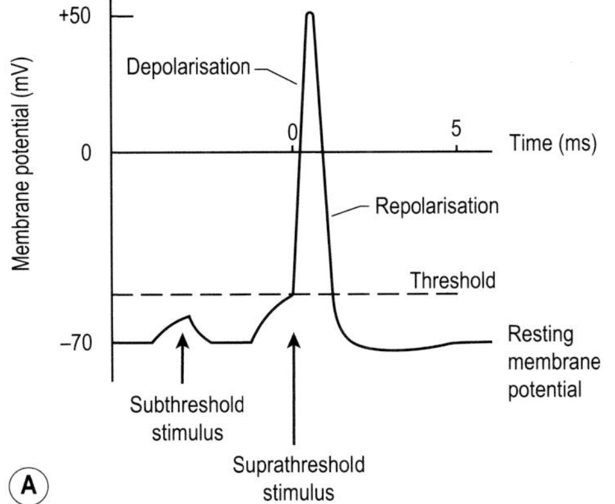

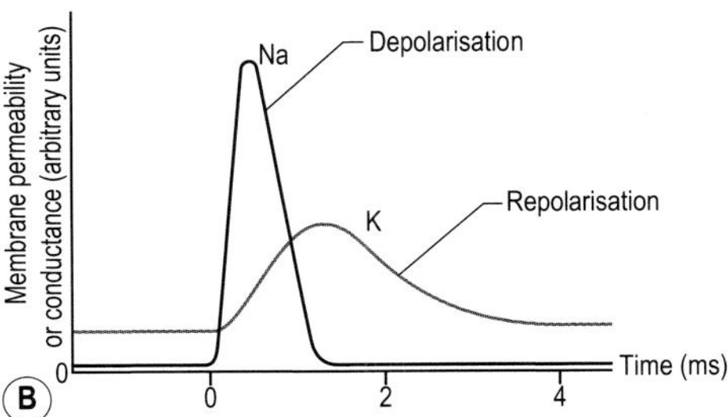

Fig. 13.5 (A) Graph illustrating the theory of the 'all-or-nothing' response to electrical stimuli. (B) The ion flows responsible for depolarization and repolarization of a nerve. (From McGeown JG. Physiology, 2nd edn. Churchill Livingstone, Edinburgh, 2002, with permission.)

- The initial depolarization is due to the rapid influx of Na^+ as the Na^+ channel opens; at the same time the K^+ channel also opens and K^+ is released into the extracellular environment.
- The Na^+ channel activates much faster than the K^+ channel. This explains the rapid influx of Na^+; the channel also closes much faster; the K^+ channel remains open over a longer period than the Na^+ channel and is responsible for repolarization as K^+ is released and the membrane potential falls back to its negative value.

Propagation of Action Potentials

- The action potential results in the inside of the cell being positive in respect to the extracellular environment; this is the opposite of the normal negative resting membrane potential; as a result, the action potential travels from positive to negative.
- The action potential is unidirectional and sets up local currents that result in the propagation of the action potential across the whole membrane; the action potential is unidirectional due to the refractory nature of the membrane, preventing further depolarization.
- The conduction velocity of action potentials is determined by two factors:
  - axon diameter: the greater the diameter the higher the conduction velocity; this effect is due to the increase in myelin causing a decrease in electrical resistance
  - myelination: myelinated cells have a much faster conduction velocity in comparison with unmyelinated cells (50–100 m/s vs 1 m/s); this effect is due to the gaps between the myelin sheath that surrounds nerves. These gaps are called the nodes of Ranvier. Action potentials are generated only at these points as the myelin acts to insulate the intervening sections; thus, the action potential jumps between the gaps. This is referred to as saltatory conduction (Fig. 13.6).

A classification of nerve fibres is shown in Table 13.1.

Synaptic Transmission

- When an action potential reaches the end of an axon it must be transmitted to the next adjacent nerve; the gap between neurons is known as the synapse.
- Transmission of the signal relies on the release of neurotransmitters; these then affect the adjacent nerve chemically to initiate another action potential.
- The action potential travels along the presynaptic nerve. The axon terminates in an expanded end; this is called the terminal bouton.
- Inside the bouton are numerous membrane-bound vesicles containing neurotransmitters.

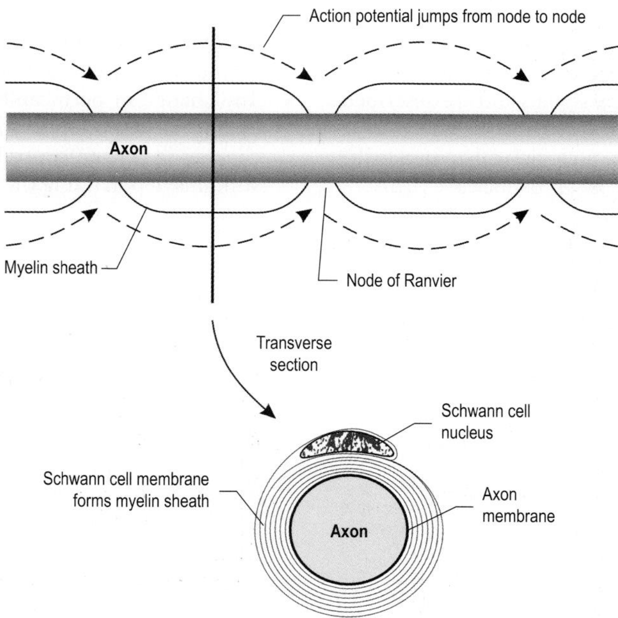

Fig. 13.6 Action potential conduction in a myelinated nerve fibre (saltatory conduction). (From McGeown JG. Physiology, 2nd edn. Churchill Livingstone, Edinburgh, 2002, with permission.)

TABLE 13.1 Different Types of Nerve Fibre, Showing Functions, Conduction Velocities and Diameters

Type	Function	Conduction Velocity (m/s)	Diameter (μm)
Aα	Motor proprioception	100	15–20
Aβ	Touch and pressure	50	5–10
Aγ	Muscle spindles	30	3–6
Aδ	Pain, temperature and touch	20	2–5
B	Autonomic	10	3
C	Pain	1	0.5–1

- The transmission of the action potential occurs by:
  - the action potential depolarizes the presynaptic membrane by opening voltage-gated Ca^{2+} channels
  - Ca^{2+} enters the axon down an electrochemical and concentration gradient
  - the increase in Ca^{2+} results in the vesicles fusing with the presynaptic membrane and releasing neurotransmitters into the synaptic cleft
  - the neurotransmitters then bind with receptors on the post-synaptic membrane
  - binding of neurotransmitters initiates secondary signals within the cell and opens ion channels, thus generating a depolarizing current
  - the transmitter is released from the receptor and is broken down by specific breakdown pathways.

Neurotransmitters

- Neurotransmitters are chemicals that are responsible for the transmission of action potentials across the synapse.
- The main neurotransmitters include:
  - acetylcholine (ACh): this is an excitatory transmitter; it is present in the brain, spinal cord, autonomic nerves and the PNS. It is broken down to acetate and choline by the enzyme acetylcholinesterase
  - amines: this group includes catecholamines (adrenaline, noradrenaline, and dopamine), 5-hydroxytryptamine (serotonin) and histamine. The catecholamines are formed from the amino acid tyrosine. Two enzymes degrade catecholamines: monoamine oxidase breaks down transmitter taken up by the presynaptic neuron; and catechol-*O*-methyl transferase breaks down catecholamines taken up by the postsynaptic neuron
  - amino acids: several amino acids act as neurotransmitters; these include:
    - glycine: inhibitory
    - glutamate: excitatory or inhibitory (can be converted to GABA)
    - aspartate: excitatory
  - peptides: examples of peptide transmitters include:
    - substance P: involved in the transmission of pain sensation
    - endorphins: inhibit pain pathways.

Pain and Sensation

- Pain is defined as an unpleasant sensory and emotional experience associated with actual or potential tissue damage.
- Pain can be classified into:
  - nociceptive: somatic and visceral
  - referred
  - neuropathic
  - psychogenic.
- Nociceptive and referred pain are the commonest types of pain encountered in the surgical patient.
- Somatic pain is defined as pain that originates from the skin, muscles, bones and joints; it tends to be sharp in nature and is well localized.
- Visceral pain is due to ischaemia, inflammation and stretching or contraction (colic) of smooth muscle in hollow viscera; it is poorly localized.
- Referred pain occurs when damage to an internal organ is associated with pain in a particular skin region; this occurs as the organ in question shares the same dermatomal innervation as the region the pain is felt. Examples of referred pain include:
  - MI and angina: pain may be referred to the neck, jaw, shoulder and left arm
  - spleen: haemoperitoneum leads to left-sided diaphragmatic irritation and left shoulder tip pain (Kehr's sign)
  - appendix: central abdominal pain in the T10 dermatome is the initial sign until peritoneal irritation localizes the pain to the right iliac fossa
  - gall bladder: cholecystitis can lead to irritation of the right hemidiaphragm and right shoulder tip pain (Boas' sign).
- Pain can also be classified according to the speed of onset; soft-tissue injury is associated with a sudden sharp pain that lasts for a few seconds and is followed by a longer-lasting dull throbbing pain. Peripheral nerves differ in their diameter and conduction velocity; this explains the different pain sensations:
  - Aδ fibres: these are myelinated nerves; as a result, they have a high conduction speed and diameter. They are responsible for the sharp initial pain

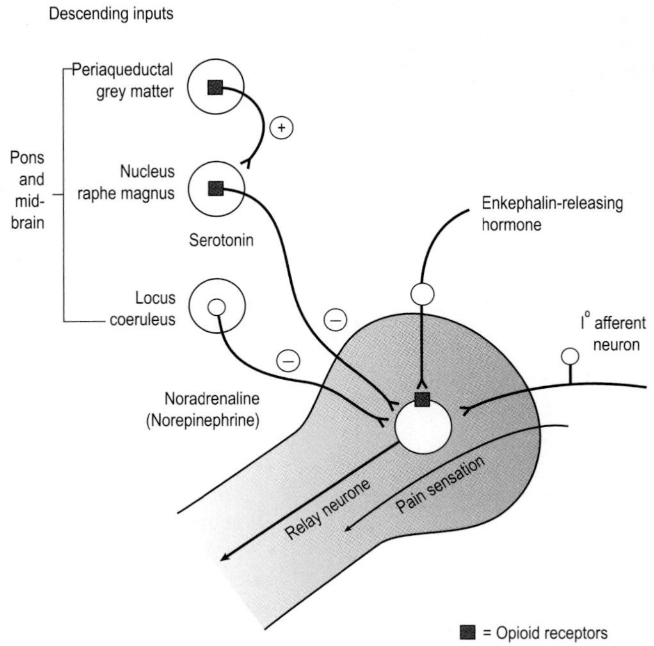

Fig. 13.7 Descending inputs modulating pain sensation.

  - C fibres: these are unmyelinated nerves and thus have a smaller diameter and lower conduction velocity. They are responsible for the longer-lasting dull pain.
- Pain transmission can be divided into:
  - transduction
  - transmission
  - modulation
  - perception.
- Transduction involves the production of electrical impulses; following tissue damage there is the release of inflammatory substances, i.e. prostaglandins, histamine, serotonin, bradykinin and substance P. These substances lead to electrical impulses that are transmitted along sensory nerves.
- Transmission of pain sensation is along Aδ and C fibres to the spinal cord; here they synapse in lamina I and III in the dorsal horn.
- The sensation of pain is then transmitted along the spinal cord where it is modulated before finally being perceived in the sensory areas of the brain.
- Modulation of pain involves the 'gate control theory' of Melzack and Wall: this theory proposes that pain impulses received in the dorsal horn can be modulated by other descending spinal inputs. These include inhibitory inputs from the periaqueductal grey matter and nucleus raphe magnus (both releasing serotonin) and the locus coeruleus (releases noradrenaline) (Fig. 13.7). In addition there is the release of the naturally occurring enkephalins and endorphins.

Drug Modulation of Pain

- There are numerous forms of analgesia used in current surgical practice; each acts on different elements in the chain of pain sensation.
- The provision of analgesia is particularly useful in the surgical patient; the effects of inadequate analgesia include:
  - respiratory:
    - ↑ chest wall splinting
    - ↓ tidal volume
    - ↓ vital capacity
    - ↓ functional residual capacity (FRC)
    - difficulty coughing and retention of secretions, leading to atelectasis and pneumonia
  - cardiovascular:
    - pain increases BP and heart rate, thus placing increased strain on the heart
  - immobilization and increased risk of thromboembolism
  - ileus
  - urinary retention
  - stress response
  - psychological stress.
- Transduction: drugs like paracetamol and NSAIDs inhibit prostaglandin production. Prostaglandins are

involved in sensitizing nociceptive receptors in injured tissues to the effects of nociceptive compounds such as bradykinin and substance P.

- Transmission: Aδ and C fibres are involved in the transmission of pain sensation. Local anaesthetics can be used to prevent the conduction of action potentials in these nerve fibres. Aβ fibres are involved in inhibiting transmission to higher centres; stimulation can thus provide analgesia. This is the basis for TENS (transcutaneous electrical nerve stimulator) machines.
- Modulation: opioids are potent analgesics. They produce their effect by combining with opioid receptors in the spinal cord and higher centres. The analgesic effect of opioids is due to:
  - combining with receptors in higher centres such as the periaqueductal grey matter and nucleus raphe magnus; here they stimulate descending inhibitory inputs to pain perception
  - binding to opioid receptors in the dorsal horn and inhibiting pain transmission; this action is believed to be related to hyperpolarizing the cell and thus decreasing the chance of propagating the pain impulse
  - inhibiting the release of substance P.
- Perception: pain perception can be influenced by factors such as fear, anxiety, depression, and activation of the 'fight or flight' mechanism.

AUTONOMIC NERVOUS SYSTEM (ANS) (Fig. 13.8)

- The autonomic nervous system is involved in the control of visceral organs, smooth muscle and secretory glands.
- It is principally involved in maintaining the internal environment by regulating cardiac, respiratory and digestive functions.
- The efferent neurons of the ANS have a two-neuron arrangement. This differs from somatic nerves. The cell body of the first neuron lies in the brainstem or spinal cord (preganglionic); the second neuron is located in the periphery in an autonomic ganglion (post-ganglionic).
- The ANS can be divided into two specific functional groups:
  - sympathetic
  - parasympathetic.

Sympathetic Nervous System

- Sympathetic neurons:
  - located in the thoracic and upper 2–3 lumbar segments of the spinal cord
  - preganglionic neurons lie in the lateral horn of the spinal grey matter
  - preganglionic axons leave via the ventral root of the spine to join the spinal nerve (see Chapter 4)
  - post-ganglionic neurons have their cell bodies either in the sympathetic chain (see Chapter 4) or in a named plexus along the aorta, i.e. coeliac, superior and inferior mesenteric.
- Spinal nerves are connected to the sympathetic chain by two small branches: the lateral white ramus communicantes (myelinated), and the medial grey ramus communicantes (unmyelinated).
- The sympathetic innervation of the head and neck is via preganglionic neurons synapsing with post-ganglionic bodies within the sympathetic chain; the post-ganglionic neurons then leave via the grey rami communicantes to join the spinal nerve.
- The sympathetic innervation of the abdominal and pelvic organs differs from that of the head and neck. Preganglionic neurons pass straight through the sympathetic chain to their individual plexuses and synapse with post-ganglionic cell bodies within the plexus.
- The neurotransmitter of the sympathetic nervous system is noradrenaline (except sweat glands; these are innervated by cholinergic fibres).

Parasympathetic Nervous System

- Preganglionic neurons lie in cranial nerve nuclei within the brainstem; the parasympathetic output is derived from the oculomotor, facial, glossopharyngeal and vagus nerves; this provides innervation to the head, neck, thorax and abdomen.
- The pelvic viscera are innervated by preganglionic neurons derived from the S2–4 spinal roots.
- The parasympathetic nervous system feeds into five ganglia before being distributed to the structures it innervates; these ganglia are:
  - oculomotor (III) nerve → ciliary ganglion
  - facial (VI) nerve → sphenopalatine ganglion and submandibular ganglion
  - glossopharyngeal (IX) nerve → otic ganglion
  - S2–4 → pelvic splanchnic nerve → pelvic ganglion.
- The cell bodies of post-ganglionic neurons lie in ganglia that are found in close proximity to the organ they innervate; an example would be the enteric nervous system (see Chapter 10). Here neurons contribute to two plexuses, the myenteric and submucosal. These are found within the bowel wall itself.
- The neurotransmitter of the parasympathetic nervous system is acetylcholine.

Functions of the Autonomic Nervous System

- The effects of the autonomic nervous system are summarized below.

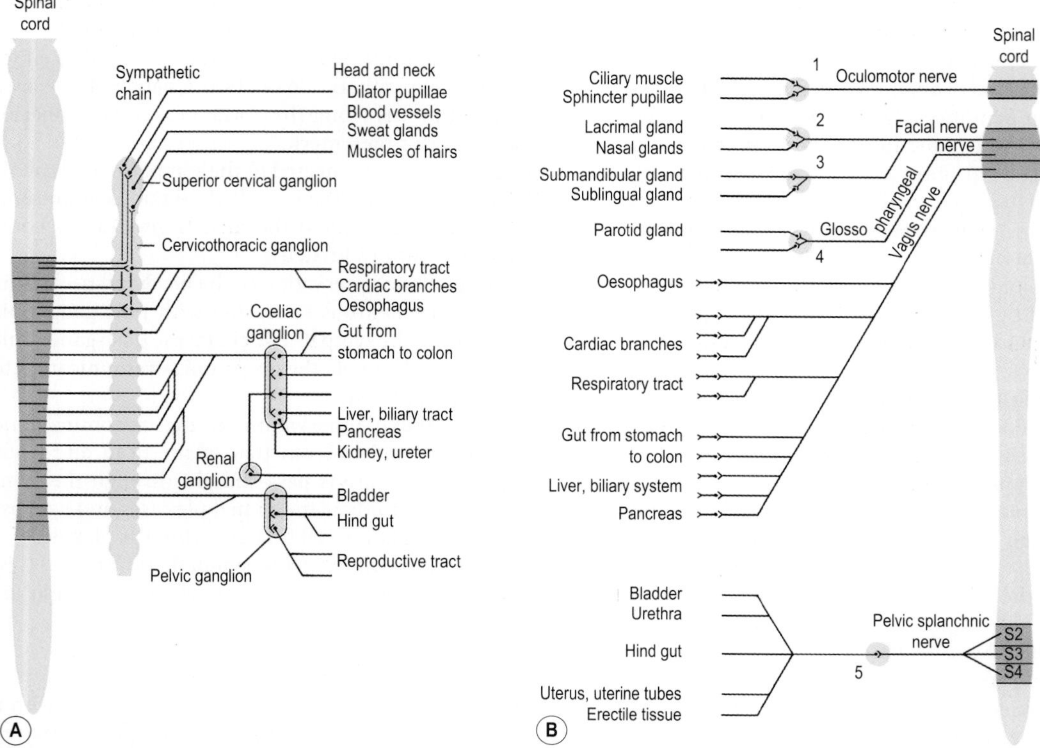

Fig. 13.8 (A) Layout of the sympathetic nervous system. (B) The parasympathetic nervous system: 1 = ciliary ganglion, 2 = sphenopalative ganglion, 3 = submandibular ganglion, 4 = otic ganglion, 5 = pelvic ganglion.

- Sympathetic system:
  - dilates pupils
  - reduces salivary secretions
  - reduces lacrimal secretions
  - increases heart rate (tachycardia)
  - increases the contractility of the heart
  - bronchodilation
  - decreases GI motility
  - increases sweat gland secretion
  - contraction of erector pili muscles in the skin.
- Parasympathetic system:
  - constricts pupils
  - increases salivary secretion
  - increases lacrimal secretion
  - decreases heart rate (bradycardia)
  - decreases the contractility of the heart
  - bronchoconstriction
  - increases GI motility.

LOCOMOTOR SYSTEM

Skeletal Muscle Physiology

Structure of Skeletal Muscle

- Muscles are composed of a number of muscle fibres; these are grouped together to form bundles called fasciculi.
- The muscle fibres are composed of numerous filamentous bundles called myofibrils.
- The myofibrils contain the contractile proteins actin and myosin; under a microscope muscle has a striated appearance due to the arrangement of actin and myosin:
  - the dark bands or A bands are composed of the thicker myosin filaments
  - the light bands or I bands are composed of the thinner actin filaments
  - the I band is divided by the Z line; the space between Z lines is called a sarcomere

  - at the Z lines the membrane of the muscle cell (sarcolemma) forms narrow tubes that traverse the sarcomere; these are called the T-tubules.
- The myosin filaments consist of a long tail and a head section; the head has a binding site for ATP.
- The actin filaments contain three different proteins:
  - actin: a thin contractile protein, arranged in a double-stranded helix
  - tropomyosin: lies in the groove between the actin filaments
  - troponin: lies at regular intervals along the filament, attached to both actin and tropomyosin; it also has binding sites for Ca^{2+} and is involved in the regulation of contraction. Troponin and tropomyosin block the myosin-binding site on actin.

Skeletal Muscle Classification

- Skeletal muscle is classified according to the speed of contraction:
  - type I or slow twitch: act as postural muscles, e.g. in the back; they are designed to perform slow, sustained contractions and resist fatigue well. They rely on aerobic metabolism and contain myoglobin
  - type II or fast twitch:
    - type IIa or fast oxidative fibres, e.g. calf muscles: they rely on aerobic metabolism and contain myoglobin; they have moderate resistance to fatigue
    - type IIb or fast glycolytic fibres, e.g. extraocular muscle: do not contain myoglobin and thus appear white; they contain a large amount of glycogen and rely on anaerobic metabolism.

Sliding Filament Hypothesis (Fig. 13.9)

- Muscle contraction is known to occur by the actin and myosin filaments sliding past each other: the sliding filament theory.
- The process of muscle contraction occurs, as the head section of myosin is able to form cross-links with actin.
- When ATP binds to the head section of myosin it dissociates from its binding site on the actin filament.
- The ATP is hydrolysed and changes the angle of the myosin head (relative to its tail); as the ATP has been hydrolysed, the myosin is again able to bind to the actin filament.
- The release of phosphate from the myosin head restores the angle and moves the actin filament along the myosin filament; this is called the power stroke.
- ATP will bind to myosin and start the process again.
- Creatine phosphate is present in very high concentrations within muscle and provides sufficient energy reserves for the above processes to take place. The enzyme creatine kinase catalyses the transfer of the phosphate group from creatine phosphate to ADP, thus replenishing ATP stores.

Excitation Contraction Coupling

- Skeletal muscle only contracts if it receives an excitatory impulse from a motor nerve (see below).
- An action potential is conducted down the motor nerve and activates an electrical signal to be conducted across the sarcolemma; this impulse is conducted deep within the cell by the invaginations in the sarcolemma (T-tubules).
- Depolarization of the cell leads to the release of Ca^{2+} from the sarcoplasmic reticulum within the cell. The rise in Ca^{2+} activates contraction by binding to troponin on the thin filaments; this leads to a conformational change and removes troponin and tropomyosin from the myosin binding site on actin.
- As the cell repolarizes, the Ca^{2+} is actively pumped back into the sarcoplasmic reticulum.
- The Ca^{2+} is removed from the troponin and thus the troponin and tropomyosin block the myosin binding site.

Neuromuscular Transmission

- Muscles are supplied by nerves from the spinal cord, known as α motor neurons; they innervate the muscle directly and lie in the anterior horn of the spinal cord grey matter.
- α motor neurons are myelinated and conduct action potentials to the muscle fibre surface; here they form a modified synapse called the neuromuscular junction.
- The motor neurons lose their myelin sheath and terminate in grooves in the muscle known as synaptic gutters; this is known as the motor end-plate. It is separated from the axon terminal of the motor neuron by a gap; this is called the neuromuscular cleft.
- Transfer of the action potential from the motor neuron to the muscle is very similar to nerve conduction described above:
  - action potential depolarizes the terminal axon of the motor neuron
  - axon membrane becomes more permeable to Ca^{2+}
  - the rise in Ca^{2+} stimulates secretory vesicles to fuse with the cell membrane and release acetylcholine (ACh) into the neuromuscular cleft
  - the ACh binds to receptors on the muscle fibres; this leads to the opening of ion channels, in turn leading to the influx of Na^+ and K^+ and depolarization of the cell; this is called the end-plate potential
  - an action potential is initiated when the threshold is reached; this leads to the impulse being propagated across the plasma membrane

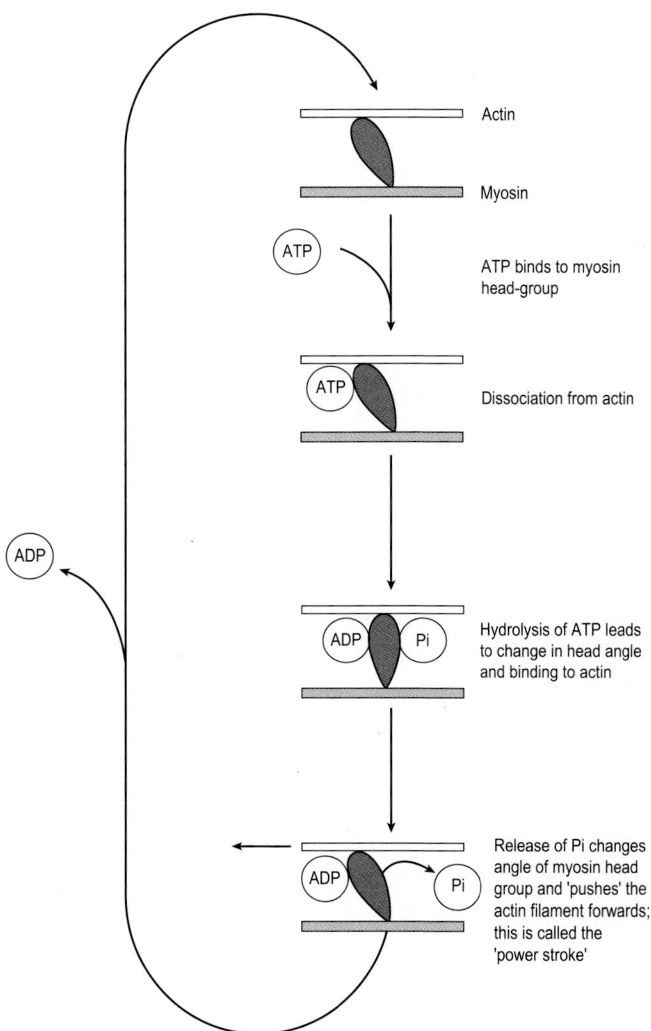

Fig. 13.9 Molecular events involved in contraction of skeletal muscle.

- acetylcholine is released from the receptor and the muscle cell repolarizes and is broken down by acetylcholinesterase.

LOCOMOTION

Spinal Cord Reflexes

- Reflex: involuntary, stereotyped response as a result of a sensory stimulus.
- The reflex pathways consist of an afferent neuron that conveys impulses from a sensory receptor, and an efferent neuron that runs from the brain to the effector organ, i.e. muscle.

Muscle Stretch Reflex (Fig. 13.10)

- Simplest reflex: it is monosynaptic and consists of the afferent input from stretch receptors in skeletal muscle and the efferent output to the stretched muscle.
- The sensory organ for the stretch reflex is the muscle spindle: this consists of intrafusal muscle fibres which lie in parallel to the skeletal muscle fibres. There are two types of intrafusal muscle fibre:
  - nuclear bag fibres
  - nuclear chain fibres.
- The muscle spindle is divided into three regions: a contractile region at either end and a receptor region in the centre.

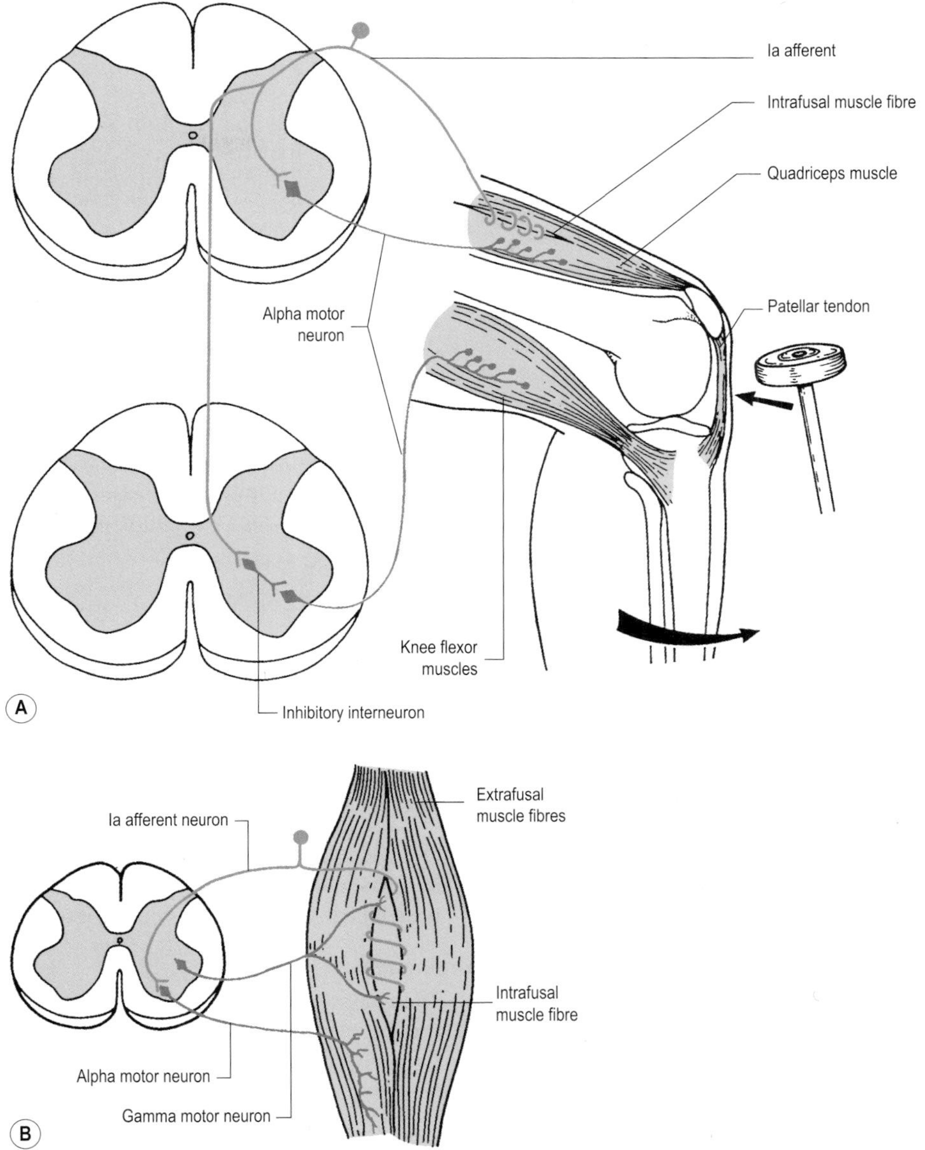

Fig. 13.10 (A) Quadriceps stretch reflex: striking the patellar tendon produces knee extension. Reciprocal innervation leads to inhibition of the knee flexors. (B) The gamma reflex loop. (From Crossman AR & Neary D. Neuroanatomy: An Illustrated Colour Text, 2nd edn. Churchill Livingstone, Edinburgh, 2000, with permission.)

- The contractile regions are supplied by γ motor neurons from the anterior horn of the spinal cord.
- The chain of events in the stretch reflex is as follows:
  - muscle spindle is stretched: this causes the receptor region to depolarize; this generates an action potential in the afferent nerve (Ia afferent)
  - the afferent impulse enters the spinal cord via the dorsal horn and synapses with an α motor neuron that supplies the stretched muscle
  - the action potential in the α motor neuron signals the muscle to contract to oppose the stretch

  - the afferent impulse also synapses with inhibitory neurons that synapse with α motor neurons that supply antagonist muscles (reciprocal inhibition). This reduces resistance to contraction of the stretched muscle.
- The anterior horn also contains γ motor neurons (innervate the contractile ends of the muscle spindle). Activation of γ motor neurons leads to contraction of the ends of the muscle spindle; this lowers the threshold for action potential generation, and thus increases the sensitivity to stretch stimuli applied to the muscle. This reflex is called the gamma reflex loop.
- The stretch reflex and gamma reflex are important for a number of reasons:
  - the control of voluntary activity: the muscle spindle is able to contract with muscle fibres and thus maintain sensory output
  - control of muscle tone: the stretch reflex resists passive changes in muscle length; this is particularly important in the maintenance of body posture, i.e. antigravity muscles of the neck, trunk and legs.
- The stretch reflex is the physiological basis underlying tendon reflexes in clinical examination:
  - biceps reflex: C5–6
  - brachioradialis reflex: C5–6
  - triceps reflex: C6–7
  - quadriceps reflex: L3–4
  - Achilles tendon reflex: S1–2.

Golgi Tendon Organ Reflex

- The Golgi tendons are another stretch receptor. They are located in the tendon of muscles and are sensitive to tension.
- The reflex they are involved in is an inhibitory response. It involves:
  - afferent impulse acting on α motor neurons that supply the contracting muscle
  - reduction in the level of active contraction (via inhibitory interneurons)
  - the reflex is protective and limits muscle/tendon stretch.

Withdrawal Reflex (Fig. 13.11)

- This is a more complex reflex; it is polysynaptic.
- The withdrawal or flexor reflex is a response to painful or noxious stimuli.
- The afferent input is from pain receptors; these synapse with several efferent neurons:
  - α motor neurons: this results in stimulation of flexors in the limb in which the painful stimulus was experienced, thus withdrawing the affected limb
  - inhibitory signals are passed to α motor neurons in the opposing extensor muscles
  - this pattern is reversed in the opposing limb: flexor muscles are inhibited and extensor muscles are stimulated; this is called the crossed extensor reflex. It enables us to balance or push away from a noxious stimuli, e.g. if you stand on a sharp object and pull away your foot, the reflex will lead to extension of the contralateral limb to maintain balance.

Control of Locomotion

- A number of areas in the brain are involved in the control of movement; these include:
  - cerebral cortex
  - brainstem
  - cerebellum
  - basal ganglia.
- Control of movement by these centres can be via descending pathways that synapse with the spinal motor neurons, or via inputs into the motor area of the cerebral cortex from the cerebellum and basal ganglia.

Cerebral Cortex

- The motor area of the cerebral cortex lies in the frontal lobe immediately anterior to the central sulcus; this area is called the precentral gyrus.
- Descending pathways leave this area to supply spinal motor neurons:
  - corticobulbar tracts: supply the motor portions of the cranial nerves
  - corticospinal tracts: supply the spinal motor neurons; they are concerned with voluntary movements.
- The descending fibres from the cerebral cortex cross the midline and innervate the opposite side of the body, i.e. the left hemisphere supplies the right (contralateral side).

Brainstem

- There are four descending inputs from the brainstem; these are:
  1. The rubrospinal tract: originates in the red nucleus and primarily innervates distal limb muscles.
  2. The tectospinal tract: fibres arise in the superior colliculus of the midbrain; it receives inputs from the visual cortex and is believed to control reflex activity in response to visual stimuli.
  3. The vestibulospinal tract: originates in the vestibular nuclei; it supplies muscles of the ipsilateral side of the body. It innervates muscles concerned with balance and posture in response to inputs from the vestibular apparatus.
  4. The reticulospinal tract: fibres are derived from the pons and medulla; they supply muscles on the ipsilateral side of the body and are important in maintaining posture and muscle tone.

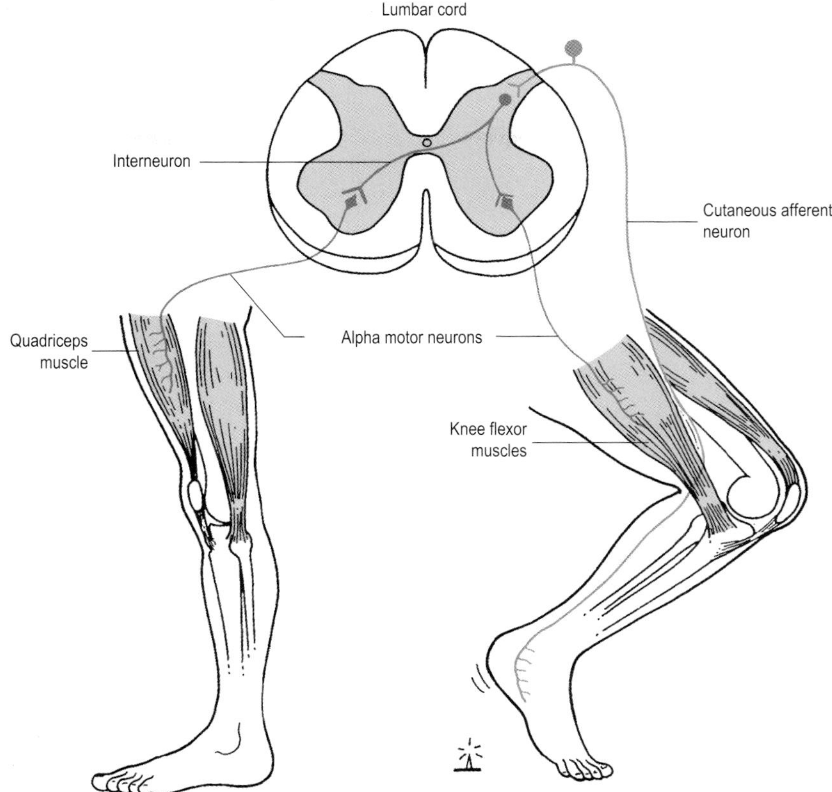

Fig. 13.11 The flexor (withdrawal) reflex and crossed extensor reflex. (From Crossman AR & Neary D. Neuroanatomy: An Illustrated ColourText, 2nd edn. Churchill Livingstone, Edinburgh, 2000, with permission.)

Cerebellum

- There are no descending pathways from the cerebellum; they influence movement via inputs directly to the motor cortex.
- The cerebellum receives information from the vestibular apparatus, visual system, corticospinal tracts and peripheral proprioceptors.
- The cerebellum collates information from these sources, and is important in maintaining balance and producing smooth, co-ordinated movements.

Basal Ganglia

- The basal ganglia have no descending tracts; they receive information from the substantia nigra, the thalamus and the motor cortex.
- The basal ganglia appear to be involved in the initiation of movement, ensuring that body posture is appropriate for a particular movement and eliminating unwanted movements.

BONE PHYSIOLOGY

- Bone is a type of connective tissue. It has an organic and inorganic component.
- The organic component is referred to as osteoid; this consists of collagen I, keratan sulfate, hyaluronic acid and glycoproteins.
- The inorganic component contains complexes of calcium and phosphate (hydroxyapatite); it also contains calcium carbonate, fluoride, magnesium and sodium ions.
- Bone has four main functions; these are:
  - mechanical support
  - locomotion (by means of joints)
  - calcium and phosphate homeostasis
  - haemopoiesis.
- Bones contain four main cell types; these are:
  - osteoprogenitor cells: undifferentiated cells
  - osteoblasts: these cells secrete the organic matrix of bone; they are also involved in mineralization

- osteocytes: mature cells; they are trapped in gaps (lacunae) after they deposit matrix. They are involved in calcium homeostasis as they are able to transport Ca^{2+} from the bone interior to the extracellular environment
- osteoclasts: these cells are responsible for the absorption of bone; this is via the release of lytic enzymes, i.e. collagenase, acid phosphatase. These cells are considered part of the mononuclear macrophage system.

Bone Formation and Reabsorption

- Bone is not an inert tissue; it is constantly remodelling in order to cope with changes in the demands placed upon it.
- 5–10% of the bone mass is recycled each week; this can be much greater in those undertaking strenuous activity. During immobility then bone mass can be rapidly lost – disuse osteoporosis.
- Remodelling of bone is a two-stage process:
  - osteoclastic reabsorption of bone
  - osteoblastic phase in which new bone is laid down.
- The control of bone remodelling is not completely understood (particularly at a cellular level); however, a number of hormones are known to be involved, including:
  - parathyroid hormone
  - calcitonin
  - thyroxine
  - oestrogen
  - vitamin D.

OSCE SCENARIOS

OSCE Scenario 13.1

An 18-year-old male is admitted to A&E following an assault. He has severe head injuries. His Glasgow coma score (GCS) is 6.

1. How is brain injury classified?
2. Describe the mechanism of compensation for an acute rise in intracranial pressure.
3. Describe the possible management options.

OSCE Scenario 13.2

A 55-year-old male presents to a pain clinic with a long history of lumbar back pain that has become more severe recently. There is no history of sciatica and there is no neurological deficit on examination. Paracetamol has been of no benefit.

1. Why is paracetamol unlikely to have been of benefit?
2. Why is ibuprofen more likely to be of benefit than paracetamol?
3. What is the mechanism of action of TENS?
4. What is the purpose of the local anaesthetic injection and what is the mechanism of action of local anaesthetics?
5. What is the mechanism of action of oramorph and what side effects might be expected?

OSCE Scenario 13.3

A 24-year-old male is in a critical condition on ITU following a road traffic accident. He has severe head injuries. The ITU consultant has discussed his poor prognosis with the family and they ask about organ donation. Answer the following questions regarding testing for brainstem death.

1. What are the pre-conditions required before diagnosing brainstem death?
2. What are the exclusion criteria?
3. Which cranial nerves are involved in the following tests:
   a. Corneal reflex
   b. Gag reflex
   c. Cough reflex
   d. Vestibulocochlear reflex

OSCE Scenario 13.4

A 75-year-old male patient is found confused during a night shift, five days following left hemicolectomy. He has past medical history of TIA, IHD and BPH. On examination, his GCS is 13/15, he appears combative and hallucinating, his temperature is 38.9°C, RR is 25/min, PR is 120/min and irregular and blood pressure is 115/65. His chest examination shows possible reduced air entry on the left side, he is diffusely tender in the abdomen, and he has a urinary catheter with urine output averaging 20/h over the last 3 h. Bedside ECG shows new fast AF. You are the night surgical SPR and asked to review the patient.

1. How would you manage this patient?
2. What is the differential diagnosis?
3. What is the most likely cause?
4. Who would you inform at this stage?

OSCE Scenario 13.5

A 65-year-old male patient has been stepped down from the high-dependency unit to the ward on day two following open repair of abdominal aortic aneurysm. As you review him on the ward round, you notice that he is comfortable in bed; however, his blood pressure is low at 95/60 and pulse rate is 58/min. He is apyrexial, his RR is 16/min and his oxygen saturation is 98% on room air. His abdominal examination is unremarkable, and his pain is well controlled, having epidural catheter in situ. The night FY1 gave him intravenous fluid challenge 2 h earlier which improved his BP reading slightly and arranged for blood tests. His Hb is 12.5 g/dL, WBC 11.2 × 10^6/dL, while the rest of his blood tests are unremarkable.

1. What are the possible causes of his low blood pressure?
2. What drugs are usually infused in epidural catheters?
3. How does epidural infusion cause hypotension?
4. Why is postoperative analgesia important for surgical patients?
5. What are the side effects and complications of epidural catheters?
6. How would you treat hypotension related to epidural catheters?

Answers in Appendix pages 458–461

Please check your eBook at https://studentconsult.inkling.com/ for more self-assessment questions. See inside cover for registration details.

SECTION III

Pathology

14 Cellular Injury

Causes of cellular injury include:

- trauma
- thermal injury – heat and cold
- chemical agents – drugs, poisons, hypoxia
- infectious organisms
- immunological mechanisms
- nutritional deficiencies
- ionizing radiation.

MECHANISMS OF CELLULAR INJURY

Cells may be damaged either reversibly or irreversibly in a variety of ways:

- Mechanical disruption:
  - trauma by direct mechanical force
  - extremes of heat and cold
  - osmotic pressure changes.
- Failure of cell membrane integrity:
  - damage to ion pumps.
- Membrane damage:
  - free radicals.
- Interference with metabolic pathways:
  - respiratory poisons and mitochondria
  - disruption of protein synthesis.
- Deficiency of metabolites:
  - hypoxia/anoxia
  - glucose (hypo- or hyperglycaemia)
  - hormones.
- DNA loss or damage:
  - ionizing radiation
  - chemotherapy
  - free radicals.

The effect of cell injury on a tissue will depend on:

- the nature of the injurious agent
- the duration of the injury
- the proportion of the type of cell affected
- the ability of the tissues to regenerate.

CELL DEATH

Cell death is the irreversible loss of the cell's ability to maintain independence from the environment. Two major forms of cell death are recognized:

- necrosis
- apoptosis.

Necrosis

Necrosis is cellular or tissue death in a living organism, irrespective of the cause. Several types of necrosis are described:

- coagulative
- colliquative
- caseous
- gangrenous
- fibrinoid
- fat.

Coagulative Necrosis

- Denaturation of intracytoplasmic proteins.
- Dead tissue will initially become firm and swollen, but later becomes soft (ventricle may rupture after myocardial infarction).
- Typically occurs in ischaemic injury (except brain).

Colliquative Necrosis

- Seen in brain, probably due to lack of supporting stroma.
- Necrotic brain tissue liquefies.
- Glial reaction at periphery with cyst formation occurs eventually.

Caseous Necrosis

- Characteristic of TB.
- Macroscopically cheese-like (caseous).
- Microscopically structureless.

Gangrenous Necrosis

- Necrosis with putrefaction of tissues due to certain bacteria, e.g. clostridia, streptococci.

- Tissue black due to iron sulfide from degraded haemoglobin.
- Ischaemic gangrene may be either 'dry' or 'wet' gangrene.
- Gas gangrene is the result of infection with *Clostridium perfringens*.
- Synergistic gangrene follows infection by a specific combination of organisms (see Chapter 21).

Fibrinoid Necrosis

- Associated with malignant hypertension.
- Necrosis of arteriole smooth muscle wall with seepage of plasma into tunica media and deposition of fibrin.
- Smudgy eosinophilic appearance in H and E sections.

Fat Necrosis

- Direct trauma to adipose tissue and extracellular liberation of fat (e.g. fat necrosis causing breast lump).
- Enzymatic lysis of fat by lipases, e.g. pancreatic lipase in acute pancreatitis. Fats split into fatty acids, which combine with calcium to precipitate as soaps (seen as white spots on the peritoneum and omentum).

Apoptosis

Apoptosis is an energy-dependent process for the deletion of unwanted individual cells. It is to be distinguished from necrosis (Table 14.1). It is a biochemically specific mode of cell death characterized by activation of endogenous endonuclease, which digests nuclear DNA into smaller DNA fragments.

Function of Apoptosis

- Morphogenesis (elimination of cells in embryonal development).
- Removal of cells which have undergone DNA damage.
- Removal of virally infected cells.
- Induction of tolerance to self-antigens by removal of autoreactive T-lymphocytes.

Mediators of Apoptosis

p53

- A tumour suppressor gene which checks the integrity of the genome prior to mitosis.
- Switches cells with damaged DNA into apoptosis.
- Loss of p53 expression is associated with poor prognosis in tumours.

bcl-2

- Inhibits apoptosis.
- Excess bcl-2 expression results in failure of initiation of apoptosis with cell accumulation.
- Overexpression in neoplasia.

fas (CD 95)

- Plasma membrane receptor which, when activated, is directly coupled to the activation of intracellular proteases, which lead to apoptosis.

Caspases

- Present in all cells and unless inhibited lead to morphological changes of apoptosis.

Morphological Features of Apoptosis

- Cell shrinkage with intact plasma membrane.
- Nuclear shrinking (pyknosis).
- Nuclear fragmentation (karyorrhexis).
- Margination of chromatin.
- Surface blebbing of cell.
- Formation of apoptotic bodies (cells break up into membrane-bound fragments).
- Fragments are either shed (if epithelial cells are involved) or phagocytosed (by neighbouring cells).

TABLE 14.1 Comparison of Apoptosis and Necrosis

Feature	Apoptosis	Necrosis
Induction	Physiological or pathological stimuli	Invariably pathological injury
Extent	Single cells	Groups of cells
Biochemical	Energy-dependent fragmentation of DNA by endogenous endonucleases Lysosomes intact	Impairment or cessation of ion homeostasis Lysosomes leak lytic enzymes
Cell membrane integrity	Preserved	Lost
Morphology	Cell shrinkage and fragmentation to form apoptotic bodies with dense chromatin	Cell swelling and lysis
Inflammatory response	None	Usual
Fate of dead cells	Phagocytosed by neighbouring cells	Phagocytosed by neutrophils and macrophages

Diseases of Increased Apoptosis

- HIV (CD4+ cells die through programmed cell death).
- Neurodegenerative diseases.

Diseases of Decreased Apoptosis

- Neoplasia.
- Autoimmune disease.

THE PROCESS OF HEALING

Regeneration and Repair

- Regeneration refers to total healing of a wound with restitution of the original tissues in their usual amounts, arrangements and with normal function.
- Repair refers to the process where the original tissue is not totally regenerated and the defect is made good to a variable extent by scar tissue.

Cell Renewal

The regenerative capacity of cells varies. Cells can be classified according to their potential for renewal:

- Labile cells:
  - good capacity for regeneration
  - e.g. surface epithelial cells constantly being replaced from deeper layers, e.g. skin, oesophagus, vagina.
- Stable cells:
  - divide at slow rate under physiological conditions
  - replaced by mitotic division of mature cells and lost cells are rapidly replaced
  - e.g. liver, renal tubular epithelium.
- Permanent cells:
  - never divide in post-natal life
  - cannot be replaced if lost
  - e.g. nerve cells, striated muscle cells, myocardial cells.

Repair

Organization is the process whereby specialized tissues are repaired by the formation of mature connective tissue, i.e. fibrous scar. Organization occurs by:

- fibrinous exudate
- removal of fibrin and dead tissue and phagocytes
- migration of fibroblasts and capillaries forming granulation tissue
- replacement of exudate by vascularized fibrous tissue
- eventually a collagen-rich scar develops.

Granulation tissue

- A combination of capillary loops and myofibroblasts.
- Capillary endothelial cells grow into the area to be repaired.
- Fibroblasts are stimulated to divide.
- Fibroblasts secrete collagen and matrix components.
- Fibroblasts acquire muscle filaments and attach to adjacent cells and become myofibroblasts.
- Myofibroblasts cause wound contraction.
- Granulation tissue appears red and granular: hence the name.
- Excessive granulation tissue protruding above the wound surface is called 'proud flesh'.

Clinical Problems with Organization and Wound Contraction

Organization

- Fibrous adhesions in the peritoneum may cause intestinal obstruction.
- Obliteration of the pericardial space with scarring may cause constrictive pericarditis.

Wound contraction

- Stenosis (narrowing at an orifice), e.g. anal stenosis after haemorrhoidectomy, pyloric stenosis after peptic ulceration.
- Stricture (a narrowing in a tube), e.g. narrowing in the colon after ischaemic colitis.
- Scarring in a muscle causing a contracture.
- Contractures following burns, especially around joints.

INJURIES TO SPECIFIC TISSUES

Skin

Healing depends upon the size of the defect. It depends on whether it is an incised wound (surgical incision) or whether there is tissue loss.

Skin Anatomy (Fig. 14.1)

- Skin is composed of epidermis and dermis.
- Beneath the dermis lie subcutaneous fat, fascia and muscle.
- The blood supply to the skin arises from blood vessels which perforate the muscle (perforator vessels) and travel through the subcutaneous tissue to form the subdermal and dermal vascular plexus.

Incised Wound (Surgical Incision) – Healing by First Intention

- Edges of incision apposed.
- Fibrin 'sticks' edges together.
- Capillaries bridge tiny gap.
- Fibroblasts invade fibrin network.
- After 10 days wound is strong and sutures can be removed.
- Remodelling occurs from then on.

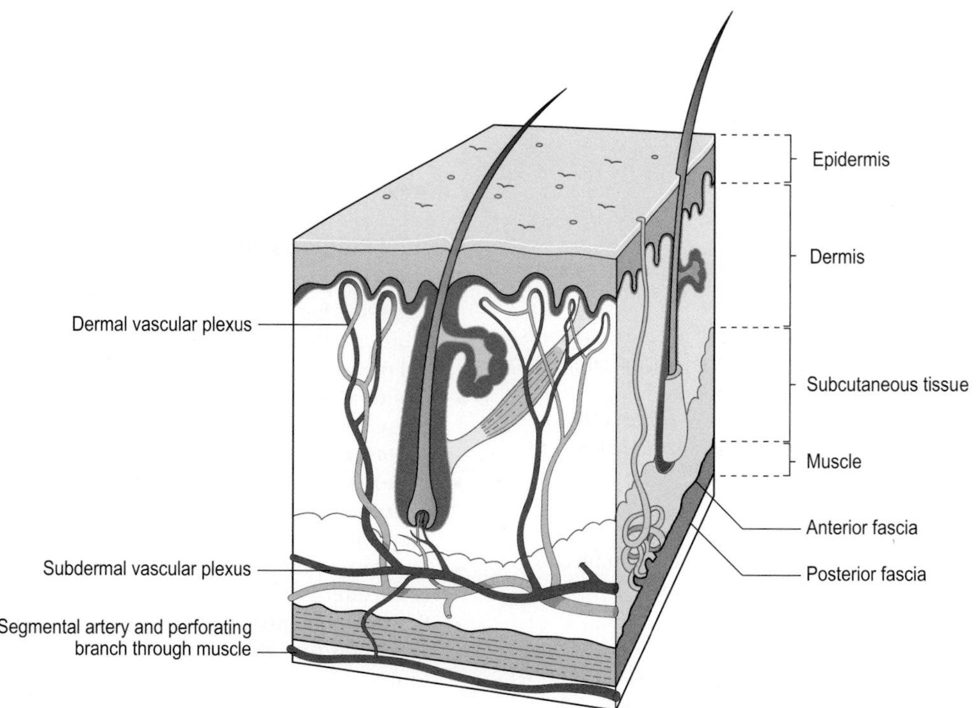

Fig. 14.1 The structure of skin with vascular plexus, fat, fascia and muscle.

Tissue Loss – Healing by Second Intention

- Tissue loss, e.g. trauma, or wound left open, e.g. grossly infected wound.
- Phagocytes remove any debris.
- Formation of granulation tissue in base of wound.
- Myofibroblasts cause wound contraction
- Centripetal growth of epithelium from wound edges (re-epithelialization) to cover defect.
- Eventually tissue deficit made good by scar tissue.
- Final cosmetic result depends on degree of tissue loss and amount of scarring.

Abnormalities of Skin Healing

Keloid

- Excessive fibroblast proliferation and collagen production.
- Particularly common in black Africans.
- Collagen deposition occurs beyond and above the wound itself.
- Occurs after surgery and injury, particularly burns.
- Covered by normal epithelium.
- Does not settle.

Hypertrophied scar

- Wound broad and raised.
- Does not extend beyond the wound itself.
- Usually settles spontaneously in up to 18 months.

Anatomy of Repair of Defects

- Wherever possible, scars from any wound should be placed in the lines of relaxed skin tension (Fig. 14.2), which are seen in the older patient as wrinkle lines.
- These lines lie perpendicular to the underlying muscle contraction.
- These are different to Langer's lines, which were anatomically derived using cadaver experiments and differ slightly due to lack of mechanical forces.

Reconstructive Ladder (Fig. 14.3)

- When assessing any wound or defect, the principles of the reconstructive ladder can be utilized.
- Employing the simplest options first, the ladder outlines different steps for closure of a wound or defect.
- The ladder can be 'climbed' as the complexity of the reconstructive situation increases.
- More recently the concept of a 'reconstructive elevator' is employed, where the appropriate reconstruction is selected for the specific defect or situation, which is not

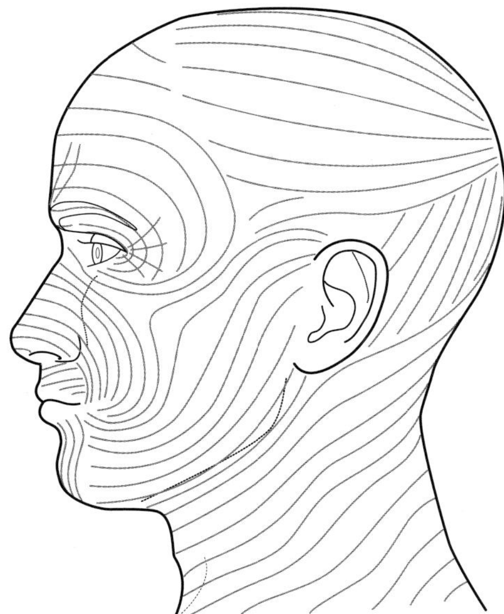

Fig. 14.2 Lines of relaxed skin tension.

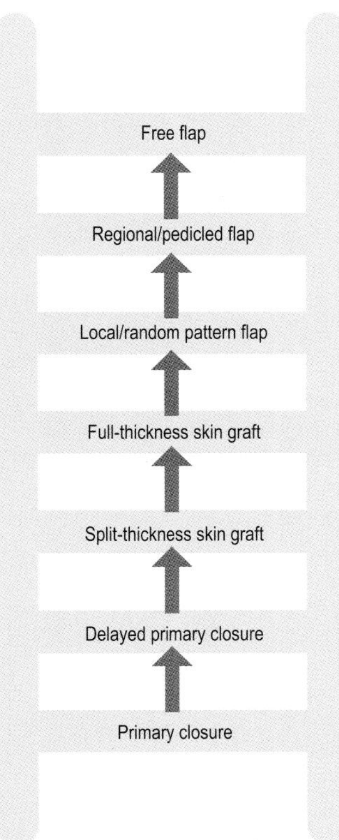

Fig. 14.3 The reconstructive ladder.

always the simplest option: e.g. a large area of exposed bone without periosteum will need a flap of some sort.

Grafts

- Common option for closure of defects that cannot be primarily closed.
- Commonly composed of skin, but may contain a variety of tissue including:
  - skin
  - cartilage
  - tendon
  - bone
  - or can be composite, using a combination of the above.
- Are not transferred with their own blood supply.
- Rely on the formation of a new vascular system at a new site.
- Different types of graft include:
  - autograft: own tissue; most common
  - allograft, e.g. cadaver bone
  - xenograft, e.g. animal tendon; rare.

Skin grafts

- A full-thickness skin graft consists of epidermis and the whole of the dermis.
- A split-thickness skin graft consists of epidermis and a variable thickness of dermis.

Mechanism of skin graft take

Skin grafts take in a series of steps, which can be broken into:

- Adherence:
  - fibrin bonds the graft to the recipient site
  - occurs in <12 h.
- Plasmic imbibition:
  - graft absorbs essential nutrients from recipient bed
  - occurs at 24–48 h.
- Inosculation:
  - revascularization of the graft via growth of vascular buds
  - occurs at 48–72 h.

Split-thickness skin grafts (Fig. 14.4)

- Common donor sites include:
  - thigh
  - buttocks.
- Result in more contraction at the recipient site.
- Can be meshed for large areas needing grafts.
- Result in pale, square scar at healed donor site (takes 10–14 days).
- Usually 'take' well as are thinner, helping them survive the imbibition phase.

Full-thickness skin grafts (Fig. 14.5)

- Common donor sites include:
  - groin
  - pre-/post-auricular areas
  - supraclavicular region.

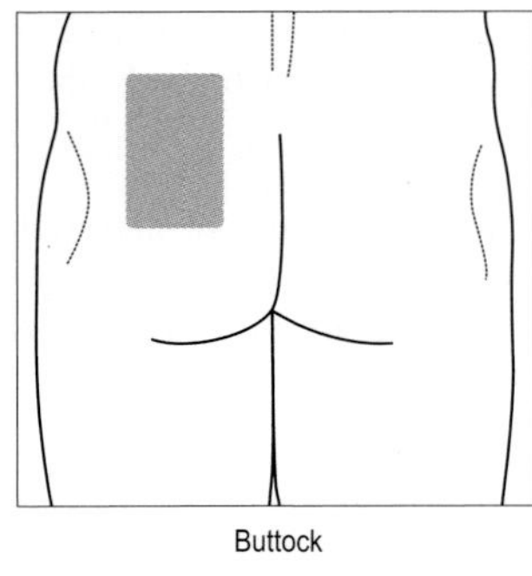

Buttock

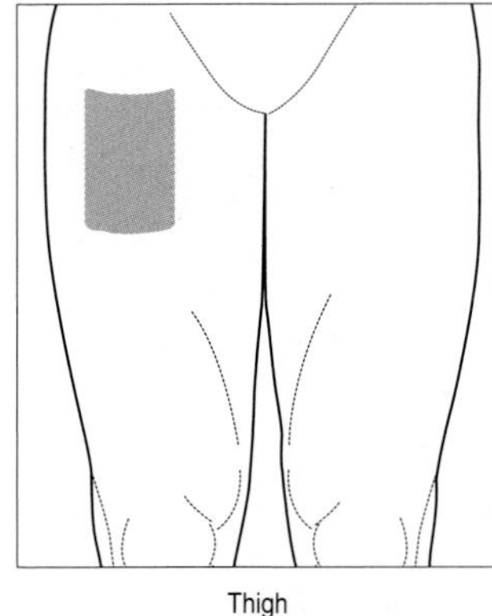

Thigh

Fig. 14.4 Split-thickness skin graft donor sites.

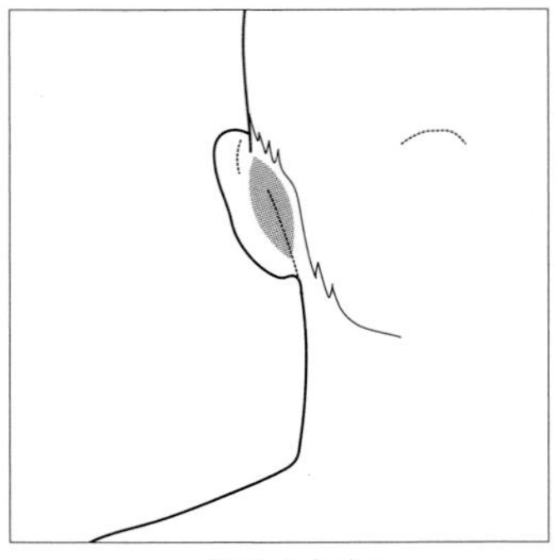

Post-auricular

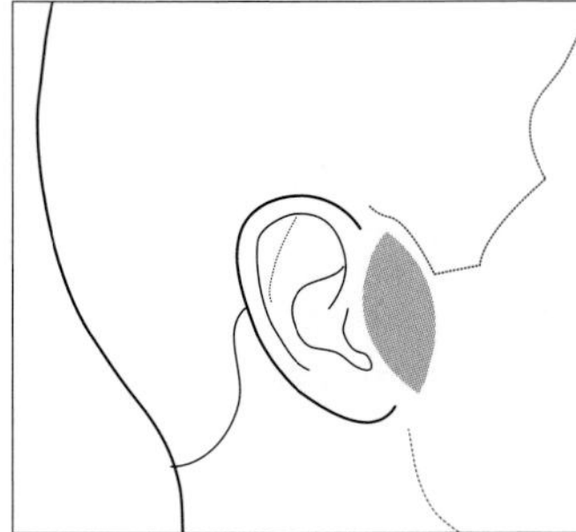

Pre-auricular

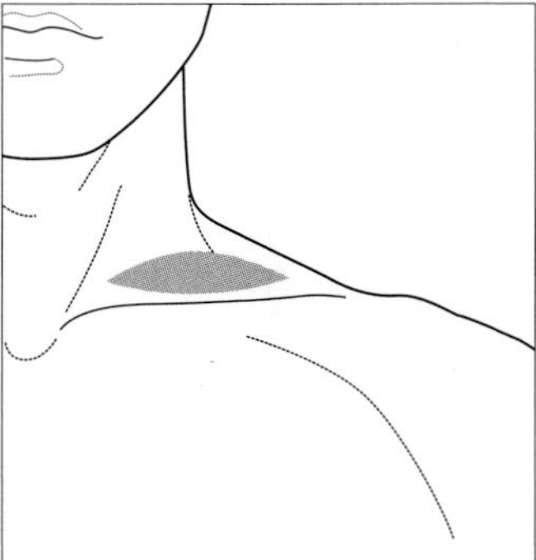

Supraclavicular

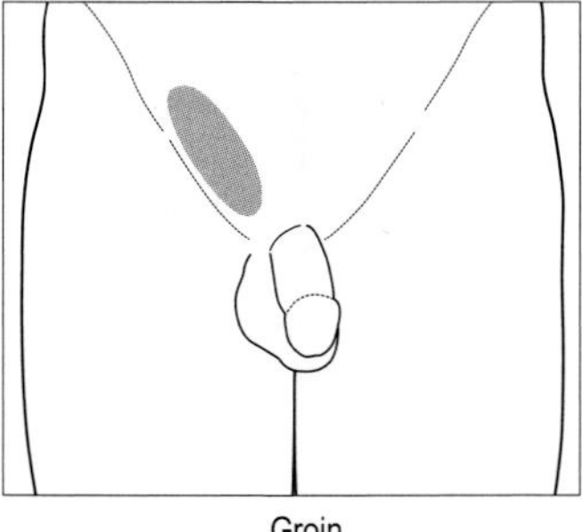

Groin

Fig. 14.5 Full-thickness skin graft donor sites.

- Result in less contraction at recipient site.
- Limited to relatively smaller areas due to direct closure of donor site.
- Result in linear scar at donor site.
- Less reliable 'take' due to thicker nature.

Flaps

- Unit of tissue transferred with its own blood supply.
- Used for:
  - large defects
  - where a graft would produce a poorer cosmetic result, e.g. face
  - where the base of a defect could not support a graft, i.e. bare bone, exposed tendon or poorly vascularized bed.

Classification

Can be classified in several ways:

- by composition: cutaneous, fasciocutaneous, myocutaneous, osteofasciocutaneous, etc. (Fig. 14.6)
- by vascular supply: random pattern, axial, island (Fig. 14.7)
- by location of donor site to defect: local, regional/pedicled, distant/free (Fig. 14.8)
- by design: transposition, Z-plasty, rotation, advancement (Fig. 14.9).

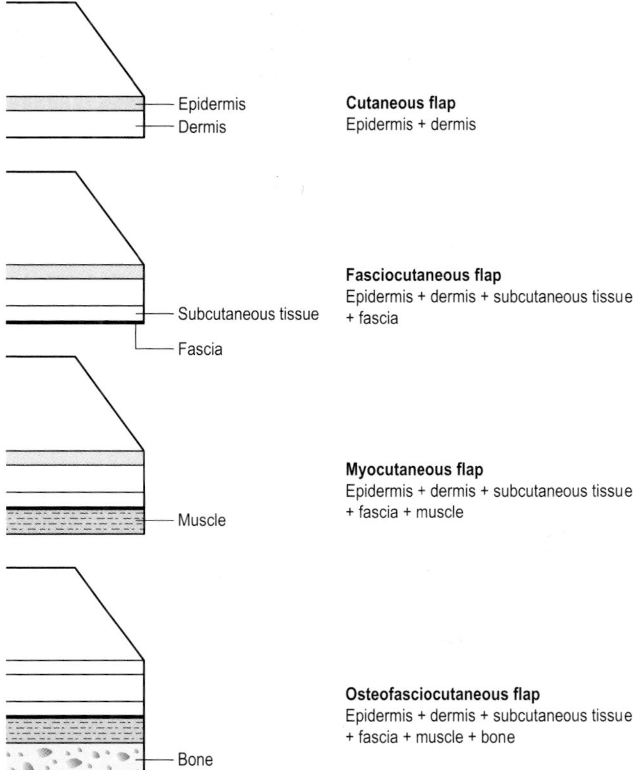

Fig. 14.6 Flaps by composition.

Local flaps

- Local flaps are composed of tissue raised adjacent to the defect to be covered.
- Can be a useful method of closing defects without tension or grafts.
- Can be utilized for scar revision, by changing the length or direction of a scar.
- This can be useful at cosmetically important sites, such as the face.

Below are some general examples of random pattern local flap options.

Transposition flap (Fig. 14.9A)

- A transposition flap can be of varying shape and is moved laterally into an adjacent defect.
- The angle of movement can be varied, but must leave significant breadth at the base of the flap to ensure vascularity.
- The transposition results in a secondary defect, which can be primarily closed, but often requires another method of closure, such as a skin graft.

Rotation flap (Fig. 14.9B)

- A rotation flap is usually a semi-circular shaped flap, which is rotated into the defect along the outer line of the semi-circle.
- This often necessitates a 'back-cut' to allow sufficient movement, but as with all flaps there must be significant width of tissue left at the base of the flap to ensure its survival.
- The rotation results in a secondary defect, which can often be primarily closed.

Advancement flap (Fig. 14.9C)

- An advancement flap moves tissue into a defect without the use of lateral transposition or rotation.
- They can be of varying shapes, some of which produce:
  - a primary defect to be closed
  - or excess tissue at the flap base which requires excision (Burow's triangles)
  - neither of the above affects the width of the flap base.

Z-plasty (Fig. 14.9D)

- A Z-plasty is composed of two interposing triangular transposition flaps.

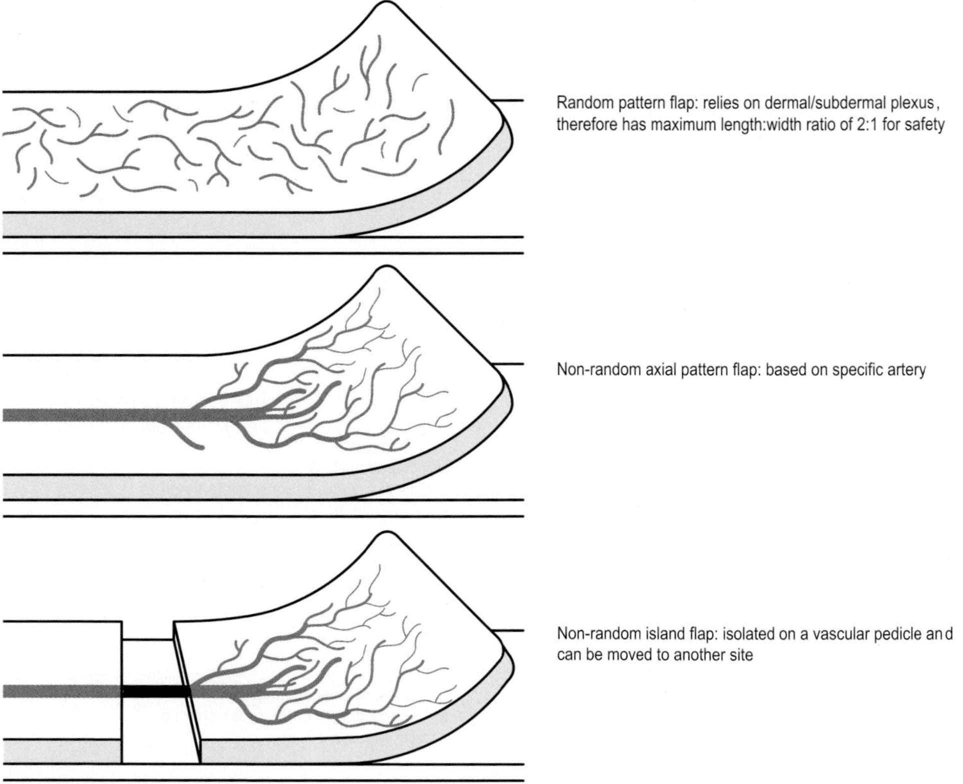

Fig. 14.7 Flaps by vascular supply.

- These can be used to alter the direction of a scar or the length of a scar contracture, depending upon the angles within the triangles of the Z-plasty.

Free flaps (Fig. 14.10)

Free flaps are used in a variety of reconstructive situations including:

- Traumatic reconstruction:
  - open fractures with soft tissue loss
  - injuries with severe degloving or tissue loss
  - burn scar revision.
- Neoplastic/cosmetic reconstruction:
  - post-cancer surgery, e.g. breast reconstruction, mandibular reconstruction
  - tissue coverage post-debridement for necrotizing infections.
- Functional reconstruction:
  - facial or limb re-animation surgery using neurotized flaps.
- Below are some common flaps used in the situations described above.

Radial forearm flap

- Vascular supply from perforating vessels of the radial artery.
- Based on the flexor aspect of the forearm.
- Donor site can be directly closed, but for larger skin requirements needs skin grafting.
- Can be taken with a segment of radius: e.g. for mandibular reconstructions.

Anterolateral thigh flap

- Vascular supply from myocutaneous/septocutaneous perforating vessels of the descending branch of the lateral circumflex artery.
- Based on a line drawn from anterior superior iliac spine to lateral patella.
- Donor site is directly closed.
- Can give large skin paddle.

Deep inferior epigastric perforator (DIEP)/transverse rectus abdominis myocutaneous (TRAM) flap

- Vascular supply from myocutaneous perforating vessels of the deep inferior epigastric artery.

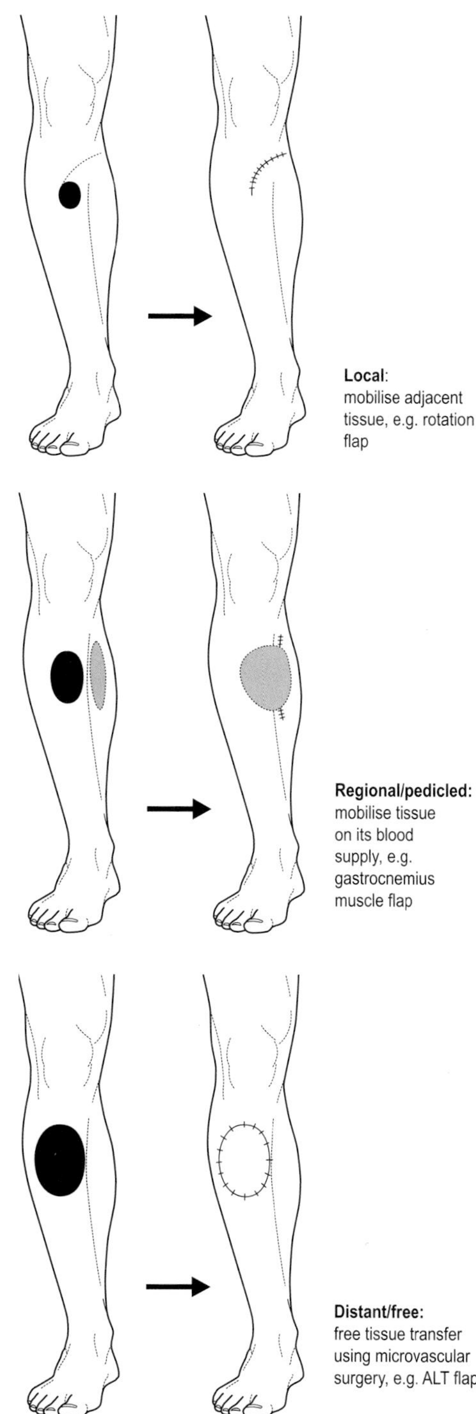

Fig. 14.8 Flaps by location.

- DIEP flap dissects out perforating vessels to preserve rectus muscle and function, in effort to reduce donor site morbidity, i.e. hernias.
- TRAM flaps take varying amount of muscle with the flap.
- Donor site is directly closed.
- Can give a large skin paddle with an acceptable abdominoplasty donor scar.

Bone

- Haematoma resulting from ruptured bone vessels and periosteal vessels forms between the ends of the fracture.
- Macrophages invade the haematoma together with polymorphs and fibroblasts; new vessels form, fibrosis occurs and by the end of the first week the clot is organized.
- Osteoblasts grow into the haematoma and form trabeculae of woven bone.
- The new bone (sometimes with islands of cartilage formed by chondroblasts) is called callus.
- Internal callus lies within the medullary cavity.
- External callus is related to the periosteum and envelops the fracture site, acting as a 'splint'.
- By 2–3 weeks the repair tissue reaches its maximum girth in long bone, but is still too weak to support weight.
- Woven bone is subsequently replaced by lamellar bone.
- Remodelling takes place according to the direction of mechanical stress.
- Restoration to normal may take up to 1 year.

Factors Affecting Bone Healing

- Movement.
- Misalignment.
- Interposition of soft tissues.
- Infection.
- Pre-existing bone disease.

Liver

- Hepatocytes have excellent regenerative capacity.
- Following surgical resection of areas of the liver for trauma, regeneration is rapid and full recovery of the organ's mass occurs and the architecture is maintained.
- When the injurious agent persists – e.g. viral damage, alcohol abuse, autoimmune disease – fibrosis occurs, cirrhosis develops and the architecture is lost.
- Damage that destroys hepatocytes only may be followed by complete restitution.
- Damage that destroys hepatocytes and the architecture may not be followed by complete restitution.

Kidney

- Epithelium can regenerate.
- Architecture cannot regenerate.

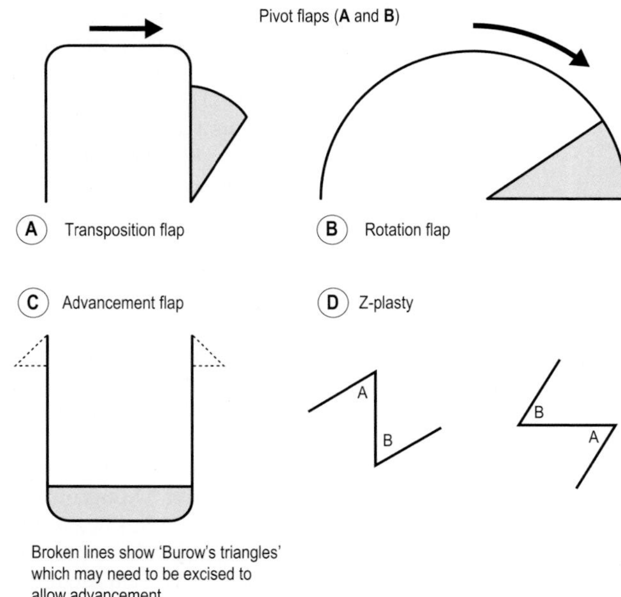

Fig. 14.9 Local flaps by design. Pivot flaps: (A) transposition flap and (B) rotation flap (these flaps are termed pivot flaps as they move around a pivot point). (C) Advancement flap. (D) Z-plasty.

- Loss of tubular epithelium, e.g. ischaemia, toxins, will recover provided enough normal epithelial cells are left to regenerate.
- Loss of glomeruli (glomerulonephritis) is likely to be permanent.

Cardiac Muscle

- Permanent cells and therefore no regeneration.
- Damaged muscle replaced by scar tissue.
- Important in myocardial infarction
- May result in ventricular aneurysm due to weakening of wall.

Neural Tissue

- Permanent cells; regeneration does not occur in the central nervous system.
- Peripheral nerves undergo Wallerian degeneration distal to the site of trauma. Recovery is variable depending upon alignment and continuity.

Peritoneum

- Sutured peritoneum may result in local ischaemia, which acts as a stimulus to adhesion formation, especially if contaminated with foreign material.
- A clean unsutured defect, no matter how large, will usually heal without adhesions.
- Perivascular connective tissue cells in the base of the defect grow towards the surface and differentiate into new mesothelial cells.
- Centripetal growth from the wound margins contributes little to mesothelial healing.
- Healing of the unsutured peritoneum is rapid and complete, irrespective of the size of the defect, and occurs with little risk of adhesion formation.

Gastrointestinal Tract

Mucosal Erosions

An erosion is loss of part of the thickness of the mucosa.

- Erosions regenerate rapidly from adjacent viable epithelial cells.
- Erosions can repair in a matter of a few hours if the cause is removed.
- Erosions can cause significant gastrointestinal (GI) bleeds but escape detection by endoscopy a few hours later as rapid healing has occurred.

Mucosal Ulcers

- Loss of full thickness of the mucosa.
- Repaired by granulation tissue in base and centripetal growth of surface epithelium.
- If cause persists, the ulcer may become chronic with considerable fibrous scarring, e.g. pyloric stenosis with chronic duodenal ulceration.

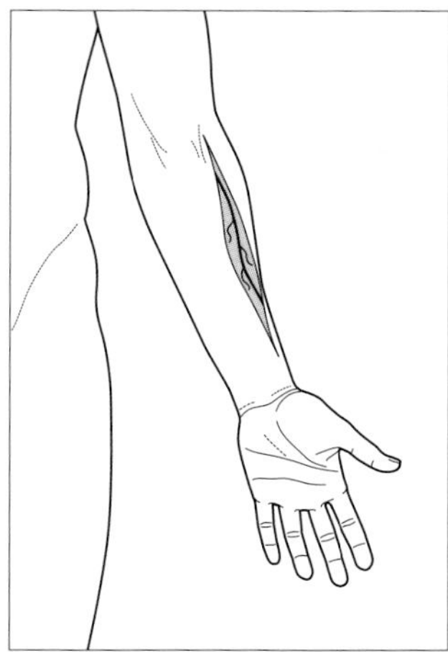

Free radial forearm flap—branches of radial artery and skin paddle

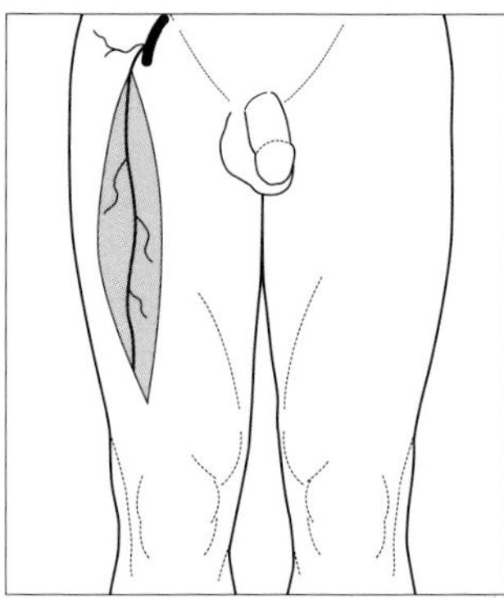

Anterolateral thigh flap—branches of lateral femoral circumflex artery and skin paddle

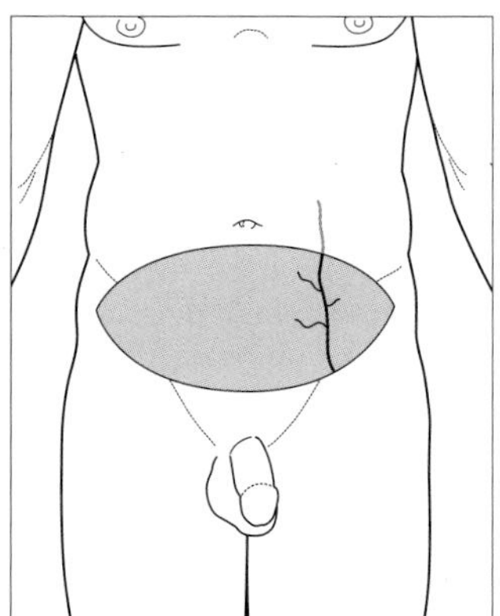

DIEP/TRAM flap—branches of the deep inferior epigastric artery and skin paddle

Fig. 14.10 Free flaps.

Gastrointestinal Anastomoses

- Healing better in upper GI tract; stomach and small bowel heal better than colon.
- Very dependent upon blood supply.
- Interrupted sutures with suturing of only the sero-muscular layers prevent ischaemia of the mucosa and allow good mucosal healing.

Factors Affecting Wound Healing

Local

- Inadequate blood supply.
- Haematoma.
- Infection.
- Early movement (especially delayed fracture healing).
- Foreign material, e.g. sutures, extraneous foreign bodies.
- Irradiation.
- Denervation, e.g. peripheral neuropathy (diabetes, neuropathic ulcers).
- Leprosy.
- Charcot's joints (joint does not repair).

Systemic

- Nutritional problems, e.g. malnutrition, vitamin C deficiency (required for collagen synthesis), zinc deficiency.
- Drugs, e.g. steroids, immunosuppressive drugs, cytotoxic agents.
- Neoplasia.
- Diabetes mellitus: affects polymorph function, microvascular disease, neuropathy.
- Age: younger patients heal better than older patients.
- Jaundice.
- Uraemia.

INJURY DUE TO IONIZING RADIATION

Biological response to irradiation depends on:

- physical factors, i.e. dose, character, time of exposure
- chemical factors, e.g. substrates for generation of free radicals
- biological factors, i.e. phase of cell cycle at time of exposure.

Individuals may be exposed to irradiation in several ways:

- Background:
    - natural sources:
        - cosmic
        - terrestrial
        - airborne
        - food sources
    - artificial sources
        - diagnostic X-rays
        - nuclear power industry.
- Accidental:
    - Chernobyl disaster.
- Occupational:
    - radiologists
    - mining of uranium.
- Medical:
    - diagnostic tests.

Mode of Action

Following the passage of ionizing radiation through tissues, several types of free radicals are formed from water in the cells. Short-lived and highly reactive free radicals (e.g. $H^•$ and $OH^•$) are formed. In well-oxygenated cells, oxygen free radicals (e.g. $HO_2^•$ and $O_2^{•-}$) are also formed. These radicals interact with macromolecules (e.g. membrane lipids and DNA) and cause damage.

The types of radiation-induced DNA damage include:

- strand breaks
- base alterations
- cross-linking.

The resulting DNA damage may have three possible consequences:

- cell death, either immediately or at the next attempted mitosis
- repair and no further damage
- a permanent change in genotype.

The outcome will depend upon the dose given and the radiosensitivity of the cell. Rapidly dividing cell populations are the most sensitive.

Effects on Tissues

These may be acute or chronic.

- Acute:
  - result in cell death
  - most marked in cells that are dividing rapidly, e.g. gut epithelium, bone marrow, skin, gonads
  - vascular endothelial damage results in fluid and protein leakage into the tissue, causing inflammation.
- Chronic:
  - damage to endothelium results in exposure of underlying collagen with platelet adherence and thrombosis
  - results in intimal proliferation and development of endarteritis obliterans
  - this results in long-term vascular insufficiency and consequent atrophy and fibrosis
  - radiation-induced mutation of the genome increases risks of neoplasia.

Effect on Individual Tissues

Bone Marrow

- Suspends renewal of all cell lines.
- Granulocytes are reduced before erythrocytes, which survive longer.
- Outcome depends on dose used.
- Varies from complete recovery to aplastic anaemia.
- Increased incidence of leukaemia in long-term survivors.

Skin

- Cessation of mitosis in epidermis with desquamation and hair loss.
- Regrowth will occur if enough basal stem cells survive.
- Damage to melanocytes results in melanin release into tissues, where it is ingested by phagocytes, which remain in the tissue, resulting in hyperpigmentation.
- Destruction of dermal fibroblasts results in inability to produce collagen, and therefore thinning of the dermis.
- Damage to small vessels results in thinning of the wall, dilatation and tortuosity, and the formation of telangiectasia.

Intestines

- Loss of surface epithelium results in diarrhoea.
- Damage of full thickness with fibrosis will result in stricture formation.

Gonads

- Extremely radiosensitive.
- Sterility may result with low doses.
- Mutations may occur in germ cells, with resultant teratogenic effect.

Lung

- Progressive pulmonary fibrosis may occur.
- Inhaled radioactive materials may induce pulmonary tumours.

Kidney

- Gradual loss of parenchyma results in impaired renal function.
- Endarteritis obliterans of small vessels will cause intrarenal renal artery stenosis and hypertension.

Whole-Body Irradiation

- As the dose increases, so does the severity and rapidity of the onset of the effects.
- Total body irradiation may be used therapeutically to ablate the bone marrow prior to marrow transplantation with either autologous stored marrow or from another donor.
- A very high dose results in CNS damage, with coma and convulsions occurring within hours. As the dose reduces, gut damage occurs within a few days; with further reduction, marrow failure can occur in weeks; and at low doses there are no immediate effects, although there is a long-term risk of neoplasia.

Ultraviolet Light

- Non-ionizing radiation does not penetrate deeply.
- Has a range of wavelengths.
- May act by inducing thymine dimers in DNA, nondimer damage, or inhibiting DNA repair processes.

- Tumours produced are basal cell carcinomas, squamous cell carcinomas and malignant melanomas.

Therapeutic Irradiation

Radiotherapy can be used therapeutically in three ways:

- With a view to a cure (radical radiotherapy).
- Adjuvant.
- Palliative.

Radical Applications

- Basal cell and squamous cell carcinoma of the skin.
- Some head and neck tumours and laryngeal tumours.
- Hodgkin's disease.
- Lymph node metastases of a testicular seminoma following orchidectomy.

Adjuvant Radiotherapy

This is aimed at clinically undetectable metastases due to spread locally or into the regional lymph nodes, e.g. carcinoma of the breast giving radiotherapy to the scar, axillary nodes, supraclavicular nodes and internal mammary nodes.

Palliative Radiotherapy

- Bony metastases: pain relief is often dramatic.
- Cerebral metastases.
- Ulcerating or fungating breast cancer: controls oozing and bleeding and allows skin healing.
- Lung cancer to prevent cough and haemoptysis.

Fractionation of Dose

- A higher dose of radiation may be given without increasing side effects if it is divided into a number of fractions and given on different days with a break in between.
- Normal cells are better able to repair than neoplastic cells.
- Results in differential cell killing of more tumour cells than normal cells.

Response Modifiers

- Low oxygen tension in tissues reduces sensitivity of tumours, probably due to fewer oxygen free radicals.
- Compounding this is the fact that tumours may be relatively avascular and the patient may be anaemic: therefore, transfusion may help.
- Radiosensitizers that enter neoplastic tissue may enhance response to radiotherapy. Experimental work with these is in progress, but none is in current clinical use.

Injury Due to Burns

- Common form of trauma in the UK:
  - approximately 250,000 burns per year, of which 70% are seen in A&E
  - approximately 300 deaths per year.
- Incidence differs between age groups:
  - 0–14 years = 30% of burns
  - 15–64 years = 60% of burns
  - 65+ years = 10% of burns.
- Aetiology differs between age groups:
  - children suffer more scalds
  - adults suffer more flame burns
  - elderly suffer more scald and contact burns.
- Repatriated military burns are an increasing group to consider.

Types of Burn

Thermal

- Flame – can be associated with inhalation injury.
- Scalds – usually hot drinks or bath water.
- Contact – often associated with loss of consciousness, medical conditions or intoxication.

Electrical

- Caused by an electrical current passing through the body; will have an 'entry' and 'exit' point.
- If the path of the electricity crosses the chest, it can affect the myocardium and produce arrhythmias.
- Low-voltage injuries are <1000 volts; usually domestic; burn the entry and exit points.
- High-voltage injuries are >1000 volts; usually industrial; can burn internal tissue, causing rhabdomyolysis.
- 'Flash' injuries occur when an arc of high-voltage electrical current occurs near to the patient, causing thermal burns, but no electrical current passes through them.

Chemical

- Caused by acids or alkalis in domestic or industrial settings.
- Can be very deep and can continue to burn unless the source is removed.
- Particular agents require specific treatments: e.g. hydrofluoric acid requires calcium gluconate, as it can cause lethal hypocalcaemia.

Causes of Burns

- Accidents:
  - domestic (most common)
  - road traffic accidents
  - industrial/workplace.
- Intoxication (alcohol/drugs).
- Suicide/self-harm.
- Assault/abuse.

Predisposing Medical Conditions

- Epilepsy.
- Dementia.

- Motor/sensory dysfunction, e.g. paralysis.
- Learning disability.
- Mental health issues.

Burn Injury Response

Burn injuries result in both local and systemic responses.

Local Response (Fig. 14.11)

Burn injury results in varying degrees of three-dimensional tissue damage, illustrated by Jackson's burn wound model:

- Zone of necrosis:
  - area of maximum damage
  - suffers rapid and irreversible cell death due to coagulation of cellular proteins.
- Zone of stasis:
  - adjacent to the zone of necrosis
  - compromised tissue perfusion due to damaged microcirculation
  - can progress to necrotic tissue if left untreated or inadequately resuscitated.
- Zone of hyperaemia:
  - outermost burn zone, adjacent to zone of stasis
  - tissue perfusion is increased due to local inflammatory mediator release
  - will usually completely recover.
- When referring to the dynamic nature of burns, it is the changeability of the zone of stasis to which we refer, i.e. the ability of a burn to progress to a deeper burn or appear more superficial.
- Factors which can influence this progression include:
  - hypoperfusion
  - infection
  - oedema.

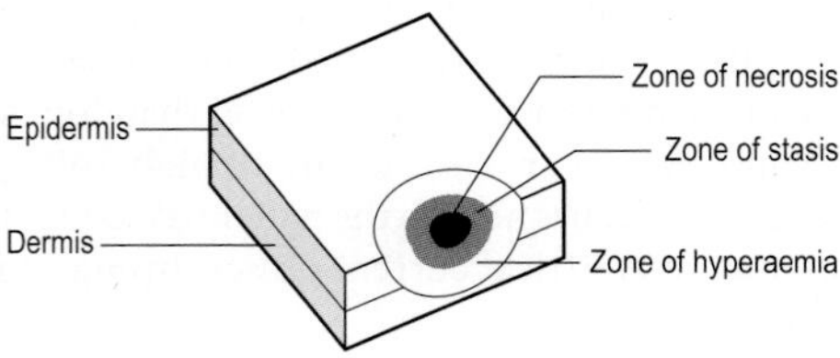

If adequately resuscitated the burn may progress to:

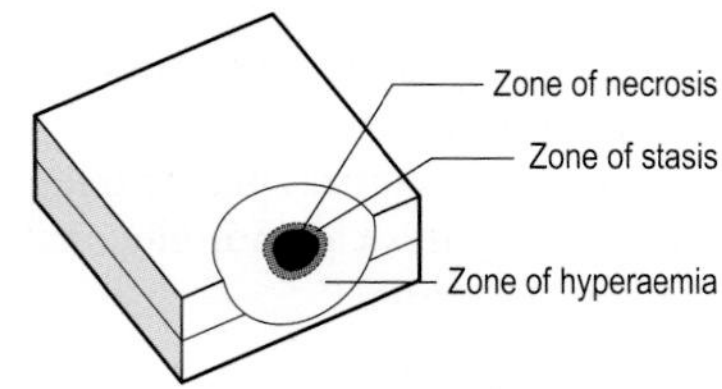

If inadequately resuscitated the burn may progress to:

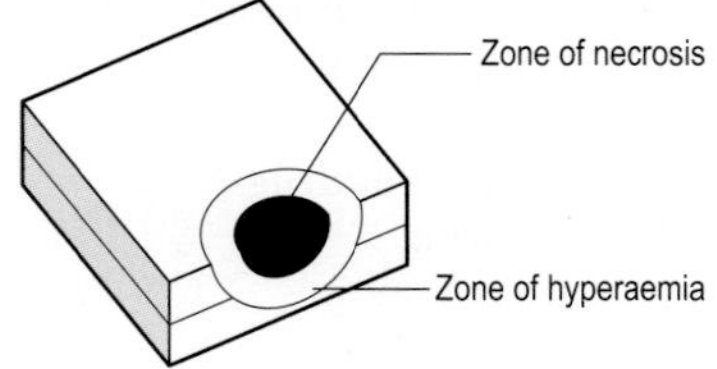

Fig. 14.11 Jackson's burn wound model and dynamic changes.

Systemic Response

Usually seen in burns of over 20%, where massive inflammatory mediator release causes changes in the following systems:

- Cardiovascular:
  - vasodilatation and increased capillary permeability cause intravascular protein loss and oedema
  - peripheral and splanchnic vasoconstriction
  - combined result of hypovolaemia, tachycardia, hypotension and increased systemic vascular resistance.
- Respiratory:
  - inhalation of hot gases causing thermal injury to the upper airways, resulting in inflammation and life-threatening airway oedema
  - inhalation of toxic combustion products (carbon monoxide, cyanide, nitrogen and sulfur oxides, etc.), causing severe respiratory compromise or acute lung injury
  - circumferential burns to the chest can restrict expansion, furthering respiratory compromise
  - inflammatory mediators create bronchoconstriction and oedema, and can lead to adult respiratory distress syndrome (ARDS).
- Metabolic:
  - basal metabolic rate can triple, causing massive catabolic changes and inducing muscle wasting
  - electrolyte disturbances, including hypo- or hypernatraemia, hyperkalaemia and hypocalcaemia.
- Musculoskeletal:
  - circumferential limb burns can compromise limb perfusion due to swelling limb contents not accommodated by inelastic eschar of burnt skin
  - compartment syndrome can follow prolonged periods of immobility due to unconsciousness or electrical injury through a limb/compartment.
- Renal:
  - hypoperfusion of kidneys due to hypovolaemia can result in acute renal failure
  - tissue injury releases myoglobin, which produces rhabdomyolysis and results in acute tubular necrosis and renal failure.

- Immunological:
  - depression of cellular and humoral immune responses, increasing risk of sepsis
  - systemic inflammatory response syndrome and resulting multi-organ failure.
- Gastrointestinal:
  - gut function impairment, leading to barrier breakdown and bacterial translocation
  - gastric ulceration due to stress response (Curling's ulcer).
- Skin:
  - barrier function of skin lost, increasing infection risk and fluid loss.

Carbon Monoxide Effects

- Colourless, odourless gas caused by incomplete oxidation of carbon.
- Detectable in blood of smokers in low levels.
- Produces different symptoms at different levels (Table 14.2).
- Has an affinity for haemoglobin 250 times that of oxygen and binds strongly to form carboxyhaemoglobin (COHb).
- Reduces the ability of the blood to transport oxygen, resulting in respiratory compromise.
- Reduces oxygen available for cytochromes, resulting in abnormal cellular functioning and occasionally encephalopathy.
- Victims seem confused, disorientated and nauseous, and can be dismissed as intoxicated.
- Treatment is by displacing COHb with oxygen – COHb has a half-life of 250 minutes in room oxygen levels and 40 minutes with 100% oxygen.

TABLE 14.2 Carboxyhaemoglobin (COHb) and Systemic Effects

COHb % in blood	Systemic effects
0–15	Nil
15–20	Confusion, headache
20–40	Disorientation, nausea, lethargy
40–60	Ataxia, hallucinations, collapse, seizures
60+	Death

Assessing a Burn

Assessment of a burn takes into account:

- the extent of body surface area burnt
- the depth of the burn.

The Extent of Body Surface Area Burnt (Fig. 14.12)

To estimate the percentage of the total body surface area of the burn (% TBSA) there are two general methods:

- The palmar surface method:
  - useful for smaller or patchy burns
  - utilizes the principle that the patient's palmar surface is roughly equal to 1% of their body surface area.
- The 'rule of nines' method:
  - divides the adult body into areas based on single or multiple 9% anatomical blocks
  - paediatric 'rule of nines' slightly altered due to different anatomical proportions; charts used
  - useful for larger burns where estimation is essential for fluid resuscitation.

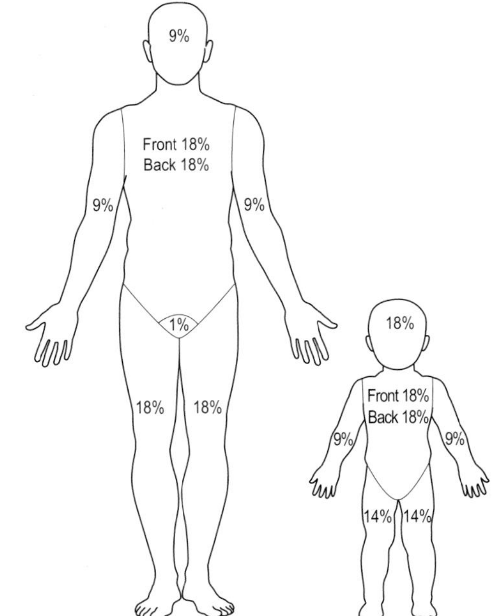

Fig. 14.12 Adult and paediatric rule of 9s.

The Depth of the Burn (Fig. 14.13)

- Estimation of burn depth can be difficult, though the clinical features of the burn can help the decision.
- Diagnostic tools can be useful, such as laser Doppler imaging to assess areas of skin perfusion.
- In practice, the majority of burns are of mixed depth, and careful, repeated assessment is needed to ensure correct depth diagnosis.
- Remember that burn depth can be dynamic, and insufficient resuscitation, infection or oedema can increase the percentage of a deep burn.

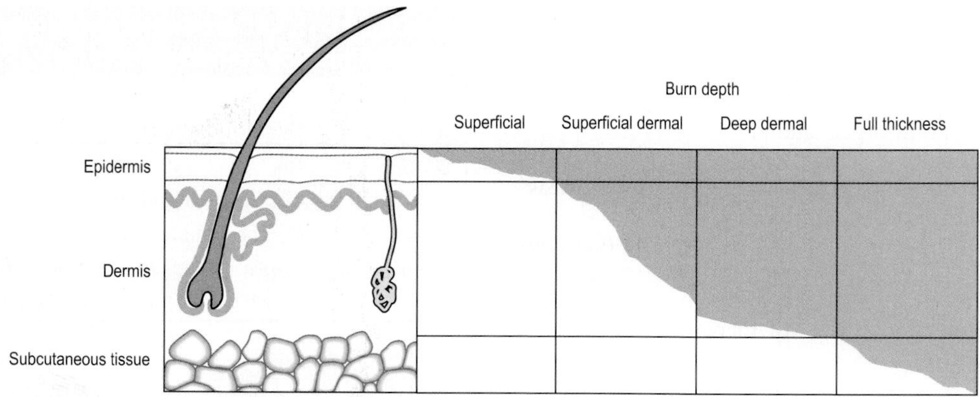

Fig. 14.13 Cross-section of skin showing depth of burn.

In general, burns can be classified from superficial to deep, depending upon the amount of epidermis, dermis and underlying tissue that has been damaged.

- Superficial epidermal burns:
  - involve the epidermis alone and are often called erythema
  - appear red but with no blistering of the skin
  - commonly caused by sunburn, superficial scalds or 'flash' burns
  - have good capillary refill on examination and intact sensation
  - can be very painful
  - will heal within 7 days from the basal epidermis, with no scarring
  - are NOT counted as part of the total body surface area burn estimation.
- Superficial dermal burns:
  - involve the epidermis and the papillary dermis
  - appear pink, oedematous and blistered
  - commonly caused by minor flame and scald burns
  - have good capillary refill on examination and intact sensation
  - can be extremely painful
  - will heal within 10–14 days from the adnexal structures, with little or no scarring
  - are counted as part of the total body surface area burn estimation.
- Deep dermal burns:
  - involve the epidermis, the papillary dermis and the reticular dermis
  - appear red and often have fixed staining or petechial points
  - commonly caused by flame, chemical, contact and scald burns
  - have reduced or absent capillary refill on examination and reduced or absent sensation
  - often not as painful as the more superficial burns
  - will not heal within 14 days and will leave significant scarring
  - are counted as part of the total body surface area burn estimation.
- Full-thickness burns:
  - involve the epidermis, the entire dermis and possibly fat, muscle and even bone
  - appear thick and can be either white or black and charred (eschar)
  - commonly caused by significant flame or chemical burns
  - have absent capillary refill on examination and absent sensation
  - are painless as all nerve endings are gone
  - will not heal within 14 days and will leave significant scarring
  - are counted as part of the total body surface area burn estimation.
- Circumferential burns:
  - on the thorax, may restrict chest wall movement
  - on the limbs, may compromise limb vascularity
  - escharotomy may be required; escharotomy placement sites and their relevant anatomy are shown in Fig. 14.14.

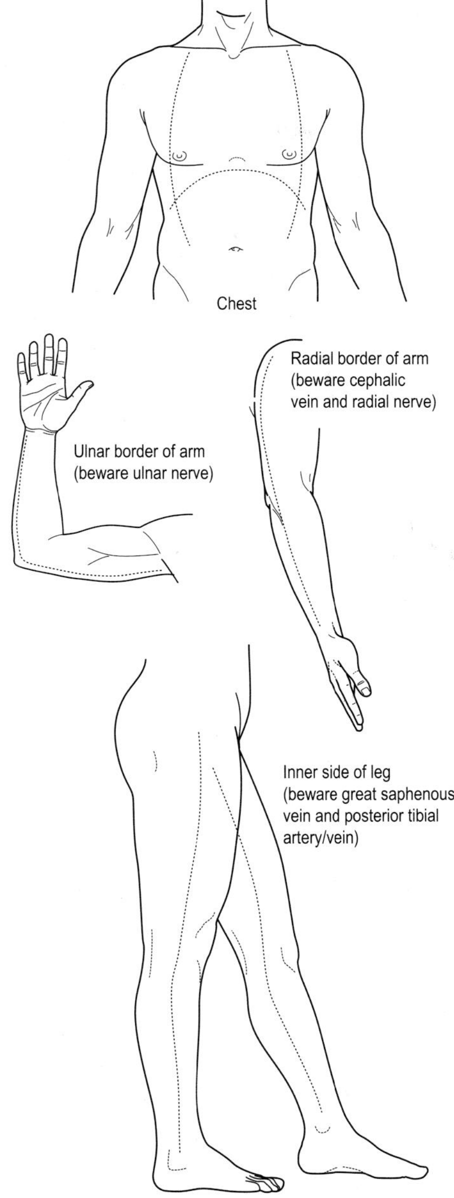

Fig. 14.14 Lines of escharotomy placement.

OSCE SCENARIOS

OSCE Scenario 14.1

A 77-year-old female presents to your clinic with a suspicious-looking lesion on her temple.

1. Outline your history, examination, investigations and management plan.
2. Draw around the lesion on the diagram (Fig. 14.1Q) to indicate your surgical margins and direction of incision. The pathology report of the lesion indicates an incompletely excised, poorly differentiated squamous cell carcinoma with ulceration. A multi-disciplinary skin cancer meeting suggests re-excision of the scar with a 1 cm margin.
3. Outline your options for closing this defect.
4. Explain the pathological findings and management plan to the patient, including her follow-up.

OSCE Scenario 14.2

You are the A&E doctor in a district general hospital at 3 am. A 33-year-old male has been trapped in a fire in his home, and had to be rescued from the house by the fire brigade, who think the fire started at around 1 am. He has superficial non-blistering burns to his face with soot around his nose, and blistering burns to the whole of his left leg and arm, including his hand. He appears confused and the ambulance crew think he may be intoxicated.

1. Approximately what percentage is this man's burn? What features would you use to assess the depth of the blistered burn?

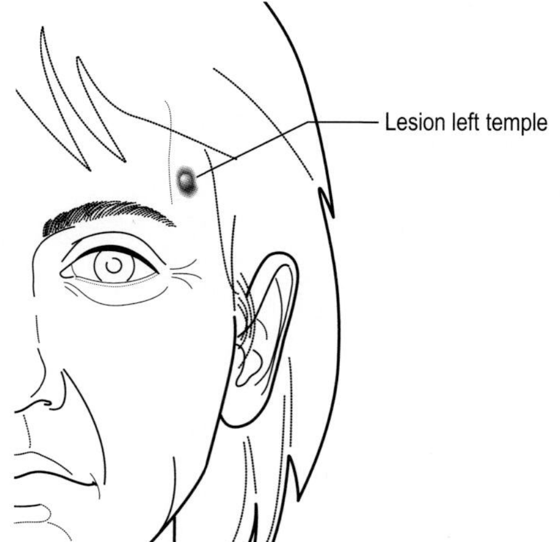

Fig. 14.1Q Indicate surgical margins and direction of incision.

2. Assuming that his facial burns are epidermal and his arm/leg burns are full-thickness, calculate this man's fluid resuscitation requirements and detail how this should be administered.
3. What acute injuries and pathology specific to burns would this man be at risk of from the above description?
4. Which allied medical staff would you like to involve?

OSCE Scenario 14.3

You see a 63-year-old male in clinic who describes a 2-year history of an ulcer on his leg. He has been self-managing the wound with dressings from the pharmacy, but recently it has become malodorous and his children encouraged him to seek medical advice.

1. What salient features from this gentleman's history would you like to know?
2. What is your differential diagnosis?
3. Describe the factors affecting wound healing.
   On further questioning the patient tells you he has previously had radiotherapy to this limb for a 'kind of skin cancer'.
4. What effects does radiotherapy have on the body? How does this change your differential diagnosis?

OSCE Scenario 14.4

A 79-year-old diabetic has neglected a foot infection and is admitted extremely unwell. The whole forefoot is black, wet and malodorous.

1. What type of necrosis has occurred in the foot?
2. What clinical term is used for this type of tissue loss?
3. What would be the clinical management of this patient?

OSCE Scenario 14.5

A 53-year-old female is in the breast cancer clinic following surgery for a right-sided breast tumour. As you are taking a history she tells you she has also had ovarian cancer and that a close relative had a brain tumour and a rare muscle tumour.

1. Do you know of any inherited condition that relates to all these tumours?
2. What does p53 normally do and how does it lead to neoplasia when genetic abnormalities occur?

Answers in Appendix pages 461–464

Please check your eBook at https://studentconsult.inkling.com/ for more self-assessment questions. See inside cover for registration details.

15

Disorders of Growth, Morphogenesis and Differentiation

GROWTH

Growth is the process of increase in size resulting from the synthesis of specific tissue components.

Physiological growth takes place by several mechanisms:

- multiplicative: increase in number of cells, e.g. in all tissues during embryogenesis
- auxetic: increase in size of cells, e.g. in growing skeletal muscle
- accretionary: increase in intercellular tissue component, e.g. growing bone
- combined patterns, e.g. in embryological development.

Cell Turnover

Growth depends on the balance between an increase in cell numbers due to proliferation and the decrease in cell numbers due to cell death. Regeneration is covered in Chapter 14.

Cell Cycle

- Cells proliferate by undergoing mitosis.
- Mitosis is only a small part of the cell cycle.
- The length of the cell cycle determines the cell kinetics of a tissue.

Phases of the Cell Cycle (Fig. 15.1)

Four main stages to the cell cycle are:

- M phase: comprising nuclear division (mitosis) and cytoplasmic division (cytokinesis).
- G_1 phase (gap 1): duration varies between cell types.
- S phase: DNA synthesis occurs.
- G_2 phase (gap 2).

Other factors involved in the cell cycle

- G_0 phase: cells can leave the cell cycle temporarily and re-enter later; said to be in the G_0 phase.
- Cells can leave the G_1 phase permanently, lose the ability to undergo mitosis, and become terminally differentiated cells.
- Differences in cell cycle times that characterize different tissues are related to the G_1 duration, which may last days or even years.
- Once a cell has passed out of G_1, the cell cycle proceeds to completion.
- S, G_2 and M phases of the cycle are remarkably constant and independent of the rate of cell division.

Control of Cell Division

- The cell cycle requires activating signals.
- Activating signals are provided by cyclins, which activate a number of proteins involved in various phases of the cycle, e.g. DNA replication, spindle formation.
- Inhibitory signals come from tumour suppressor genes, e.g. p53 and cyclin-dependent kinase inhibitors.
- Removal of the growth-inhibiting action of the retinoblastoma gene allows growth to proceed.
- Protein growth factors direct the proliferation of different types of cell, regulating cell population densities, e.g.:
  - epidermal growth factor (EGF)
  - platelet-derived growth factor (PDGF)
  - insulin-like growth factor (IGF-1).
- Growth factors act on cells in G_0 phase, leading to DNA synthesis followed by cell division.

Therapeutic Interruptions of Cell Cycle (Fig. 15.2)

- Various cancer chemotherapeutic agents act at specific parts of the cell cycle.
- Attack rapidly dividing cancer cells.
- May attack rapidly dividing normal cells, e.g. bone marrow, lymphoid tissue, resulting in anaemia, thrombocytopaenia and immunosuppression.

Factors Affecting Growth

Normal growth requires a number of factors whose absence may result in limited or abnormal growth. These include:

- genetic factors
- hormones
- nutrition
- blood supply
- oxygen supply
- nerve supply
- growth factors.

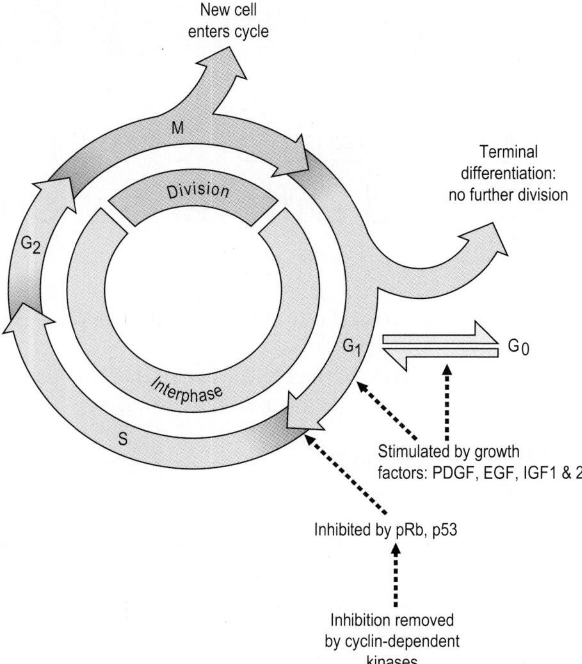

Fig. 15.1 The cell cycle. The four main stages of the cell cycle are the M phase (mitosis and cytokinesis, i.e. cell division) and the interface stages G_1 (gap 1), S phase (DNA synthesis) and G_2 (gap 2). Cells may enter a resting phase, G_0, which may be of variable duration, followed by re-entry into the G_1 phase. Some cells may terminally differentiate from the G_1 phase, with no further cell division and death at the end of the normal lifetime of the cell. The sites at which growth factors and inhibitors act are shown. (From Underwood JCE (ed). General and Systematic Pathology, 4th edn. Churchill Livingstone, Edinburgh, 2004, with permission.)

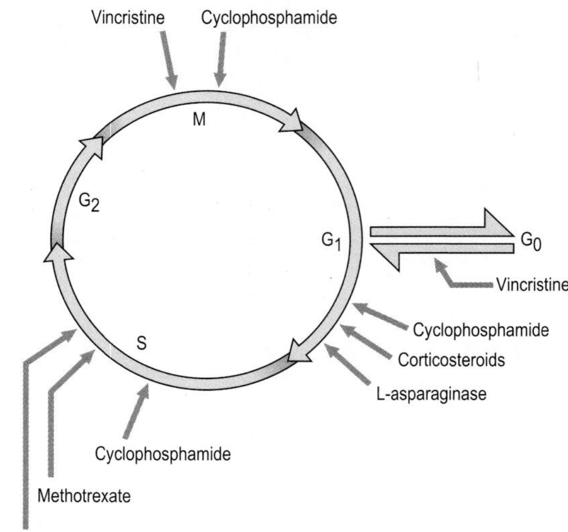

Fig. 15.2 Pharmacological interruption of the cell cycle: the sites of action in the cell cycle of drugs that may be used in the treatment of cancer. (From Underwood JCE (ed). General and Systematic Pathology, 4th edn. Churchill Livingstone, Edinburgh, 2004, with permission.)

Genetic Factors

- Achondroplasia (dwarfism): a primary disturbance of endochondral ossification occurring in early fetal life. An autosomal dominant condition.
- Beckwith–Wiedemann syndrome: increased growth due to duplication of short arm of chromosome 11 where the genes for insulin and somatomedin IGF-2 reside, resulting in excessive growth.

Hormones

- General body size is controlled by growth hormone (GH) from the anterior pituitary gland.
- GH release is stimulated by hypothalamic growth hormone releasing factor (GHRF) and inhibited by somatostatin.
- GH stimulates release of somatomedin IGF-1 and IGF-2 from the liver; these act on target tissue such as muscle and bone.
- Reduced growth may be due to:
  - reduced GH production resulting in proportionate dwarfism, which is corrected by GH injections prior to puberty (when skeletal growth arrests due to epiphyseal fusion)
  - reduced GH receptors (Laron dwarfism): circulating GH is high but the liver is insensitive to GH; treatment with GH does not increase growth rate
  - reduced thyroid hormone secretion causes reduced hepatic IGF-1 secretion. Dwarfism results with stunted limbs because bone ossification is reduced. GH injections do not help, but thyroxin given before puberty is corrective.
- Increased growth may be due to:
  - increased pituitary GH. Before puberty this results in gigantism; after puberty (after epiphyseal fusion), acromegaly results.

Nutrition

- General catabolic states may cause poor growth.

- Starvation in the form of kwashiorkor (protein deprivation) or marasmus (protein and total calorie deprivation) disturb growth.

Blood Supply

- Maldevelopment of a vessel can lead to non-development of the organ it should supply.
- Epidermal atrophy occurs in the skin of the lower limbs with chronic ischaemia due to arterial disease.
- Increased blood flow, e.g. arteriovenous fistula, may cause increase in size of a limb.

Oxygen Supply

- Infants born at altitudes of 15,000 feet have a 16% lower birth weight due to reduced intrauterine oxygen availability.

Nerve Supply

- Loss of muscle innervation causes muscle atrophy, e.g. poliomyelitis, nerve injury.
- Loss of whole limb innervation causes disuse atrophy of bone.

Growth Factors

- PDGF, EGF and IGFs act locally in healing skin by stimulation of basal cell division.

Increased Growth

Growth may occur in relation to physiological or pathological stimuli by the following mechanisms:

- Hypertrophy: increase in cell size without cell replication.
- Hyperplasia: increase in cell number due to cell division.
- A combination of the two.
- The stimuli for hypertrophy and hyperplasia are similar.
- In permanent cells, hypertrophy is the only adaptive option as the cells cannot divide.
- A decreased cell loss by apoptosis is an important component of hyperplasia.
- Hyperplasia and hypertrophy are reversible when the stimulus is removed.
- Hyperplasia and hypertrophy may be physiological or pathological.

Physiological Hypertrophy and Hyperplasia

Examples include:

- muscle hypertrophy in athletes
- hyperplasia of bone marrow at high altitude
- hyperplasia of breast tissue, e.g. puberty, pregnancy, lactation
- hypertrophy and hyperplasia of uterus in pregnancy
- thyroid hyperplasia as result of increased metabolic demands at puberty and pregnancy.

Pathological Hypertrophy

- Myocardial hypertrophy and hypertension.

Pathological Hyperplasia

- Grave's disease.
- Endometrium exposed to excess oestrogen.

Atrophy

Atrophy is a decrease in size due to loss of cells or reduction in size of individual cells. It may be reversible when stimulus returns, with certain exceptions, e.g. heart muscle, neurons. Organ atrophy may be due to:

- reduction in cell size
- reduction in cell numbers
- both of these.

For atrophy to occur there must be:

- cessation of growth
- reduction in cell size and/or cell numbers mediated by apoptosis.

Atrophy may be physiological or pathological.

Physiological (Box 15.1)

- Occurs any time from early embryological life to old age.

BOX 15.1 Tissues Involved in Physiological Atrophy and Involution

Embryo and fetus
Branchial clefts
Notochord
Thyroglossal duct
Müllerian duct (males)
Wolffian duct (females)

Neonate
Umbilical vessels
Ductus arteriosus
Fetal layer adrenal cortex

Early adult
Thymus

Late adult and old age
Uterus, endometrium (females)
Testes (males)
Bones (particularly females)
Gums
Mandible (particularly edentulous)
Cerebrum
Lymphoid tissue

Pathological

- Decreased function, e.g. muscle atrophy of limb after immobilization for fracture treatment.
- Loss of innervation, leading to muscle and bone atrophy (osteoporosis), e.g. poliomyelitis, spinal cord injuries.
- Loss of blood supply, e.g. following tissue hypoxia, epidermal atrophy is seen in the skin of lower limbs in chronic ischaemia.
- Pressure atrophy, e.g. destruction of skin and subcutaneous tissue as in bed sores.
- Lack of nutrition, e.g. cachexia in severe starvation, gut atrophy in starvation.
- Loss of endocrine stimulation, e.g. hypophysectomy results in adrenal atrophy due to lack of stimulation from ACTH.
- Hormone-induced atrophy, e.g. oestrogens and testicular atrophy, corticosteroids and adrenal atrophy (via 'negative feedback' reduction of ACTH).

Decreased Growth (Hypoplasia)

Hypoplasia is the failure of an organ to attain its normal size. It is a failure of morphogenesis, although closely related to atrophy and pathogenesis. Examples include:

- congenital adrenal hypoplasia associated with anencephaly or pituitary hypoplasia (no ACTH)
- failure of lower limb development in spina bifida.

DIFFERENTIATION

This is the process whereby a cell develops a specialized function that was not present in the parent cell. Differentiation is an important part of morphogenesis; growth also plays an important part in morphogenesis.

Control of Differentiation

In the fetus, differentiation is controlled by:

- genes
- systemic hormones
- local growth factors
- position within the fetus
- matrix proteins.

Differentiation and morphogenesis may be disturbed by environmental factors, e.g. teratogens, such as:

- irradiation
- drugs
- infections.

During embryonic development, cell determination and differentiation occur by transcriptional modifications to genomic expression. There is no increase or decrease in the number of genes present.

MORPHOGENESIS

Morphogenesis is a highly complex process of development of structural form and shape of organs, limbs, etc., from primitive cell masses during embryogenesis. It involves cell growth and differentiation and relative movement of cell groups. Unwanted features are removed by apoptosis.

Congenital Disorders of Differentiation and Morphogenesis

Chromosomal Abnormalities Affecting Whole Chromosomes

- Autosomal chromosomes, e.g. trisomy 21 (Down's syndrome).
- Sex chromosomes, e.g. Klinefelter's syndrome (47 XXY), Turner's syndrome (45 X).

Chromosomal Abnormalities Affecting Parts of Chromosomes

- Cri-du-chat syndrome (46 XX 5p–, or 46 XY 5p–, i.e. deletion of short arm of chromosome 5).

Single Gene Alterations

- Enzyme defects:
  - decreased enzyme synthesis
  - defective enzyme synthesis, e.g.
    - accumulation of phenylalanine, causing mental retardation due to phenylalanine hydroxylase deficiency (phenylketonuria)
    - albinism caused by absent melanin production due to tyrosinase deficiency.
- Defects in receptors or cellular transport, e.g.
  - insensitivity of tissues to androgens due to loss of androgen receptors can lead to pseudohermaphroditism
  - cystic fibrosis in which there is a defective cell membrane transport system across exocrine secretory cells.
- Non-enzyme protein defects, e.g.
  - abnormal haemoglobin in sickle cell disease
  - defective collagen in Marfan's syndrome and Ehlers–Danlos syndrome.
- Adverse reaction to drugs, e.g.
  - G6PD deficiency and haemolysis after administration of the antimalarial drug primaquine.

Functional Aspects of Developmental Disorders

- Embryo division abnormalities, e.g. Siamese twins, fetus in fetu.
- Exposure to teratogens: organ development occurs in first 4–8 weeks of intrauterine life and teratogens have major effects at this time (Box 15.2).

BOX 15.2 Teratogens and Their Effects

Teratogen	Teratogenic Effect
Irradiation	**Microcephaly**
Drugs	
Thalidomide	Amelia/phocomelia (absent/rudimentary limbs; heart, kidney, gastrointestinal and facial abnormalities)
Folic acid antagonists, e.g. 4 amino PGA	Anencephaly, hydrocephalus, cleft lip/palate, skull defects
Anticonvulsants	Cleft lip/palate, heart defects, minor skeletal defects
Warfarin	Nasal/facial abnormalities
Testosterone and synthetic progestogens	Virilization of female fetus, atypical genitalia
Alcohol	Microcephaly, abnormal facies, oblique palpebral fissures, growth disturbance
Infections	
Rubella	Cataracts, microphthalmia, microcephaly, heart defects
Cytomegalovirus	Microcephaly
Herpes simplex	Microcephaly, microphthalmia
Toxoplasmosis	Microcephaly

- Failure of cell and organ maturation, e.g.
  - Kartagener's syndrome: defect in ciliary motility affects cell mobility during organogenesis, resulting in situs inversus; in later life results in bronchiectasis and infertility (due to sperm immobility)
  - Hirschsprung's disease: absence of ganglion cells in Meissner's and Auerbach's plexuses due to defective migration of cells from neural crest
  - undescended testis (cryptorchidism): often isolated anomaly, but may be associated with Klinefelter's syndrome.

Anomalies of Organogenesis

These include:

- agenesis: failure of development of an organ or structure
- atresia: failure of development of a lumen in a normally tubular structure
- hypoplasia: failure of an organ to attain its normal size
- dysgenesis: failure of normal organ differentiation or persistence of primitive embryological structures
- ectopia: development of mature tissue at an inappropriate site.

Agenesis (Aplasia)

- Renal agenesis:
  - may be unilateral or bilateral
  - failure of mesonephric duct to give rise to ureteric bud, with failure of induction of metanephric blastema.
- Thymic agenesis (di George syndrome):
  - resulting in absent T-cells and deficiency of cell-mediated immunity.
- Anencephaly:
  - absence of cerebrum due to neural tube defect; fatal.

Atresia

- Oesophageal atresia:
  - failure of separation of trachea and oesophagus from primitive foregut
  - may be associated with tracheo–oesophageal fistula.
- Biliary atresia:
  - absence of bile ducts; obstructive jaundice in infancy.

Hypoplasia

- Developmental dysplasia of the hip.
  - failure of development of bone of acetabulum, causing dislocation of hip due to flattened acetabular roof.

Dysgenesis (Dysplasia)

- Renal dysgenesis due to anomalous metanephric differentiation.

Ectopia (Heterotopia)

- Gastric mucosa in a Meckel's diverticulum.

Acquired Disorders of Differentiation and Growth

These include:

- metaplasia

- dysplasia
- polyps
- neoplasia.

Metaplasia

Metaplasia is the reversible transformation of one type of terminally differentiated cell into another fully differentiated cell type.

Metaplasia:

- may affect epithelial or mesenchymal cells
- often represents an adaptive response of tissues to environmental stress
- is due to activation and/or repression of genes involved in maintenance of cellular differentiation
- metaplastic tissue is better able to withstand adverse environmental changes
- itself does not progress to malignancy, but may undergo further indirect transformation to neoplasia via dysplasia.

Examples of metaplasia in epithelial tissue include:

- squamous metaplasia in ciliary epithelium of bronchus in smokers
- squamous metaplasia in transitional epithelium in the bladder in schistosomiasis
- replacement of squamous epithelium in the oesophagus with columnar glandular epithelium in patients with reflux (Barrett's oesophagus)
- transformation of the columnar lining of the gall bladder to squamous epithelium in the presence of gallstones and chronic inflammation
- squamous metaplasia in the nose, bronchi and urinary tract associated with vitamin A deficiency.

Examples of metaplasia in mesenchymal tissues include:

- bone formation (osseous metaplasia):
  - calcium deposition in atheromatous arterial walls
  - in bronchial cartilage.

Dysplasia

Dysplasia is a premalignant condition characterized by increased cell growth, cellular atypia and decreased differentiation.

Dysplasia:

- may be caused by long-standing irritation of tissues by chronic inflammation or exposure to carcinogens
- in the early phases may be reversible if the initial stimulus is removed
- if severe, will progress to malignancy unless adequately treated.

Dysplasia may be recognized by:

- Evidence of increased growth:
  - increased tissue bulk
  - increased mitotic activity.
- Cellular atypia:
  - pleomorphism
  - high nuclear–cytoplasmic ratio
  - hyperchromatic nuclei (denser staining due to increased nuclear DNA).
- Decreased cellular differentiation:
  - cells more primitive than normal.

Other features of dysplasia:

- May be present for many years before malignancy develops.
- May occur in tissue which has coincidental metaplasia, e.g.
  - dysplasia in metaplastic squamous epithelium in the bronchus of smokers
  - dysplasia in metaplastic glandular epithelium in Barrett's oesophagus.
- May develop without coexisting metaplasia, e.g.
  - squamous epithelium of uterine cervix
  - glandular epithelium of the stomach.

Polyps

A polyp is a sessile or pedunculated protrusion from a body surface.

Polyposis is a term used to describe a condition or syndrome where there are multiple polyps in an organ or organ system, e.g.

- organ: polyposis coli of large bowel
- organ system: Peutz–Jeghers syndrome: hamartomatous polyps throughout the gastrointestinal tract.

The term polyp:

- is purely descriptive of the shape of a lesion
- does not imply any specific underlying pathological process, e.g. hyperplasia, neoplasia
- is a result of focal tissue expansion at a site, at or near a body surface, which, when enlarging, takes the line of least resistance, i.e. outwards to a surface or lumen rather than inwards.

Pathological Processes Causing Polyps

These may be either non-neoplastic or neoplastic.

- Non-neoplastic:
  - inflammation
  - hyperplasia
  - metaplasia
  - dysplasia.
- Neoplastic:
  - epithelial
  - mesenchymal
  - lymphoid.

Non-neoplastic and most neoplastic polyps are common and benign, but a small proportion of malignant neoplasms have a polypoid appearance, e.g. polypoid adenocarcinoma of the colon, lymphomatous polyps of GI tract.

Symptoms of Polyps

Polyps may be asymptomatic or may produce symptoms:

- haemorrhage
- local trauma
- torsion
- inflammation
- ulceration
- anaemia:
  - ulceration
- mechanical effects:
  - obstruction
  - intussusception.

Examples of Polyps

Polyps occur in many organ systems. Accurate diagnosis is essential and histopathological examination is required to determine a precise pathological diagnosis. Examples of polyps include:

- Nasal:
  - very common
  - due to chronic infective or allergic inflammation
  - consist of oedematous masses of connective tissue with inflammatory cells and glands.
- Uterine (endometrial):
  - hyperplastic/metaplastic polyps
  - found in perimenopausal women
  - caused by inappropriate response of endometrium to oestrogenic stimuli
  - malignant change is rare.
- Uterine (cervical):
  - epithelial non-neoplastic polyps
  - common
  - consist of columnar mucus-secreting epithelium with oedematous stroma
  - no malignant potential.
- Colonic:
  - the large bowel is by far the most common site for gastrointestinal polyps. Types of polyps occurring in the large intestine are shown in Table 15.1.

Neoplasia

Neoplasia have the following characteristics:

- abnormal and excessive cell growth uncoordinated with that of normal tissues
- persist after the initiating stimulus has been withdrawn
- associated with genetic alteration
- influence behaviour of normal cells by production of hormones (a paraneoplastic effect) and growth factors.

  Neoplasia are covered in detail in Chapter 18.

TABLE 15.1 Polyps of the Large Intestine

Type	Benign	Malignant
Epithelial	**Neoplastic**	Adenocarcinoma
	• adenoma	Carcinoid
	• tubular adenoma	
	• tubulo-villous adenoma	
	• villous adenoma	
	Inflammatory	
	• pseudopolyp, e.g. ulcerative colitis	
	Hamartomas	
	• juvenile polyp	
	• Peutz–Jeghers syndrome	
	Metaplastic	
	• adenoma	
Mesenchymal	Lipoma	Sarcomas
	Leiomyoma	Lymphomatous polyps
	Fibromas	
	Haemangiomas	

OSCE SCENARIOS

OSCE Scenario 15.1

A 66-year-old male is admitted through A&E with painless red bleeding per rectum. He has no past medical history and a subsequent colonoscopy shows multiple benign-looking polyps only, which have been biopsied. He is anxious and worried about his condition and has asked to speak to a doctor.

1. Answer the patient's questions about polyps and rectal bleeding. Explain the different types of polyps and the need for the biopsy, avoiding medical jargon.

The patient then explains that several members of his family have had 'camera tests' in their bowel, and you notice some small dark dots on his lower lip.

2. Name the most likely condition causing this patient's polyps.
3. Explain to the examiners the type of polyps caused by this condition, any risks from the polyps and any screening procedures that need to be in place.

OSCE Scenario 15.2

A 40-year-old-male presents to your orthopaedic outpatient clinic having been referred by his GP for 'tingling' sensations in his hands. He complains of the symptoms progressing over the last nine months. He is a carpenter by trade and is starting to drop things due to weakness in his grip. He has no past medical history and takes no medications. He is concerned about his hands, as being self-employed his inability to work is impacting upon him financially.

1. Take a brief history regarding this patient's symptoms and examine his hands.
2. What is the diagnosis?

The patient then explains that he has seen his GP for headaches recently, which he feels are stress-related due to his worry about his job.

3. In view of this new information and your previous diagnosis, what condition are you now concerned about?
4. Explain to the examiners the other symptoms and signs you would now check for in this patient, and briefly outline the investigations and management.

OSCE Scenario 15.3

A nurse in your clinic asks you to see a very distressed 50-year-old gentleman regarding the result of a biopsy performed on his cheek two weeks ago. He attended the outpatient clinic earlier today, and was informed by a different doctor that he had 'dysplasia' 'but it was completely removed and nothing to worry about' and was told to come back in three months. He has spent the last two hours near to tears in the hospital canteen and tells you he is worried he has cancer.

1. Explain the diagnosis of dysplasia to this gentleman, being sensitive to his heightened emotional state.
2. Tell the examiners what risk factors exist for oral cavity tumours and the names of any pre-malignant conditions you know of.
3. How would you draw this consultation to a close and ensure the patient felt supported?

OSCE Scenario 15.4

A 35-year-old man with a long-standing history of gastro-oesophageal reflux undergoes endoscopy which reveals suspicion of Barrett's oesophagus. Biopsy confirms the diagnosis, and the patient attends outpatient clinic to discuss the results.

1. Describe to the patient the diagnosis and pathogenesis.
2. What is the significance of Barrett's oesophagus?
3. The patient does not attend any further medical appointments and after 15 years presents with history of dysphagia and weight loss. Investigations reveal advanced lower oesophageal cancer. Palliative chemotherapy is advocated. Describe the phases of cell cycle and the relationship to chemotherapy.
4. As you discuss potential side effects of chemotherapy, explain to the patient the reason for the likelihood of hair loss, developing anaemia and the susceptibility to infection and bleeding.

OSCE Scenario 15.5

A 15-year-old boy attends the outpatient clinic with his parents after getting concerned regarding bilateral breast enlargement over the past year. This is causing embarrassment and he would like to understand its aetiology. Following assessment, you conclude that the findings are consistent with physiologic changes during puberty.

1. Explain to the patient and his family the underlying pathogenesis.
2. Give other examples of organs that can undergo physiologic changes during early adulthood.
3. What are the other causes of gynaecomastia that you need to exclude?

Answers in Appendix pages 464–467

Please check your eBook at https://studentconsult.inkling.com/ for more self-assessment questions. See inside cover for registration details.

16

Inflammation

Inflammation is the local physiological response to injury.

CLASSIFICATION

- Acute inflammation: the initial and often transient reaction to injury.
- Chronic inflammation: the subsequent and often prolonged tissue reaction to injury.

Acute Inflammation

- Vascular phase:
  - change in vessel calibre
  - increased vascular permeability
  - formation of fluid exudates.
- Exudative cellular phase:
  - adhesion of neutrophils
  - neutrophil migration
  - diapedesis
  - neutrophil chemotaxis.
- Outcome:
  - resolution
  - suppuration
  - organization
  - chronic inflammation.

Causes of Acute Inflammation

- Microbial infections:
  - pyogenic bacteria
  - viruses.
- Hypersensitivity reactions:
  - parasites
  - tubercle bacilli.
- Chemical agents:
  - corrosives
  - acids
  - alkalis
  - toxins.
- Physical agents:
  - trauma
  - ionizing radiation
  - heat
  - cold.
- Tissue necrosis:
  - ischaemia
  - infarction.

Macroscopic Signs and Symptoms of Acute Inflammation

- Redness (rubor):
  - small vessel dilatation.
- Heat (calor):
  - increased blood flow in skin.
- Swelling (tumour):
  - oedema.
- Pain (dolor):
  - stretching and tissue distortion
  - pus under pressure in abscess
  - chemical mediators, e.g. prostaglandins, bradykinins.
- Loss of function (functio laesa):
  - conscious and reflex inhibition of movement by pain
  - swelling may physically immobilize tissues.

Stages of Acute Inflammation

- Change in vessel calibre.
- Increased vascular permeability.
- Formation of cellular exudates.

Changes in Vessel Calibre

- Changes described by Lewis in 1927 as 'triple response to injury': flush, flare, weal.
- If a blunt instrument is drawn across the skin the following changes take place:
  - transient white line due to arteriolar vasoconstriction
  - flush: dull red line due to capillary dilatation
  - flare: red irregular zone due to arteriolar dilatation
  - weal: zone of oedema due to fluid exudate in to the extravascular space.

Increased Vascular Permeability

- Capillary hydrostatic pressure increased in acute inflammation.
- More fluid leaves vessels than returns to them.
- Formation of an exudate: a protein-rich fluid.
- Fluid exudates:
  - protein content up to 50 g/L
  - contains immunoglobulins: destruction of invading micro-organisms
  - coagulation factors: fibrinogen converted to fibrin in fibrinous exudates.
- Removal of exudate by lymphatic channels and replacement with new exudate if stimulus to inflammation persists.

Formation of Cellular Exudate

- Margination of neutrophils.
- Neutrophil adhesion:
  - interaction between paired adhesion molecules on leucocyte and endothelial surfaces
  - leucocyte surface adhesion molecule expression increased by:
    - complement C5a
    - leukotriene B4
    - tumour necrosis factor (TNF).
  - endothelial expression of adhesion molecules increased by:
    - interleukin-1 (IL-1)
    - endotoxins
    - TNF.
- Neutrophil migration.
- Amoeboid movement through venules (C5a and leukotriene B4).
- Diapedesis:
  - escape of red cells from capillaries
  - passive; depends on hydrostatic pressure.
- Neutrophil chemotaxis:
  - leukotriene B4
  - IL-8.

Chemical Mediators of Acute Inflammation

- Histamine:
  - source: mast cell, basophil, eosinophil, platelets
  - release stimulated by C3a, C5a, neutrophil lysosomal protein
  - action: vasodilatation transiently increases vascular permeability.
- Lysosomal compounds:
  - source: neutrophils
  - release stimulated by bacteria, damaged tissue
  - action: increased vascular permeability
  - activate complement.
- Prostaglandins:
  - source: platelets, endothelium, monocyte/macrophage, other cells
  - action: different actions:
    - potentiate increase in vascular permeability
    - platelet aggregation (pA_2)
    - platelet disaggregation (pI_2).
- Leukotrienes:
  - synthesized from arachidonic acid
  - synthesis occurs in neutrophils, mast cells, basophils, some macrophages
  - SRS-A (slow reacting substance of anaphylaxis) is a mixture of leukotrienes involved in type I hypersensitivity.
- Cytokines:
  - source: many cells
  - action: attract various types of leucocyte to site of inflammation, e.g. IL-8 mainly specific for neutrophils.
- Nitric oxide:
  - source: endothelium, macrophage, short-lived free radicals
  - action: toxic to bacteria; major factor in endotoxic shock.

Plasma Factors

- Complement.
- Kinins.
- Coagulation system.
- Fibrinolytic system.

Complement System

- Cascade of enzymatic proteins.
- Series of 20 proteins synthesized in liver and macrophages.
- Activated during acute inflammatory response:
  - enzymes released from dying cells during tissue necrosis
  - infection
  - products of kinins, coagulation and fibrinolytic system.
- Products of complement activation important in inflammation are:
  - C5a: chemotactic for neutrophils; increase vascular permeability, release of histamine from mast cells
  - C3a: similar action to C5a but less active
  - C5, 6, 7: chemotactic for neutrophils
  - C5, 6, 7, 8, 9: cytolytic activity
  - C4b, 2a, 3b: opsonization of bacteria and facilitate phagocytosis by macrophages.

Kinin System

- Activated by coagulation factor XII.
- Converts prekallikrein to kallikrein.

- Kallikrein cleaves kininogen to release bradykinin.
- Bradykinin controls vascular permeability and is a chemical mediator of pain.

Coagulation System

- Protein synthesized in liver in inactive form.
- System responsible for conversion of fibrinogen to fibrin, a major component of the inflammatory response.
- Coagulation factor XII is activated by exposed basement membranes and various proteolytic enzymes of bacterial origin. In turn it activates coagulation, kinin and fibrinolytic systems.

Fibrinolytic System

- Protein synthesized in liver.
- Negative feedback arm that limits coagulation.
- Plasmin (released by action of activated factor XII), lyses fibrin to fibrin degradation products (FDP).

Role of Macrophages

- Stimulated by local infection or injury.
- Produce IL-1 and TNF-α which stimulate endothelial cells to produce adhesion molecules which bind and activate neutrophils.

Role of Lymphatics

Terminal lymphatics are blind-ended endothelium-lined tubes present in most tissues in similar numbers to capillaries.

- Lymphatics drain into collecting lymphatics, which have valves and propel lymph passively to lymph nodes.
- Gaps open passively between lymphatic endothelial cells, allowing large protein molecules to enter.
- In acute inflammation lymphatic channels become dilated as they drain away oedema fluid of inflammatory exudates.
- This tends to limit the extent of tissue oedema.
- Important in the immune response to infecting agents as antigens are carried to regional lymph nodes for recognition by lymphocytes.

Role of Neutrophil Polymorphs

- Characteristic cell of acute inflammatory exudates.
- Movement: amoeboid movement in a directional response (chemotaxis) to chemicals of acute inflammation.
- Bind to micro-organisms which have been opsonized by immunoglobulins or complement components.
- Phagocytosis: facilitated by opsonization. Cells ingest particle into vacuole, which fuses with lysosome, resulting in killing of micro-organism.
- Release of lysosomal products: damage local tissues by proteolysis, e.g. elastase and collagenase. Some compounds released increase vascular permeability, while others are pyrogens causing systemic fever.

SPECIAL TYPES OF INFLAMMATION

1. Serous

- Abundant protein-rich fluid with low cellular content.
- Inflammation of serous cavities, e.g. peritonitis (peritoneal cavity), synovitis (synovial joint).
- Vascular dilatation apparent to naked eye, e.g. conjunctivitis.

2. Catarrhal

- Hypersecretion of mucus in acute inflammation of a mucous membrane, e.g. coryza (common cold).

3. Fibrinous Inflammation

- Exudate contains much fibrinogen.
- Fibrin forms a thick coating, e.g. acute pericarditis, fibrinous peritonitis.

4. Haemorrhagic Inflammation

- Accompanied by vascular injury or coagulopathy.
- Examples include acute haemorrhagic pancreatitis due to proteolytic digestion of vessel walls; and meningococcal septicaemia, resulting from associated disseminated intravascular coagulation (DIC).

5. Suppurative Inflammation

- Production of pus, i.e. dying and degenerate neutrophils, organisms and liquefied tissues.
- May become walled-off by fibrin or fibrous tissue to produce an abscess, i.e. a localized collection of pus.
- May form an empyema (a collection of pus in a hollow viscus, e.g. gall bladder).

6. Membranous Inflammation

- Epithelium coated with a membrane of fibrin, desquamated epithelial cells and inflammatory cells.
- Example: grey membrane seen in pharyngitis due to diphtheria.

7. Pseudomembranous Inflammation

- Superficial mucosal inflammation and ulceration with sloughing of mucosa, fibrin, mucus and inflammatory cells.
- Example: pseudomembranous colitis due to *Clostridium difficile*.

8. Necrotizing Inflammation

- Tense oedema may cause vascular occlusion and thrombosis, resulting in septic necrosis.
- Example: gangrenous appendicitis.

Effects of Acute Inflammation

Beneficial Effects (Exudate)

- Dilution of toxins.
- Arrival of antibodies.
- Transport of drugs.
- Fibrin formation.
- Delivery of oxygen and nutrients.
- Stimulation of immune response.

Harmful Effects (Release of Lysosomal Enzymes)

- Digestion of normal tissue.
- Swelling.
- Inappropriate inflammatory response, e.g. type I hypersensitivity reactions.

Sequelae of Acute Inflammation

- Resolution.
- Suppuration.
- Organization.
- Chronic inflammation.

Resolution

- Resolution is complete restoration of tissues to normal.

  Conditions favouring resolution

  Include:
- Minimal tissue damage.
- Occurrence in organ with regenerative capacity, e.g. liver, rather than one that cannot regenerate, e.g. brain.
- Rapid destruction of causal agents, e.g. bacterial phagocytosis.
- Rapid removal of fluid and debris.

  Sequence of events leading to resolution
- Phagocytosis of bacteria.
- Fibrinolysis.
- Phagocytosis of debris by macrophages.
- Resolution of vascular dilatation.

Suppuration

- The formation of pus.
- Pus is a mixture of living, dead and dying bacteria and neutrophils with cellular debris and liquefied tissue.
- The causative organisms are usually pyogenic bacteria, e.g. *Staphylococcus aureus*, *Staph. pyogenes*, coliforms and *Neisseria* spp.
- The causative stimulus is usually persistent.
- An accumulation of pus in the tissues becomes surrounded by a 'pyogenic membrane', i.e. capillaries, neutrophils and occasional fibroblasts.
- Bacteria within abscess cavities are relatively inaccessible to antibiotics and antibodies; hence the need to drain pus.

Organization

- Organization is replacement of the tissue by granulation tissue.

  Circumstances favouring organization
- Excess fibrin formation with swamping of the fibrinolytic system.
- Substantial volume of necrotic tissue.
- Exudate and debris cannot be removed or discharged.

  Sequence of organization
- Capillaries grow into the inflammatory tissue.
- Fibroblasts proliferate under the influence of TGF-β, resulting in fibrosis.
- Example: after peritonitis a fibrinous exudate covers the bowel and loops stick together in a fibrinous adhesion. Failure to remove the fibrin results in its invasion with capillaries accompanied by fibroblasts, which lay down collagen resulting in a permanent fibrous adhesion between loops of bowel.

Progress to Chronic Inflammation

- Acute inflammation may progress to chronic if the causative agent is not removed.
- The tissues become organized and the cellular exudate changes with lymphocytes, plasma cells and macrophages, and multinuclear giant cells replacing polymorphs.

Systemic Effects of Inflammation

- Pyrexia.
- Weight loss.
- Constitutional symptoms, e.g. malaise, nausea, anorexia.
- Haematological changes:
  - increased ESR
  - leucocytosis.
- Reactive hyperplasia:
  - lymphadenopathy
  - splenomegaly.
- Anaemia:
  - loss of blood into exudates, e.g. acute pancreatitis
  - haemolysis, e.g. bacterial toxin
  - 'anaemia of chronic disease' – bone marrow depression.
- Amyloidosis (secondary or reactive):
  - long-standing chronic inflammation, e.g. TB, rheumatoid arthritis, bronchiectasis.

CHRONIC INFLAMMATION

Chronic inflammation implies that the process has extended over a long period of time; however, the term 'chronic' applied to inflammation indicates a cellular infiltrate that differs from acute inflammation, i.e. lymphocytes, plasma cells and macrophages predominate in chronic inflammation. Chronic inflammation is usually primary but occasionally follows acute inflammation.

Features of Chronic Inflammation

- Lymphocytes, plasma cells and macrophages predominate.
- Usually primary but may follow acute inflammation.
- Granulomatous inflammation is a specific type of chronic inflammation.
- May be complicated by secondary amyloidosis.

Causes of Chronic Inflammation

- Primary chronic inflammation.
- Progress from acute inflammation.
- Recurrent episodes of acute inflammation.
- Transplant rejection.

Primary Chronic Inflammation

- Resistance of infective agents to phagocytosis and intracellular killing, e.g. tuberculosis, leprosy, viral infections.
- Foreign body reactions:
  - endogenous materials, e.g. necrotic bone, uric acid crystals
  - exogenous materials, e.g. asbestos fibres, suture materials, implanted prostheses.
- Autoimmune diseases, e.g. Hashimoto's thyroiditis, chronic gastritis of pernicious anaemia, rheumatoid arthritis.
- Specific diseases of unknown aetiology, e.g. chronic inflammatory bowel disease – ulcerative colitis.
- Primary granulomatous disease, e.g. Crohn's disease, sarcoidosis.

Progression from Acute Inflammation

- Commonest variety of acute inflammation to progress to chronic inflammation is the suppurative type.
- Inadequate drainage of pus which is deep-seated, e.g. chronic abscess of osteomyelitis or chronic empyema thoracis.
- Foreign-body reactions may develop into granulomatous reactions, e.g. suture material, wood, metal, glass, implanted prosthesis.

Recurrent Episodes of Acute Inflammation

- Recurring cycles of acute inflammation and healing eventually result in chronic inflammation.
- Best example of this in clinical practice is chronic cholecystitis due to gallstones. Multiple recurrent episodes of acute inflammation lead to replacement of the gall bladder muscle with fibrous tissue.

Transplant Rejection

- Cellular rejection of renal transplants involves chronic inflammatory cell infiltration.

Macroscopic Appearances of Chronic Inflammation

- Chronic ulceration:
  - venous stasis ulcer
  - peptic ulcer.
- Chronic abscess:
  - osteomyelitis.
- Caseating granulomatous inflammation:
  - pulmonary tuberculosis.
- Thickening of a hollow viscus:
  - chronic cholecystitis
  - Crohn's disease.
- Fibrosis:
  - distortion, e.g. pyloric stenosis after peptic ulceration.

GRANULOMATOUS DISEASE

A granuloma is an aggregate of epithelioid histiocytes.

Epithelioid histiocytes

- Named because of vague histological resemblance to epithelial cells.
- Arranged in clusters.
- Little phagocytic activity.
- Produce angiotensin-converting enzyme (raised in sarcoidosis).
- Caseous necrosis may occur in granulomas, e.g. tuberculosis.
- Histiocytes may be converted into multinucleate giant cells.

Types of Giant Cell

- Histiocytic:
  - form where particulate matter is indigestible by macrophages, e.g. silica, tubercle bacilli.
- Langhans:
  - horseshoe arrangement of peripheral nuclei at one pole of cell
  - characteristically seen in tuberculosis.
- Foreign body:
  - large cells with nuclei randomly scattered throughout cytoplasm
  - seen in relation to particulate foreign body material.
- Touton:
  - ring of central nuclei
  - clear peripheral cytoplasm with accumulated lipid, seen at sites of adipose tissue breakdown and in xanthomas.

Causes of Granulomatous Disease

- Specific infections:
  - mycobacteria, e.g. tuberculosis
  - fungi
  - parasites.
- Foreign bodies:
  - endogenous, e.g. keratin, necrotic bone, uric acid crystals
  - exogenous, e.g. talc, silica, suture materials, silicone.
- Specific chemicals:
  - beryllium.
- Drugs:
  - hepatic granulomatous due to allopurinol, phenylbutazone, sulphonamides.
- Unknown:
  - Crohn's disease
  - sarcoidosis
  - Wegener's granulomatosis.

OSCE SCENARIOS

OSCE Scenario 16.1

A 16-year-old male presents to your clinic with a 6-month history of weight loss and vague abdominal pain with intermittent rectal bleeding.

1. Outline your history, examination and investigations.
2. What is your differential diagnosis?
   The colonic mucosal biopsy shows chronic inflammation with focal colitis and granulomas. The patient is currently well but is worried as he does not know what this means.
3. Explain the findings and diagnosis to the patient.

OSCE Scenario 16.2

A 19-year-old male is admitted with a history of central abdominal pain localizing to the right iliac fossa after 12 h. It is now five days since the onset of symptoms. On admission to A&E he has a temperature of 38.5°C with a tachycardia of 120, and abdominal examination reveals a tender mass in the right iliac fossa. A clinical diagnosis of appendix abscess is made and this is confirmed by CT scan.

1. What is suppuration? Why in some cases does acute appendicitis perforate and cause peritonitis while in others abscess formation occurs?
2. Why do abscesses require drainage?
3. What organisms are likely to be cultured from the pus?
4. What sequelae other than suppuration may follow acute inflammation?The patient is re-admitted to hospital 1 year later with vomiting, central abdominal colicky pain, abdominal distension and constipation. Plain abdominal X-ray shows dilated loops of small bowel and a diagnosis of small bowel obstruction is made.
5. Why is this likely to have occurred? Explain the pathology of the condition.

OSCE Scenario 16.3

You see an 8-year-old girl along with her mother in A&E who fell over earlier today and banged her arm, which is slightly pink and swollen. The child is happy and playing with her arm in a sling, with normal observations and no evidence of serious injury or infection. The patient's mother explains that the nurse practitioner performed an X-ray, which showed no fracture but that she doesn't understand why it is red and sore if it isn't infected or broken. She asks if her daughter needs antibiotics.

1. Explain to this worried parent the difference between inflammation, fractures and infection and answer her question regarding antibiotics.
2. Explain to the examiners the stages of acute inflammation and the key cells and mediators involved.
3. Explain to the examiners what factors in the presentation of a child to A&E would make you think of non-accidental injury (NAI)?

OSCE Scenario 16.4

A 44-year-old female is brought in unwell with severe central abdominal pain radiating through to her back with nausea and vomiting. Her amylase is 3400 U/L.

1. What is the diagnosis?
2. Five days later she has clinically deteriorated and is hypotensive and anaemic. A CT scan has shown considerable bleeding in and around the pancreas. What is this type of inflammation called and why does it occur?
3. Do you know any common causes of pancreatitis?

OSCE Scenario 16.5

A 48-year-old man has accidently been given IV penicillin – he is known to have a severe allergy to all penicillin-based antibiotics. He is very unwell and has collapsed on the ward, he is struggling to breathe, his arm is swollen and he is profoundly hypotensive.

1. What type of shock does he have?
2. Explain why he is having difficulty breathing and is hypotensive.
3. How would you treat this patient?

Answers in Appendix pages 467–470

Please check your eBook at https://studentconsult.inkling.com/ for more self-assessment questions. See inside cover for registration details.

17

Thrombosis, Embolism and Infarction

THROMBOSIS

A thrombus is defined as a solid mass formed in the living circulation from the components of the streaming blood.

This is to be distinguished from clotting, which is solidification of the blood when it is:

- static
- outside a blood vessel
- outside a body
- within a vessel in a dead body.

Causes of Thrombosis

Several factors contribute to thrombus formation and these are usually grouped together as Virchow's triad, i.e.

- changes in the vessel wall
- changes in blood flow
- changes in the constituents of the blood.

Damage to Vessel Wall

- Arteries: atherosclerotic plaques or synthetic grafts.
- Heart: congenital abnormalities or artificial valves.
- Veins: local injury caused by pressure on the calves from bed or operating table.

Arterial thrombosis

- The commonest cause is atherosclerosis.
- Vessels most commonly affected are the coronary arteries, abdominal aorta, mesenteric arteries, cerebral arteries, renal arteries and arteries of the lower limb.
- Arterial thrombosis is more associated with damage to the vessel wall, as compared with venous thrombosis, which is most associated with blood flow disturbances.
- Factors increasing the risk of atherosclerosis and thus indirectly of thrombosis:
  - family history
  - male sex
  - smoking
  - hypertension
  - hypercholesterolaemia
  - diabetes mellitus
  - homocysteinaemia.

Venous thrombosis

- The commonest cause is stasis.
- Mechanical damage due to pressure on calf veins during surgery may be contributory.
- The main sites of venous thrombosis are calf veins and pelvic veins.
- Emboli occur to the lungs via the right side of the heart.

Alterations in Blood Flow

Normal laminar flow may change to a turbulent pattern. This may occur with:

- prolonged inactivity following surgery, trauma or myocardial infarction
- cardiac failure
- proximal occlusion of venous drainage, e.g. pregnancy, pelvic tumour.

Alterations of the Constituents of the Blood

These include:

- increased number of platelets and increased adhesiveness of platelets following surgery or injury
- dehydration, which may increase viscosity
- thrombophilia: abnormal balance of clotting factors and natural anticoagulants.

Stages in the Development of Thrombosis

- Thrombus may develop in heart, arteries or veins.
- First stage involves platelets sticking to damaged endothelium.
- A dense layer of fibrin and leucocytes adheres to the surface of the platelets.
- Blood clot (fibrin and red cells develop on this layer of leucocytes and platelets).
- A secondary layer of platelets collects on the surface of the blood clot.
- Gradual extension of thrombosis leads to a propagated or consecutive thrombus.
- Organization then begins, with adherence to the vessel wall as mural thrombus.

- A second stage develops, with a further batch of platelets laid down over the initial aggregate, and then a further layer of blood clot.
- In this way, alternate layers of platelets and blood clots form a lamina arrangement.
- This causes a differential contraction of platelets and fibrin and gives a rippled appearance, reminiscent of rippling of sand on a beach.
- Ridges on the surface of the thrombi are known as the lines of Zahn.

Fate of Thrombi

- Lysis (resolution): the thrombolytic system may remove thrombi completely, especially if they are small.
- Recanalization: following organization, new vessels may grow through the thrombus, eventually forming a single or several new channels.
- Propagation: because the thrombus itself results in slowing of the blood flow, it may cause further thrombosis and the clot may increase in length.
- Embolization: part of the thrombus or the whole thrombus may become dislodged and move through the circulation until arrested in a vessel which is of similar size to itself, causing that vessel to be occluded.

EMBOLISM

An embolus is an abnormal mass of undissolved material which passes in the bloodstream from one part of the circulation to another, impacting in blood vessels too small to allow it to pass.

Emboli may consist of:

- thrombus
- gas (air and nitrogen)
- fat
- tumour
- amniotic fluid
- foreign body, e.g. i.v. cannula, particulate matter with i.v. drug abuse
- therapeutic emboli, e.g. gel, foam and steel coils.

Thromboembolism

Venous Thromboembolism

- Venous thromboembolism gives rise to pulmonary embolism.
- The overwhelming majority of emboli arise from thrombi in the veins of the lower limb.
- They travel through the inferior vena cava to the right side of the heart and impact in the pulmonary artery or one of its major branches, depending upon the size of the embolus.
- The effect of the embolism depends on its size:
  - small emboli may be thrown off in showers and are asymptomatic until their cumulative effect limits respiration
  - medium emboli may cause dyspnoea, respiratory distress and chest pain
  - large emboli may occlude both pulmonary arteries and cause sudden death.
- If only one major pulmonary vein is blocked, severe shortness of breath and circulatory collapse may occur. This may be due to a vagal reflex inducing spasm of the coronary and pulmonary arteries associated with peripheral vasodilatation.

Arterial Thromboembolism

- Systemic emboli from arteries deposit in arteries more distally along the arterial tree.
- Total occlusion of such arteries may produce relative ischaemia. A collateral supply may be available.
- If there is no collateral supply, infarction will take place.
- Arterial thromboembolism may come from the following:
  - heart, e.g. left auricular thrombus in atrial fibrillation, mural thrombus following myocardial infarction
  - valvular disease, including prosthetic valves
  - proximal atherosclerotic plaques
  - aneurysms
  - paradoxical: from the venous system via a right-to-left shunt, e.g. patent interatrial septum.

Gas Embolism

Gas must be free within the bloodstream and not in solution. There are two main causes of gas embolism: i.e. gas entering the bloodstream usually as air, and gas dissolved in the blood coming out of solution.

Gas entering the bloodstream:

- injection of air (100 mL or more)
- trauma to neck veins: low pressure during inspiration causes air to flow in, especially with patient in erect sitting position.

Nitrogen embolism may occur in decompression sickness when a diver ascends too rapidly:

- Nitrogen (previously in solution under high pressure) forms bubbles within the circulation as pressure is rapidly reduced.
- Bubbles may also be found in ligaments and joints, causing severe pain which causes the patient to lie and bend double in an attempt to relieve the pain; hence, 'the bends'.

Fat Embolism

- Most commonly associated with long bone fractures.
- Initially thought to be due to entry of globules of fat into the circulation from the bone marrow, but now

considered more probably to be due to metabolic changes.
- Can be demonstrated in about 90% of multiple fracture cases, although significant clinical consequences are rare.
- The emboli may pass through the pulmonary vessels and into the systemic circulation, where they may become impacted in the capillaries of brain, kidneys, skin and other organs.
- Symptoms consist of fever, respiratory distress and cerebral symptoms. Occasionally brain damage is sufficient to cause coma and death.
- Haemorrhagic skin eruptions may occur as may subconjunctival and retinal haemorrhages.

Tumour Emboli

- All malignant tumours tend to invade blood vessels at an early stage, and isolated malignant cells are commonly present in the circulation.
- Various factors are responsible for survival of metastatic tumours within the bloodstream, and for the ability to escape to surrounding tissues and to grow following impaction within a vessel bed of small enough calibre to impede its further progress (see Chapter 18).

Amniotic Fluid Embolism

- Occurs in labour when the placenta is detached from the uterine wall and amniotic fluid enters the maternal circulation.
- Rare event 1 : 50 000 deliveries.
- Effects may be produced by thromboplastins in amniotic fluid.
- Onset is indicated by severe respiratory difficulty with shock and fits.
- Death is due to disseminated intravascular coagulation in many cases.

Foreign Body Embolism

- Pieces of cannulae may break off during i.v. instrumentation.
- Intravenous injection with undissolved drugs may also be involved in i.v. drug abusers.
- Accidental intra-arterial injection may occur with arterial embolus and thrombosis.

Therapeutic Embolism

- Therapeutic emboli such as gel, foam or steel coils may occasionally be used to:
  - stop haemorrhage
  - thrombose aneurysms
  - reduce vascularity of a tumour prior to surgical removal
  - treat arteriovenous fistulae.

Non-Thromboembolic Vascular Insufficiency

Causes include:

- atheroma
- torsion
- spontaneous vascular occlusion, e.g. spasm in Raynaud's disease
- 'steal' syndrome, i.e. redirected blood supply
- external pressure occlusion, e.g. tumours, tourniquets, fractures, tight plasters.

Atheroma

- Tends to occlude the lumen of arteries progressively.
- Risk of thrombosis occurring on atheromatous plaque.
- With thrombus formation, total occlusion may occur, with development of gangrene.

Torsion

- May affect testis, ovary, bowel.
- As organ rotates on pedicle or mesentery, venous return is affected first.
- Arterial supply unaffected initially and continues to pump blood into organ, which becomes engorged and swollen.
- Eventually with oedema, venous pressure equals arterial pressure, flow ceases and there is impending infarction.

Spontaneous Vascular Occlusion

- May be due to vascular spasm.
- Spasm may occur in such vessels as coronary arteries (myocardial infarction), peripheral arteries (Raynaud's disease).
- Spasm occurs due to contraction of smooth muscle in vascular wall.

'Steal' Syndrome

- Occurs when blood is redirected preferentially along one branch of a vessel to the detriment of the end territory of the branch.
- May be seen with proximal arteriovenous fistula (usually created for dialysis) in the proximal part of a limb, e.g. between brachial artery and cephalic vein at the elbow. The flow from the brachial artery goes preferentially through the cephalic vein with very little blood passing down the ulnar and radial arteries to the hand.

External Pressure Occlusion

- May be caused by tumours, tourniquets or tight plaster of Paris cast.
- May also be caused by fractures, e.g. super-condylar fracture of the femur where the distal fragment is drawn backwards, compressing and damaging the popliteal artery.

ISCHAEMIA, INFARCTION AND GANGRENE

Ischaemia

Ischaemia is the condition of an organ or tissue where the supply of oxygenated blood is inadequate for its metabolic needs.

Causes

General

- Ischaemia may follow a sudden fall in cardiac output.
- Myocardial infarction occasionally results in symmetrical gangrene of the extremities.
- Different tissues are affected with different degrees of severity, e.g. the brain is the most sensitive to ischaemia.

Local

- Arterial obstruction:
    - atherosclerosis
    - intra-arterial thrombosis
    - embolism
    - external pressure
    - compartment syndrome.
- Venous obstruction:
    - tissues become engorged with blood such that eventually arterial pressure and venous pressure equate and arterial blood flow ceases
    - strangulated hernias
    - mesenteric venous thrombosis
    - phlegmasia cerulea dolens: a severe form of deep vein thrombosis with venous engorgement such that venous gangrene may supervene.
- Small vessel obstruction:
    - spasm, e.g. Raynaud's phenomenon
    - vasculitis
    - frostbite
    - microembolism
    - precipitated cryoglobulins
    - thrombocythaemia.

Severity of Ischaemia

This depends upon:

- speed of onset
- the extent of obstruction
- the extent and patency of collateral circulation
- the metabolic requirements of the tissues.

Infarction

Infarction is death of the tissue following acute ischaemia when irreparable damage has occurred.

Sequence of Events

- Dead tissue undergoes progressive autolysis of parenchymal cells and haemolysis of red cells.
- Living tissue surrounding the infarct undergoes an acute inflammatory response.
- Demolition phase: when there is an increase in the polymorphs, and after a few days, macrophage infiltration.
- Repair phase: gradual ingrowth of granulation tissue and the infarct is eventually organized into a fibrous scar.
- Infarcts may either be described as red or white (pale).
- White infarcts are usually due to arterial occlusion of 'end' arteries in solid tissues, e.g. heart, spleen, kidneys.
- Red infarcts are due to venous infarcts and occur in loose tissues, e.g. the lung, where the bronchial arteries continue to pump in blood.
- In the long term, dystrophic calcification may occur in some infarcts.

Systemic Effects of Infarcts

- Fever.
- Leucocytosis.
- Raised erythrocyte sedimentation rate (ESR).
- Rise in certain specific enzymes according to the tissue affected, e.g. creatine kinase (CK) raised in myocardial infarction.

Low-flow infarction

In some tissues, infarction may be due to impaired blood flow (or oxygenation), rather than complete cessation of flow. Areas involved include:

- 'watershed' areas
- splenic flexure of the colon, which is situated between the territories of the superior and inferior mesenteric arteries (ischaemic colitis)
- the deep myocardium between the subendocardial myocardium, oxygenated directly from the blood of the ventricles and the remainder, which is perfused by the coronary arteries
- tissues perfused by a portal vasculature, e.g. the anterior pituitary, which is perfused by blood that has already perfused the hypothalamus
- tissues distal to pathological arterial stenoses, e.g. arteriosclerotic narrowing of arteries may be sufficient to allow distal perfusion in normotensive individuals, but in hypotension, the blood flow falls and the distal tissue may become infarcted
- metabolically active tissues, e.g. cerebral neurons, in which irreversible damage can occur within a few minutes of cessation of blood flow and oxygenation.

Gangrene

This is the death of tissue.

Two types of gangrene are recognized:

- Dry gangrene:
    - tissue dies
    - becomes mummified
    - healing occurs above it

- eventually the dead area drops off below a line of demarcation (auto-amputation), e.g. gangrenous toes in diabetes.
- Wet gangrene:
  - bacterial infection and putrefaction occur
  - gangrene spreads proximally
  - there is no line of demarcation
  - proximal amputation is required where the blood supply is better
  - death may occur from overwhelming sepsis.

Specific Forms of Gangrene

- Gas gangrene.
- Meleney's gangrene.
- Fournier's gangrene.
- Necrotizing fasciitis.

These conditions are dealt with in Chapter 21.

OSCE SCENARIOS

OSCE Scenario 17.1

A 42-year-old female on your ward develops a painful calf five days after having a mastectomy and free flap reconstruction for breast cancer. She has a body mass index (BMI) of 25, is otherwise fit and well, and takes no medications.

1. Take a brief history from this patient.
2. What is your diagnosis?
3. What specific risk factors does this patient have for a deep vein thrombosis (DVT)?
4. What venous thromboembolism prophylaxis measures would you check that she had received?
5. Outline your assessment and any investigations you would perform.

The vital signs and blood tests were all unremarkable; however, the duplex Doppler reveals a DVT in the popliteal vein of the affected calf.

6. Outline your management plan.

OSCE Scenario 17.2

A 69-year-old male presents to A&E an hour after developing acute pain in his left buttock, thigh and calf. He has a history of angina and hypertension, and admits to episodes over several months of cramp-like pain in the left buttock, thigh and calf when walking uphill. On examination, his left leg is paler and cooler and he complains of a 'pins and needles' sensation in it.

1. What is the likely diagnosis?
2. An arteriogram is carried out (Fig. 17.2Q). What abnormalities are shown? Is there evidence that this is acute-on-chronic rather than simply acute?
3. Outline your immediate management plan to the examiners.

OSCE Scenario 17.3

You are asked to see a 60-year-old male in ICU who has been intubated and ventilated for two days after a cardiac arrest – attributed to a myocardial infarction. He had approximately 45 minutes of CPR before a heartbeat was restored. The intensivists are concerned as he has a rising serum lactate and acidosis despite good cardiac output and no obvious evidence of infection. He has reduced bowel sounds, though no abdominal distension exists. He has a temperature of 38.1°C. His WCC is 14.2×10^9/L and his lactate is 5.6 mmol/L.

1. What is your differential diagnosis?
2. A plain AXR is non-contributory and a CT scan is carried out and is shown below (Fig. 17.3Q).
3. What other investigation could be carried out to establish the diagnosis?
4. Outline your management plan.
5. Explain to the examiners the likely cause of this patient's pathology.

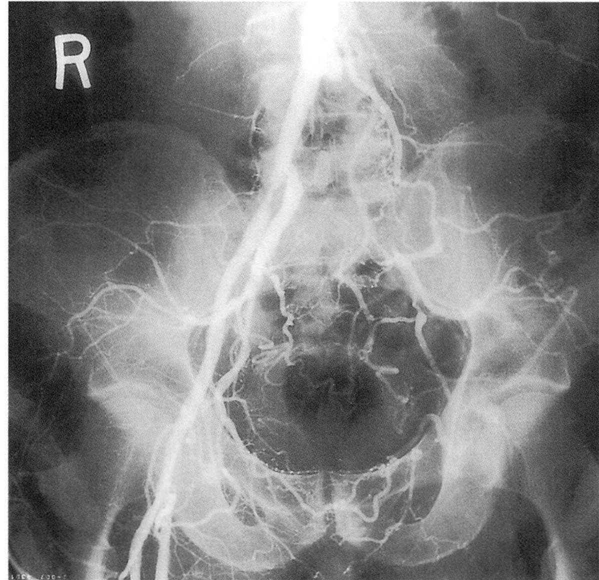

Fig. 17.2Q The patient's arteriogram.

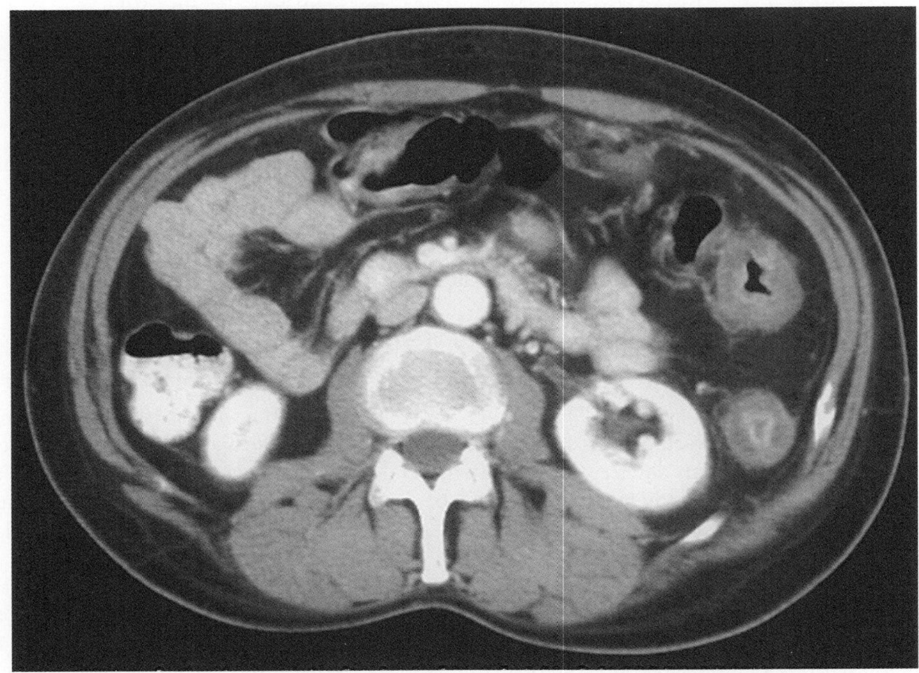

Fig. 17.3Q The patient's CT scan. (From Pretoris ES, Solomon JA. Radiology Secrets Plus, 3rd edn. Mosby, 2011, with permission.)

OSCE Scenario 17.4

A 65-year-old smoker is referred to you due to episodes of unsteadiness, blurred vision in the left eye and a numb left arm. During your history you find out he is a painter and these symptoms occur only when he is painting or using his arm for other physical tasks. He is left-handed.

1. What is the potential diagnosis?
2. Would you expect to find a difference in the blood pressure of each arm and why? Are there any other significant examination findings?
3. Can you explain his symptoms given the diagnosis?
4. You order a duplex ultrasound scan; can you describe the findings you would expect to see?

OSCE Scenario 17.5

A 29-year-old man is involved in a road traffic accident and has a badly fractured right femur, a splenic haematoma and broken right wrist. He is taken to theatre early the next morning and has had his femur nailed to fix the fracture. You are called by the nurse caring for him to tell you he is very confused – he is pulling away when the nurse has tried to take a blood gas; he is making noises and opens his eyes when you speak. In addition, his SpO_2 is 88% and his chest is covered in a petechial rash.

1. What is the likely diagnosis and what is the cause? What differential diagnosis should you consider?
2. What tests would you order?
3. How would you treat this patient?
4. What is his GCS score?

Answers in Appendix pages 470–473

Please check your eBook at https://studentconsult.inkling.com/ for more self-assessment questions. See inside cover for registration details.

18

Neoplasia

A neoplasm is a lesion resulting from abnormal growth of a tissue, which is partly or completely autonomous of normal growth controls, and persists after the initiating stimulus has been removed.

CLASSIFICATION OF TUMOURS

- Behavioural classification: benign or malignant.
- Histogenetic classification: cell of origin.

Behavioural Classification

The behavioural classification divides tumours into:

- benign
- malignant.

The pathological criteria for classifying a tumour as benign or malignant are shown in Box 18.1.

Histogenetic Classification

- Classification by cell of origin.
- Histologically determined.
- Degree of histological resemblance allows tumour to be graded.
- Grading correlates with clinical behaviour.

Major Categories of Tumour Origin

- From epithelial cells.
- From connective tissue cells (mesenchymal).
- From lymphoid and haemopoietic tissue.

Differentiation

The degree to which the tumour histologically resembles its cell or tissue of origin. Degree of differentiation determines the tumour grade.

- Well-differentiated: resembles parent tissue more than poorly differentiated tumours.
- Poorly differentiated: may be so poorly differentiated that they lack easily recognizable histogenetic features. They are more aggressive than well-differentiated tumours.

BOX 18.1 Behavioural Classification

Benign	Malignant
Slow growing	Rapidly growing
Low mitotic rate	High mitotic rate
Resembles parent tissue	Differs from parent site
Non-infiltrating	Infiltrating
Cells normal	Cells abnormal
Never metastasizes	Frequently metastasizes
Often circumscribed or encapsulated	Often poorly defined or irregular
Rarely ulcerates	Frequent ulceration on skin/mucosal surfaces
Rarely undergoes necrosis	Necrosis common
Only fatal if damaging vital function, e.g. cerebral tumour	Always fatal if untreated

- Moderately differentiated: intermediate between well- and poorly differentiated tumours.
- Tumours defying histogenetic classification are called anaplastic.

NOMENCLATURE OF TUMOURS

- All have the suffix '-oma'.
- Benign epithelial tumours are either papillomas or adenomas.
- Benign connective tissue tumours have a prefix denoting the cell of origin, e.g. lipoma (fat), osteoma (bone).
- A carcinoma is a malignant epithelial neoplasm.
- A sarcoma is a malignant connective tissue neoplasm.

Examples of tumour nomenclature are shown in Table 18.1.

TABLE 18.1 Examples of Tumour Nomenclature

Tissue of origin	Benign	Malignant
Epithelium		
Glandular	Adenoma	Adenocarcinoma
Squamous	Squamous cell papilloma	Squamous cell carcinoma
Transitional	Transitional cell papilloma	Transitional cell carcinoma
Mesenchyme		
Fat	Lipoma	Liposarcoma
Striated muscle	Rhabdomyoma	Rhabdomyosarcoma
Smooth muscle	Leiomyoma	Leiomyosarcoma
Bone	Osteoma	Osteosarcoma (osteogenic sarcoma)
Cartilage	Chondroma	Chondrosarcoma
Blood vessel	Angioma	Angiosarcoma
Fibrous tissue	Fibroma	Fibrosarcoma

Epithelial Tumours

Benign Tumours

- Papilloma: benign tumour of non-glandular or non-secretory epithelium, e.g. transitional or stratified squamous epithelium.
- Adenoma: benign tumour of glandular or secretory epithelium, e.g. colonic adenoma.

Malignant Tumours

- Carcinoma: malignant tumour of epithelium, e.g. squamous cell carcinoma.
- Adenocarcinoma: malignant tumour of glandular epithelium, e.g. adenocarcinoma of the stomach.

Carcinoma In Situ

A lesion with all the cytological features of cancer but no evidence of invasion through the epithelial basement membrane, e.g. ductal carcinoma in situ (DCIS) of the breast.

Connective Tissue Tumours

Tumours of connective tissue are named according to the cell of origin and behavioural classification.

Teratomas

A teratoma is a germ cell neoplasm representing all three germ cell layers, i.e. ectoderm, mesoderm and endoderm. Ovarian teratomas tend to be benign and cystic. Testicular teratomas tend to be malignant and solid.

Embryonal Tumours (Blastomas)

These bear a histological resemblance to the embryonic form of the organ from which they arise.

- Nephroblastoma: Wilms' tumour; kidney.
- Neuroblastoma: adrenal medulla, autonomic ganglia.
- Retinoblastoma: eye (inherited predisposition).
- Hepatoblastoma: liver.

Apudomas and Carcinoid Tumours

- APUD (amine content and/or precursor uptake and decarboxylation).
- Describes cells of diffuse (neuro-) endocrine system.
- Examples of apudomas and their clinical manifestations are:
  - insulinoma: episodes of hypoglycaemia
  - gastrinoma: extensive peptic ulceration (Zollinger–Ellison syndrome)
  - phaeochromocytoma: paroxysmal hypertension
  - carcinoid: if metastases are present, flushing, palpitations and pulmonary valve stenosis.

Mixed Neoplasm

A neoplasm showing more than one neoplastic component; usually both epithelial and mesenchymal, e.g. pleomorphic adenoma of the parotid (glandular tissue in a cartilaginous or mucinous matrix), fibroadenoma of the breast. Carcinosarcomas are most common in the female genital tract.

Hamartomas

A hamartoma is a tumour-like lesion which lacks autonomy but in which the elements are fully differentiated and are normally found in the tissue of origin. They usually contain two or more mature cell types native to the organ of origin but the constituent parts are abnormally organized, e.g. pigmented naevi, pulmonary hamartomas, which consist of a mixture of cartilage and bronchial epithelium.

Poorly Named Tumours (Misnomas!)

- Lymphoma: malignant, therefore lymphosarcoma.
- Hepatoma: malignant, therefore hepatocellular carcinoma.
- Melanoma: malignant, therefore melanocarcinoma.

TUMOUR GROWTH PATTERNS

- Sessile, polypoid and papillary tumours are likely to be benign (but not always).
- Fungating, ulcerating, annular and infiltrating tumours are likely to be malignant.
- Ulcerated tumours can often be distinguished from benign ulcers. The latter have sloping edges while the former have rolled, everted edges, e.g. squamous cell carcinoma.
- Encapsulated tumours tend to be benign. Beware the false capsule of compressed connective tissue, e.g. pleomorphic adenoma of the parotid. 'Shelling out' this tumour would leave residual tumour.

Histological Pattern

Malignant features include:

- loss of differentiation
- disordered growth pattern
- variability in cell size
- variability in nuclear size
- high nuclear:cytoplasmic ratio
- increased mitotic activity
- abnormal nucleoli may be multiple
- abnormal chromatin pattern.

CARCINOGENESIS

- This is the process by which normal cells are converted into cells capable of forming neoplasms.
- A carcinogen is an agent known or suspected to participate in the causation of tumours. Such agents are said to be carcinogenic (cancer-causing) or oncogenic (tumour-causing). Strictly speaking, carcinogenesis applies to the causation of malignant tumours, whereas oncogenesis includes all tumours, benign and malignant.
- The main classes of carcinogen are:
    - chemicals
    - radiation
    - viruses
    - hormones
    - bacteria, fungi, parasites
    - other agents.

Chemicals

- Polycyclic aromatic hydrocarbons:
    - scrotal cancer in chimney sweeps due to exposure to polycyclic aromatic hydrocarbons in soot (of historical interest)
    - 3,4-benzpyrene in tobacco smoke. Carcinogenic on direct contact, e.g. smoking, but absorbed into bloodstream, which may explain why smokers have higher incidence of cancer at other sites, e.g. kidney, bladder
    - carcinogenic components of tar, which can cause skin cancers by direct contact.
- Aromatic amines:
    - β-naphthylamine: high incidence of bladder cancer in dye and rubber industry.
- Nitrosamines:
    - gut cancers in animals.
- Azo dyes:
    - bladder and liver cancers in animals.
- Alkylating agents, e.g. cyclophosphamide:
    - small risk of leukaemia in humans.

Radiation

- UV light is a major cause of skin cancer.
- Exposure to ionizing radiation is associated with increased risk of cancer at many sites, e.g.
    - carcinoma of the thyroid after childhood irradiation of the neck
    - increased incidence of leukaemia and carcinoma of breast, lung and thyroid after nuclear explosions at Hiroshima and Nagasaki during the Second World War
    - cancer of thyroid after Chernobyl disaster, which released radioactive iodine
    - leukaemia and liver neoplasms developing years after exposure to thorium-containing contrast medium (thorotrast)
    - angiosarcoma developing at the sites of previous radiotherapy treatment for breast cancer

Viruses

- HPV:
    - common wart
    - cervical carcinoma, strong association with HPV type 16 and 18.
- EBV:
    - Burkitt's lymphoma
    - nasopharyngeal carcinoma
    - B-cell lymphoma in immunosuppressed patients.
- Hepatitis B virus:
    - hepatocellular carcinoma.

- HIV:
  - Kaposi's sarcoma.
- HTLV-1:
  - T-cell lymphoma/leukaemia.

Hormones

- Experimentally, oestrogens can be shown to promote formation of breast and endometrial carcinoma.
- Increased incidence of endometrial carcinoma in postmenopausal women treated with oestrogen-containing compounds.
- Androgenic and anabolic steroids are known to induce hepatocellular tumours in humans.

Bacteria, Fungi, Parasites

- *Helicobacter pylori* implicated in the pathogenesis of gastric lymphoma.
- Aflatoxins (B1) produced by *Aspergillus flavus* have been linked to high incidence of hepatocellular carcinoma in certain areas of Africa.
- *Schistosoma* is strongly implicated in the high incidence of bladder cancer where infection (schistosomiasis) is rife, e.g. Egypt.
- *Clonorchis sinensis* (liver fluke): dwells in bile ducts where it may cause cholangiocarcinoma.

Other Agents

- Asbestos:
  - mesothelioma (strong association)
  - carcinoma of the bronchus.
- Metals:
  - nickel exposure is associated with nasal and bronchial carcinoma.
- Betel nut:
  - chewing betel nut is associated with increased risk of neoplasms of oral cavity.

HOST FACTORS AND CARCINOGENESIS

- Race.
- Diet.
- Inherited predisposition.
- Age.
- Sex.

Race

- Precise role unknown due to coincidence with diet, habit and location.
- Incidence of oral cancer high in India and South East Asia, but probably related to chewing betel nut.
- High incidence of hepatocellular carcinoma in Africa and South East Asia, but is probably related to exposure to dietary carcinogens and viral hepatitis.
- Immigrant groups tend eventually to assume the disease profile of their adopted country.

Diet

- Aflatoxins and hepatocellular carcinoma.
- Diet low in fibre in colorectal cancer.
- High dietary fat in breast cancer.

Inherited Predisposition

- Some diseases appear to run in families ('cancer families').
- A woman whose mother and one sister have breast cancer stands a 50% probability of developing the disease.
- Examples of familial cancer are shown in Table 18.2.

Age

- The incidence of cancer increases with age.
- This reflects the cumulative effects of exposure to carcinogens with age.
- Effects of immune defences may be lost with old age.

TABLE 18.2 Examples of Familial Cancer Syndrome

Syndrome	Gene Affected	Resultant Neoplasms
Li–Fraumeni	p53	Breast and ovarian carcinomas, astrocytomas, sarcomas
Retinoblastoma	Rb1	Retinoblastoma, osteosarcoma
Familial polyposis coli	APC	GI tract carcinomas; mainly colon
von Hippel–Lindau	VHL	Renal carcinoma, phaeochromocytoma, haemangioblastoma
Multiple endocrine neoplasia syndromes (I–III)	RET, others	Tumours of pituitary parathyroids, thyroid, pancreas, adrenal glands (combination depends on which syndrome)
Familial breast cancer	BRCA1, BRCA2	Breast, ovarian syndrome, prostatic carcinomas

BOX 18.2 Commonest Cancers by Sex

Male	Female
Carcinoma of the prostate	Carcinoma of the breast
Bronchopulmonary carcinoma	Bronchopulmonary carcinoma
Colorectal adenocarcinoma	Colorectal adenocarcinoma
Urinary tract carcinoma	Uterine carcinoma

- Familial neoplasms occur at a younger age than sporadic neoplasms.
- Individual neoplasms have their own specific age distribution, e.g. fibroadenoma of the breast (18–35 years), carcinoma of the breast (more common after the menopause), neuroblastoma (childhood).

Sex

- Carcinoma of the breast is 200 times more common in women than in men.
- The commonest tumours in men and women differ, and current statistics can be seen in Box 18.2.

PREMALIGNANT DISEASE

A premalignant lesion is a discrete identifiable lesion associated with an increased risk of progression to a malignant neoplasm.

Examples include:

- benign neoplasms that can become malignant, e.g. colorectal adenoma–carcinoma sequence (Fig. 18.1)
- dysplasia/in situ malignancy
- metaplasia–dysplasia sequence (Table 18.3).

A premalignant condition is a non-neoplastic condition which is associated with an increased risk of developing malignant tumours. Examples of premalignant lesions and conditions are shown in Box 18.3.

Carcinogenic Process

Multistep Theory

- Latency: the causal event is usually followed by a variable but usually lengthy delayed period. This is because:
  - more than one effect is required for cancer to develop (multistep)
  - it takes time for the mutated cell to produce a clone of a significant number of cells to produce signs and symptoms.
- Initiation: exposure of cell/tissue to carcinogen and induction of lesion in cell's genome bestowing neoplastic potential; irreversible.
- Promotion: the event stimulating clonal proliferation of the initiated transformed cell. A promoter is a substance that will cause cancer in an initiated cell but not a normal cell, e.g. croton oil in experimental skin cancers initiated by methylcholanthrene.
- Persistence: initiators and promoters no longer required. The tumour becomes autonomous with vascular ingrowth, increased growth rate, invasiveness and metastasis.

Genetics of Cancer

An increased predisposition to development of malignant neoplasm may be inherited as:

- part of a clinical syndrome with other diagnostic features in addition to the increased risk of malignancy, e.g. acute leukaemia in Down's syndrome
- an increased likelihood of neoplasia developing as the only manifestation, e.g. familial retinoblastoma syndrome.

Inherited syndromes associated with an increased risk of malignancy are:

- syndromes with a major chromosomal abnormality, e.g. Down's syndrome and acute leukaemia
- syndromes determined by single gene defects, e.g. familial polyposis coli and colorectal cancer.

Evidence for Genetic Alterations Causing Cancer

- Translocations: part of one chromosome becomes attached to another, e.g. Philadelphia chromosome and chronic myeloid leukaemia (CML), Burkitt's lymphoma.
- Extra chromosomes: usually trisomies (i.e. three copies of a chromosome rather than two), e.g. trisomy 21 (Down's syndrome), acute leukaemia.
- Familial aggregations, e.g. retinoblastoma.
- Increased risk of malignancy associated with incapacity to repair damaged DNA, e.g. xeroderma pigmentosum and skin cancers.
- Association between chemical mutagens and their carcinogenic effects (see above).
- Evidence that mutation or unregulated expression of certain genes converts normal cells to malignant cells.

Genetic Mechanisms in Carcinogenesis

Two important genetic mechanisms leading to neoplasia are:

- abnormal or excessive expression of dominant stimulatory genes – oncogenes
- loss or inactivation of recessive inhibitory genes – tumour suppressor genes.

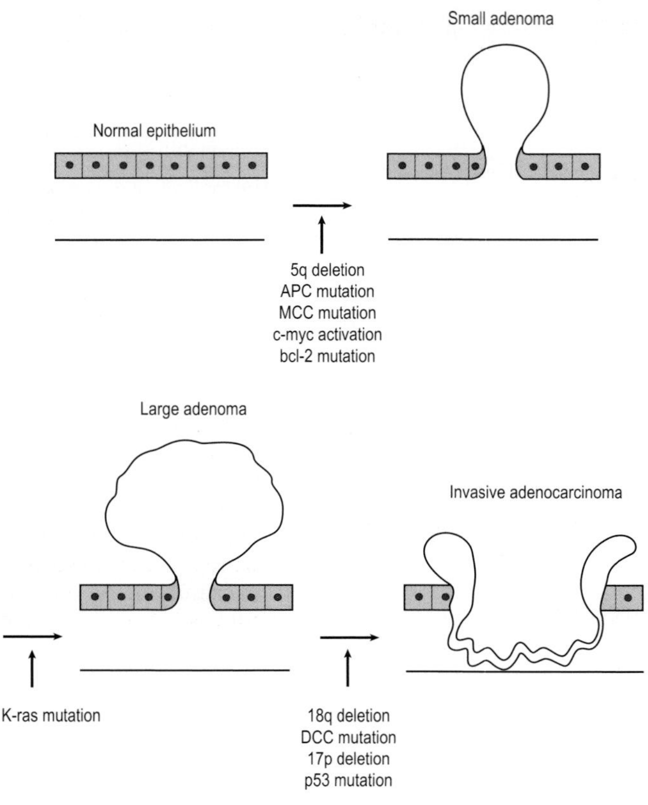

Fig. 18.1 Molecular genetics of the adenoma–carcinoma sequence.

TABLE 18.3 Examples of Metaplasia–Dysplasia Sequence

Organ	Metaplasia Undergoing Dysplasia	Resulting Malignancy
Oesophagus	Barrett's oesophagus (intestinal metaplasia)	Oesophageal adenocarcinoma
Stomach	Intestinal metaplasia (associated with achlorhydria)	Gastric adenocarcinoma
Bronchus	Squamous metaplasia (smokers)	Bronchogenic squamous cell carcinoma
Cervix	Squamous metaplasia	Squamous cell carcinoma
Kidney (renal pelvis)	Squamous metaplasia (stone or chronic infection)	Squamous cell carcinoma of renal pelvis

Abnormal expression of oncogenes drives normal cells towards a neoplastic state. Loss of tumour suppressor gene function allows neoplastic transformation as a result of oncogene expression.

Oncogenes

- Genes whose presence in certain forms and/or activity can stimulate the development of cancer.

- Oncogenes contribute to the development of cancer by instructing cells to make proteins that stimulate excessive growth and cell division.
- Oncogenes are related to normal genes called proto-oncogenes.
- Proto-oncogenes are a family of normal genes that code for proteins involved in the normal growth-control pathway of a cell.
- Growth factors, receptors, signalling enzymes and transcription factors are encoded by proto-oncogenes.
- Oncogenes arise from mutations of proto-oncogenes.
- Oncogenes code for altered versions or excessive quantities of growth-controlled proteins that disrupt the growth-signalling pathway of the cell.
- The growth-signalling pathway becomes hyperactive and cells grow and divide more rapidly.

BOX 18.3 Examples of Premalignant Conditions

Premalignant Lesion/ Condition	Cancer Risk
Colorectal adenomatous polyp	Colorectal adenocarcinoma
Epithelial hyperplasia of the breast	Carcinoma of the breast
Cervical epithelial dysplasia	Carcinoma of the cervix
Ulcerative colitis	Colorectal adenocarcinoma
	Bile duct carcinoma
Xeroderma pigmentosum	Skin cancer
Cirrhosis of the liver	Hepatocellular carcinoma
Paget's disease of bone	Osteogenic sarcoma

- A cancer cell may contain one or more oncogenes, such that one or more components of the pathway may be abnormal.

Examples of oncogenes and their products are shown in Table 18.4.

Tumour Suppressor Genes

- Normal genes whose absence can lead to the development of cancer.
- Tumour suppressor genes are categorized according to their mechanism of action (Table 18.5):
  - caretaker genes maintain the integrity of the genome by repairing DNA damage
  - gatekeeper genes inhibit proliferation, or promote the death of cells with damaged DNA.
- If a pair of tumour suppressor genes are lost from a cell, or inactivated by mutation, cancer can result.
- Individuals who inherit an increased risk of developing cancer are often born with a defective copy on one tumour suppressor gene.
- Because genes come in pairs, an inherited defect in one copy will not cause cancer if the other normal copy is functional.
- If the second copy undergoes mutation, then cancer may occur because there is no longer a functional copy of the gene.

Examples of Tumour Suppressor Genes

Rb gene and retinoblastoma

- Individuals with an inherited predisposition to develop retinoblastoma are born with absence of one of normally paired Rb1 suppressor genes. Only one further mutational loss of the remaining Rb1 gene is required for retinoblastoma to develop. High risk of bilateral familial retinoblastoma.

TABLE 18.4 Examples of Oncogenes

Oncogene	Protein Produced	Abbreviated From
Growth factors and their receptors		
sis	Platelet-derived growth factor	Simian sarcoma virus
erb-B	Epidermal growth factor receptor	Erythroblastosis virus
fms	Macrophage colony-stimulating factor receptor	Feline McDonagh Sarcoma virus
Signal transduction molecules		
ras	G-protein	Rat Sarcoma virus
abl	Tyrosine kinase	Abelson murine leukaemia virus
Transcription factors		
myc	DNA binding proteins	Myelocytomatosis virus

TABLE 18.5 Tumour Suppressor Genes and Associated Tumours

Category	Gene	Tumour Susceptibility if Mutation	Other Associations
Gatekeepers	p53	Li–Fraumeni syndrome (predisposed to wide range of tumours, e.g. breast, ovary, sarcoma)	Mutated in 50% of human epithelial cancers
	Rb1	Familial retinoblastoma	
	APC	Familial adenomatous polyposis	Often mutated in sporadic colorectal cancers
Caretakers	BRCA1	Familial breast and ovarian cancer	Rarely mutated in sporadic breast cancers
	BRCA2	Familial breast cancer	

- Individuals with paired Rb1 genes have a low incidence of retinoblastoma because two mutational losses in the same cell or daughter cells would be required; hence, sporadic retinoblastoma is very rare. Risk of unilateral retinoblastoma.

p53 tumour suppressor gene

- Situated on short arm of chromosome 17.
- Most frequently mutated of the class of genes.
- Normal functions are:
  - repair of damaged DNA before S phase of cycle by arresting cell cycle in G phase until damage is repaired
  - apoptotic cell death if DNA damage is extensive.
- Inherited germ line mutations of p53 occur in the rare Li–Fraumeni syndrome, giving an inherited predisposition to a wide range of tumours.

BEHAVIOUR OF TUMOURS

Invasion

Invasion is the sole most important criterion for malignancy. Metastases are a consequence of invasion. Invasion demands that tumours should be removed in continuity with a wide margin of apparently normal tissue.

Factors influencing tumour invasion include:

- Abnormal or increased motility:
  - malignant cells are more mobile than their normal counterparts.
- Secretion of proteolytic enzymes:
  - matrix metalloproteinases are secreted by malignant cells
  - they digest surrounding connective tissue, e.g. interstitial collagenases degrade collagens Type I, II and III.
- Decreased cellular adhesion:
  - loss of surface adhesion molecules, e.g. cadherins enable migration of individual cells.

Clinical Consequences of Local Invasion

Clinical consequences of local invasion depend upon the site of the tumour. Box 18.4 indicates some of the clinical consequences of local invasion of bronchial carcinoma.

BOX 18.4 Clinical Consequences of Local Invasion of Bronchial Carcinoma

Structure Invaded	Consequence
Oesophagus	Dysphagia
Thoracic major vessels	Massive haemoptysis
Superior vena cava	Facial oedema/cyanosis
Recurrent laryngeal nerve	Hoarseness
Sympathetic chain	Horner's syndrome
Brachial plexus	Pancoast syndrome (also Horner's syndrome and unilateral recurrent laryngeal nerve palsy)
Phrenic nerve	Paralysis of hemidiaphragm
Pericardium	Pericardial effusion

Metastasis

Metastasis is the process whereby malignant tumours spread from their site of origin (primary) to form other tumours (secondary) at distant sites. Metastasis is tumour spread in discontinuity as distinct from invasion, which is spread in continuity.

Steps in the Metastatic Cascade

- Detachment of tumour cells.
- Invasion of surrounding tissues to reach vessels.
- Intravasation into lumen of vessels (blood and lymphatics).
- Evasion of host defence mechanisms.
- Adherence to endothelium at remote location.
- Extravasation from vessel lumen into surrounding tissue.
- Survival and growth within the tissue.
- Establishment of own blood supply.

Routes of Metastasis

- Lymphatic: regional lymph nodes.
- Haematogenous: via the bloodstream.
- Transcoelomic: across peritoneal, pleural and pericardial cavities.
- Seeding or implantation during surgery.

Lymphatic

- Most carcinomas spread via lymphatics.
- May remain discrete in lymph nodes or invade outside nodes, involving adjacent nodes and connective tissue when they become matted together.
- Melanomas may permeate lymphatics and appear as black streaks in subcutaneous tissue.
- Lymphatic blockage causes lymphoedema of tissues; in the breast it is associated with peau d'orange.

Haematogenous

- Bone is a favoured site for haematogenous spread from five carcinomas: lung, breast, thyroid, kidney and prostate.
- Other favoured sites are lung, liver and brain.
- Sarcomas spread by the bloodstream and NOT lymphatics.

Transcoelomic

- Spread of carcinoma of stomach to ovaries (Krukenberg tumours).
- Spread of ovarian cancer to omentum and peritoneum (ascites).
- Spread of bronchial carcinoma to pleura (pleural effusion).

Seeding or Implantation at Surgery

- Tumour grows in sites of surgical incision or investigation, e.g. FNA.

CLINICAL EFFECTS OF TUMOURS

These may be:

- local
- systemic
- paraneoplastic
- metabolic
- others.

Local

- Mass.
- Bleeding due to ulceration: haematemesis, haematuria.
- Pain.
- Obstruction: hollow tube, e.g. large bowel obstruction with carcinoma.
- Irritation at tissue of origin, e.g. cough due to bronchial tumour.
- Pressure on adjacent structures, e.g. nerves, blood vessels, bile ducts (cancer of head of pancreas and obstructive jaundice).

Systemic

Effects of Metastases

- Enlarged lymph nodes: may be discrete or hard, irregular and matted.
- Hepatomegaly: primary tumour in stomach, colon, bronchus or breast.
- Jaundice: nodes in porta hepatis with primary tumour in stomach, pancreas or colon.
- Ascites: ovarian or any gastrointestinal (GI) malignancy.
- Abdominal mass due to omental secondaries often in association with ascites.
- Pathological fractures due to bony metastases: breast, bronchus, thyroid, prostate or kidney.
- Pleural effusion: bronchial carcinoma and breast cancer.
- Fits, confusion, personality change from cerebral metastases, e.g. breast, bronchus or malignant melanoma.
- Anaemia – pancytopenia: bone marrow deposits.

Paraneoplastic Effects

These are effects that occur in the presence of a neoplasm which are not directly caused by the tumour itself or metastases. They can be divided as follows:

- humoral (mediated by a tumour-secreted product)
- immunological (usually autoimmune).

Humoral

- Bronchial carcinoma and Cushing's syndrome due to inappropriate secretion of adrenocorticotrophic hormone (ACTH).
- Bronchial carcinoma and inappropriate secretion of antidiuretic hormone (ADH, vasopressin).
- Hypercalcaemia of malignancy caused by secretion of parathyroid hormone-related peptide.
- Carcinoid syndrome with liver metastases from a carcinoid tumour due to 5-hydroxytryptamine (5HT, serotonin).

Immunological

- Autoimmune disease may be triggered by malignancy.
- Dermatomyositis developing in later life may be due to an underlying malignancy.
- Membranous glomerulonephritis can be initiated by an underlying malignancy.

Metabolic Effects

These are usually hormonal and reflect appropriate secretion of hormones:

- thyrotoxicosis from thyroid adenoma
- Cushing's syndrome from adrenal cortical adenoma

- hyperparathyroidism from parathyroid adenoma
- insulin from an insulinoma.

Others

- Cachexia: all tumours; probably multifactorial.
- Pyrexia of unknown origin (PUO): lymphoma, hypernephroma.
- Hypertrophic pulmonary osteoarthropathy associated with bronchial carcinoma.
- Thrombophlebitis migrans associated with visceral cancer, usually carcinoma of the head of the pancreas.
- Acanthosis nigricans associated with carcinoma of the pancreas.

Tumour Markers

Neoplastic cells often have quantitative and qualitative abnormalities of protein synthesis. They may either overproduce a normal product or they may produce a substance which is abnormal for their tissue of origin. Protein production by some tumours has been utilized clinically as tumour markers. Examples of tumour markers are shown in Box 18.5.

A tumour marker:

- May be a substance which is secreted into the blood or other body fluid or expressed on the cell surface of malignant cells in larger quantities than in normal counterparts.
- Detection is by measuring the concentration of the marker in the body fluids, usually by immunoassay.
- Some markers may be detected in histological sections using immunohistochemistry.
- Tumour markers are rarely sufficiently specific to be of absolute diagnostic value.

BOX 18.5 Examples of Tumour Markers

Tumour	Marker
Prostatic adenocarcinoma	Prostate-specific antigen (PSA)
Hepatocellular carcinoma	α-fetoprotein
Testicular cancer	β-Human Chorionic Gonadotropin (HCG), α-fetoprotein, placental alkaline phosphatase
Choriocarcinoma	β-HCG
Ovarian carcinoma	CA 125
Colorectal cancer	Carcinoembryonic antigen (CEA)

- The main value of tumour markers is in following the course of a malignant disease and monitoring the response to treatment and hence prognosis.
- Tumour markers can also be used for tumour localization and antibody-directed therapy.

TUMOUR DEPENDENCY

Although the growth of tumours is autonomous, some retain a requirement for growth factors/endocrine support. Good examples of those requiring endocrine support are carcinomas of the breast, prostate and thyroid.

Breast

- A large proportion of breast carcinomas express oestrogen receptors.
- The degree of oestrogen-receptor expression correlates well with the response of the tumour to oestrogen blockade, e.g. with the selective oestrogen receptor-modulating drug tamoxifen.
- Oestrogen-receptor-positive tumours tend to be of a lower grade and have a better prognosis than oestrogen-receptor-negative tumours.

Prostate

- Prostatic epithelium is dependent on androgenic stimulation.
- Castration results in apoptosis of prostate epithelial cells and partial involution of the gland.
- Many prostatic carcinomas retain the above characteristics, allowing their growth to be inhibited by androgen blockade.
- Androgen blockade can be achieved by:
  - orchidectomy
  - oestrogens (side effects unacceptable)
  - luteinizing hormone (LH) released from pituitary stimulates androgen production by Leydig cells. LH production can be inhibited by luteinizing hormone releasing hormone (LHRH), which, after transient stimulation, causes long-term depression of LH release.
- After a period of time, androgen sensitivity is lost and therefore the above treatments are not curative.

Thyroid

- Papillary and follicular carcinoma respond in the same way as normal thyroid epithelium to thyroid-stimulating hormone (TSH).
- TSH suppression with thyroxine, in conjunction with surgery and radioiodine therapy, is used to treat these neoplasms.

PROGNOSIS OF TUMOURS

This depends on:

- type of tumour
- stage (extent of spread)
- grade (degree of differentiation)
- surface receptors, e.g. oestrogen receptors in breast cancer
- gene expression
- sensitivity to treatment modalities
- age
- nutritional status
- immune status and human leucocyte antigen (HLA) type.

Tumour Staging

This represents the extent of spread. Staging can be assessed as follows:

- clinical assessment
- imaging techniques
- histopathological examination of resected specimen.

Some types of staging rely on one of the above alone (e.g. Dukes' classification) and some rely on a combination (TNM). Staging is designed to define prognosis.

Dukes' Classification

A pathological classification drawn up by Cuthbert Dukes (pathologist) originally to stage rectal cancer but now extrapolated to colorectal cancer.

- Dukes A: invasion into, but not through, the bowel wall.
- Dukes B: invasion through the bowel wall.
- Dukes C: involvement of regional lymph nodes.
- Dukes D was not in the original classification but was added later: indicates distant metastases.

TNM Classification

- T: primary tumour. Number suffix indicates tumour extent or size.
- N: lymph nodes. Number suffix indicates number of lymph nodes or groups of lymph nodes involved.
- M: metastases. Number suffix indicates presence or absence.
- Example: TNM classification for carcinoma of the breast:
  - Tis: carcinoma in situ
  - T0: no primary located
  - T1: tumour <2 cm
  - T2: tumour 2–5 cm
  - T3: tumour >5 cm
  - T4: extension to chest wall ± skin
  - N0: no nodal involvement
  - N1: mobile ipsilateral axillary nodes
  - N2: fixed ipsilateral axillary nodes
  - N3: ipsilateral supraclavicular nodes
  - M0: no metastases
  - M1: distant metastases
  - MX: metastases suspected but not confirmed.

Other Staging

- Malignant melanoma:
  - Breslow's classification (the distance between the stratum granulosum and the deepest part of the melanoma). Directly related to survival:
    - <0.76 mm: very good prognosis
    - >4.0 mm: very poor prognosis and high risk of metastases
  - Clark's classification (defined according to anatomical boundaries) relates to anatomical area of penetration, e.g. level 1: confined to epidermis, to level 5: tumour cells present in the subcutaneous tissue.

Breslow's classification is more widely used, and has an influence on the surgical margins taken. These margins are a source of controversy and vary between countries, but current UK guidance states that if a lesion is less than or equal to 1 mm thick, then a 1 cm margin is taken; 1.01–4.0 mm, then a 2 cm margin is taken; and >4 mm, then a 3 cm margin is taken.

SCREENING

Population screening programmes are aimed at reducing morbidity and mortality from a particular disease within an entire population. Screening should be directed at an asymptomatic population at risk. The principles underlying screening depend on the following:

- for screening to be cost-effective, the cancer must constitute a major health risk, i.e. high incidence and high mortality rate
- it must be a relatively common disease, e.g. breast cancer in the UK; gastric cancer in Japan
- there must be an established and effective treatment for the disease
- it must be demonstrated that early diagnosis and treatment do increase the cure rate
- there must be a diagnostic test available that can be applied to a large number of people
- the test must have a high level of sensitivity and specificity
- the test should not cause harm to the individual being tested
- the cost of screening large populations must be justified by the yields.

Screening Programmes

Breast

- Mammographic screening.
- Women aged 50–70 years old (currently being extended to women aged 47–73 years old in some areas of the UK as a trial extension of the programme).
- Repeated 3-yearly.

Cervix

- Exfoliative cytology.
- Identification of cervical intraepithelial neoplasia (CIN).
- Co-ordinated national screening programme in the UK.
- Women aged 25–49 years old, screened every 3 years; women aged 50–64 years old, screened every 5 years.

OSCE SCENARIOS

OSCE Scenario 18.1

A 32-year-old female attends your clinic after triple assessment has shown her breast lump to be a benign cyst. She remains very anxious. Although she has no family history of breast cancer, her sister-in-law has just been diagnosed with ductal carcinoma in situ (DCIS) and is due to have a mastectomy. She wishes to know about the screening programme for breast cancer and to discuss any risk factors she has.

1. Answer this patient's questions about cancer and carcinoma in situ.
2. Answer her questions about risk factors for cancer, in particular breast cancer.
3. Explain the breast screening programme to her.

OSCE Scenario 18.2

A 58-year-old female with known breast cancer is admitted with pain in the back and ribs which has been present for several weeks but has suddenly become much worse. She is in obvious pain but has no neurological symptoms. A bone scan had been carried out 1 week previously (Fig. 18.2Q).

1. What is your suspected diagnosis? What does the bone scan show?
   The patient is admitted for pain relief and a CT scan shows liver and bone metastases. She has completed her surgery and chemotherapy and understands that her disease has spread. She wishes to go home as soon as possible as her eldest daughter is getting married in 3 weeks.
2. After ruling out any fractures, what multidisciplinary treatment plan may be appropriate for her now? What specific treatment may help her back pain?
3. How does therapeutic radiotherapy work? On which tissues does it work best?
4. What side effects can radiotherapy have in the short and long term?

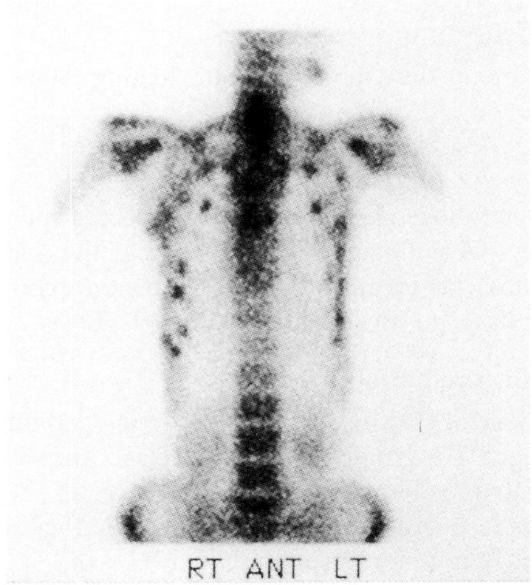

Fig. 18.2Q The patient's bone scan.

OSCE Scenario 18.3

A 22-year-old male attends your clinic after referral by his GP for testicular discomfort. He describes a vague history of trauma during football several weeks ago. Examination reveals a firm, painless mass near the superior pole of the testis but no other clinical abnormalities.

1. What is your differential diagnosis?
2. What other clinical features would you look for on examination?
3. Explain to the examiners some known risk factors for testicular cancer and the most common pathological types.
4. How should this man be investigated? How are these tumours staged?

OSCE Scenario 18.4

A 70-year-old smoker has had a cough for the last six months and has been losing weight due to a poor appetite. The GP does some baseline blood tests and sends the patient for a chest X-ray. The blood tests come back before the chest X-ray and show a sodium of 120 mmol/L.

1. What are you concerned about?
2. What further tests would you need to do to secure the diagnosis?

3. What type of lung condition is it most often associated with?
4. What is this type of condition called and can you name any others?

OSCE Scenario 18.5

A 30-year-old male is seen in the general surgery clinic with a history of rectal bleeding and abdominal pain. In the process of your history-taking you discover his father died from bowel cancer at a young age. At colonoscopy you find hundreds of colorectal polyps.

1. What is the diagnosis?
2. What gene is abnormal and what group of genes is it part of? Describe how these genes cause cancer when they are abnormal.
3. Can you name another group of genes involved with cancer and describe how abnormalities in these genes can give rise to cancers? Give some examples.

Answers in Appendix pages 473–476

Please check your eBook at https://studentconsult.inkling.com/ for more self-assessment questions. See inside cover for registration details.

19

Immunology

IMMUNITY

Immunity is a body defence mechanism characterized by specificity and memory.

Defence against infection is accomplished by two systems:

- innate (non-specific/natural) immunity
- adaptive (specific/acquired) immunity.

Innate Immunity

- Physical barriers:
  - skin
  - mucous membranes.
- Mechanical factors:
  - coughing
  - ciliary action in respiratory tract.
- Humoral factors:
  - secretions with antibacterial activity, e.g. lysozyme in tears
  - complement and interferons.
- Cellular factors:
  - phagocytic cells, e.g. polymorphs, macrophages, mast cells and basophils: produce soluble mediators in inflammatory response
  - natural killer (NK) cells: kill infected tissue cells in non-specific manner (non-MHC–restricted killing).

Adaptive Immunity

Adaptive immune responses are more effective than innate ones. They are mediated by lymphocytes and antibodies, which amplify and focus responses and provide additional effector functions.

Essential Features of the Immune System

- Specificity.
- Diversity.
- Memory.
- Recruitment of other defence systems.

Specificity

- Immune responses in mammals have specificity for one particular antigen.
- No cross-over reaction with closely related antigens.
- Many infection antigens are similar and specificity of response is essential.

Diversity

- Immune system encounters many different antigens in a lifetime.
- Likely to encounter antigens for which it has no programme.
- Immune system must therefore have diversity to respond to a great range of antigens that are new to it.

Memory

- The first time an antigen is encountered the response may be slow and relatively non-specific as the antigen reacts with a clone of immunologically competent cells.
- During the process memory cells are produced so that the second and subsequent times the antigen is presented, the immune response is rapid and specific.
- This forms the basis of active immunization procedures.

Recruitment of Other Defence Mechanisms

- The immune system on its own cannot destroy and remove all foreign material.
- Chemical messengers are therefore recruited, e.g. polymorphs, macrophages, mast cells, kinins, complement, lytic enzyme.

Antigen

An antigen is any substance capable of producing an immune response. More precisely, it is a substance binding specifically to an antibody or T-cell antigen receptor.

The immune system can respond to an antigen in two ways:

- cell-mediated immunity (CMI)
- humoral immunity.

Both are dependent upon specifically responsive lymphocytes, which recognize and react to the presented antigen:

- CMI is attributable to T-lymphocytes

- humoral immunity is attributable to immunoglobulin produced by plasma cells derived from B-lymphocytes
- T-lymphocytes can help and suppress B-lymphocyte activity.

HUMORAL IMMUNITY

The production of antibodies, which are small, soluble globulin proteins (immunoglobulins, Ig).

- The production of antibodies is dependent on the differentiation of B-lymphocytes into plasma cells.
- Immunoglobulin molecules comprise light chains (κ or λ) and heavy chains (γ, μ, α, δ, ε).
- Molecules can be enzymatically separated into fragment antigen-binding (Fab) or fragment crystallizable (Fc). Some leucocytes have receptors for Fc.
- One plasma cell produces antibody of one class reactive with only one antigen.
- Antibodies by binding to antigens can cause:
  - lysis of bacteria
  - neutralization of toxins
  - opsonization (i.e. surface coating of foreign material by complement to promote engulfment by phagocytic cells which have cell surface receptors for complement)
  - antibody-dependent cell-mediated cytotoxicity.

Antibody Production

- Antibodies are produced by plasma cells in lymph nodes, bone marrow and spleen.

The basic structure of any immunoglobulin is shown in Fig. 19.1.

- There are five classes of immunoglobulin: IgG, IgM, IgA, IgD and IgE, characterized by differences in structure of their heavy chains. Structure and roles of immunoglobulins are shown in Table 19.1.
- The antigen-binding site of an IgG molecule is at the N-terminal end of the Fab polypeptide chain.
- Huge numbers of combining sites exist to recognize the vast number of antigenic epitopes.
- Diversity in antibodies is due to variability of the amino acid sequences at the N-terminal regions.
- The amino acid sequences of the N-terminal regions vary between different antibody molecules and are known as variable regions (V).
- Most of the differences reside in three hypervariable regions in the molecule. In the folded molecule the hypervariable chains come together with their counterparts on the other pair of heavy and light chains to form the antigen-binding site.
- In any individual, 10^6 different antibody molecules could be made up by 10^3 different heavy chain variable regions associated with 10^3 different light chain variable regions.

Cell-Mediated Immunity

- Cells responsible are T-lymphocytes.
- T-cells are characterized by antigen-specific T-cell receptors (TCR).

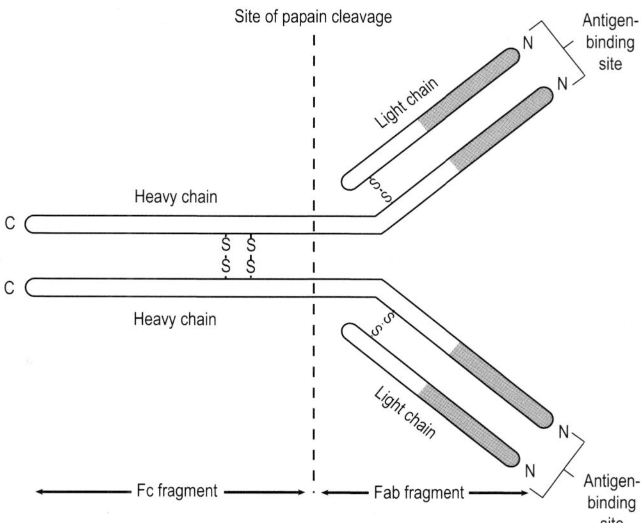

Fig. 19.1 Basic structure of an immunoglobulin molecule showing the four polypeptide chains, the variable regions (shaded), and the fragments produced by enzyme (papain) cleavage.

TABLE 19.1 Properties and Functions of Immunoglobulins

Ig Class	Heavy Chain	Molecular Weight	Plasma Level (g/L)	Antigen-Binding Sites	Complement Activation	Role
IgG	γ	150 000	5–15	2	Yes	Crosses placenta (only one to do so) Characteristic of secondary immune response Neutralizes toxins opsonization
IgA	α	380 000 (dimer in secretions)	1.5–5	4	No	Principal immunoglobulin in secretions of respiratory and GI tracts Secreted locally in tears, saliva, sweat, mucus Dimers of Ig joined by a J chain Major immune protection for mucosal surfaces
IgM	μ	900 000 (pentamer)	0.5–2	10	Yes	Characteristic of primary immune response Powerful agglutinator (of bacteria) and opsonin
IgE	ε	185 000	$2–4 \times 10^{-7}$	2	No	Binds to mast cells and basophils Anaphylactic hypersensitivity Antiparasitic by degranulating mast cells and attracting eosinophils
IgD	δ	185 000	0–0.5	2	No	Lymphocyte membrane receptor Involved in B-cell differentiation

- TCRs are membrane-bound and are made of two pairs of polypeptide chains: TCR1 (γ and δ chains), TCR2 (α and β chains).
- Leucocytes are differentiated by their cell surface molecules known as clusters of differentiation (CD), which are identified by monoclonal antibodies.
- CD3 is closely linked to the receptor and is responsible for transduction of the signal into the interior of the T-cell.
- Two main sets of T-lymphocytes exist:
  - helper T-cells (CD4+)
  - cytotoxic T-cells (CD8+).
- Helper T-cells respond to antigenic stimulus by producing cytokines, which activate T-cells (cytotoxic CD8+ T-cells), B-cells and macrophages.
- Cytotoxic T-cells, once activated (CD25+ T-cells), destroy allogenic or infected target cells.
- Both CD4+ and CD8+ T-cells can suppress immune response through production of suppressive cytokines, negative regulation of signal transduction and via idiotypic network.

Major Histocompatibility Complex Antigens (MHC)

- MHC is a set of genes encoding cell surface glycoproteins.
- MHC antigens play a fundamental role in the immune response by presenting antigenic peptides to T-cells.
- TCR of an individual T-cell will only recognize antigen as part of a complex of the antigenic peptide and the individual's MHC complex.
- The process of dual recognition of peptide plus MHC is known as MHC restriction, since the MHC molecule restricts the ability of the T-cell to recognize antigen.
- MHC genes are carried on the short arm of chromosome 6 and code for three classes of molecules:
  - class I are divided into three different groups: A, B, C; they are present on virtually all nucleated cells and signal to cytotoxic T-cells
  - class II loci are known as DP, DQ and DR; they are restricted to a few cell types (i.e. B-cells, activated T-cells, macrophages) and signal to T-helper cells
  - class III are genes for components of the complement system.

BOX 19.1 Some HLA-Associated Diseases

HLA Antigens	Disease
B 27	Ankylosing spondylitis Reiter's disease
DR 2	Goodpasture's syndrome
DR 3	Addison's disease Hashimoto's disease Myasthenia gravis
DR 4	Insulin-dependent diabetes

- MHC restriction allows antigens in different intracellular compartments to be captured and presented to CD4+ or CD8+ cells.
- Endogenous antigens (including viral antigens) are presented by MHC class I-bearing cells exclusively to CD8+ T-cells (cytotoxic T-cells).
- Exogenous antigens are presented by MHC class II-bearing cells to CD4+ T-cells (helper T-cells).
- HLA (human leucocyte antigen) subtypes are important in determining matching in transplantation.
- HLA subtypes are statistically related to certain diseases, e.g. B27 and ankylosing spondylitis (see Box 19.1).

THE STRUCTURE OF THE IMMUNE SYSTEM

- All lymphoid cells originate from a pluripotential stem cell in the bone marrow.
- Lymphoid progenitor cells destined to become T-cells migrate from the bone marrow to thymus.
- B-cell development occurs in the bone marrow.
- The thymus and bone marrow are primary lymphoid organs.
- Lymph nodes, spleen and MALT are secondary lymphoid organs.

Lymph Nodes

- Lymph node architecture is well adapted to function (Fig. 19.2).
- Afferent lymphatics penetrate the capsule, and lymph enters into the marginal sinus.
- A branching network of sinuses passes through the cortex and medulla to efferent lymphatics.
- The sinus network provides a filtration system for antigens entering the node.
- Cortex contains primary follicles of B-lymphocytes surrounded by T-cells in the paracortex.
- Cortex also contains dendritic cells, which form a mesh within the follicles, i.e. antigen presenting cells (APC).
- Primary follicles develop into secondary follicles on antigenic stimulation. Secondary follicles contain germinal centres comprising B-cells and a few helper T-cells.
- B-cells in secondary follicles are antigen activated.
- Activated B-cells migrate from the follicle to the medulla, where they develop into plasma cells in the medullary cords and release antibodies into the efferent limb.
- Interdigitating dendritic cells (IDC) are found in the paracortex. They stimulate T-cells within the paracortex.

Spleen

- Responds to antigens in the blood.
- Lymphoid tissue is in the white pulp, arranged around arterioles.
- T-cells surround the central arteriole.
- B-cells are eccentrically placed within the white pulp; they may form germinal centres when stimulated.

Mucosa-Associated Lymphoid Tissue (MALT)

- Responds to antigens at mucosal surfaces.
- Important in transport of immunoglobulins to luminal surfaces.
- Consists of three components in the gut:
  - Peyer's patches: dense aggregates of lymphoid tissue in the terminal ileum. The flattened epithelium over these aggregates contains M-cells, which are capable of antigen binding and processing. They pass antigenic material to adjacent T-helper cells
  - lamina propria cells: T-helper cells
  - intraepithelial cells: T-suppressor cells; may be important in maintaining tolerance to food antigens.

The Immune Response (Summary)

- Presentation of antigen to lymphocytes is performed by specialized antigen presenting cells (APCs), which can be dendritic cells, macrophages or B cells.
- Antigen presentation can be direct (unprocessed antigen presentation by donor cells) or indirect (processed antigen presentation by recipient helper T cells).
- Processed antigen is presented to T-cells alongside MHC class II antigen on the APC surface because T-cells do not recognize processed antigen alone.
- Each B-lymphocyte is committed to the production of an antibody with a unique antigen-binding site, i.e. idiotype.
- Antibody production usually requires the intervention of T-helper cells.
- T-helper cells are divided into two subgroups according to the cytokines which they produce:
  - Th1-cells secrete TNF and IFN-γ, and mediate cellular immunity
  - Th2-cells secrete IL-4, IL-5, IL-10 and IL-13, and stimulate antibody production by B-cells.

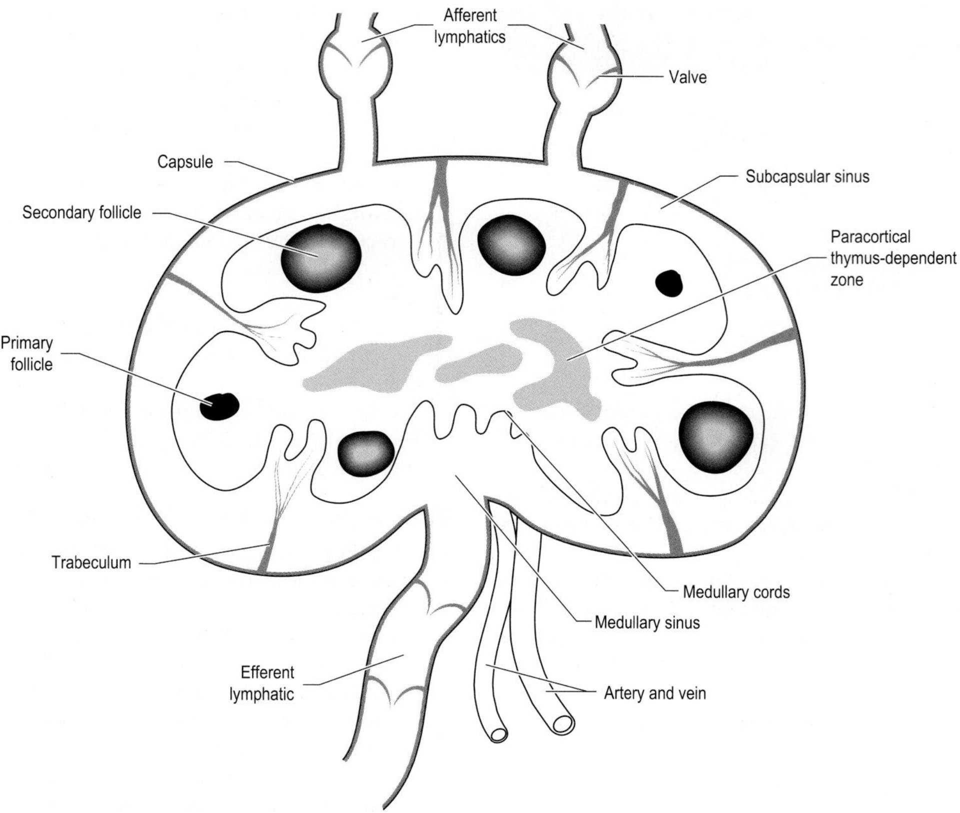

Fig. 19.2 The structure of a normal lymph node.

- The efficiency of the secondary antibody response is due to clonal expansion.
- T-lymphocytes can directly kill virus-infected cells or release cytokines which contribute to inflammation.

COMPLEMENT

- Complement is a complex series of proteins that act as an enzymatic cascade. Activation occurs in a stepwise cascade, each activated component having the ability to activate several molecules of the next protein in the cascade.
- Complement can be activated by antigen–antibody complexes, i.e. the classical pathway, or by bacterial cell surfaces, i.e. the alternative pathway (Fig. 19.3).
- In both pathways the outcome is the production of a membrane attack complex.
- Functions of complement include:
  - bacterial killing or target cell killing by membrane lysis
  - opsonization promoting phagocytosis
  - removal of immune complexes
  - mediation of vascular and cellular components of acute inflammation.

IMMUNE DEFICIENCY

- Immune deficiency can be classified as:
  - specific deficiencies: defects in the immune system itself, i.e. primary and secondary
  - non-specific deficiencies, e.g. neutrophil deficiency, complement deficiencies.
- Specific deficiencies are divided into:
  - primary: due to an intrinsic defect in the immune system (usually genetic)
  - secondary: due to an underlying condition.

Primary Immune Deficiency

- Rare.
- May affect different cell types:

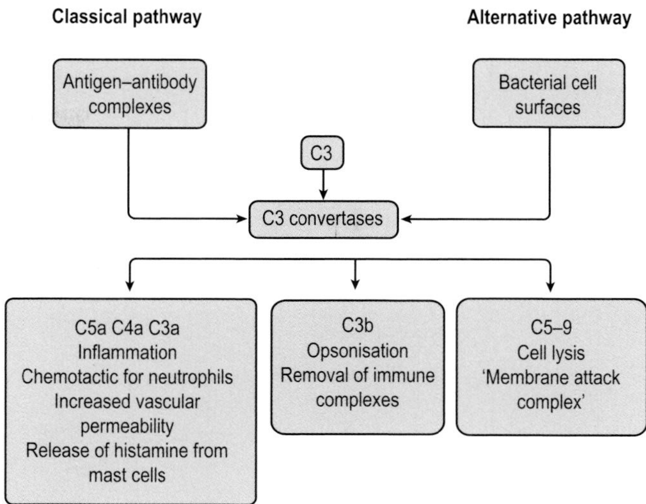

Fig. 19.3 Pathways of complement activation.

- several types of cell, i.e. reticular dysgenesis – failure of stem cells, severe combined immunodeficiency (SCID) – T- and B-cells affected
- predominantly T-cells, e.g. di George syndrome, Nezelof syndrome
- predominantly B-cells, e.g. agammaglobulinaemia.

Secondary Immune Deficiency

- Age: relative lack of immune response in infancy and old age.
- Malnutrition: defect in antibody and, in severe cases, T-cell function.
- Neoplastic disorders of immune system, e.g. Hodgkin's disease, B-cell lymphoma, myeloma, chronic lymphocytic leukaemia.
- Iatrogenic, e.g. drugs to prevent allograft rejection, splenectomy.
- Infection: immunodeficiency extreme with HIV, may occur transiently with cytomegalovirus (CMV), rubella, infectious mononucleosis and viral hepatitis.

Infections characteristic of the different types of immunodeficiency are shown in Fig. 19.4.

HYPERSENSITIVITY REACTIONS

Hypersensitivity is an altered immunological response in which a severe and harmful reaction occurs to extrinsic antigens.

There are four types of hypersensitivity reaction:

- type I: immediate hypersensitivity or 'allergy' due to overproduction of IgE on mast cells and basophils (anaphylactic or immediate)
- type II: antibody to cell-bound antigen (cytotoxic)
- type III: immune complex reaction
- type IV: delayed hypersensitivity mediated by T-cells.

Type I

- Overproduction of IgE on mast cells and basophils.
- Release of vasoactive substances, e.g. histamine, chemokines, leading to vasodilatation.
- Anaphylactic shock, e.g. bee and wasp venom, antibiotics (penicillin), peanuts.
- Atopic diseases (individuals producing an excessive reaction to antigens are termed atopic), e.g. asthma, hayfever, allergic rhinitis.

Type II

- Circulating antibodies (IgG or IgM) react with antigen on cell surface.
- Death of cells occurs via:
  - lysis of cell membrane due to complement activation
  - phagocytosis of cell to which antibody is bound
  - promotion of killer cell cytotoxicity.
- Examples of Type II hypersensitivity include:
  - transfusion reactions
  - rhesus incompatibility
  - autoimmune haemolytic disease
  - idiopathic thrombocytopaenic purpura
  - myasthenia gravis
  - Goodpasture's syndrome.

Type III

- Deposition or formation of immune complexes in the tissues.

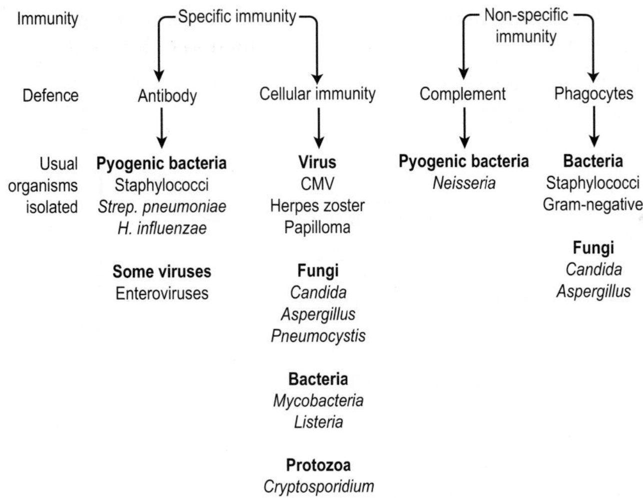

Fig. 19.4 Infections characteristic of types of immunodeficiency.

- Free antigen and antibody (IgG or IgM) combine in the presence of complement and precipitate as immune complexes, causing tissue destruction.
- Tissue destruction results from:
  - release of lysosomal enzymes by neutrophils
  - vasoactive amines released by platelet aggregates
  - platelet aggregates occlude circulation.
- Examples include:
  - endogenous antigens, e.g. serum sickness, drug-induced haemolytic anaemia (quinine)
  - microbial antigens, e.g. post-streptococcal glomerulonephritis
  - autologous antigens, e.g. rheumatoid arthritis, systemic lupus erythematosus, polyarteritis nodosa.

Type IV

- Cell-mediated hypersensitivity involving specifically primed T-lymphocytes.
- Release of lymphokines.
- Reaction takes 2–3 days to develop.
- Examples include:
  - microbial agents, e.g. tuberculosis, viruses and fungi
  - tuberculin test
  - rejection of tissue and organ grafts
  - contact dermatitis.

Type 'V' (Not Part of the Original Gell & Coombs Classification)

- Some IgG antibodies stimulate cells against which they are directed.
- Example: TSH receptor antibody results in prolonged hypersecretion of thyroid hormone in Graves' disease.

AUTOIMMUNITY

- Autoimmunity is an immune response against a self-antigen, i.e. loss of tolerance to 'self'.
- Autoimmune disease results in tissue damage or disturbed function resulting from an autoimmune response.
- Autoimmune responses can occur without resulting disease.
- Autoimmune disease may attack a single organ, i.e. organ-specific; or involve autoantigens widely distributed throughout the body, i.e. non-organ-specific.

Possible Mechanisms of Autoimmunity

- Genetic factors.
- Antigenic abnormality.
- Dysregulation of the immune response.

Genetic Factors

- Association of disease with specific alleles of MHC class II (HLA-D region) (see Box 19.1).

Antigenic Abnormality

- Surface antigens modified by drugs, e.g. haemolytic anaemia due to antibodies against e-antigen of rhesus system with methyldopa.
- Cell antigens modified by inflammation or disease processes when new antigens are formed, e.g. Epstein–Barr virus.

BOX 19.2 Examples of Autoimmune Disease

Examples of Autoimmune Disease	Autoantibodies Present Against
Organ-specific	
Hashimoto's thyroiditis	Thyroglobulin, thyroid peroxidase
Graves' disease	TSH receptor
Pernicious anaemia	Parietal cells, intrinsic factor
Goodpasture's syndrome	Glomerular and lung basement membrane
Myasthenia gravis	Acetylcholine receptor
Non-organ-specific	
Systemic lupus erythematosus (SLE)	Nuclear antigens, DNA, smooth muscle
Rheumatoid arthritis	IgG (rheumatoid factor)
Scleroderma (CREST variant)	Centromere

- Microbial antigens crossreacting with host tissues, e.g. β-haemolytic streptococcus and antigen in cardiac muscle, resulting in rheumatic fever.
- Exposure of previously secluded antigens, e.g. sympathetic ophthalmitis with penetrating eye injuries, sympathetic orchidopathia and testicular damage (torsion, mumps).

Immune Dysregulation

- Abnormal presence/activity of autoreactive T-cells.
- Failure of regulatory cells.
- CD4+ cell activity increased.

Examples of self-antigens and autoimmune disease are shown in Box 19.2.

ORGAN TRANSPLANTATION

Types of Graft

- Autograft: tissue is transferred from one area of the body to another in the same individual, e.g. skin graft.
- Isograft: tissue is transferred between genetically identical individuals, e.g. monozygotic twins.
- Allograft: tissue is transferred between genetically dissimilar individuals of the same species, e.g. deceased donor renal transplant.
- Xenograft: tissue is transferred between different species.

Major Histocompatibility Complex (MHC)

- Located on short arm of chromosome 6.
- Group of antigens governing rejection are part of the human leucocyte antigen (HLA) system.

HLA Class I: Coded at A, B, C Loci

- To date, 1381 alleles for HLA-A, 1927 for HLA-B and 960 for HLA-C have been identified.
- HLA-A and HLA-B induce formation of complement-fixing cytotoxic antibodies, and act as cell surface recognition markers for cytotoxic T-cells.
- In kidney grafts, class I antigens are present on vascular endothelium, interstitial cells, mesangial cells and tubular epithelium.

Class II

- HLA-D locus: DR (927 alleles), DP (170 alleles) and DQ (162 alleles).
- Class II antigens are expressed on the surface of B-cells, macrophages, activated T-cells and antigen-presenting cells.
- Class II molecule recognition activates CD4+ T-helper cells, which begin the process of clonal expansion, and also support cytotoxic T-cell clonal expansion by stimulating the CD4+ lymphocyte generation of regulatory cytokines.
- Matching of class II antigens is the most important factor in predicting the outcome of transplantation.

Immunological Pathology of Graft Rejection

The alloimmune response or rejection process has two phases (Fig. 19.5):

- afferent (sensitization) phase
- efferent (effector) phase.

Afferent Phase

- Allorecognition may occur in the graft itself, or in the lymphoid tissue of the recipient.
- Donor MHC molecules found on donor graft tissue are recognized by recipient CD4+ T-cells, i.e. allorecognition (direct pathway).
- Recipient helper T-cells recognize donor MHC molecules that have been processed by APCs of recipient origin (indirect pathway).
- Following antigen presentation, binding of the co-stimulation molecules present on the APC and T-cell receptor activates the intracellular signalling pathways, leading to IL-2 gene transcription, translation and release. IL-2 binds to CD25, resulting in T-cell proliferation.

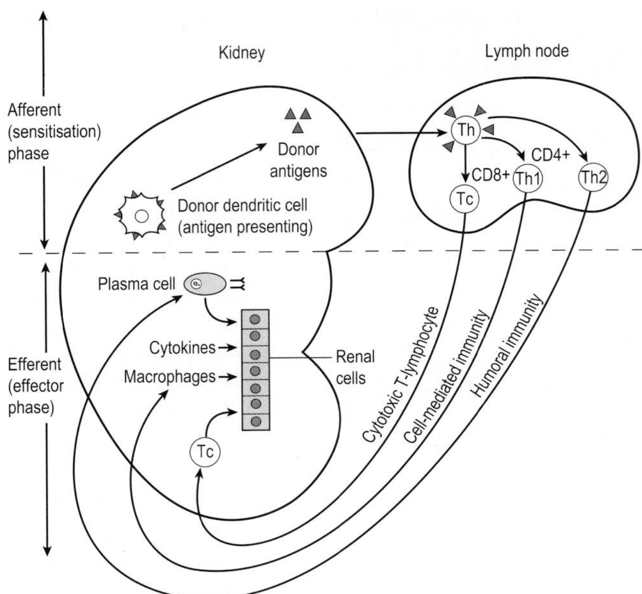

Fig. 19.5 Immunopathology of graft rejection.

Efferent Phase

- CD4+ T-cells (helper cells) enter the graft and recruit cells responsible for the tissue damage of rejection.
- Cells recruited include B-lymphocytes, macrophages, natural killer cells, CD8+ T-cells (cytotoxic T-cells).
- Activated cytotoxic cells damage the graft cells by proteolytic action (granzyme B and perforin).
- Cytokines important in graft rejection are IL-2 and gamma interferon.

Clinical Rejection

There are four types of clinical rejection:

- hyperacute
- accelerated acute
- acute
- chronic.

Hyperacute

- Rare.
- Occurs within minutes to hours.
- Occurs during operation and in the case of the kidney it is seen to be flaccid, cyanotic, and eventually thromboses.
- Occurs with ABO incompatibility or preformed cytotoxic antibodies as a result of failed transplant, pregnancy or blood transfusion.
- Preformed cytotoxic antibody reacts with MHC class I antigen in donor organ.
- Activation of complement: influx of polymorphs, platelet aggregation, obstruction of blood vessels, ischaemia.
- IgG and C3 bound to endothelial cells.
- No successful therapy.
- Graft loss occurs.

Accelerated Acute

- Occurs within 2–4 days.
- Previous sensitization to donor antigens often due to previous transplant.

Acute Rejection

- Cell-mediated or antibody-mediated
- Common.
- Treatable.
- Occurs between 1 week and 3 months post-transplant, but is commonest around 7–10 days.
- Patient may have several episodes of acute rejection in first 3 months post-transplant.
- Early diagnosis is essential, as prompt treatment curtails organ damage.
- Histology of cell-mediated rejection shows infiltration of tubules and interstitium by cytotoxic T-cells, which destroy the graft in the absence of treatment.
- In antibody-mediated rejection, there are detectable donor-specific antibodies (DSA) in recipient blood, and histology of the kidney shows intimal arteritis and

thrombosis of blood vessels with deposition of C4d in the peritubular capillaries.

Chronic Rejection

- Characterized by slow loss of organ function over a period of months or years. In kidneys, there is associated hypertension and proteinuria.
- Histological findings include thickening of the glomerular basement membrane, hyalinization of glomeruli, intimal hyperplasia, tubular atrophy and interstitial fibrosis.
- Both immunological and non-immunological factors are implicated in the process.
- Chronic allograft injury (CAI) is the latest nomenclature because the aetiology is poorly understood.
- Chronic rejection is untreatable; however, modulation of risk factors prolongs allograft survival.

Transplant Tolerance

- Induction of tolerance (unresponsiveness) to donor antigen and elimination of the requirement of maintenance immunosuppression remains the ultimate goal.
- Still remains in experimental stage.
- Regulatory T-cells (Tregs) suppress the responses of activated T-cells in tolerance.
- Co-stimulation blockade for the induction of tolerance using belatacept is under investigation.

IMMUNOSUPPRESSION

Prevention of rejection requires:
- good matching between donor and recipient HLA
- suppression of the immune system of the recipient.

Immunosuppressive Drugs

These have the following indications:
- Induction therapy:
  - given prior to transplantation and in the early postoperative period in order to avoid or delay acute rejection episodes
  - examples include anti-IL-2R monoclonal antibodies (basiliximab and daclizumab), anti-thymocyte globulin (ATG). Orthoclone anti-CD3 monoclonal antibody (OKT3) is seldom used these days because of the severe side-effects from cytokine release syndrome
  - combination of immunosuppressive agents are commenced immediately following transplantation
  - combinations are used to allow reduction in dose of each agent in attempt to reduce toxicity
  - examples of acute rejection prophylaxis combination therapy include: calcineurin inhibitor (tacrolimus or ciclosporin) in combination with an antimetabolite (mycophenolate mofetil or azathioprine) and prednisolone.
- Maintenance therapy:
  - drugs used as prophylaxis against acute rejection are usually continued as maintenance therapy
  - the dose is gradually reduced over a period of time
  - in some cases, one of the drugs may be eliminated with time, e.g. steroids, to prevent long-term complications
  - sirolimus is used to substitute CNIs if intolerance or nephrotoxicity develops.
- Anti-rejection therapy:
  - cell-mediated acute rejection is treated with three intravenous pulses of steroids (methylprednisolone); steroid-resistant cell-mediated rejection is treated with ATG
  - antibody-mediated acute rejection is treated with plasmapheresis to remove anti-HLA antibodies, intravenous immunoglobulin to neutralize the circulating antibodies, and rituximab (anti CD-52 monoclonal antibody) to suppress further production of antibodies by B cells.

Immunosuppressive Drugs

Corticosteroids

- Mainstay of immunosuppression since the 1950s.
- Interfere with antigen presentation.
- Inhibit T-cell activation by blocking IL-1, IL-2, IL-6 and IFN-γ.
- Exert anti-inflammatory effects as well as immunosuppressive effects.
- Inhibit neutrophil phagocytic activity.

Antiproliferative Drugs

These include azathioprine, mycophenolate mofetil (MMF) and mycophenolate sodium (MPS).
- Azathioprine:
  - interferes with nucleic acid
  - affects cells that are actively replicating, i.e. T-cells undergoing clonal expansion
  - non-specific and affects all proliferating cells.
- MMF and MPS:
  - inhibit enzyme in pathway of purine synthesis through inhibition of inosine monophosphate dehydrogenase (IMPDH)
  - more effective than azathioprine in prevention of acute rejection
  - more selective than azathioprine
  - block proliferation of T- and B-cells, inhibit antibody formation, inhibit generation of cytotoxic T-cells

- prevent smooth muscle cell proliferation, which might have additional benefit for chronic rejection.

Calcineurin Inhibitors (CNI)

These include ciclosporin and tacrolimus.

- Both drugs are fungal products.
- CNIs inhibit T-cell activation through inhibition of IL-2 gene transcription, thereby inhibiting generation of cytotoxic T-lymphocytes.
- Both drugs are nephrotoxic at high dose so blood concentrations require measurement.

Other Drugs

Sirolimus (Rapamycin) and Everolimus

- Macrolide antibiotic.
- Engages a protein-designated mammalian target of rapamycin (mTOR) and its inhibition reduces cytokine-dependent cellular proliferation at G_1 to S phase of cell division cycle, thereby blocking T-cell activation.
- Non-nephrotoxic.
- Impairs wound healing.

Antilymphocyte Globulin (ALG) and Antithymocyte Globulin (ATG)

Both prepared by immunizing animals with lymphocytes, which increases the risk of anaphylaxis.

- Thymocytes are used to prepare ATG.
- Used to treat steroid-resistant rejection episodes.
- May be used prophylactically in highly sensitized patients.

Monoclonal Antibodies

These include anti-CD3 monoclonal antibody and anti-IL-2R monoclonal antibody.

- Anti-CD3 (OKT3):
  - directed against CD3 complex of T-cell receptor
  - also blocks the function of killer T-cells
  - can be used to treat steroid-resistant rejection.
- Anti-IL-2R (basiliximab and daclizumab):
  - targeted against IL-2 receptors
  - designed to prevent, but not treat, acute rejection episodes.

Drugs Under Evaluation

- Belatacept: costimulation blockade.
- Alemtuzumab: anti-CD52 monoclonal antibody.
- Bortezomib: proteosome inhibitor.
- Eculizumab: anti-C5 monoclonal antibody.
- Sotrastaurin: protein kinase C inhibitor.

Side Effects of Immunosuppression

Apart from side effects specific to the different drugs, the general side effects of immunosuppression include infection and neoplasia.

Infection

- Patients are prone to infection, particularly with opportunistic organisms.
- Opportunistic infections include:
  - bacterial, e.g. TB and urinary tract infection
  - viral, e.g. cytomegalovirus, herpes simplex, herpes zoster and BK virus infections
  - fungal, e.g. *Candida*, *Aspergillus*, *Pneumocystis jirovecii*
  - protozoal, e.g. toxoplasmosis.

Neoplasia

- Skin tumours, e.g. squamous cell carcinoma.
- Post-transplant lymphoproliferative disease (PTLD), e.g. B-cell lymphoma.
- Kaposi's sarcoma.
- Other cancers have up to a 100-fold increase compared with age-matched controls.

Graft-Vs-Host Disease

- Occurs when immunocompetent lymphocytes are introduced into an immunocompromised host in sufficient numbers.
- Complication of bone marrow transplantation when immunocompetent cells recognize the host as foreign and start an immunological attack.
- Clinical manifestations include fever, weight loss, rash, hepatosplenomegaly, diarrhoea.
- Mortality severe: 70% of those with severe disease die.

OSCE SCENARIOS

OSCE Scenario 19.1

A 17-year-old female presents to your trauma service with an infected dog bite to her right arm, with associated lymphangitis. Whilst on the ward awaiting theatre for washout and debridement, she is started on intravenous antibiotics. Shortly after, the staff nurse in the patient's bay calls for help, and you find that the patient is flushed, anxious and you can hear a slight wheeze when she is breathing.

1. What is the most likely diagnosis?
2. What type of immune reaction is this?

3. What other signs/symptoms may be present in this type of reaction?
4. Briefly outline your immediate management.
5. Before the patient is discharged, what actions would you ensure had been taken?

OSCE Scenario 19.2

A 20-year-old male undergoes a first renal transplant from a well-matched deceased donor. He has no preformed cytotoxic antibodies.

1. What immunosuppressive regime would you commence in the post-operative period?

The serum creatinine falls to 130 µmol/L by the 6th post-operative day. On the 8th post-operative day, there is reduced urine output and the creatinine has risen to 200 µmol/L. The ciclosporin level in the blood is within therapeutic limits.

2. What are the possible diagnoses?
3. Name two investigations which you would perform to confirm the diagnosis. In which order would you perform them?
4. What histological features suggest the diagnosis of acute rejection?
5. If cell-mediated rejection is confirmed, how would you treat it?
6. If the kidney fails to respond to planned treatment, what further treatment would you institute?

OSCE Scenario 19.3

You have recently incised and drained an abscess on the neck of a 48-year-old man, which did not exhibit the usual features of an inflamed abscess. The microbiologist reports seeing acid- and alcohol-fast bacilli on the Gram stain.

1. What infection does this suggest? When you see the patient in clinic he tells you he has recently had a cough and shortness of breath. An X-ray and sputum culture performed by his GP has revealed a *Pneumocystis* pneumonia.
2. What possible underlying condition do you now suspect?
3. Summarize the immune response.
4. Explain to the examiners the difference between the humoral and cell-mediated immune systems.
5. What is complement?

OSCE Scenario 19.4

A 42-year-old male is having a blood transfusion following a major colorectal procedure; the nurse looking after him comes to tell you that the patient has just finished the first bag of blood but he has a temperature of 38°C and is very flushed and complaining of back and flank pain.

1. What is the possible diagnosis?
2. Explain how it occurs and what type of immune reaction it is.
3. What is a Coombs test? Which will be the most relevant in this case?

OSCE Scenario 19.5

A 27-year-old female visits you in the transplant clinic; she is very upset regarding some unwanted facial hair growth, acne and excess growth of her gums. She had a cadaveric renal transplant four months ago and it has been functioning very well.

1. Which immunosuppressant drug has these side effects?
2. Explain how this drug works to prevent graft rejection.
3. Another patient attends who has had a working transplant for over 15 years. They are complaining of fevers, night sweats and palpable lumps in the right side of their neck. What is the likely diagnosis and how has the drug mentioned in question 1 led to this complication?

Answers in Appendix pages 476–478

Please check your eBook at https://studentconsult.inkling.com/ for more self-assessment questions. See inside cover for registration details.

20

Haemopoietic and Lymphoreticular System

HAEMOPOIESIS

Haemopoiesis is the production of blood cells. Sites of haemopoiesis include:

- fetus: bone marrow, spleen and liver
- at birth: marrow
- adult life: red marrow remains only in axial skeleton, ribs, skull and proximal ends of humerus and femur.

Red Blood Cell (Erythrocyte)

- Non-nucleated blood cells that are biconcave and deformable.
- Most abundant blood cell, forming 45% of the total blood volume, i.e. haematocrit or packed-cell volume (PCV).
- Function: to carry oxygen.
- Mature erythrocytes survive for 18–120 days in the circulation before being removed by macrophages in the spleen and, to a lesser extent, bone marrow and liver.
- Within the macrophage the erythrocyte is broken down to haem and globin.
- Amino acids of globin enter the general amino acid pool of the body.
- Haem is broken down with release of iron, which attaches to transferrin.
- Transferrin is an iron-binding beta globulin responsible for iron transport and delivery to receptors on erythroblasts or to iron stores. The remainder of the haem is converted to bilirubin.
- Renal secretion of erythropoietin stimulates red cell production to keep pace with rate of destruction.
- Erythropoiesis requires an adequate dietary intake of iron, vitamin B_{12} and folate: depletion of these will reduce erythropoiesis.

Reticulocytes

- About 1% of red cells in the circulation are reticulocytes, which stain purplish because of residual RNA.
- The proportion of reticulocytes in the bloodstream increases when bone marrow production of erythrocytes increases, e.g. after haemorrhage.

ANAEMIA

Anaemia is the reduction of the concentration of haemoglobin in the circulation below the normal range. The normal range for a male is 13–18 g/dL and for the female 11.5–16.5 g/dL. There are three main causes of anaemia:

- blood loss
- haemolysis
- impairment of red cell formation/function.

Blood Loss

- Immediately after acute haemorrhage the haemoglobin level is normal.
- In the absence of i.v. fluid replacement there is a slow expansion in plasma volume over the next 2–3 days.
- Acute haemorrhage results eventually in a normochromic, normocytic anaemia.
- Reticulocytosis occurs; maximal at 1 week.
- There is a mild neutrophil leucocytosis with occasional metamyelocytes.
- Chronic blood loss leads to hypochromic microcytic iron deficiency anaemia.

Haemolysis

Haemolytic anaemias are a group of diseases in which red cell life span is reduced.

- Haemolysis is usually associated with increased erythropoiesis.
- Laboratory evidence of increased red cell destruction is demonstrated by:
  - increased serum unconjugated bilirubin
  - reduced serum haptoglobin
  - morphological evidence of red cell damage, e.g. spherocytes, red cell fragments, sickled cells
  - reduced life span of red cells, e.g. demonstrated by tagging with radioactive chromium.
- Laboratory evidence of increased erythropoiesis is demonstrated by:
  - reticulocytosis in peripheral blood
  - erythroid hyperplasia in the bone marrow.

Clinical Features of Haemolytic States

These result from:

- red cell destruction
- compensatory erythropoiesis.

Red cell destruction results in:

- pallor
- mild jaundice
- pigment stones may form in the gall bladder
- splenomegaly may occur.

Haemolytic states may result in:

- expansion of marrow cavities with thinning of cortical bone in congenital forms
- frontal bossing of the skull may occur, due to widening of the marrow space between inner and outer tables of the skull.

There are a number of haemolytic conditions but only two, which are surgically relevant, will be described here, i.e. sickle cell anaemia and hereditary spherocytosis.

Sickle Cell Anaemia

- Due to presence of haemoglobin variant HbS in red cells.
- Deoxygenated HbS is 50 times less soluble than deoxygenated HbA; polymerizes on deoxygenation into long fibres, which deform the red cell into the typical sickle shape.
- The presence of HbS is the result of a defect in gene coding for glutamic acid, the latter being replaced by valine.
- In heterozygous individuals, both HbA and HbS are formed, and the individual has sickle-cell trait. Patients with sickle-cell trait are usually haematologically normal and usually asymptomatic.
- In the presence of sickle-cell trait, red cells do not usually sickle until the oxygen saturation falls below 40%, which is rarely reached in venous blood.
- In surgical practice, the anaesthetist needs to be aware of the trait so that hypoxia is avoided intra-operatively.
- In homozygous individuals, HbA is not formed. The red cells readily deform and sickle cell anaemia develops.
- In the homozygous form, cells sickle at the oxygen tension normally found in venous blood.
- Increased rigidity of the cells causes them to plug small blood vessels with infarction and painful crises.
- Patients may develop acute abdominal and chest pain that mimics other intra-abdominal and thoracic catastrophes.
- Bone pain and priapism may also occur.
- The anaemic patient responds poorly to infection; septicaemia and osteomyelitis may develop, the latter being attributable on occasion to salmonella.
- The spleen may calcify and atrophy due to repeated infarction.
- Pigment gallstones may occur.

Hereditary Spherocytosis (Congenital Acholuric Jaundice)

- Due to defect in red cell membrane.
- Spherocytes are identified by blood film.
- Clinical features include family history, pallor, mild jaundice and splenomegaly.
- Raised serum bilirubin and increased reticulocyte count.
- Cholecystitis may occur as result of pigment stones.
- Splenectomy is the treatment of choice, being delayed until after the age of 10 years, as post-splenectomy sepsis is less after this age.
- Splenectomy does not cure spherocytosis but prevents the abnormally shaped cells being destroyed by the spleen.
- Following splenectomy:
  - haemoglobin level rises
  - jaundice disappears
  - the life span of red cells increases to near-normal levels.

Impairment of Red Cell Formation/Function

This may arise as a result of:

- deficiency of essential haematinics, e.g. iron, folate, vitamin B_{12}
- chronic disorders, e.g. infections (TB), renal disease, liver disease, neoplasia, collagen disease
- marrow infiltration, e.g. carcinoma, myeloma, lymphoma, myelofibrosis
- endocrine disease, e.g. hypothyroidism
- cytotoxic and immunosuppressive agents.

Classification of Anaemia

Anaemias may be classified by the morphological appearance of erythrocytes in the stained blood smear.

- Normocytes: red cells with a normal diameter.
- Microcytes: red cells with a reduced diameter.
- Macrocytes: red cells with an increased diameter.
- Normochromic: normal staining of a red cell with a central area of pallor.
- Hypochromic: reduced staining with a large central area of pallor.
- Haematocrit or PCV: percentage of packed cells in relation to the total volume of blood; normally 45%.

Other important parameters in assessing anaemia are:

- Mean corpuscular volume (MCV), measured in femtolitres (fL):

$$\frac{\text{haematocrit (L/L)}}{\text{red cell concentration } (\text{L}^{-1})} = 78 - 98 \text{ fL}$$

- Mean corpuscular haemoglobin (MCH), in picograms (pg):

$$\frac{\text{haemoglobin concentration (g/dL)}}{\text{red cell concentration } (\text{L}^{-1})} = 26 - 33 \text{ pg}$$

TABLE 20.1 Morphological Classification of Anaemia

Morphology	Values	Cause
Microcytic	MCV <78	Iron deficiency
Hypochromic	MCH <28	Thalassaemia
Macrocytic	MCV >98	Folate deficiency, vitamin B_{12} deficiency, alcoholism
Normocytic Normochromic	MCV normal MCH normal	Acute blood loss Haemolytic anaemia Chronic disorders Leucoerythroblastic anaemias

- Mean corpuscular haemoglobin concentration (MCHC), in grams per decilitre (g/dL):

$$\frac{\text{haemoglobin concentration (g/dL)}}{\text{haematocrit (L/L)}} = 30 - 35\ \text{g/dL}$$

A morphological classification of anaemia is shown in Table 20.1.

Polycythaemia

Polycythaemia is an increase in the concentration of red cells above normal level. There is a rise in both total blood volume and PCV; the latter may be as high as 60%. Features of polycythaemia include:

- Hb concentration rises to above 18 g/dL
- blood viscosity is high
- polycythaemia may be a primary condition, i.e. polycythaemia rubra vera, or may be secondary, relative or due to inappropriate secretion of erythropoietin (Box 20.1)
- increase in blood viscosity results in a sluggish blood flow through heart, brain and limbs, leading to myocardial infarction, stroke and ischaemic limbs
- splenomegaly occurs in 75% of cases
- haemorrhagic lesions may be a feature, especially in the gastrointestinal tract
- peptic ulceration is common in polycythaemia rubra vera but the reason is unknown.

BOX 20.1 Causes of Polycythaemia

- True
  - polycythaemia rubra vera
- Secondary: chronic hypoxia stimulates erythropoietin
  - high altitude
  - respiratory disease
  - cyanotic heart disease
  - smoking
  - haemoglobinopathy.
- Relative: reduced plasma volume, normal red cell mass
  - vomiting
  - diarrhoea
  - burns
  - inadequate fluid intake.
- Inappropriate: increase of erythropoietin
  - kidney disease, e.g. carcinoma
  - renal transplantation
  - hepatocellular carcinoma
  - giant uterine fibroids
  - cerebellar haemangioblastoma

WHITE BLOOD CELLS (LEUCOCYTES)

White blood cells form part of the body's defence mechanisms. They are divided into two main groups:

- phagocytes, which engulf and destroy bacteria and foreign matter
- lymphocytes, which are responsible for the immune response.

Types of White Blood Cell

Neutrophils

- Develop from myeloblasts in red bone marrow.
- Have a scavenging function and are important in defence against bacterial infection.
- Possess a segmented nucleus and abundant cytoplasmic granules containing enzymes, e.g. alkaline phosphatase and lysozyme.
- Spend 14 days in the bone marrow, whereas their life span in blood is 6–12 h.
- Enter tissues by penetrating the endothelium.

Lymphocytes

The role of lymphocytes is described in Chapter 19.

Monocytes

- Develop in red bone marrow from myeloblasts.
- Largest blood cells.
- Function is similar to that of neutrophils.
- Enter the tissues, and phagocytose and digest foreign and dying material.

Eosinophils

- Important in the mediation of the allergic response.
- Important in defence in parasitic infections.

Basophils

- Least frequent leucocytes in blood.
- Have similar function to tissue mast cells.
- Important in immediate hypersensitivity reactions, when they release histamine.

Changes in White Cells in Disease

Leucocytosis

- Leucocytosis is an increase in the number of circulating white cells. The normal reference range is shown in Box 20.2.
- Leucocytosis may involve any of the white cells, but polymorphonuclear leucocytosis is the most common, i.e. neutrophilia.
- The causes of leucocytosis are shown in Box 20.3.

Leucopenia

Leucopenia is a reduction in circulating leucocytes. In practice the most common form is neutropenia, i.e. deficiency of neutrophil granulocytes. Neutropenia may be selective or part of a pancytopenia (Box 20.4).

Neutropenia

- Neutrophil counts of $<0.5 \times 10^9$/L may result in:
  - severe sepsis, e.g. oral or oesophageal candida, septicaemia, opportunistic infections
  - this type of disease is seen in patients receiving chemotherapy for malignant disease or immunosuppressive therapy for organ transplantation.

Platelets

- Platelets are discoid, non-nucleated, granule-containing cells that form in the bone marrow by fragmentation of the cytoplasm of megakaryocytes.
- Concentration in normal blood is $160–450 \times 10^9$/L.
- Survive in circulation for 8–10 days.
- Contractile and adhesive cells which are important in haemostasis.
- Adhere to exposed subendothelial tissues, aggregate and form haemostatic plug.
- Take part in repair process after vascular injury.
- Platelet-derived growth factor is mitogenic for smooth muscle and fibroblasts; it may also be involved in the development of atherosclerosis.
- A reduction in the number of platelets is called thrombocytopenia (Box 20.5).

BOX 20.2 Reference Range for White Cell Concentrations

Cell	Count (10^9/L)
Total white cell count	4–11
Neutrophils	2.0–7.5
Lymphocytes	1.0–3.0
Monocytes	0.15–0.6
Eosinophils	0.05–0.35
Basophils	0.01–0.10

BOX 20.3 Causes of Leucocytosis

Cell	Cause
Neutrophils	Sepsis, e.g. acute appendicitis
	Trauma, e.g. major surgery
	Infarction, e.g. myocardial infarction
	Mesenteric infarction
	Malignant disease
	Acute haemorrhage
	Steroid therapy
Lymphocytes	Viral infections, e.g. glandular fever, CMV, rubella, influenza, hepatitis
	Bacterial infections, e.g. pertussis, TB, brucellosis
	Chronic lymphocytic leukaemia
	Post-splenectomy (temporary)
Monocytes	Sepsis
	Chronic infection, e.g. TB
	Malignant disease
Eosinophils	Allergy, e.g. asthma
	Parasitic infection
	Malignant disease, e.g. Hodgkin's disease

HAEMOSTASIS

Haemostasis is the physiological process by which bleeding is controlled. It consists of four components:

- vasoconstriction
- platelet activation
- coagulation mechanism
- fibrinolytic system.

BOX 20.4 Causes of Neutropenia

Type	Cause
Pancytopenia	Bone marrow depression, e.g. cytotoxic drugs
	Malignant infiltration
	Severe vitamin B_{12} or folate deficiency
	Hypersplenism
Selective	Overwhelming sepsis, e.g. septicaemia
	Autoimmune
	Drug-induced, e.g. indomethacin, chloramphenicol, co-trimoxazole

BOX 20.5 Causes of Thrombocytopenia

Type	Cause
Reduced production	Aplastic anaemia
	Drugs, e.g. tolbutamide, alcohol, cytotoxic agents
	Viral infections, e.g. EBV, CMV
	Myelodysplasia
	Bone marrow infiltration, e.g. carcinoma, leukaemia
	Myeloma, myelofibrosis
	Megaloblastic anaemia
	Hereditary thrombocytopenia
Decreased platelet survival	
Immune	Idiopathic thrombocytopenic purpura
	Drugs, e.g. heparin, quinine, sulphonamides, penicillins, gold
	Infections
	Post-transfusion
Non-immune	Disseminated intravascular coagulation
	Thrombotic thrombocytopenic purpura
Hypersplenism	Sequestration of platelets

Vasoconstriction

- Due to smooth muscle contraction mediated by:
  - local reflexes
  - thromboxane A2 released by activated platelets
  - serotonin released by activated platelets.

Platelet Activation

- Vascular damage promotes haemostasis if the endothelial lining of blood vessels is disrupted.
- Platelets adhere to the site of damage, aggregate there, and ultimately form a platelet plug.

Adherence

- Injury to vessel wall results in loss of endothelium and exposes subendothelial collagen.
- Platelets adhere to the damaged area and there is activation of the intrinsic pathway of coagulation.
- Damaged endothelial cells release von Willebrand's factor, which is necessary for platelet adhesion; tissue thromboplastin is also released, which activates the intrinsic pathway of coagulation.
- Simultaneously, platelet granules release ADP, which initiates platelet aggregation.

Aggregation

- Thromboxane A2 is produced from arachidonic acid released from platelet phospholipids.
- Thromboxane A2 induces further ADP release, causing further platelet aggregation.

Platelet Plug

- Aggregated platelets act as catalysts of coagulation with local generation of thrombin and conversion of fibrinogen to fibrin.
- Aggregated platelets, thrombin and fibrin fuse to form platelet plug.

Coagulation Mechanism

- End-point of blood coagulation is conversion of soluble fibrinogen to insoluble fibrin by thrombin.
- Coagulation mechanism involves two interacting systems: intrinsic and extrinsic pathways.
- Activation of Factor X is the result of preceding enzyme reactions in the two pathways.
- The intrinsic pathway involves normal blood components.
- The extrinsic pathway requires tissue thromboplastin, released by damaged cells.
- The pathways are shown in Fig. 20.1.
- All soluble coagulation factors are manufactured in the liver, with the exception of Factor VIII (endothelium), calcium, platelet factors and thromboplastin.

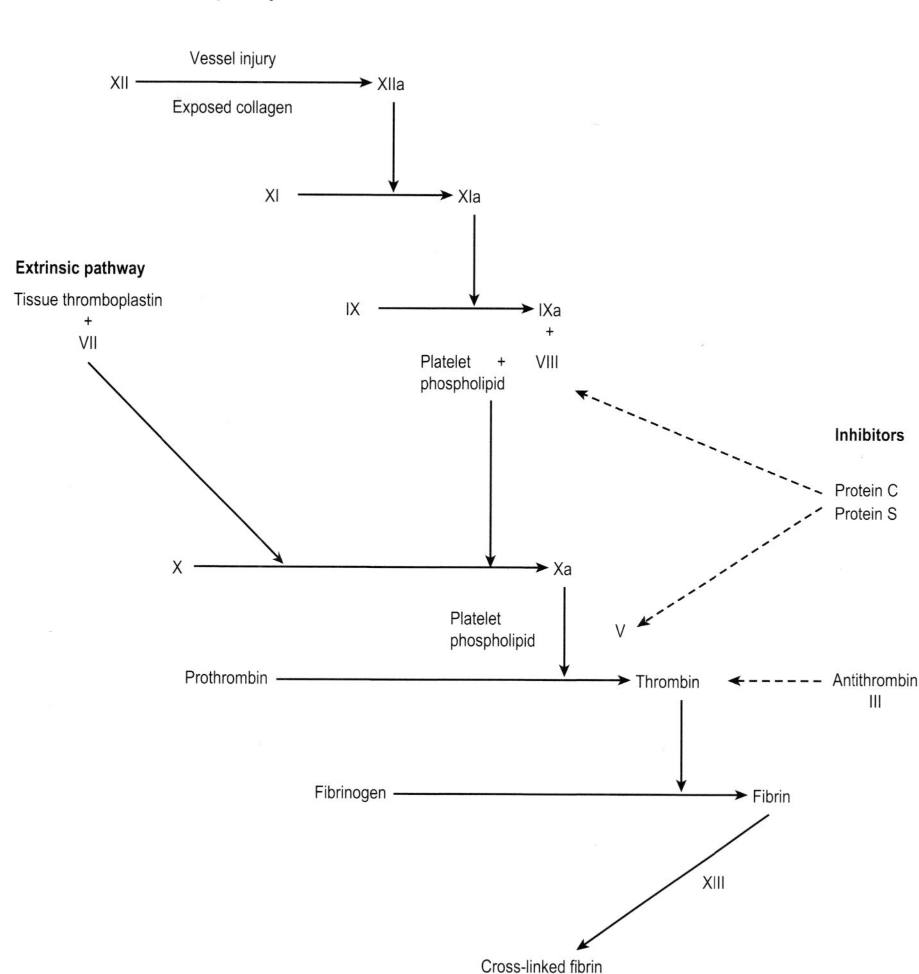

Fig. 20.1 The coagulation mechanism.

Fibrinolytic System

- Fibrin is removed by the fibrinolytic system during the repair process in blood vessels and healing wounds (Fig. 20.2).
- Fibrin is broken down to soluble fibrin degradation products by plasmin.
- Plasmin is derived from inactive precursor plasminogen by action of plasminogen activators.
- Tissue plasminogen activator is released from endothelial cells.
- Control of activation of plasminogen is provided by plasminogen-activator inhibitor 1 (PAI-1).
- PAI-1 is released by endothelial cells and rapidly inactivates tissue plasminogen activator.

Assessment of Coagulation System

Platelet Count

- Normal range $160–450 \times 10^9$/L.
- Thrombocytopenia exists with counts of less than 100×10^9/L.
- Counts of 70×10^9/L are usually adequate for surgical haemostasis.
- Spontaneous bleeding occurs with counts of less than 20×10^9/L.

Bleeding Time

- Time for a small puncture wound in the skin made by standard technique to stop bleeding.
- Time varies from 1 to 8 min.

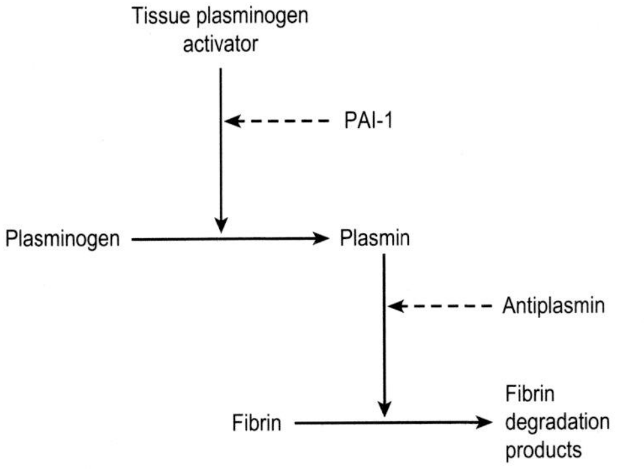

Fig. 20.2 The fibrinolytic mechanism (PAI-1 = plasminogen-activator inhibitor 1).

BOX 20.6 Assessment of Bleeding States

Test result	Conclusion
APTT and PT normal	Platelet or vessel defect
APTT and PT abnormal	Deficit in common pathway
APTT normal and PT abnormal	Factor VII deficiency
APTT abnormal and PT normal	Deficit in intrinsic system

Note: APTT tests the intrinsic system; PT tests the extrinsic system.

- A time within this range implies:
  - adequate platelet count
  - normal platelet function
  - normal vascular response to injury.
- A prolonged bleeding time implies:
  - thrombocytopenia
  - platelet defects
  - failure of vascular contraction.

Whole-Blood Clotting Time

- Blood clots in glass tube in 5–15 min.
- A clotting time within this range requires:
  - integrity of the intrinsic system
  - adequate final common pathway
  - normal platelet function.

Prothrombin Times (PT)

- Tests the integrity of the extrinsic pathway and final common pathway.
- Deficiencies of Factors I, II, V, VII and X will be detected.

Activated Partial Thromboplastin Time (APTT)

- Tests the intrinsic system, i.e. all factors except Factor VII.

Kaolin-Cephalin Clotting Time (KCCT)

- Independent of platelet count.
- Tests intrinsic pathway and common pathway.

Thrombin Time (TT)

- Increased if there is an inadequate concentration of fibrinogen.
- Prolonged by heparin and presence of fibrin degradation products.

Fibrin Degradation Products (FDPs)

- Products released from fibrinogen and fibrin by plasmin.
- Increased in disseminated intravascular coagulation (DIC).

Assessment of the different pathways involved in coagulation may be made with two simple tests:

- APTT for intrinsic system
- PT for extrinsic system.

Test results and the conclusions that may be drawn from them are shown in Box 20.6.

DISORDERS OF HAEMOSTASIS

Platelet Disorders

Thrombocytopenia

This may be due to:

- failure of platelet production
- increased destruction or sequestration of platelets.

The causes of thrombocytopenia are shown in Box 20.5.

Abnormal Platelet Function

- May cause bleeding despite a normal platelet count.
- Abnormal platelet function may occur with:
  - drugs, e.g. aspirin, non-steroidal anti-inflammatory drugs; carbenicillin, ticarcillin
  - uraemia
  - septicaemia
  - von Willebrand's disease.

Blood Vessel Wall Abnormalities

These are rare and may be due to:

- scurvy (vitamin C deficiency)
- steroids

- Cushing's syndrome
- Henoch–Schönlein purpura.

Disorders of Coagulation

Congenital Coagulation Disorders

These are uncommon, the commonest being haemophilia A and von Willebrand's disease.

Haemophilia A

- Inherited deficiency of Factor VIII.
- X-linked recessive disorder affecting males and carried by females.
- Severity of the disease depends upon the degree of Factor VIII deficiency.
- Prothrombin time (PT) normal but activated partial thromboplastin time (APTT) prolonged.

von Willebrand's disease

- Due to deficiency of von Willebrand's factor.
- Transmitted as autosomal dominant condition.
- Vascular endothelium releases decreased amounts of Factor VIII.
- Platelet count usually normal, but platelet interaction with endothelium is defective because of deficiency of von Willebrand's factor.

Acquired Disorders of Coagulation

Vitamin K deficiency

- Vitamin K is present in green vegetables and is synthesized by intestinal bacteria.
- It is fat soluble and requires bile for absorption.
- It is required for formation of Factors II, VII, IX and X.
- Vitamin K deficiency may occur in the surgical patient as a result of:
  - obstructive jaundice
  - antibiotic therapy, which alters normal intestinal flora
  - prolonged parenteral nutrition without vitamin K supplements.

Liver disease

- Commonly associated with coagulation defects due to failure of clotting factor synthesis and the production of abnormal fibrinogen.
- Vitamin K will not help if there is hepatocellular failure.
- In addition, there may be thrombocytopenia due to hypersplenism.

Disseminated intravascular coagulation (DIC)

- Results from simultaneous activation of coagulation and fibrinolytic systems.
- Activation of coagulation system leads to formation of microthrombi in many organs with the consumption of clotting factors and platelets.
- This in turn leads to haemorrhage.
- DIC may arise as the result of the following disorders:
  - septicaemia
  - malignancy
  - trauma
  - shock
  - liver disease
  - acute pancreatitis
  - obstetric problems, e.g. toxaemia, amniotic fluid embolism.
- Clinically there is widespread haemorrhage.
- Diagnosis confirmed by presence of:
  - thrombocytopenia
  - decreased fibrinogen
  - elevated fibrin degradation products.

Natural Anticoagulants

Antithrombin III

- Inhibitor of thrombin.
- Action potentiated by heparin.
- Congenital antithrombin III deficiency is inherited in an autosomal dominant fashion.
- Heterozygotes may suffer from recurrent deep vein thrombosis (DVT), pulmonary embolism (PE) and mesenteric thrombosis.
- Homozygotes present in childhood with severe arterial and venous thrombosis.

Protein C and Protein S

- Both synthesized in the liver and dependent on vitamin K.
- Protein C degrades Factors Va and VIIIa, and promotes fibrinolysis by inactivating plasminogen-activator inhibitor 1.
- Protein S is a cofactor for protein C and enhances its activity.
- Hereditary protein C deficiency may occur, patients being more susceptible to:
  - pulmonary embolism
  - superficial thrombophlebitis
  - cerebral venous thrombosis.

Anticoagulant Drugs

The two most commonly used in surgical practice are heparin and warfarin. Many newer anticoagulants have been developed; the most commonly encountered of these in surgical practice are clopidogrel and the most recently launched new oral anticoagulants (NOACs; e.g. rivaroxaban).

Heparin

- Heparin potentiates the action of antithrombin III.

- Standard unfractionated heparin is administered intravenously or subcutaneously and has a half-life of about 1 h.
- Low-molecular-weight heparin (LMWH) is used subcutaneously, has a longer biological half-life and does not require monitoring but is contraindicated in severe renal failure and cannot be reversed. This is now the standard treatment for DVT/PE or to reduce the risk of DVT or PE in patients undergoing major surgery or patients who are on prolonged bed-rest, e.g. post-myocardial infarction or orthopaedic patients.
- Intravenous heparin is used in patients with thromboembolic disease with severe renal failure precluding LMWH, or in cases where rapid reversal of heparin anticoagulation is required, as this can be performed by stopping the heparin infusion and administering protamine sulphate intravenously.
- Dosage is monitored by performing APTT, which should be maintained at 2–2.5 × normal.
- Heparin does not cross the placenta and is therefore the drug of choice when anticoagulation is required during pregnancy.
- Side-effects of heparin include:
  - thrombocytopenia
  - hypersensitivity reactions
  - alopecia
  - osteoporosis (when used long term).

Warfarin

- Coumarin derivative which is administered orally.
- Vitamin K antagonist – in effect induces a state analogous to vitamin K deficiency.
- Interferes with the activities of Factors II, VII, IX and X.
- Delays thrombin generation, thus preventing the formation of thrombi.
- Usual to give a loading dose (10 mg) and to determine the international normalized ratio (INR; prothrombin ratio standardized by correcting for the sensitivity of the thromboplastin used) about 15–18 h later.
- Subsequent doses are based on monitoring of INR.
- Warfarin is usually administered for 3–6 months following DVT or PE.
- Life-long warfarin therapy is required for:
  - recurrent venous thromboembolic disease
  - some prosthetic heart valves
  - congenital deficiency of antithrombin III
  - deficiency of protein C or protein S
  - patients with lupus anticoagulant
  - valvular heart disease complicated by embolism or atrial fibrillation.
- Bleeding is controlled by stopping warfarin and administering fresh frozen plasma or vitamin K, depending on the degree of urgency.
- If vitamin K is used, there is a period of resistance to warfarin and control may be difficult initially when the patient is restarted on warfarin.
- A number of drugs may interfere with the control of warfarin; these are:
  - antibiotics
  - laxatives (interfere with vitamin K absorption)
  - phenylbutazone (interferes with binding of warfarin to albumin)
  - cimetidine (inhibits hepatic microsomal degradation).
- Warfarin crosses the placenta and is teratogenic, and therefore should be avoided particularly in the first trimester of pregnancy.

Clopidogrel

- Antiplatelet agent administered orally.
- Used in patients with ischaemic heart disease, cerebrovascular disease and to prevent thromboembolic events where warfarin is contraindicated.
- It inhibits activation and aggregation of platelets by blocking the glycoprotein IIa/IIIb pathway.
- Needs to be stopped for 7 days to reverse the effect.
- No coagulation monitoring test or specific reversal agent exists.

NOACs (New Oral Anticoagulants, e.g. Rivaroxaban)

- Direct inhibitors of activated Factor X.
- They are administered orally.
- Used for treatment and prophylaxis of venous thromboembolism and in patients with cerebrovascular disease.
- Effects are mostly reversed (i.e. can perform minor procedures) within 24 h of stopping the drug and totally reversed in 48 h.
- No coagulation monitoring test or specific reversal agent exists.

LYMPHOID SYSTEM

Lymph Nodes

Normal Structure and Function

- Lymph nodes are discrete encapsulated, usually kidney-shaped, structures, and range in diameter from a few mm to several cm.
- Situated along the course of lymphatic vessels and are numerous where these vessels converge, e.g. the root of the limbs, the neck, the pelvis, the mediastinum.
- Structure of a lymph node is shown in Fig. 19.2.
- There are three distinct microanatomical regions within a lymph node; these are:
  - the cortex: contains either primary or secondary lymphoid follicles

- the paracortex: the T-cell-dependent region of the lymph node
- the medulla: contains the medullary cords and sinuses; also contains lymphocytes, which are much less densely packed than in the cortex, together with macrophages, plasma cells and a small number of granulocytes.

Cortex

- Consists of primary lymphoid follicles, which are unstimulated follicles, spherical in shape, containing densely packed lymphocytes.
- Secondary follicles are present after lymphocytes have been stimulated antigenically.
- Secondary follicles have an outer ring of small B-lymphocytes surrounding the germinal centre which contains largely dividing lymphoblasts, macrophages and dendritic cells.
- Antigen is trapped upon the surface of the dendritic cells and presented to 'virgin' B-lymphocytes in the presence of T-helper cells.
- These B-cells subsequently undergo a series of morphological and functional changes.
- The function of germinal centres is to generate immunoglobulin-secreting plasma cells in response to antigenic challenge.

Paracortex

- T-cell-dependent region of the lymph node.
- When a T-cell response occurs there is marked proliferation of cells in this area.
- Paracortex contains large number of T-lymphocytes with the predominance of helper/inducer cells.
- Cluster of differentiation (CD4) is expressed by helper/inducer T-cells.

Medulla

- Lymph enters the marginal sinus of the node and drains to the hilum through the sinuses, which converge into the medullary region.
- Sinuses are lined by macrophages that phagocytose foreign or abnormal particles from lymph passing through the node, i.e. filtering function.
- Between the sinuses in the medulla lie the medullary cords, which contain numerous plasma cells and are one of the main sites of antibody production within the lymph node.

The immunological function of lymph nodes is discussed in greater detail in Chapter 19.

LYMPHATIC SYSTEM

- A network of blind-ending lymphatic capillaries line the interstitial space near blood capillaries.
- Spaces between endothelial cells in lymphatic capillaries are larger than those in blood capillaries, making them readily permeable to protein and lymph fluid.
- Lymph collects in thin-walled lymph vessels, which eventually drain on the left side into the thoracic duct and subsequently into the subclavian vein.
- Lymph from the right upper part of the body drains into the right lymphatic duct.
- Lymph is composed of fluid and lymphocytes.
- Plasma protein that leaks out of capillaries and fluid that is not reabsorbed into capillaries are returned to the circulatory system via lymphatics.
- Lymphatics also act as pathway of absorption of fat from the gut.
- Lymph flow is aided by the rhythmical contractions of smooth muscle in the wall of lymphatic vessels, retrograde flow being prevented by valves.

Obstruction to Lymphatics (Lymphoedema)

Lymphoedema is the accumulation of tissue fluid due to lymphatic obstruction or defective lymphatic drainage. If the lymphatics are obstructed, protein and excess fluid in the interstitial fluid cannot return to the vascular system and accumulate behind the obstruction, producing local oedema.

Lymphoedema may be:

- primary
- secondary.

Primary Lymphoedema

- Due to aplasia or hypoplasia of lymphatics.
- There are three types:
  - congenital lymphoedema or Milroy's disease: presents shortly after birth
  - lymphoedema praecox: presents at puberty
  - lymphoedema tarda: presents around age 30.

Secondary Lymphoedema

- May be secondary to result of damage to lymphatic channels by:
  - infection
  - surgery
  - radiotherapy
  - malignant infiltration
  - trauma.
- Blockage of inguinal lymphatics by filarial parasites frequently causes oedema of the legs and, in the male, the scrotum also (elephantiasis).
- Blockage of lymphatic drainage from the small intestine usually occurs because of tumour involvement, causing malabsorption of fats and fat-soluble substances.
- Blockage of lymphatic drainage at the level of the thoracic duct causes chylous effusions in the pleura and

peritoneal cavities – fluid opalescent at paracentesis or thoracocentesis because of presence of tiny fat globules (chyle).

Lymphadenopathy

Lymphadenopathy is the enlargement of lymph nodes. Causes are shown in Box 20.7.

SPLEEN

Gross anatomy of the spleen is covered in Chapter 2.

BOX 20.7 Causes of Lymphadenopathy

Primary infection	
Viral	Infectious mononucleosis
	HIV
	CMV
	Rubella
	Measles
Bacterial	TB
	Syphilis
	Brucellosis
	Cat scratch disease
	Septicaemia
Protozoal	Toxoplasmosis
Parasitic	Filariasis
Secondary infection	E.g. tonsillitis with cervical lymphadenitis, abscess with regional lymphadenitis
Primary malignancy	Acute lymphoblastic leukaemia
	Chronic lymphatic leukaemia
	Hodgkin's disease
	Non-Hodgkin's lymphoma
	Myeloproliferative disorders
Secondary malignancy	Metastases from local and distant malignancy
Others	Sarcoidosis
	SLE
	Rheumatoid arthritis

Internal Structure (Fig. 20.3)

When a fresh spleen is cut across, two areas can be identified on the cut surface:

- islands of pale areas, 1–2 mm in diameter, which are white and are known as white pulp
- deep red background, which is known as red pulp.

White Pulp

- Consists of central arteries ensheathed by lymphocytes and lymphoid nodules.
- T-lymphocytes are located in the immediate vicinity of the central artery.
- Nodules contain mostly B-lymphocytes.
- Activated lymphocytes migrate to periphery of nodule, the marginal zone between red and white pulp, and differentiate into plasma cells.
- Plasma cells circulate in the red pulp and enter sinusoids.

Red Pulp

- Forms most of the spleen.
- Contains sinusoids which trap defective or effete red cells, which are destroyed by adjacent macrophages.

Functions of the Spleen

The two main functions are:

- production of antibodies
- filtration of blood and disposal of defective blood cells.

The two functions are architecturally distinct, lymphoid function occurring in the white pulp and phagocytic activity in the red pulp.

Filtering Function

- Removal of old or abnormal red cells.
- Removal of abnormal white cells.
- Removal of normal and abnormal platelets and cellular debris.

Immunological Function

- Opsonization: while opsonized bacteria can be removed from the circulation by the entire reticulo-endothelial system, the spleen is well suited to removing poorly opsonized or encapsulated pathogens.
- Antibody synthesis: occurs chiefly within the white pulp.
- Protection from infection: splenectomy leaves patients more prone to certain types of infection (see below).

Disorders of the Spleen

Hypersplenism

Hypersplenism is splenomegaly associated with the following:

- any combination of anaemia, leucopenia or thrombocytopenia

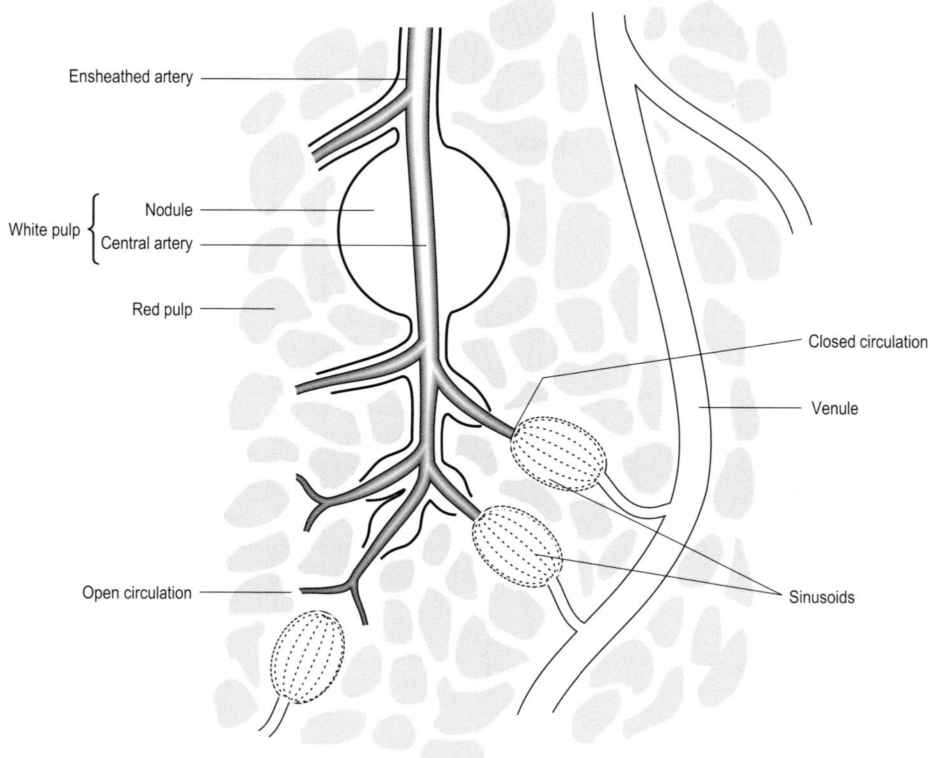

Fig. 20.3 The structure of the spleen showing the circulation.

- compensatory bone marrow hyperplasia
- improvement after splenectomy.

There is an exaggerated destruction or sequestration of circulating blood elements, which can affect red cells, white cells and platelets. The condition may be either primary or secondary.

Primary hypersplenism

- Essentially a diagnosis of exclusion, where all causes of secondary hypersplenism have been excluded.
- Rare condition of unknown aetiology, mainly affecting women.
- May be massive splenomegaly and accompanying pancytopenia, especially leucopenia.
- There may be recurring fevers and infection.
- Splenectomy results in good haematological response, although some patients remain leucopenic.

Splenomegaly

- The spleen must be enlarged to about three times its normal size to become clinically palpable.
- The spleen may be so massive in size that it is palpable in the right iliac fossa. Massive splenomegaly is likely to be due to:
  - chronic myeloid leukaemia
  - myelofibrosis
  - lymphoma.
- Splenomegaly may lead to hypersplenism, i.e. pancytopenia, as cells become trapped and destroyed in an overactive spleen.

The causes of splenomegaly are shown in Box 20.8.

Effects of Splenectomy

Haematological Effects

- Reduction in the capacity of the spleen to remove immature or abnormal red cells from the circulation.
- Red cell count does not change but red cells with cytoplasmic inclusion, e.g. Howell–Jolly bodies, may appear.
- Granulocytosis occurs immediately after splenectomy but is replaced in a few weeks by lymphocytosis and monocytosis.

BOX 20.8 Causes of Splenomegaly

Infective	
Bacterial	Typhoid
	Typhus
	TB
	Septicaemia
	Abscess
Viral	Glandular fever
Spirochaetal	Syphilis
	Leptospirosis
Protozoal	Malaria
Parasitic	Hydatid cyst
Inflammatory	Rheumatoid arthritis
	Sarcoidosis
	Lupus
	Amyloid
Neoplastic	Leukaemia
	Lymphoma
	Polycythaemia vera
	Myelofibrosis
	Primary tumours
	Metastases
Haemolytic disease	Hereditary spherocytosis
	Acquired haemolytic anaemia
	Thrombocytopenic purpura
Storage diseases	Gaucher's disease
Deficiency diseases	Pernicious anaemia
	Severe iron-deficiency anaemia
Splenic vein hypertension	Cirrhosis
	Splenic vein thrombosis
	Portal vein thrombosis
Non-parasitic cysts	

- The platelet count is usually increased and may stay at levels of 400 000–500 000 × 10^9/L for over a year.
- A thrombocytosis in excess of 1000 × 10^9/L may occur – not an indication for anticoagulation, but antiplatelet agents such as aspirin may help prevent thrombosis.

Post-Splenectomy Sepsis

- Following splenectomy, individuals are susceptible to fulminant bacteraemia, which is potentially life-threatening but is largely preventable.
- Risk is greatest in young children, especially in the first 2 years after surgery.
- Risk is also greater when splenectomy is undertaken for disorders of the reticuloendothelial system rather than for trauma.
- Lethal sepsis is more common in children and is indeed rare in adults.
- The most common infection is pneumococcal infection (mortality up to 60%), followed by *H. influenzae* type b (less common but significant in children) and *N. meningitides*.
- Other infections include *E. coli*, malaria, babesiosis and *Capnocytophaga canimorsus* (associated with dog bites).
- A distinct clinical syndrome starts with mild non-specific symptoms followed by high pyrexia and septicaemic shock, which may ultimately be fatal.
- Risk of fatal sepsis is less after splenectomy for trauma, possibly due to splenosis, i.e. multiple small implants of splenic tissue which result from dissemination and auto-transplantation following trauma.
- Patients undergoing splenectomy should have the following vaccinations:
  - polyvalent pneumococcal vaccine (PPV). Children under the age of 2 have a reduced ability to mount an antibody response to polysaccharides and are at particular risk of vaccine failure. The newer conjugate 7-valent vaccine produces a better response in this group
  - vaccination against *H. influenzae* type b (Hib)
  - vaccination against meningococci A and C. A combination of MenC vaccine and MenACWY conjugate vaccine is used according to protocol for different age groups. MenACWY conjugate vaccine is particularly recommended in the under-2s
  - influenza vaccination is recommended annually.
- All vaccinations should be given at least 2 weeks before a planned splenectomy. Following emergency splenectomy, functional antibody responses are better with delayed (14-day) vaccination. Re-immunization of asplenic patients is currently recommended every 5 years.
- Antibiotic prophylaxis with penicillin (or erythromycin for penicillin-sensitive patients) should be given in the first 2 years post-splenectomy, especially in children under 2 years. Some authorities consider that they should be given until age 18 years. Others recommend life-long prophylactic antibiotics. Antibiotic prophylaxis may need to be altered depending on knowledge

of local antibiotic resistance patterns. Patients developing infection, despite prophylactic measures, must be admitted to hospital and given systemic antibiotics.
- Asplenic patients should be strongly advised of the increased risk of severe falciparum malaria, should take all anti-malarial precautions/prophylaxis, and ideally should avoid holidays in malaria-endemic areas.

THYMUS

Disorders of the Thymus

- Agenesis results in immunodeficiency syndromes.
- Histological abnormalities of the thymus, such as lymphoid hyperplasia or tumours, may be seen in association with:
  - myasthenia gravis
  - systemic lupus erythematosus
  - dermatomyositis
  - aplastic anaemia.

Thymic Tumours

- These include:
  - thymoma
  - Hodgkin's disease
  - non-Hodgkin's lymphoma
  - teratoma
  - thymolipoma
  - thymic carcinoma.
- Thymoma is rare.
- Many thymomas are asymptomatic and detected on chest X-ray performed for other reasons.
- Some cases are detected when myasthenia gravis develops.
- Patients may present with signs of local disease such as cough, dyspnoea, stridor or superior vena caval obstruction.
- Majority of thymomas are benign and well encapsulated.
- Malignant tumours are locally invasive, spreading by direct invasion of adjacent structures.

BLOOD GROUPS

ABO System (Table 20.2)

- Consists of three allelic genes: A, B and O.
- A and B are responsible for converting a basic substance H, present in every red cell, into A or B substances, thus converting the cells to group A or group B.
- gene has no effect on H substance.
- Thus, there are six genotypes and four phenotypes.
- An individual inherits one of three ABO antigen groups (agglutinogen) from each parent: A, B or neither.
- Individuals inherit antibodies (agglutinins), which react against red cells of groups other than their own, i.e. anti-A, anti-B. There is no anti-O.
- Blood group O is the universal donor because there are no A or B antigens on the red cell membrane.
- Blood group AB is the universal recipient because there is no anti-A or anti-B in the serum.
- Individuals with blood group A have A antigens on the red cells and B antibodies in the plasma.
- Individuals who are blood group B have B antigens on the surface of the red cells and A antibodies in the plasma.
- Individuals who are blood group AB have both A and B antigens on the red cells and no A or B antibodies in the plasma.
- Individuals who are blood group O have neither A nor B antigens on the red cells but have both A and B antibodies in the plasma.

Principles of Grouping and Cross-Matching

- Grouping:
  - individuals have antibodies against those red cell antigens they lack
  - when red cells carrying one or both antigens (A, B) are exposed to corresponding antibodies, they agglutinate or clump together
  - blood is mixed with reagents including different antibodies, i.e. anti-A and anti-B
  - agglutination indicates that the blood has reacted with a certain antibody and therefore is not compatible with blood containing that kind of antibody
  - if agglutination does not take place it indicates that the blood does not have the antigens binding to that specific antibody in the reagent

TABLE 20.2 The ABO Blood Group System

Genotype	Phenotype	Agglutinogen on Cell	Natural Agglutinins in Plasma	% Phenotypic Frequency (UK)
OO	O	Nil (or H substance)	Anti-A, Anti-B	46
AA, AO	A	A	Anti-B	42
BB, BO	B	B	Anti-A	9
AB	AB	A, B	None	3

- grouping is checked by determining whether anti-A or anti-B is present in the recipient serum by adding known group A and B cells.
- Cross-matching:
  - antibodies to the A, B antigens are naturally occurring, whereas antibodies to other red cell antigens (e.g. Rhesus, Kell, Duffy) appear only after sensitization by transfusion or pregnancy
  - group-compatible red cells from a donor pack of blood are mixed with recipient serum and examined for agglutination, i.e. that there is no antibody present in the recipient's serum that will react with any antigen on the donor's cells
  - cross-matching will also rule out any errors that may have occurred in the determination of the donor and recipient blood groups
  - compatibility of transfusions between various groups is shown in Table 20.3.

Rhesus Group

- There are a number of Rh antigens, of which group D (RhD) is the most important agglutinogen.
- 15% of the population have no RhD antigens and are therefore Rh negative.
- There is no preformed Rh agglutinin (i.e. anti-D).
- An Rh-negative individual can make anti-D only after sensitization with Rh positive.
- Rh typing is carried out using an agglutinating IgM anti-D.
- An Rh-negative individual has 50% chance of developing anti-D after the transfusion of a single unit of Rh-positive blood. It is important therefore that Rh-negative individuals receive Rh-negative blood. A universal donor therefore should be O Rh negative.
- The major importance of the Rh system is to avoid the danger of RhD incompatibility between mother and fetus.

Rhesus Incompatibility

- An Rh-negative mother and Rh-positive father may produce an Rh-positive fetus.
- If fetal red cells enter the maternal circulation, anti-D will be produced (IgG).
- If these IgG antibodies cross the placenta in future pregnancies they will destroy the fetal red cells, resulting in haemolytic disease of the newborn.
- Sensitization can be prevented by administering a single dose of anti-Rh antibodies in the form of Rh immunoglobulin during the post-partum period after the birth of an Rh-positive baby. This will destroy the fetal red cells, preventing maternal sensitization.

BLOOD PRODUCTS (Fig. 20.4)

Over 90% of donated blood is separated into its various constituents so that individual components can be administered.

Whole Blood

- Less readily available because of demand for blood products.
- Most blood for transfusion is essentially red cells alone.
- Whole blood is product of choice for massive transfusion.
- In practice, concentrated red cells with colloid or crystalloid are given following considerable haemorrhage.
- Whole blood may be stored for up to 42 days.
- Granulocytes and platelets lose their function in a few days.
- Clotting Factors V and VIII are rapidly lost.
- Increasing content of lactate, phosphate and potassium in stored blood is usually clinically insignificant, except in massive transfusion.

Red Cell Concentrates

- Red cell concentrates or packed cells consist of whole blood from which plasma has been removed.
- Treatment of choice for anaemia without hypovolaemia.
- Shelf life 42 days at 4°C.
- Storage changes include:
  - increased lactate
  - increased potassium
  - increased phosphate

TABLE 20.3 Compatible Transfusions

Blood Group	Antigens	Antibodies	Can Donate to	Can Receive From
O	None	A, B	AB, A, B, O	O
A	A	B	A, AB	A, O
B	B	A	B, AB	B, O
AB	A, B	None	AB	AB, A, B, O

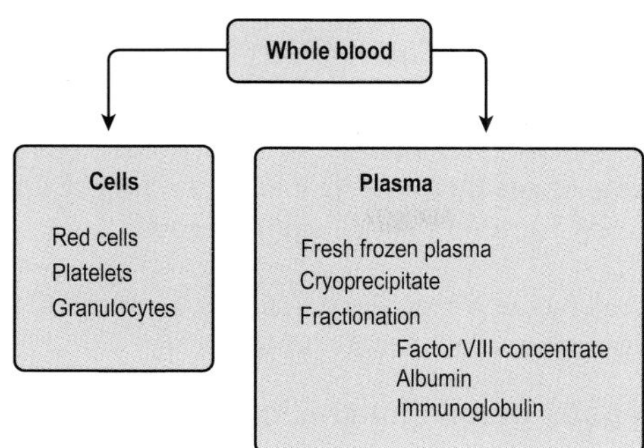

Fig. 20.4 Blood products.

- decrease in pH
- haemolysis
- microaggregation of dead cells
- loss of granulocyte and platelet function
- loss of Factors V and VIII.

Indications for Blood Transfusion

- Significant anaemia, e.g. Hb <7 g/dL.
- Significant haemorrhage leading to hypovolaemia.

Platelet Concentrates

- Platelets suspended in plasma.
- Shelf-life 3 days at room temperature.
- Should be ABO compatible.

Indications for Platelet Transfusion

- Haemorrhage in the presence of thrombocytopenia.
- Thrombocytopenia prior to invasive procedures.
- Consumptive coagulopathy, e.g. DIC.
- Counts of $50\,000 \times 10^9$/L are adequate for haemostasis.

Administration

- Four hours or less before procedure.
- Infuse rapidly via short-giving set with no filter.
- Usual adult dose is 6 units, which should raise the count by $40\,000 \times 10^9$/L.
- Counts should be checked 10 min to 1 h post-transfusion.
- Failure of the count to rise may be due to platelet antibodies, post-transfusion purpura or DIC.

Granulocytes

- Very short shelf-life (<24 h) at room temperature.
- Effect of infusion short-lived; expensive; induces pyrexial response; role remains controversial.
- Granulocyte-colony stimulating factor (G-CSF) is now used to stimulate bone marrow response.

Fresh Frozen Plasma (FFP)

- Separated from fresh blood and frozen at −30°C.
- Contains all clotting factors.
- Shelf-life 1 year at −30°C.
- Use within 1 h of thawing.

Indications for FFP Transfusion

- Used to replace clotting factors following major haemorrhage (due to poor clotting ability of stored blood).
- Patients short of clotting factors, e.g. liver disease or rapid reversal of warfarin.
- DIC in conjunction with platelets and cryoprecipitate.
- Prophylaxis or treatment of haemorrhage in patients with specific clotting defects for which the specific factor is unavailable.

Administration

- Group-compatible FFP should be used.

Cryoprecipitate

- Concentrate prepared by freeze-thawing plasma from a single donor.
- Rich in Factor VIII, fibrinogen and von Willebrand's factor.

Indications for Cryoprecipitate Transfusion

- Haemophilia.
- Von Willebrand's disease.
- Fibrinogen deficiency, e.g. DIC.

Factor VIII Concentrate

- Used for treatment of haemophilia A.

Complications of Blood Transfusion

Haemolytic Transfusion Reactions

Immediate

- ABO incompatibility.
- Symptoms and signs:
  - pyrexia
  - dyspnoea
  - chest pain
  - severe loin pain
  - collapse
  - hypotension
  - haemoglobinuria
  - oliguria (often proceeding to acute renal failure)
  - jaundice
  - DIC with spontaneous bruising and haemorrhage.

Delayed

- Low-titre antibody too weak to detect in cross-match and unable to cause lysis at the time of transfusion.
- Occurs 5–10 days post-transfusion.
- Symptoms and signs:
  - pyrexia
  - anaemia
  - jaundice
  - haemoglobinuria.

Reaction to white blood cells

- Febrile reaction.
- Relatively common in patients who have had previous transfusions or pregnancy.
- Fever and flushing soon after starting transfusion.
- Due to recipient leucocyte antibodies.
- If patient known to have previous similar reaction, washed red cells should be given.

Infection

Infection is unlikely with the present testing in the UK but may be a problem where testing is not carried out. Causes include:

- HIV
- hepatitis B
- hepatitis C
- CMV
- malaria
- syphilis
- prion disease, e.g. Creutzfeldt–Jakob disease.

Complications of Massive Blood Transfusion

- Fluid overload.
- Cardiac arrhythmias due to cold blood.
- Citrate toxicity with resulting hypocalcaemia.
- Hypothermia.
- Hyperkalaemia.
- Metabolic acidosis because of acidity of stored blood.
- Haemorrhage due to coagulopathy unless FFP and platelets are administered simultaneously.
- DIC.
- ARDS (acute respiratory distress syndrome)/TRALI (transfusion-related acute lung injury).

Autologous Blood Transfusion

Methods of reducing blood bank transfusion involve 'recycling' of patient's own blood (autotransfusion). Autotransfusion may be carried out in several ways:

- Predonation:
  - blood is taken from the patient at weekly intervals prior to elective surgery (up to 4 units over 4 weeks).
- Normovolaemic haemodilution:
  - collect blood immediately prior to surgery and replace with colloid
  - up to 2 L can be removed safely from adults without cardiac disease
  - blood is fresh; contains viable platelets and clotting factors.
- Intraoperative blood salvage techniques:
  - blood spilled at operation is collected by suction, processed and reinfused (using a 'cell saver')
  - blood is anticoagulated and returned to the patient via a fine filter
  - useful when massive bleeding occurs in an uncontaminated operative field, e.g. ruptured aortic aneurysm, liver trauma
  - unsuitable where contamination occurs, e.g. in abdominal surgery where the bowel is breached.

OSCE SCENARIOS

OSCE Scenario 20.1

A 73-year-old female is seen in pre-assessment clinic as she is due to have a hip replacement in 4 weeks' time. Her bloods show a haemoglobin of 6.7 g/dL and an MCV of 69 fL with a normal clotting screen.

1. What type of anaemia is shown in the test results?
2. What are the common causes of this type of anaemia? Which is the most likely in this case?

You discuss the case with the operating surgeon, who asks you to take a full history and arrange any investigations required.

3. Ask the patient relevant questions about her health status, and explain what the next investigations you would suggest will involve. You should also introduce the possibility of her hip operation needing to be delayed.

OSCE Scenario 20.2

You are fast-bleeped to a surgical ward by the nursing staff as a 68-year-old male patient has become pyrexial, short of breath and hypotensive. The staff nurse informs you that the patient is normally fit and well, on no medications and had an uncomplicated hip replacement yesterday. This morning he was prescribed 2 units of blood as his haemoglobin was 6.9 g/dL and his transfusion was commenced about 5 min before the onset of these symptoms. The patient cannot answer your questions due to his dyspnoea.

1. What is your differential diagnosis?

The nurse in charge shows you that the first name and date of birth on the detail label on the partially transfused bag of blood do not match those on the patient's wristband.

2. Outline your immediate actions.

OSCE Scenario 20.3

A 19-year-old female patient is admitted with a femoral fracture after a road traffic accident. When preparing her for theatre she tells you that she is a Jehovah's Witness and does not want blood under any circumstances, even if it would mean her death, and informs you she has an Advanced Decision recorded in her medical notes and wallet stating the same. You assess her as having full capacity, confirmed by a senior colleague.

1. If this patient required a life-saving transfusion during her operation, should you administer it?
2. What if she was unconscious?
3. What if she was three years old?
4. What methods can be employed to reduce the need for transfusion?

OSCE Scenario 20.4

A 38-year-old male has been involved in a high-speed motorbike accident. He has multiple injuries and has been in theatre for some time, having received 12 units of blood. He has returned to the ITU following surgery.

1. One of the nurses on ITU calls you an hour later and says that every time the blood pressure cuff goes up the hand of the patient spasms. What do you think this might be due to and what is the cause?
2. While you are examining the patient you notice the ECG looks odd and the T waves are very high and peaked. What is the cause of this and what would be the urgent treatment?
3. Unfortunately, despite managing the above problems, after 3–4 h the patient starts to ooze from his nose, operative wounds and various different cannula sites. What could be the potential causes of this and how could you prevent it?

OSCE Scenario 20.5

A 78-year-old male is seen in clinic for potential total hip replacement; he tells you he is on warfarin for a prosthetic heart valve – it is metallic.

1. Describe how you will manage this patient's warfarin prior to surgery.
2. On the evening before the operation the INR has come back as 1.9; you tell your consultant who says it must be below 1.5 and asks if you will kindly sort this out. Describe what you can do to lower the INR and why it will work given the method of action of warfarin.
3. Imagine the patient has presented with an INR of 6 and has small bowel obstruction and needs urgent surgery, describe what options you have to reverse the action of warfarin.

Answers in Appendix pages 478–481

Please check your eBook at https://studentconsult.inkling.com/ for more self-assessment questions. See inside cover for registration details.

21

Basic Microbiology

SOURCES OF SURGICAL INFECTION

Hospital-acquired infections (nosocomial infection) occur in about 10% of hospitalized patients. Of these, 75% occur in surgical patients. Most postoperative infection arises from the patient's own flora.

The commonest sites of infection are:

- urinary tract
- respiratory tract
- wound
- skin and soft tissue.

Predisposition to hospital-acquired infections include:

- age: the extremes of life
- susceptible patient, e.g. immunocompromised, diabetes, prosthetic implants
- modes of treatment, e.g. intravenous lines, indwelling catheters.

The origin of bacterial infection may be divided into two main sources:

- endogenous: patient's own flora
- exogenous: from other people or objects in the environment.

Endogenous Infection

Endogenous infection occurs when organisms are carried by the patient as:

- part of normal flora
- part of 'replacement' flora, i.e. organisms that colonize various sites when the patient is treated with antimicrobial drugs.

Normal Body Flora

- Skin: coagulase-negative staphylococci, diphtheroids.
- Nostrils: *Staphylococcus aureus*.
- Oral cavity: streptococci, anaerobes.
- Upper respiratory tract: viridans streptococci, diphtheroids, anaerobes, commensal neisseria.
- Lower gastrointestinal (GI) tract: coliforms, faecal enterococci, anaerobes (*Bacteroides* and clostridia).
- Anterior urethra: skin flora (as above), faecal flora (as above).

Commensal Organisms

- Potential pathogens.
- Infection may result if balance is disturbed by breach of body defences or if an organism gains access to a site where it is not a commensal, e.g. *Escherichia coli* (normal in the colon) gaining access to the urinary tract and causing a urinary tract infection (UTI).
- Normal flora may be altered by broad-spectrum antibiotics, allowing overgrowth of resistant bacteria, which may result in serious infection.
- 'Replacement' organisms (conditional pathogens) resulting from antibiotic therapy may cause infection, e.g. *Klebsiella* may colonize the upper respiratory tract after a course of antibiotics and give rise to a chest infection, especially in intubated, ventilated patients.

Prevention of Endogenous Infection

This involves:

- disinfection of skin
- bowel preparation
- appropriate antibiotic prophylaxis.

Exogenous Infection

This is derived from either people or objects in the environment.

- People:
  - medical staff
  - nursing staff
  - other patients with infection, subclinical infection, or asymptomatic carriers.
- Inanimate objects (fomites):
  - surgical instruments
  - anaesthetic equipment
  - ventilators
  - humidifiers
  - parenteral fluids (especially if drugs are added under non-sterile conditions).
- Other sources:
  - floors
  - blankets

- bedside curtains
- urine bottles
- toilets
- dust
- air
- air-conditioning systems.

Methods of Spread of Infection

- Contact, e.g. hands, clothing.
- Airborne:
  - droplets and respiratory tract infection
  - dust
  - scales shed from skin
  - aerosols
  - nebulizers
  - air conditioning.
- Ingestion:
  - food poisoning
  - overcrowded wards (especially psychiatric and geriatric)
  - faecal–oral spread
  - poor kitchen hygiene
  - carriers.

Sources of Wound Contamination

- Direct inoculation:
  - Patient's residual flora
  - Patient's skin contamination
  - Surgeon's hands
  - contaminated instruments
  - contaminated dressings
  - contaminated procedure
  - drains, catheters, i.v. lines.
- Airborne contamination:
  - skin of staff and patient
  - air flow in operating theatre.
- Haematogenous spread:
  - i.v. lines
  - sepsis at other sites.

Prevention and Control of Hospital-Acquired Infection

The following are important factors in the prevention and control of hospital-acquired infection:

- Education of staff; hand washing; correct disposal of waste, e.g. soiled dressings; good nursing care; safe environment, e.g. appropriate space between beds, clean toilets, etc.; good theatre technique; good aseptic surgical technique.
- Skin infection and antisepsis.
- Sterilization and disinfection.
- Prophylactic antibiotics.
- Protective clothing.
- Isolation of patients with established infection or colonized with pathogens.
- Appropriate design of hospital buildings.
- Staff health:
  - exclude staff suffering from infection from contact with patient
  - protect staff, e.g. hepatitis B immunization
  - surveillance, e.g. infection control
  - monitoring of infection rates
  - careful tracking of potentially dangerous bacteria
  - appropriate policy-making.

Control of Staphylococcal Outbreaks

- Exclude personnel with skin sepsis or skin lesions from the surgical team.
- Exclude and treat carriers of *Staphylococcus aureus*.
- Personnel should wear:
  - protective theatre clothing
  - caps to cover hair
  - clean theatre clothes
  - gowns
  - masks.
- Alcohol hand rubs before and after patient contact.
- Wear gloves.
- Theatre environment:
  - correct direction of air flow
  - keep floors clean
  - horizontal surfaces, e.g. trolleys, should be reduced to a minimum as they act as dust traps
  - clean walls and ceilings on regular basis
  - operating lights should be kept clean and dust-free.
- Patient:
  - bed linen and clothes must not be allowed in theatre area
  - shaving must be carried out immediately prior to surgery and not some time before, which allows staphylococci to colonize small lacerations in skin
  - skin at and around the operation should be disinfected
  - wounds should be isolated from surroundings by sterile drapes.

Fig. 21.1 shows how staphylococcal infection may spread.

Meticillin (Methicillin)-Resistant Staphylococcus aureus (MRSA)

- MRSA is a major nosocomial pathogen.
- Causes severe morbidity and mortality.
- Infection/colonization rates vary with time and place.
- 10–40% of nosocomial *S. aureus* infections may be meticillin-resistant.

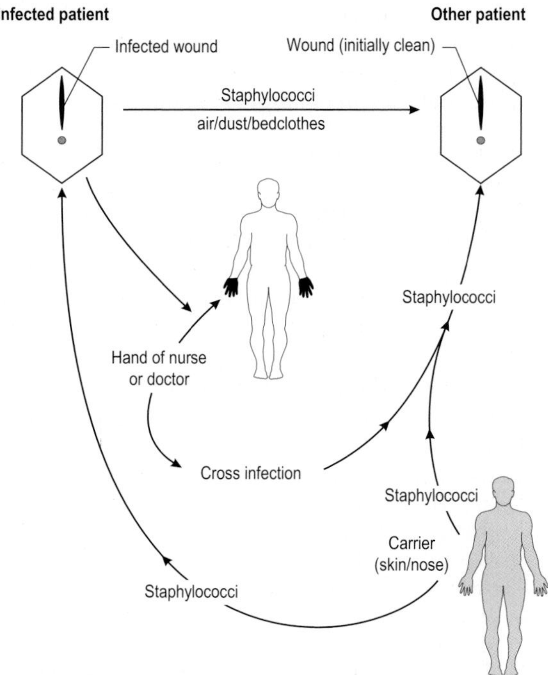

Fig. 21.1 The spread of staphylococcal infection.

- Many inpatients are colonized or infected.
- Hospital personnel may be carriers.
- Located in inguinal, perineal, axillary or anterior nares areas.
- Spread by hands, usually of nursing or medical staff.

Risk Factors for Colonization

- Advanced age.
- Previous hospitalization.
- Length of hospitalization.
- Stay in intensive treatment unit (ITU).
- Chronic illness.
- Prior and prolonged antibiotic therapy.
- Presence of wound.
- Exposure to colonized or infected patient.
- Presence of invasive indwelling devices.

Clinical Presentation

- Pneumonia.
- Line sepsis.
- Surgical site infection.
- Intra-abdominal sepsis.
- Osteomyelitis.
- Toxic shock syndrome.

Infection Control

- Screening of patients and sometimes staff.
- If MRSA suspected, take swabs from:
  - hairline
  - nose
  - axilla
  - groin
  - perineum.
- Alcohol hand rubs.
- Use of gowns and gloves when appropriate.
- Isolation of infected or colonized patient (barrier nursing).
- Environmental cleaning.

Management

Carriers

- Application of antiseptics, e.g. mupirocin, to nose and skin.
- Use antiseptic soaps and shampoos.
- May need 3 weeks' treatment.
- Check swabs at 3 days and 3 weeks after use of antiseptics.

Patients with MRSA

- Nurse in isolation.
- Vancomycin or teicoplanin are most often used.
- Co-trimoxazole or tetracycline are useful if no resistance.
- Linezolid, quinupristin and dalfopristin are newer alternatives.

SURGICALLY IMPORTANT MICROORGANISMS

Surgically important microbes may be divided into:

- conventional pathogens: those that may cause infection in the previously healthy person
- conditional pathogens: those that cause infection in those who have a predisposition to infection
- opportunistic pathogens: those that are usually of low virulence but will cause infection in the immunocompromised patient.

Examples of the above are shown in Box 21.1. Microorganisms that are of the greatest significance in surgery are usually bacteria. They may be classified as follows:

- Shape:
  - bacilli: rod-shaped
  - cocci: spherical.
- Gram staining:
  - Gram-positive: blue
  - Gram-negative: pink.
- Growth requirements:
  - aerobic
  - anaerobic
  - facultatively anaerobic.

BOX 21.1 Microbial Infections

Conventional
Staphylococcus aureus: wound infection
Haemophilus influenzae: chest infection
Neisseria gonorrhoeae: gonorrhoea

Conditional
Pseudomonas aeruginosa: wound infection
Klebsiella: urinary tract infection

Opportunistic
Pneumocystis carinii: chest infection
Candida albicans: oesophagitis
Aspergillus fumigatus: aspergillosis

Gram-Positive Cocci

Staphylococci

- Arranged in grape-like clusters.
- Divided into coagulase-positive and coagulase-negative.
- Coagulase-positive staphylococci are called *Staphylococcus aureus*.
- *S. aureus* are responsible for the following:
  - superficial infections, e.g. boils, abscesses, styes, conjunctivitis, wound infections
  - deep infection, e.g. septicaemia, endocarditis, osteomyelitis, pneumonia
  - food poisoning
  - toxic shock syndrome.
- Coagulase-negative staphylococci, e.g. *Staphylococcus epidermidis*, are of lower pathogenicity, and rarely cause infection in healthy people.
- *S. epidermidis* forms part of the normal skin flora.
- *S. epidermidis* and other coagulase-negative staphylococci may be responsible for infection in association with foreign bodies, e.g.
  - prosthetic cardiac valves
  - implanted pacemakers and defibrillators
  - prosthetic joints
  - intravenous lines
  - continuous ambulatory peritoneal dialysis
  - vascular grafts.
- These infections may lead to septicaemia and endocarditis, and become life-threatening.
- Treatment with antibiotic is usually inadequate and the prosthesis nearly always requires removal.
- *S. saprophyticus*, a commensal, may cause UTIs in sexually active women.

PVL-producing *Staphylococcus aureus* (Panton–Valentine leukocidin)

- PVL is a toxin produced by some strains of *S. aureus*.
- It is a virulence factor and usually causes cellulitis and abscesses.
- It is associated with community-acquired infections and spread by close contact (sports, gyms) and shared items (towels, razors).
- Infections are managed as per normal *S. aureus* and decolonized as per MRSA.

Antibiotic sensitivity

- *S. aureus* appears in multiple resistant forms in hospital practice.
- Recently there has been an increase in MRSA, posing a major threat to surgical patients.
- Antibiotics that may be active against *S. aureus* include:
  - penicillin (90% of hospital strains are resistant)
  - flucloxacillin (active against β-lactamase-producing organisms but not MRSA)
  - erythromycin
  - clindamycin
  - fusidic acid
  - cephalosporins
  - vancomycin.

Streptococci and Enterococci

- Spherical or oval cocci occurring in chains or pairs.
- Classified by their ability to lyse red blood cells present in blood-containing culture medium.
- Further divided by serology into Lancefield groups on the basis of polysaccharide antigens on their surface.
- Species responsible for sepsis are β-haemolytic strains where colonies completely lyse the blood cells on a cultured plate.
- These β-haemolytic types include Lancefield groups A, B, C and G.

Lancefield group A

Streptococcus pyogenes causes:

- tonsillitis and pharyngitis
- peritonsillar abscess (quinsy)
- otitis media
- mastoiditis
- wound infection with cellulitis and lymphangitis
- erysipelas
- necrotizing fasciitis.

Antibiotic sensitivity

- All strains are sensitive to penicillin.
- Patients sensitive to penicillin should be treated with erythromycin, but some strains are resistant.
- At present clindamycin is a good second-line or additional anti-streptococcal agent.

Lancefield group D

- Includes enterococci.
- *Enterococcus faecalis* is the most important, surgically, in this group.

- *E. faecalis* may cause UTIs and abdominal wound infections, and may be isolated from the bile in acute cholecystitis.

Antibiotic sensitivity

- Enterococci are sensitive to ampicillin.
- Moderately resistant to penicillin.
- Resistant to cephalosporins.

Viridans streptococci

- Alpha-haemolysis on blood-containing culture plates with a green discoloration (hence, viridans).
- Most human strains are commensals of the upper respiratory tract and of low pathogenicity.
- May be responsible for endocarditis.
- *Streptococcus milleri* may be classified with this group but is more often now classified with pyogenic streptococci; it may cause liver, lung, or brain abscesses.

Streptococcus pneumoniae (pneumococcus)

- *S. pneumoniae* consists of encapsulated diplococci.
- Virulence correlates with presence of capsule, probably because this prevents or inhibits phagocytosis.
- *S. pneumoniae* is responsible for the following:
  - lobar pneumonia
  - chronic bronchitis
  - meningitis
  - sinusitis
  - conjunctivitis
  - septicaemia (especially in splenectomized patients).

Antibiotic sensitivity

- Most streptococci are sensitive to penicillin but some strains of *S. pneumoniae* show resistance.

Gram-Positive Rods

Anaerobic Gram-positive rods are mainly soil saprophytes, but a few are pathogens.

- *Clostridium perfringens* (gas gangrene).
- *C. tetani* (tetanus).
- *C. botulinum* (botulism).
- *C. difficile* (pseudomembranous colitis).

Clostridium difficile

- Anaerobic Gram-positive bacillus that occasionally presents in normal adult bowel.
- It has become a major problem in hospital-acquired infections and its prevention is a major aim of all NHS trusts.
- It produces a cytotoxin.
- Carriage is often asymptomatic.
- Spectrum of illness from mild diarrhoea to fulminant pseudomembranous colitis.
- Diagnosis is by detection of toxin in stool.
- Main susceptibilities are advanced age, chronic illness, cancer and surgery.
- Illness precipitated, and spread promoted by antibiotics.
- Parenteral cephalosporins, quinolones and clindamycin known to be especially risky.
- Recent high rates of morbidity and mortality in European and North American hospitals.
- Spread is faecal–oral and hands are very important in spread.
- As alcohol-resistant spores – washing with soap is the appropriate mode of hand hygiene.
- Control requires tight restriction of antibiotic use, improvement in infection control and detection, isolation and treatment of cases.
- Treatment is by metronidazole in mild cases and oral vancomycin in the sick or high risk.

Gram-Negative Cocci

- *Neisseria* (pairs).
- *N. meningitidis* (meningococcus): meningitis and septicaemia.
- *N. gonorrhoeae* (gonococcus): gonorrhoea.
- *N. gonorrhoeae* may cause fever and severe lower abdominal pain (salpingitis in females), or be the cause of a urethral discharge in males.
- Gram stain from a smear of a high vaginal swab in the female or urethral discharge in the male may confirm diagnosis by demonstrating the presence of Gram-negative intracellular diplococci. It is imperative to perform culture or molecular detection.

Gram-Negative Bacilli

This is a large group of microorganisms of surgical importance.

Facultative Anaerobes (Enterobacteria, Coliforms)

Escherichia coli

- Normal inhabitant of human intestine.
- Some strains produce powerful toxins.
- An important cause of sepsis and diarrhoea.
- Examples of sepsis include:
  - UTIs
  - wound infection, along with anaerobes, especially after surgery on the lower GI tract
  - peritonitis – along with anaerobes
  - biliary tract infections
  - septicaemia.
- Examples of diarrhoeal illnesses include:
  - infantile gastroenteritis
  - traveller's diarrhoea
  - haemorrhagic diarrhoea can present as rectal bleeding and can cause haemolytic-uraemic syndrome.

Klebsiella

- *Klebsiella* spp. inhabit the human intestine.
- Some strains are saprophytic in soil, water and vegetation.
- *Klebsiella* causes:
  - UTIs
  - septicaemia
  - pneumonia (rare).

Proteus

- *Proteus* spp. cause:
  - UTIs
  - wound infections, e.g. burns, pressure sores
  - septicaemia.

Salmonella

- Inhabit animal GI tract.
- Predominantly animal pathogens which can produce disease in humans.
- *Salmonella typhi* differs from other species in that man is the only natural host.
- Foodstuffs from animal sources are the usual source of transmission of infection.
- They cause:
  - enteric fever, typhoid or paratyphoid; these are due to *S. typhi* and *S. paratyphi* A, B, C
  - gastroenteritis (food poisoning), usually due to *S. enteritidis* or *S. typhimurium*
  - osteomyelitis (rare)
  - septic arthritis (rare).
- *Salmonella typhi* may survive in symptomless carriers and persist in the gall bladder.
- Faecal carriage may occur via biliary tract colonization.
- Epidemics may occur, especially if the carrier is a food-handler.

Shigella

- Intestinal parasite in man.
- Causes dysentery.
- *Shigella dysenteriae* produces exotoxin, which causes most severe illness.
- *Shigella sonnei* is most common cause of dysentery in the UK.

Yersinia

- Animal parasite which occasionally causes disease in humans.
- *Yersinia pseudotuberculosis* and *Y. enterocolitica* are the most common, causing food poisoning and possibly mesenteric adenitis.

Other enterobacteria

- These include *Enterobacter*, *Citrobacter*, *Providencia*, *Morganella* and *Serratia*.
- Human and animal intestinal parasites, but some strains are saprophytes.
- Moist hospital environments may act as reservoirs.
- Often multi-resistant to antibiotics.
- They may cause the following:
  - UTIs
  - wound infection after abdominal surgery
  - respiratory infections in hospitalized patients
  - septicaemia.

Antibiotic sensitivity

- Sensitivity should be determined, as some strains may be resistant to the more commonly used antibiotics.
- Antibiotics used against enterobacteria include ampicillin, amoxicillin, trimethoprim, aminoglycosides, ciprofloxacin, cephalosporins (second- and third-generation) and chloramphenicol.
- For UTIs the antimicrobial drugs trimethoprim and nitrofurantoin may be appropriate.

Aerobic Gram-Negative Bacilli

Pseudomonas aeruginosa

- Inhabits water and soil.
- Organism survives in moist environments in hospitals, and may also survive in aqueous antiseptics and other fluids.
- Important cause of hospital-acquired infections.
- It has a characteristic green appearance of exudate on dressings and an unpleasant odour.
- Particularly affects patients with serious underlying conditions, e.g. burns, malignancies.
- Affects patients with urinary catheters, endotracheal tubes.
- Frequent cause of sepsis in the immunocompromised patient.
- Is a pathogen in the following conditions:
  - UTIs, especially with indwelling catheters
  - burns
  - wound infections
  - septicaemia
  - pressure sores
  - venous stasis ulcers
  - chest infections, especially patients on mechanical ventilation and those with cystic fibrosis
  - eye infections (it may contaminate certain types of eye drops).

Antibiotic sensitivity

- Presence of *P. aeruginosa* is not necessarily an indication for antibiotic therapy, especially if isolated from a superficial site.
- Clinical and bacteriological assessment in the individual patient is appropriate before prescribing antibiotics.
- *P. aeruginosa* is resistant to most common antibiotics.
- The most suitable antibiotics are aminoglycosides, certain β-lactams, e.g. penicillins (ticarcillin, piperacillin), ciprofloxacin, cephalosporins (ceftazidime).

Anaerobic Gram-Negative Bacilli

Bacteroides

- Found in lower GI tract, female genital tract, and mouth.
- Important in abdominal and gynaecological sepsis.
- Often found along with other organisms, notably coliforms.
- Also important in dental and oropharyngeal disease.

Antibiotic sensitivity

- *Bacteroides fragilis* (most important in surgery). It is penicillin-resistant due to β-lactamase production.
- *Bacteroides* are sensitive to metronidazole.

Other Gram-Negative Bacilli

Campylobacter

- Curved or spiral rods which are microaerophilic.
- Found in various animal species, including chickens, domestic animals and seagulls.
- *Campylobacter* is the most common cause of bacterial food poisoning in the UK.

Haemophilus influenzae

- Found mainly in the respiratory tract.
- Often part of the normal flora.
- May cause respiratory disease, especially community-acquired respiratory disease.
- Exists in non-capsulated and capsulated strains.
- Non-capsulated strains are responsible for exacerbations of chronic bronchitis and bronchiectasis.
- Capsulated strains cause severe infections in young children, e.g. meningitis, acute epiglottis, osteomyelitis, arthritis and orbital cellulitis.
- Septicaemia with *H. influenzae* may occur as part of post-splenectomy sepsis.
- A vaccine is available against *H. influenzae* type b (Hib).

Antibiotic sensitivity

H. influenzae is sometimes sensitive to ampicillin, tetracycline, ciprofloxacin, cephalosporins (second- and third-generation and co-trimoxazole). Chloramphenicol should be reserved for severe infections, e.g. meningitis and acute epiglottitis.

Pasteurella multocida

- Small, ovoid, Gram-negative bacillus.
- Inhabits respiratory tract of many animals, notably dogs and cats.
- In man it may cause septic wounds after animal bites.
- Sensitive to penicillin, tetracycline, erythromycin and aminoglycosides.

Helicobacter pylori

- Gram-negative spiral, motile, microaerophilic bacterium.
- Transmission by faecal–oral, oral–oral or iatrogenic (endoscopes and endoscopists).
- Associated with gastritis, peptic ulceration, gastric lymphoma, gastric cancer.
- Diagnostic tests include:
  - urea breath test
  - mucosal biopsy (*Campylobacter*-like organism [CLO] test)
  - histopathological examination
  - serology.
- Eradication therapy involves triple therapy with a 1-week course of a proton pump inhibitor plus amoxicillin plus clarithromycin (in penicillin-sensitive patients, metronidazole is substituted for amoxicillin).

PATHOPHYSIOLOGY OF SEPSIS

The incidence of sepsis has been increasing over the last 25 years; it is the commonest cause of death in ITU.

Systemic Inflammatory Response Syndrome (SIRS)

Development of SIRS is manifest by two or more of:

- temperature >38°C or <36°C
- tachycardia >90 beats/min
- tachypnoea >20 breaths/min or $PaCO_2$ < 4.25 kPa
- WBC $>12 \times 10^9$/L or $<4 \times 10^9$/L.

Note: immunocompromised patients can be septic without eliciting an inflammatory response.

Systemic Inflammatory Response Syndrome and Multi-Organ Dysfunction Syndrome (MODS)

Primary precipitating event → inflammatory response → SIRS → MODS → multi-organ failure (MOF)

Primary Precipitating Event

The main causes are:

- localized or generalized sepsis
- peritonitis (especially associated with pancreatitis)
- burns
- trauma
- haemorrhage.

Inflammatory Response

The immune system responds to tissue damage by instituting an inflammatory response. Initially this is protective, but later may become destructive, resulting in the detrimental effects observed in SIRS.

Three stages in the development of SIRS have been described.

Stage I

As a result of local insult, the local environment produces cytokines which:

- provoke an inflammatory response
- promote wound repair
- recruit reticuloendothelial cells.

Stage II

- Cytokines are released into the circulation to enhance local response.
- Macrophages and platelets are recruited.
- Growth factor production is stimulated.
- Acute phase response, which is controlled by a simultaneous decrease of pro-inflammatory mediators and release of endogenous antagonists.
- These mediators hold the initial inflammatory response in check until the wound is healed, infection resolves and homeostasis is restored.

Stage III

- This occurs if homeostasis is not restored.
- Massive systemic reaction with cytokines becomes destructive.
- Loss of integrity of microcirculation.
- Dysfunction of various distant organs.

Mediators of SIRS include:

- endotoxin
- tumour necrosis factor (TNF)
- interleukins, chiefly IL-1, IL-6
- cells, e.g. endothelial cells, neutrophils
- secondary inflammatory mediators
- arachidonic acid metabolites, e.g. prostaglandins, thromboxane
- nitric oxide
- platelet activating factor (PAF)
- stress hormones, catecholamines, steroids, insulin
- other mediators, e.g. histamine, bradykinin, serotonin.

Clinical Definition of Sepsis Syndrome

This involves the progression from:

SIRS → sepsis → severe sepsis → septic shock (refractory shock) → death

- Sepsis: SIRS resulting from documented infection.
- Severe sepsis: sepsis associated with evidence of end-organ dysfunction, hypoperfusion, hypotension.
- Septic shock: severe sepsis with refractory hypotension (in spite of adequate volume resuscitation).

Clinical Effects of Sepsis Syndrome

These depend upon the precipitating cause, degree of organ involvement and severity. They include:

- overt or occult infection
- flushed, warm periphery
- hypotension
- tachycardia
- tachypnoea
- hypoxia
- metabolic acidosis
- deranged clotting function (abnormality of clotting cascade in inflammatory response).

Septic shock (refractory shock)

- Peripheral vascular failure.
- Persistent hypotension resistant to vasoconstrictors.
- Usually high output due to low systemic vascular resistance (SVR) and increased heart rate.
- Usually myocardial depressant factor.
- Cardiac dysfunction also due to:
  - metabolic acidosis
  - hypoxaemia.
- Microcirculatory changes due to:
  - vasodilatation
  - A–V shunting (maldistribution of flow)
  - increased capillary permeability
  - interstitial oedema
  - decreased O_2 extraction.
- Defect of O_2 utilization at cellular level.

Multi-Organ Dysfunction Syndrome

- Progression from SIRS.
- Results in end-organ dysfunction.
- Diagnosed dysfunction of two or more organ systems.
- Results from hypoperfusion and ischaemia of tissues.
- The clinical picture depends on organ systems affected.

Factors Leading to Multi-Organ Failure

- Excessive release of endogenous mediators, including TNF-α, IL-1, IL-6.
- Impaired local microvascular perfusion interfering with O_2 delivery to tissues, with disruption of cellular metabolic functions.
- Impaired intestinal barrier function, with bacterial translocation releasing endotoxins into the portal circulation.
- Damage to reticuloendothelial function.
- Immune depression with T- and B-cell depression.
- T-suppressor cell stimulation resulting in increased vulnerability to infection.

Clinical Picture of Multi-Organ Dysfunction

The clinical picture depends on the organ systems involved.

Respiratory

- Acute respiratory distress syndrome (ARDS) may follow SIRS.
- Hypoxia.
- Signs and symptoms of respiratory failure.
- Nosocomial pneumonia in 70% of patients.

Cardiovascular

- Endothelial damage, leading to interstitial oedema.
- Vasodilatation, leading to hypotension.
- Tissue hypoxia.
- Lactic acidosis.
- Myocardial dysfunction due to effects of inflammation, circulating myocardial depressant factor, endotoxin.

Renal

- Oliguria (<0.5 mL/kg/h urine production).
- Elevated urea and creatinine.

Hepatic

- Reduced drug metabolism.
- Reduced hormone metabolism.
- Poor control of glucose homeostasis.
- Failure of synthesis, e.g. clotting factors.
- Failure to conjugate bilirubin (hyperbilirubinaemia).

Gastrointestinal tract

- Atrophy of mucosa due to hypoperfusion and ischaemia.
- Increased risk of bacterial translocation into portal system, stimulating liver macrophages to produce cytokines with amplification of SIRS.

Cerebral

- Confusion.
- Agitation.
- Stupor.
- Coma.
- Above due to hypoperfusion, septic encephalopathy, metabolic encephalopathy.

Haematological

- Anaemia.
- Leucopenia.
- Thrombocytopenia.
- Leucocytosis.
- Abnormal coagulation; APPT ↑, PT ↑, frank disseminated intravascular coagulation (DIC).

Metabolic

- Hyperglycaemia due to sepsis and catecholamines (both cause insulin resistance).
- Lactic acidosis, generalized catabolic state.

If MODS continues unchecked, then organ dysfunction will become irreversible (MOF). This is potentially preventable with appropriate treatment.

Failure of individual organs in MOF often follows a predictable pattern: first respiratory failure; then hepatic, intestinal and renal; and finally cardiac failure.

Principles of Treatment of Sepsis Syndrome

These include:

- eradication of source of infection
- treatment of sepsis-associated metabolic, cardiovascular and multi-organ disturbances
- inhibition of toxic mediators, e.g. activated protein C is used.

Mortality is related to the number of organs that are failing:

- 1 organ: 70% survival
- 2 organs: 50% survival
- 4 organs: mortality approaches 100%.

Prognosis is affected by:

- older age
- previous compromise of organ function.

SURGICAL SEPSIS

The term 'sepsis' covers several purulent infections, which the surgeon may encounter in surgical practice.

Skin Infections

Boils, Styes and Carbuncles

- Definitions:
  - boil (furuncle): an infection of a hair follicle
  - stye (hordoleum): an infection in a hair follicle on an eyelid
  - carbuncle: a group of boils interconnected in the subcutaneous tissue by tracts.
- These infections are painful but not serious.
- Antibiotics are rarely indicated for boils and styes, but may be appropriate for carbuncles.
- Infection is usually due to *S. aureus*, which is usually an endogenous strain carried in the nose or skin.
- Boils may be recurrent, appearing in crops over several weeks or months.
- May be a presenting sign of diabetes.
- Antibiotic therapy is indicated only for certain cases, e.g. boils on the 'dangerous area' of the face where venous drainage is to the cavernous sinus and where cavernous sinus thrombosis may result; also in immunocompromised patients.

Erysipelas

- Spreading infection of the skin due to *S. pyogenes*.
- Presents as a raised, red, indurated area of skin which is sharply demarcated.
- Patient may present with high fever and may appear toxic.
- Rare condition at present; responds well to penicillin.

Cellulitis

This is the spread of infection of the subcutaneous tissue.

Acute Pyogenic Cellulitis

- Usually due to *S. pyogenes*.
- Presents as a red, painful swelling, usually of a limb, being commonly associated with lymphangitis and lymphadenitis.
- Likely to appear in a lymphoedematous limb.
- Treatment is with penicillin and/or clindamycin.

Anaerobic Cellulitis

- Rare.
- Usually due to anaerobes or clostridia, but more often is due to synergistic infection with both aerobes and anaerobes.

- Causative organisms are usually a combination of anaerobes (*Bacteroides*, clostridia, anaerobic cocci) and aerobes (coliform, *P. aeruginosa* and *S. pyogenes*).
- Clinically, redness and oedema present around a wound (surgical or traumatic).

Anaerobic cellulitis may progress in two ways:

- Bacterial gangrene:
  - skin becomes purple and ischaemic, and eventually undergoes necrosis
  - Fournier's gangrene of the scrotum and Meleney's gangrene are examples (see below).
- Necrotizing fasciitis:
  - in this condition the skin remains normal in the early stages while the infection spreads along fascial plains, causing extensive necrosis
  - later, the overlying skin becomes deprived of its blood supply, losing its sensation, eventually becoming purple-black and undergoing necrosis
  - necrotizing fasciitis is a life-threatening condition in which the patient is seriously ill with fever, toxaemia and occasionally septic shock
  - wide excision of the area of necrosis and infection is required, together with appropriate antibiotics
  - the mortality rate is high.

Fournier's Gangrene

- Rapidly progressive gangrene of scrotum of spontaneous onset.
- Elderly diabetics particularly prone, but may occur in otherwise healthy young men.
- Caused by synergy between faecal bacteria and anaerobes.

Meleney's Gangrene

- Occurs at site of abdominal surgery or at site of accidental abrasion of the skin.
- Originally attributed to synergy between a microaerophilic, non-haemolytic streptococcus and *S. aureus*; however, other bacteria may be involved.
- Best considered as infection caused by a combination of anaerobic and aerobic bacteria which forms a cellulitis followed by gangrene.

Fournier's gangrene and Meleney's gangrene probably have similar aetiological factors, and only the site of infection distinguishes the two.

Lymphangitis and Lymphadenitis

- Definitions:
  - lymphangitis: a non-suppurative infection of lymphatic vessels that drain an area of cellulitis
  - lymphadenitis: infection of the regional lymph nodes as a result of infection in an area which they drain.
- Lymphadenitis usually, but not always, results from cellulitis and lymphangitis.
- Occasionally the lymph nodes suppurate and form an abscess.
- Lymphangitis produces red, tender streaks along the lines of lymphatics extending from the area of cellulitis towards regional lymph nodes.
- Lymphadenitis is represented by enlarged, tender regional lymph nodes.
- Occasionally the overlying skin is red and the glands are fluctuant.
- Treatment of both lymphadenitis and lymphangitis depends on isolation of the appropriate infecting organism.

Gas Gangrene

- Rare disease in peacetime, but closely associated with grossly contaminated wounds due to war injuries.
- Clostridial spores are widely distributed in the environment.
- May enter traumatic or surgical wounds.
- Contamination may also occur from the patient's own faecal flora (*C. perfringens* is a normal bowel inhabitant).
- May occur after elective surgery, e.g. GI tract, lower limb amputation, vascular surgery on ischaemic limb.
- In case of trauma it is due to contamination of wounds by dirt and soil containing clostridia derived from animal faeces.
- Infection favoured by extensive wounds with presence of necrotic tissue, which provide an anaerobic environment for clostridia to proliferate.
- Anaerobic environment initiates conversion of spores to vegetative, toxin-producing pathogens.
- Clostridia proliferate and produce toxins that diffuse into surrounding tissue.
- Toxins destroy local microcirculation.
- This allows further invasion, which can advance extremely rapidly.
- Alpha toxin of *C. perfringens* kills muscle cells and destroys fat.
- Gas formation occurs.
- As disease advances, toxins are released into systemic circulation.

Clinical features

- Patients are generally toxic and unwell.
- Exhibit pallor, restlessness, delirium, tachycardia, jaundice, and ultimately septic shock and death.
- Local signs of gas gangrene include:
  - myositis or myonecrosis
  - gas formation with palpable crepitus
  - mottled discoloration of overlying skin.

- Plain X-ray shows gas in subcutaneous tissue and fascial plains.

Diagnosis

- Clinical features.
- Specimens of exudate and tissue for Gram staining when typical Gram-positive bacilli are seen.

Treatment

- Adequate resuscitation.
- Debridement or amputation should be considered to remove all affected tissue or limb.
- Organisms are usually sensitive to penicillin.
- Hyperbaric oxygen may be helpful.

Prevention

- Benzylpenicillin antibiotic prophylaxis in those with:
  - contaminated wounds
  - amputations
  - diabetics undergoing elective peripheral vascular surgery.

Tetanus

- Rare condition in UK: <100 cases reported each year.
- Caused by *C. tetani*, an anaerobic Gram-positive bacillus, which produces a neurotoxin.
- Found in soil and faeces.
- Neurotoxin enters peripheral nerves and travels to spinal cord, where it blocks inhibitory activity of spinal reflexes.
- Disease follows the implantation of spores into deep, devitalized tissues.

Clinical features

- Neurotoxic blockade of inhibitory activity of spinal reflexes results in characteristic features of disease.
- Facial muscle spasm produces trismus.
- Typical facial appearance, i.e. risus sardonicus (lockjaw).
- Spasm in back muscles produces opisthotonos (arching of the neck and back due to spasm).
- Stiffness in the neck, back and abdomen follows, together with generalized spasm, which may cause asphyxia.
- Muscles remain in spasm between convulsions.
- Death may also occur from inhalation of vomit with aspiration pneumonia.

Diagnosis

- Diagnosis is usually clinical.
- Attempts at bacteriological confirmation often fail.

Prevention

- Tetanus is rare because of active immunization programmes in childhood with tetanus toxoid.
- All children should be immunized; this is carried out at 2, 3 and 4 months; preschool; and between 13 and 18 years of age.
- After the 5th dose, immunity remains for life and further boosters are not required.

Treatment

Preventative.

- Patients attending A&E with new trauma, however mild, should have a booster dose of tetanus toxoid if they have not had a full course.
- Contaminated and penetrated wounds should be debrided.
- Prophylactic penicillin should be administered.
- Those with contaminated wounds should be given human antitetanus immunoglobulin.

Treatment in suspected case

- Passive immunization with antitetanus immunoglobulin.
- Adequate wound debridement.
- Intravenous benzylpenicillin.
- Intensive care support.
- Despite the supportive measures, mortality is about 50%.

Abscesses

- A localized collection of pus.
- Walled off by a barrier inflammatory reaction (pyogenic membrane). Fibrosis occurs, 'encapsulating' the abscess.
- Therefore, impossible to treat abscesses satisfactorily with antibiotics alone.
- Surgical drainage is necessary.
- Without treatment abscesses tend to 'point' spontaneously to the nearest epithelial surface, e.g.:
  - skin (boil)
  - gut (pelvic abscess to rectum)
  - bronchus (lung abscess).
- Spontaneous drainage often leads to healing, provided the initiating stimulus has been eliminated.
- If spontaneous drainage does not eliminate the initiating stimulus, a chronic abscess forms, often resulting in a continuously discharging sinus which intermittently develops, discharges and heals, e.g. stitch abscess and stitch sinus which does not settle until the stitch is removed.
- Treatment of abscesses inappropriately with antibiotics alone may halt expansion of the abscess and sterilize the pus, giving rise to a sterile abscess or 'antibioma'.
- Pyogenic abscesses are caused by a wide variety of bacteria and occur at many different sites (Table 21.1).
- Abscesses do not necessarily form at the site of primary infection, but may form at a distant site, e.g. pelvic or subphrenic abscesses after perforated appendicitis.
- 'Metastatic' abscesses may form as a result of haematogenous spread or 'pyaemic' spread of infected thrombi, e.g. portal pyaemia following appendicitis may result in liver abscesses; infective endocarditis may result in cerebral abscesses.

TABLE 21.1 Common Sites of Abscesses

Site	Source of Infection	Organism
Skin (boil)	Hair follicle	*Staphylococcus aureus*
Breast	Breast feeding	*S. aureus*
Pelvic	Abdominal or pelvic sepsis, e.g. salpingitis, appendicitis	Coliforms, *Bacteroides*, *Streptococcus faecalis*
Subphrenic	Abdominal or pelvic sepsis, e.g. peritonitis	Coliforms, *Bacteroides*, *S. faecalis*
Tubo-ovarian	Pelvic sepsis, gonorrhoea	Genital flora, *Neisseria gonorrhoeae*
Ischio-rectal	Spread from perianal glands	Coliforms
Perinephric	Acute pyelonephritis	Coliforms
Hepatic	Cholangitis, portal pyaemia	Coliforms
Lung	Aspiration pneumonia, bronchiectasis, bronchial obstruction, *S. aureus* pneumonia	*Streptococcus pneumoniae*, anaerobes, *S. aureus*
Cerebral	Haematogenous, e.g. bronchiectasis, infective endocarditis, sinusitis, otitis media	Streptococci, *S. aureus*, *Bacteroides*

SURGICAL SITE INFECTION (SSI)

Bacteria enter a wound by one or more of the following ways:

- airborne bacteria-laden particles
- direct inoculation from surgical equipment and operating theatre personnel
- from the patient's skin
- from the flora of the patient's internal viscera (e.g. large bowel, biliary tract)
- blood-borne.

Important factors in the prevention of SSIs include:

- operating environment
- minimizing infection from operating theatre personnel
- skin preparation (see below)
- sterilization of surgical instruments and other equipment (see below)
- prophylactic antibiotics (see below)
- surgical technique (the reader is referred to a textbook of surgery).

Operating Environment

Factors influencing airborne operating theatre infection rates include:

- concentration of organisms in the air
- size of bacteria-laden particles
- duration of exposure of an operating wound.

The first two of these are influenced by theatre design and air flow, the third by avoiding unnecessarily long procedures.

Theatre Layout

There are four main zones:

- Protective 'outer' zone:
  - reception and waiting areas connected to the main hospital
  - changing rooms.
- Clean 'inner' zone:
  - used to transfer from protective to sterile zone
  - personnel should wear clean scrub suits and surgical footwear
  - consists of clean corridor, anaesthetic room, scrub room, exit bay, staff room, storage area for equipment and supplies.
- Sterile 'theatre' zone:
  - preparation room
  - operating room
  - scrubbed and gowned personnel
  - minimum essential staff only.
- Disposal zone:
  - disposal area
  - sluice
  - connects with disposal corridor.

Air Flow in Theatre

- Maintain positive pressure.
- Maintain at least 15 air changes per hour, at least 3 of which are fresh air.
- Filter all air. Most theatres use high-efficiency particulate air (HEPA) filters that help minimize airborne spread of bacteria and small particles (down to 0.3 micron), e.g. skin particles shed by staff.

- Introduce air at ceiling level and exhaust near floor. To help with outward flow of air, the operating room is cooler than the corridors – the warmer corridor air rises, with the cooler theatre air replacing it.
- Consider ultra-clean air for orthopaedic implant surgery. Ultra-clean air delivery systems are used for joint replacement surgery. Laminar air flow systems can reduce infection rates up to fourfold. A strong downward flow of air from above the operating table sweeps particles away from the operating site and into return ducts below.
- Enclosure of the patient in a sterile tent (Charnley tent) in which surgeons wear a space-type suit (body exhaust suit) can reduce infection rates by up to a further 5%.
- Keep theatre doors closed as far as possible.
- Limit staff in theatre to essential personnel. Movement of excess personnel increases infection risk.

Minimizing Infection from Operating Theatre Personnel

- Wear a mask that fully covers the mouth and nose throughout the operation.
- Wear a cap or hood to cover hair on head and face.
- Wear sterile gloves, if a member of the scrub team.
- Use gowns and drapes that resist liquid penetration.
- Change scrub suits when visibly soiled.

For further information on SSIs and their prevention, the reader is referred to NICE clinical guideline 74, *Surgical site infection* (October 2008, reviewed 2014).

PREVENTION OF INFECTION

Principles of Asepsis and Antisepsis

- Definitions:
  - asepsis: the exclusion of organisms from tissues
  - antisepsis: the attempt to prevent growth and multiplication of the microorganisms that cause sepsis.

Risk Factors Contributing to Sepsis

These are shown in Box 21.2

BOX 21.2 Risk Factors Contributing to Sepsis

Patient-related
Age
Diabetes
Intercurrent illness, e.g. cardiac, respiratory, renal
Immunosuppression
Nutritional status
Obesity

Injury- or disease-related
Location
Extent

Treatment-related
Length of preoperative stay
Duration of surgery
Emergency vs elective surgery
Poor surgical technique

Environment-related
Contamination
Superinfection
Long-term stay on ITU

Wound Infection

Classification of Wounds

Wounds may be classified by their potential for infection:

- Clean wound: an operation carried out through clean, non-infected skin under sterile conditions, where the GI tract, genitourinary (GU) tract or respiratory tract are not breached, e.g. hernia repair, varicose vein surgery; risk of wound infection should be <2%.
- Clean contaminated wounds: an operation carried out under sterile conditions with breaching of a hollow viscus other than the colon, where contamination is minimal, e.g. cholecystectomy, hysterectomy; the risk of wound infection should be <8%.
- Contaminated wound: an operation carried out where contamination has occurred, e.g. by opening the colon, an open fracture, or animal or human bites; the risk of wound infection is around 15%.
- Dirty wounds: an operation carried out in the presence of pus or a perforated viscus, e.g. perforated diverticulitis, faecal peritonitis; the risk of wound infection is >25%.

Factors Influencing the Development of Wound Sepsis

These are shown in Box 21.3.

Preoperative Skin Preparation

Skin Shaving

- Makes surgery, suturing and dressing removal easier.
- Wound infection rate lowest when performed immediately prior to surgery.
- Infection rate increased if performed more than 12 h prior to surgery.
- Abrasions or lacerations caused by shaving can become colonized with skin organisms and increase risk of wound infection.
- Clippers or depilatory creams may reduce infection rates to less than 1%.

Skin Preparation

- Alcohol:

BOX 21.3 Factors Influencing the Development of Wound Sepsis

Type of surgery
Clean or contaminated
Prosthesis or foreign body
Drain
Duration of surgery
'Place' on list

Surgical team
Skill of surgeon
Aseptic technique
Carriage of *Staphylococcus aureus*

Age and general condition of patient

Precautions taken against possibility of infection
Preoperative duration of stay
Adequate antisepsis of hands
Adequate skin preparation
Preparation of bowel
Antibiotic prophylaxis
Adequate ventilation

Ward factors postoperatively

- acts by denaturing proteins
- broadest spectrum at 70% concentration
- effective against Gram-positive and Gram-negative organisms
- some antiviral activity
- relatively inactive against spores and fungi
- inflammable, especially if pooling, therefore ensure dryness before using diathermy
- may irritate sensitive areas, e.g. genitalia.

- Chlorhexidine:
  - quaternary ammonium compound
  - causes bacterial cell wall disruption
  - bactericidal
  - more effective against Gram-positive organisms
  - moderate activity against Gram-negative bacteria
  - has long duration of action (up to 6 h)
  - non-toxic to skin and mucous membranes in aqueous solution
  - used in local antisepsis as 0.5% solution
  - used as surgical scrub in 4% solution in detergent (Hibiscrub)
  - chlorhexidine–cetrimide mixture (Savlon) is used for contaminated wounds
  - 0.5% chlorhexidine in 70% alcohol is used for local antisepsis; much more effective than aqueous preparations but risk of fire with diathermy.
- Povidone–iodine:
  - broad-spectrum against bacteria, spores, fungi, viruses (hepatitis B and HIV)
  - bactericidal
  - rapidly inactivated by organic material such as blood, faeces, pus
  - patient and operating staff skin sensitivity is occasionally a problem
  - stains skin and fabrics
  - used for preoperative skin disinfection
  - used for wound antisepsis
  - used as surgical scrub.

Occlusive adhesive drapes

- No evidence that they reduce infection rate.
- May trap bacteria under drape, increasing skin bacterial count during surgery.

DISINFECTION

This is a process used to reduce the number of viable microorganisms. It fails to inactivate some bacterial spores and some viruses. Disinfection has to be distinguished from cleaning, which is a process that physically removes contamination but does not necessarily inactivate microorganisms.

Efficacy

Depends on several factors:

- length of exposure
- presence of blood, faeces, or other organic matter, which may reduce the efficacy of the disinfection process.

Examples of Disinfectants

- Hypochlorite (Milton, Eusol):
  - wide antibacterial spectrum, also viruses
  - inactivated by organic matter.
- Povidone–iodine (Betadine): see under 'Skin preparation' earlier.
- Chlorhexidine: see under 'Skin preparation' earlier.
- Alcohols: see under 'Skin preparation' earlier.
- Quaternary ammonium salts (cetrimide):
  - active against Gram-positive bacteria
  - no action against *Pseudomonas*
  - weak disinfectant.
- Formaldehyde:
  - wide antibacterial spectrum, including spores
  - hazardous substance
  - irritant to eyes, respiratory tract and skin
  - aqueous 10% formaldehyde can be used to disinfect contaminated surfaces
  - if used as gas, needs to be in air-tight cabinet.
- Glutaraldehyde:
  - wide antibacterial spectrum; also viruses

- kills spores slowly
- penetration is poor
- irritant and may cause hypersensitivity.
- Boiling water:
  - efficient disinfection process
  - kills bacteria including TB; some viruses including HBV and HIV; and some spores
  - items for disinfection must be thoroughly cleaned and totally immersed in boiling water
  - suitable for proctoscopes and rigid sigmoidoscopes.
- Pasteurization:
  - used for foodstuffs such as milk
  - milk is held at 63–66°C for 30 min
  - All non-spore-forming pathogenic bacteria, including *Mycobacterium tuberculosis, Brucella, Campylobacter and Salmonella*, are killed.

STERILIZATION

- This is the complete destruction of all viable microorganisms, including spores, cysts and viruses.
- May be used for inanimate objects only.

Physical

Heat

Moist heat (autoclave)

- Steam under pressure attains a higher temperature than boiling water, the final temperature being directly related to pressure.
- Sterilization by steam under pressure is the most commonly used method in hospitals.
- Carried out in an autoclave where steam is heated to 121°C.
- Steam condenses on the surface of the instruments in the autoclave, giving up a large amount of latent heat of vaporization required for its production.
- Sterilizing cycle must be long enough to ensure adequate sterilization.
- Holding times depend on temperature and pressure, e.g. 121°C for 15 min at pressure of 15 lb/in^2; 134°C at 30 lb/in^2 for 3 min.
- Entire cycle is longer, allowing for heating up and cooling down time.
- Continuous recordings should be made of the temperature in the autoclave and all sterilizers should have a preset automatic cycle that cannot be interrupted until the cycle is completed.
- Monitoring of efficacy of sterilization is carried out by a Browne's tube placed among the instruments: a glass tube containing fluid that changes from red to green after appropriate exposure.
- Sterile packs can be identified as appropriately sterilized by changing colour of heat-sensitive inks on the pack (Bowie–Dick test).
- Bacteria, fungi, spores and viruses are destroyed.
- Prions are difficult to destroy and will need longer times.
- Moist heat is more effective than dry heat because it penetrates materials better and denatures protein of the cell walls of microorganisms.

Dry heat

- The efficacy of dry heat depends on the initial moisture of the microbial cells.
- Dry heat at 160°C with 'hold-time' of 2 h will kill all microorganisms.
- Many articles will not withstand these high temperatures.
- Unsuitable for materials that are denatured or damaged at required temperature, e.g. plastics.
- Not suitable for aqueous fluids, e.g. i.v. fluids.
- Suitable for solids, non-aqueous liquids, and to sterilize objects that will stand the heat in enclosed (airtight) containers.
- All items must be thoroughly cleaned and dried before placing in hot-air ovens.

Irradiation

- Sterilization by ionizing radiation is an industrial process.
- Used commercially for large batches of suitable objects.
- Heat-labile articles and single-use items, e.g. catheters, syringes, i.v. lines.

Filtration

- Bacteria and spores may be removed from heat-labile solutions by filtration.
- Efficiency of sterilization determined by pore size.
- Used by pharmaceutical industry for sterilization of drugs for injection.

Chemicals

Ethylene oxide

- Highly penetrative agent.
- Active against vegetative bacteria, spores and viruses.
- Highly explosive and used under strictly controlled conditions.
- Used to sterilize heat-labile articles.
- Ideal for electrical equipment, fibre-optic endoscopes, sterilization of single-use items, e.g. dialysis lines (not condoned, but necessitated by financial expediency in some countries).
- Penetrates well into rubber and plastics.
- Toxic, irritant, mutagenic and possibly carcinogenic.

Glutaraldehyde

- Immersion in 2% glutaraldehyde used to sterilize endoscopes and other instruments containing plastic or rubber.
- Inactivation of microbes varies and different times are required, e.g. 60 min for TB.
- Exposure of at least 3 h kills all microbes.
- Toxic: may cause irritation to skin, eyes and lungs.

Formaldehyde

- Dry, saturated steam in combination with formaldehyde kills vegetative bacteria, spores and most viruses.
- Used for heat-labile instruments, e.g. cystoscopes, as sterilization can be achieved at low temperature, i.e. 73°C for 2 h.
- Items contaminated with body fluids are excluded as proteins will be fixed and deposited on the equipment.

MODERN ANTIBIOTIC USAGE

Commonly Used Antibiotics

This section deals with antibiotics, particularly their use in the surgical patient.

Penicillins

Benzylpenicillin

- Active against streptococci, pneumococci, clostridia, *N. gonorrhoeae* and *N. meningitidis*.
- Few staphylococci are now sensitive.
- Main surgical indications:
  - prophylaxis of gas gangrene
  - prophylaxis of tetanus
  - streptococcal wound infections.
- May be given parenterally either i.v. or i.m.

Phenoxymethylpenicillin (penicillin V)

- Administered orally.
- May follow a course of intravenous benzylpenicillin to complete a course of treatment.
- Used prophylactically following splenectomy to prevent pneumococcal septicaemia, especially in children.
- May be used for prophylaxis in patients with rheumatic heart disease.

Flucloxacillin

- Indicated for penicillinase-resistant *S. aureus*.
- Used as adjunct to drainage of abscesses, especially in diabetics or immunosuppressed patients.
- Administered either orally, i.m. or i.v.

Amoxicillin and ampicillin

- Usually given for chest infections and some UTIs.
- Many staphylococci and coliforms produce β-lactamase and are therefore resistant.
- Amoxicillin and ampicillin are active against enterococci and many *H. influenzae* strains.
- May be administered either orally, i.m. or i.v.

Co-amoxiclav (Augmentin)

- Contains amoxicillin and potassium clavulanate.
- Clavulanate is inhibitory to β-lactamase and extends the spectrum of amoxicillin.
- Active against coliforms, staphylococci and *Bacteroides*.
- Often a first choice in animal and human bite injuries due to broad cover.
- Useful in surgery as prophylaxis in bowel, hepatobiliary and GU surgery.
- Useful as prophylaxis when prosthetics are being implanted.
- May be administered either orally or i.v.

Piperacillin (Tazocin)

- Only now available in combination with tazobactam – a β-lactamase inhibitor.
- Active against *Bacteroides*, coliforms, *Klebsiella* and *P. aeruginosa*.
- Often used in combination with an aminoglycoside for life-threatening infections.

Precautions when administering penicillins

- Check for previous allergy.
- Exercise caution in asthmatics and others with history of allergic conditions.
- Hypersensitivity reactions usually manifested by urticarial rash, although anaphylaxis may occur.
- Cross-allergy between different penicillins.
- About 10% of patients who are allergic to penicillin are also allergic to cephalosporins.
- Most penicillins are relatively non-toxic; therefore large doses may be given.
- Caution must be exercised in patients with renal and/or cardiac failure as injectable forms contain potassium and sodium salts.
- Convulsions may occur in rare cases after giving high doses i.v. or following intrathecal injection.

Cephalosporins

Cefradine and cefalexin

- First-generation cephalosporins.
- Active against a wide range of Gram-positive and Gram-negative organisms, including some *E. coli, Klebsiella, Proteus* and *S. aureus* (unless meticillin-resistant).
- Not active against enterococci, *P. aeruginosa* or many anaerobes.
- Useful as a second-line drug for treatment of infections of the urinary tract, respiratory tract, skin and soft tissue.
- Most commonly used orally.

Cefuroxime

- Second-generation cephalosporin.
- Broad-spectrum antibiotic against Gram-positive and Gram-negative organisms.

- Not active against *Pseudomonas* or many anaerobes.
- Widely used in prophylaxis, especially in combination with metronidazole in colorectal and biliary surgery.
- May be given orally, i.m. or i.v.

Cefotaxime and ceftazidime

- Third-generation cephalosporins.
- Broad-spectrum similar to second-generation drugs but ceftazidime is also active against *Pseudomonas*.
- Normally reserved for serious sepsis due to susceptible aerobic Gram-negative bacilli.
- Cefotaxime is used to treat meningitis.
- May be administered i.m. or i.v.

Precautions when administering cephalosporins

- <10% of patients who are penicillin-allergic are also allergic to cephalosporins.
- Rashes and fevers may occur.
- In patients with renal failure, dose reduction is required.
- Mild transient rises in liver enzymes may occur.

Sulfonamides and Trimethoprim

Co-trimoxazole (sulfamethoxazole + trimethoprim)

- Used for treatment of UTIs and respiratory infections.
- Active against Gram-positive and Gram-negative organisms.
- *Pseudomonas aeruginosa* is resistant.
- May be used for *Pneumocystis* pneumonia.
- Nausea, vomiting, rashes and mouth ulcers may occur.
- Leucopenia and thrombocytopenia occur rarely.
- May be given orally or i.v.

Trimethoprim

- Used for UTIs and respiratory infections.
- Should be avoided in pregnancy.
- Nausea, vomiting, rashes, stomatitis and marrow suppression may occur.
- Potentiates the action of warfarin and phenytoin.
- May be administered orally or by slow i.v. infusion.

Macrolides

Erythromycin and clarithromycin

- Use in surgical patients limited.
- Usually a second-line drug in patients with penicillin allergy.
- Active against streptococci, staphylococci, clostridia and *Campylobacter*.
- Used for infections of skin, soft tissue and respiratory tract.
- Valuable in atypical pneumonia, legionnaires' disease and *Campylobacter*.
- Chief side-effect when given orally is diarrhoea.
- Chief side-effect for erthyromycin when given i.v. is phlebitis at the site of infusion.
- May potentiate warfarin and ciclosporin.
- Usually administered orally or i.v. by slow infusion.

Aminoglycosides

These are first-choice drugs for severe Gram-negative infections usually given in combination with a β-lactamase antibiotic.

Gentamicin

- Active against coliforms, *P. aeruginosa* and staphylococci.
- Streptococci and anaerobes are resistant.
- Usually given i.v. but can be given i.m.

Amikacin

- Reserved for life-threatening infections with gentamicin-resistant organisms with proven amikacin sensitivity.

Precautions when administering aminoglycosides

- Chief side-effects of aminoglycosides are ototoxicity (vertigo or deafness) and nephrotoxicity.
- Therapeutic levels depend on renal function.
- Serum levels must be monitored.

Quinolones

Ciprofloxacin

- Broad-spectrum antibiotic against Gram-negative bacteria, including *P. aeruginosa* and staphylococci.
- Many anaerobes are resistant.
- Used in UTIs, especially those that are catheter-related, prostatitis, skin and soft tissue infections with *P. aeruginosa*.
- Used also for chest infections, particularly those with Gram-negative organisms.
- Side-effects include nausea, diarrhoea and vomiting.
- CNS side-effects include anxiety, nervousness, insomnia and rarely convulsions.
- Ciprofloxacin potentiates warfarin.
- Promotes colonization, infection and cross-infection with MRSA and *Clostridium difficile*.
- Usually given orally or i.v.

Other Antibiotics and Microbials

Metronidazole

- Widely used in surgery, both prophylactically and therapeutically.
- Active against anaerobic bacteria, e.g. *Bacteroides* and clostridia.
- Also active against protozoal organisms, *Entamoeba histolytica* and *Giardia lamblia*.
- Used for intraperitoneal sepsis and gynaecological sepsis.
- Used prophylactically in appendicitis and colorectal surgery to prevent wound infection.
- Used for giardiasis, intestinal amoebiasis and amoebic liver abscess.
- Side-effects include anorexia, sore tongue, unpleasant metallic tastes and alcohol intolerance.
- Potentiates warfarin.
- May be given orally, i.v. or rectally.

Tetracycline and doxycycline

- Limited use in surgery.
- May be used in chronic bronchitis, non-specific urethritis and atypical pneumonia.

Fusidic acid

- Used for serious staphylococcal infections in combination with other agents.
- Tissue concentrations are good.
- May be administered orally or i.v. (i.v. route can cause cholestatic jaundice).

Vancomycin

- Active against staphylococci (including meticillin-resistant strains), streptococci and clostridia.
- Used for severe infections and intraperitoneal administration in CAPD peritonitis.
- Side-effects include 'red man syndrome' when given i.v., ototoxicity and nephrotoxicity.
- Serum levels must be monitored to control dosage.
- May be administered orally, i.v. or intraperitoneally diluted in continuous ambulatory peritoneal dialysis (CAPD) fluid.

Teicoplanin

- Bactericidal glycopeptide active against both aerobic and anaerobic Gram-positive bacteria.
- Active against *S. aureus* and coagulase-positive staphylococci (sensitive or resistant to meticillin), streptococci, enterococci, *Listeria monocytogenes*, micrococci and Gram-positive anaerobes including *C. difficile*.
- Teicoplanin is chemically related to vancomycin, with similar activity and toxicity.
- It is usually administered i.v. or may be given i.m.

Carbapenems

- Parenteral β-lactams – meropenem, imipenem and ertapenem.
- Not destroyed by most current β-lactamases, including extended-spectrum β-lactamases (ESBLs).
- Very broad spectrum – Gram-negatives, anaerobes and Gram-positives, except for MRSA.
- Drugs of last resort; should be used very sparingly.
- Resistance of Gram-negatives to carbapenems now appearing worldwide and emergence of multi-resistant carbapenemase-producing organisms (CPOs).

Clindamycin

- A lincosamide antibiotic.
- Effective against Gram-positive bacteria and anaerobes.
- Ineffective against Gram-negative bacteria.
- Used in skin and soft tissue infections where penicillin is not an option or severe streptococcal cellulitis, including necrotizing infections.
- Very good oral bioavailability.
- It can be taken during pregnancy and breastfeeding.

Antibiotics in Surgery

- Antibiotics are never a substitute for sound surgical technique.
- Dead tissue and slough need removing.
- Antibiotics should be used carefully and only with positive indication.
- Prolonged or inappropriate use of antibiotics may encourage emergence of resistant strains.
- Except in straightforward cases, advice should be sought from a microbiologist before prescribing.

Principles of Antibiotic Therapy

Selection of antibiotic

The following sequence of events is usually appropriate in selection of an antibiotic.

- A decision is made on clinical grounds that an infection exists.
- Based on signs, symptoms and clinical experience, a 'best guess' is made at the likely infecting organism.
- The appropriate specimens are taken for microbiological examination, i.e. culture and sensitivity.
- The safest and most effective drug or combination of drugs effective against the suspected organism is given.
- The clinical response to treatment is monitored.
- The antibiotic treatment is altered, if necessary, in response to laboratory reports of culture, and sensitivity and clinical progress.
- Occasionally the response of the infection to an apparently appropriate antibiotic is poor. Possible causes for this include:
  - failure to drain pus, excise necrotic tissue or remove foreign bodies
  - failure of the drug to reach the tissues in therapeutic concentration, e.g. ischaemic limb
  - the organism isolated is not the one responsible for the infection
  - after prolonged antibiotic therapy, new organisms cause infection
  - inadequate dosage
  - inappropriate route of administration.

Treatment with a combination of antibiotics

- A combination of antibiotics may be appropriate in the following circumstances:
  - as a temporary measure during the investigation of unknown illness
  - to achieve a synergistic effect
  - to prevent the development of bacterial resistance
  - to treat mixed infections
  - to allow reduction in dosage of a potentially toxic drug.
- Use of a bactericidal and a bacteriostatic drug together may be antagonistic.

- Two bacteriostatic drugs used in combination may be simply additive.
- The use of two bactericidal drugs in combination may achieve a synergistic effect.

Route of administration

- In severe illnesses antibiotics should be administered i.v.
- Some antibiotics can only be given by the parenteral route, e.g. gentamicin.
- Following GI surgery, antibiotics are best given parenterally until GI function resumes.
- It is best to avoid the i.m. route as it is uncomfortable for the patient and in shocked patients absorption would be inadequate.

Duration of therapy

- Depends on the individual's response and laboratory investigations.
- Duration will depend on the site and infecting organism, and should be as short as possible.
- A clinical cure is the most appropriate response, but this should be taken in conjunction with microbiological data.

Dosage

- Dosage may need to be modified in renal and hepatic disease.
- In renal failure, the dosage of drugs eliminated by the kidney may require major adjustment, e.g. aminoglycosides or vancomycin.

Penetration of tissue

- The drug must penetrate to the site of infection, e.g. in meningitis the antibiotic must pass into the cerebrospinal fluid (CSF).
- Deep abscesses are a particular problem and an important cause of antibiotic failure.
- An antibiotic cannot penetrate through the wall of an abscess to a collection of pus, but may allow healing around the pus and may create an 'antibioma'.
- The importance of draining pus cannot be overemphasized.

Hypersensitivity

- Most often due to penicillins.
- May manifest by the development of a rash, but may also manifest in the form of life-threatening anaphylaxis.
- A clear history of antibiotic sensitivities must be sought.

Drug toxicity

- Some antibiotics are toxic: e.g. ototoxicity and nephrotoxicity with aminoglycosides; bone marrow depression with chloramphenicol.

Superinfection

- Superinfection may occur with antibiotic-resistant microorganisms, e.g. yeasts.
- Most commonly occurs in immunosuppressed patients.
- Antibiotic-associated pseudomembranous colitis may occur in any patients taking antibiotics (β-lactamase antibiotics are most often involved).

Prophylactic Antibiotics

Indications include:

- implantation of foreign bodies, e.g. cardiac prosthetic valves, artificial joints, prosthetic vascular grafts
- amputation, especially for ischaemia or crush injuries where there is dead muscle. The risk of gas gangrene is high, especially in a contaminated wound; penicillin is the antibiotic of choice
- patients with diabetes
- immunosuppressed patients
- organ transplantation
- compound fractures and penetrating wounds
- surgical incisions where there is a high risk of bacterial contamination, i.e. clean contaminated wounds or frankly contaminated wounds (e.g. bowel preparation for colonic surgery)
- patients with certain forms of pre-existing cardiac disease are no longer routinely offered antibiotic prophylaxis for defined interventional procedures. Any benefit from prophylactic antibiotics needs to be weighed against the risks of adverse effects for the patients and the development of antibiotic resistance. The reader is referred to NICE clinical guideline 64, *Prophylaxis against infective endocarditis* (March 2008).

Indications for prophylactic antibiotics are shown in Table 21.2, though local guidance will vary.

Antibiotic Resistance

This may be either:

- Intrinsic (innate): occurs when the organism lacks the target site for the agent or is impermeable to the antibiotic.
- Acquired: refers to organisms that were previously susceptible to the agent in question.

Acquiring Resistance

Resistance may be acquired in several ways:

- Altered target site: results in lower affinity for antibiotic.
- Altered uptake: involves decreasing the amount of drug reaching the target by either decreasing permeability or by actively pumping the drug out of the cell.
- Antibiotic-inactivating enzymes, e.g.
  - β-lactamase against penicillins
  - aminoglycoside-modifying enzymes
  - chloramphenicol acetyl transferases.

Spreading Resistance

Resistance may spread between bacteria in three genetic ways:

- chromosomal mutation causing an altered protein

TABLE 21.2 Typical Prophylactic Antibiotic Regimens

Clinical Situation	Likely Organism(s)	Prophylactic Regimen
Appendicectomy	Anaerobes	Metronidazole (single dose per rectum 1 h preop.)
Biliary tract surgery	Coliforms	Co-amoxiclav (i.v. immediately preop. and for 24 h postop.)
Colorectal surgery	Coliforms, anaerobes	Co-amoxiclav (i.v. immediately preop. and for up to 48 h postop.) or metronidazole + cephalosporin (i.v. immediately preop. and for up to 48 h postop.)
GU surgery Open surgery	Coliforms	Co-amoxiclav (1–2 doses i.v. preop.) or gentamicin (single i.v. dose immediately preop.). Cephalosporin (i.v. immediately preop. and for 24–48 h postop.) or gentamicin (single i.v. dose immediately preop.)
Insertion of prosthetic joints	*Staphylococcus aureus, Staphylococcus epidermidis*	Flucloxacillin (i.v. immediately preop. and for 24 h postop.)
Amputation of limb	*Clostridium perfringens*	Penicillin (i.v. immediately preop. and for 24 h postop.)
Vascular surgery with prosthetic	*S. aureus, S. epidermidis*, coliforms	Cephalosporin (i.v. immediately preop. and for 24 h postop.)
Prevention of tetanus in contaminated wound (+ immunoprophylaxis)	*Clostridium tetani*	Penicillin (i.v. or i.m. on presentation)
GU instrumentation	Coliforms	Co-amoxiclav + gentamicin (i.v. immediately preop.)

- genes on transmissible plasmids
- transposons.

Chromosomal mutation causing an altered protein

- Single mutation:
  - ribosomal protein (streptomycin resistance)
  - altered enzyme (sulfonamides).
- Series of mutations:
  - changes in penicillin-binding proteins in penicillin-resistant pneumococci.
- In the presence of antibiotic, spontaneous mutants survive and outgrow the susceptible population. They spread to other sites in the same patient or by cross-infection to other patients.

Genes on transmissible plasmids

- Transmissible plasmids (small circular DNA units) replicate independently of the chromosome and transfer between cells.
- Some plasmids cross the species barrier and the same resistant gene is therefore found in widely different species; e.g. TEM-1 – the most common plasmid-mediated β-lactamase in Gram-negative bacteria – also accounts for penicillin resistance in some *N. gonorrhoeae* and ampicillin resistance in *H. influenzae*.

Transposons

- Transposons, or 'jumping' genes, are capable of integration into the chromosomes or plasmids.
- Transposons jumping from chromosomes to plasmids allow chromosomal genes to be disseminated more rapidly.
- Can also move from plasmid to plasmid, again accelerating dissemination.

Predictable Sensitivity

After identification is made, the sensitivity pattern of an organism is often predictable. Predictability of sensitivity may change and will have local variations; hence, the need to discuss treatment with local microbiologists.

Examples of organisms and antibiotics for which sensitivity is usually predictable include:

- streptococci: penicillin, erythromycin, clindamycin, vancomycin
- staphylococci: flucloxacillin, clindamycin, fusidic acid, vancomycin
- *Escherichia coli*: gentamicin, co-amoxiclav, ciprofloxacin
- *Haemophilus influenzae*: co-amoxiclav, tetracycline
- *Bacteroides fragilis*: metronidazole, co-amoxiclav.

Examples of organisms and antibiotics for which resistance is usually predictable include:

- staphylococci: most penicillins (except meticillin)
- *Escherichia coli*: penicillin, vancomycin, metronidazole
- anaerobes: aminoglycosides.

Clinical Factors Leading to the Emergence of Resistant Strains

The unnecessary use, misuse and abuse of antibiotics have led to the development of antibiotic-resistant strains. The most common misuse and abuse of antibiotics include:

- inappropriate and indiscriminate use of antibiotics by medical practitioners
- prescribing of antibiotics for viral infections; increases susceptibility to developing resistant strains which can live and multiply unhindered
- use of prophylactic antibiotics where they are inappropriate, e.g. attempted prevention of infection of indwelling urinary catheters
- use of topical antibiotics.

When prescribing antibiotics, it is appropriate to:

- use a single agent
- use the narrowest spectrum appropriate for the likely organism
- use specific prophylaxis
- use the shortest effective course
- avoid topical agents – infections involving superficial structures are best treated systemically (except conjunctivitis); use on the skin may encourage resistant strains
- avoid fixed combinations of antibiotics
- critically read advertising literature that may lead to the erroneous belief that newer, broader-spectrum antibiotics are always better.

Surgery and Blood-Borne Viruses

The surgeon, and indeed any medical, nursing or paramedical personnel, is at risk from three main viral infections: hepatitis B (HBV), hepatitis C (HCV) and human immunodeficiency virus (HIV).

Hepatitis B

- Double-stranded DNA virus.
- Incubation period 6 weeks to 6 months.
- Period of infectivity is from 6 weeks before onset of symptoms and possibly indefinitely thereafter.
- 10% of infected adults become chronic carriers.
- Seen particularly in intravenous drug users (IVDUs); heterosexual men and women and homosexual men (men-who-have-sex-with-men [MSMs]) with multiple partners; renal dialysis patients; those born in high-endemicity areas (sub-Saharan Africa, Central and South East Asia) and their children; and occasionally healthcare workers.

Hepatitis B may be transmitted by:

- blood transfusion
- inoculation via sharps injuries from blood or blood products
- droplet transmission including saliva, semen and cervical secretions onto mucosal surfaces
- IVDUs sharing needles, syringes or other drug paraphernalia
- unprotected sexual intercourse with an infected partner (in particular MSM/bisexual)
- tattooing, body piercing, etc., with unsterile equipment.

Clinical presentation

- Asymptomatic infection (common)
- Acute hepatitis with clinical recovery and subsequent immunity (90–95%).
- Acute fulminating hepatitis with death (<1%).
- Chronic active hepatitis with risk of developing cirrhosis and hepatocellular carcinoma (80% are caused by HBV).

Serology

There are three viral antigens:

- HBsAg: hepatitis B surface antigen
- HBcAg: hepatitis B core antigen (not detectable in peripheral blood)
- HBeAg: hepatitis B 'e' antigen.

Following infection, antibodies are formed against all three viral antigens, but there are important clinical consequences of their identification:

- infected persons and carriers have HBsAg and anti-HBcAg, but lack anti-HBsAg (HBs antibody)
- the 'e' antigen is found only in HBsAg-positive sera and appears during the incubation period
- the presence of HBeAg implies high levels of circulating viral DNA and therefore high infectivity
- on recovery from infection, HBsAg disappears from the blood and anti-HBsAg becomes demonstrable together with anti-HBcAg (IgG anti-HBcAg) and anti-HBeAg
- presence of anti-HBsAg in isolation generally represents previous vaccination.

Surgeons who possess the 'e' antigen or high levels of HBV DNA may infect their patients during 'exposure-prone procedures' (EPPs). As effective treatment is available for HBV, all individuals with acute or chronic infection should be referred to local hepatitis services for further management following diagnosis.

Hepatitis C

- Single-stranded RNA virus.
- Incubation period 2 weeks to 6 months.
- UK prevalence of chronic HCV infection is 0.4%.
- Transmission by blood-borne route from viraemic carriers of infection.
- Routes of transmission:
  - IVDUs sharing needles, syringes and other paraphernalia; 20% seroconversion/year
  - recipients of blood transfusions before September 1991
  - recipients of pooled plasma products (including Factor VIII and immunoglobulin) manufactured prior to 1986
  - transplant recipients and haemodialysis patients, particularly if performed overseas
  - healthcare workers from occupational sharps injuries
  - vaccination, cultural rituals, tattooing and acupuncture with unsterile equipment
  - mother-to-child transmission (3–10% transmission at birth without intervention)
  - transmission by sexual contact may occur but is rare.

Clinical presentation

- Often asymptomatic.
- Only about 25% become symptomatic and jaundiced.
- Severity of symptoms does not necessarily equate to extent of liver disease.

Serology

- Antibody test used for screening.
- 15–40% of people infected with HCV will clear the virus in the acute stage but will remain antibody-positive.
- PCR to detect HCV RNA will identify if infection is still active.

Outcome

Of the 60–85% of patients who do not clear the virus in the acute stage (within 6 months from infection):

- some will never develop liver damage
- many will develop only moderate liver damage with or without symptoms
- 20% will progress to cirrhosis within 20 years
- of these, 25% will progress to end-stage liver disease (oesophageal varices, ascites and/or hepatic encephalopathy) or develop hepatocellular carcinoma.

Effective treatment is available for HCV infection using combination treatment with interferon-α and ribavirin. Patients newly diagnosed with HCV infection should be referred to a specialist hepatitis service for further assessment and management.

HIV

- Single-stranded RNA retrovirus.
- Produces DNA via the enzyme reverse transcriptase.
- DNA integrated into host cell genome (integrase).
- During replication, this proviral DNA is transcribed into mRNA and translated into viral proteins. These are cleaved into constituent parts by protease enzyme.
- These enzymes act as potential targets for antiretroviral therapy (ART).
- HIV infection results in widespread immunological dysfunction by replicating in and eventually exhausting CD4+ T-helper cells, macrophages and antigen presenting cells.
- Loss of immune function causes:
  - increased risk of infection (see below) and opportunistic infections
  - increased risk of cancer – all types (both HIV- and non-HIV associated)
  - patients infected with HIV also have higher rates of cardiovascular disease, endocrine abnormalities, renal dysfunction and osteoporosis.
- HIV may be transmitted by:
  - sexual intercourse (MSM and heterosexual – fastest rate of increase is among heterosexual white couples in UK)
  - blood transfusion
  - intravenous drug abuse and needlestick injuries
  - mother-to-child transmission (MTCT).
- The following are therefore at risk of becoming HIV positive:
  - anyone of any age who is sexually active
  - commercial sex workers (CSWs), both male and female
  - intravenous drug users (IVDUs)
  - haemophiliacs or recipients of blood products before routine testing of donated blood became available, i.e. October 1995
  - sexual partners of the above
  - children of infected mothers, particularly in high-endemicity areas.

Natural history

- During acute infection, rapid viral replication occurs.
- The patient may be asymptomatic for 4–8 weeks prior to the development of a 'seroconversion illness'.

- This is a flu-like or glandular fever-like illness with symptoms including fever, lymphadenopathy, pharyngitis and rash.
- Patients are highly infectious during this period and their CD4 cell count may fall sufficiently to allow the development of opportunistic infections.
- Subsequently an asymptomatic ('plateau') phase occurs; HIV antibodies are present, controlling viral replication; CD4 count low normal; may continue for many years.
- HIV often progresses within 5–10 years from infection.
- When CD4 count falls <350 cells/mm^3, treatment should be initiated (current recommendations).
- When CD4 count falls <200 cells/mm^3, risk of developing opportunistic infection and HIV-associated malignancy increases.
- These used to be termed AIDS-defining conditions, and are important indicators of underlying potential HIV infection (see below).
- Without treatment, net median survival time in developed countries is 9–11 years.

HIV tests

- HIV antibody tests will be negative until seroconversion occurs (the window period).
- Modern 4th-generation tests look for both antibody and antigen (the p24 antigen) to shorten this to about 4 weeks. If the patient is at 'on-going' risk then repeat testing should be performed.
- Only verbal consent is required to perform a routine HIV test, and can be obtained by any medical/surgical practitioner. Higher-risk patients should be counselled by those with training to do so (health advisors, ID/GU department).
- Measurement of CD4 count in those presenting with surgical complaints may be useful to determine risk of opportunistic infection/malignancy and (if relevant) treatment compliance.

HIV indicator diseases

HIV testing is **strongly** recommended when the following conditions are suspected (RCP Guidelines):

- Any unusual manifestation of bacterial, fungal or viral disease, i.e.
  - tuberculosis infection (any site including pulmonary)
  - suspected *Pneumocystis jirovecii* (formerly *carinii*) pneumonia
  - suspected cerebral toxoplasmosis
  - oral/oesophageal candidiasis
  - oral hairy leucoplakia
  - persistent genital ulceration
  - presence of blood-borne or sexually transmitted infection, e.g. syphilis, HBV
  - suspected primary seroconversion illness
  - also anyone with **recurrent** bacterial infections (see list below).
- Unusual tumours, i.e. cerebral lymphoma, non-Hodgkin's lymphoma or Kaposi's sarcoma.
- Unexplained thrombocytopenia or lymphopenia.
- Unusual skin problems, including severe seborrhoeic dermatitis, atypical psoriasis or extensive molluscum, and recurring shingles or shingles in a young person.
- Persistent lymphadenopathy or unexplained lymphoedema.
- Neurological problems including peripheral neuropathy or focal signs due to a space-occupying intracerebral lesion.
- Unexplained weight loss or diarrhoea, night sweats, or pyrexia of unknown origin.
- Any other unexplained ill health or diagnostic problem.

Sites of bacterial infection in those with underlying HIV infection may include:

- recurrent pneumonia
- boils, carbuncles, cellulitis
- anorectal abscesses
- empyema thoracis
- necrotizing fasciitis
- osteomyelitis
- septic arthritis
- epididymo-orchitis
- pelvic inflammatory disease.

Precautions in Hepatitis B, Hepatitis C and HIV Patients

Sources of infection are:

- contact: blood, urine, faeces, saliva, tears, CSF, etc.
- aerosol: use of power tools
- inoculation: sharps injuries – needlestick, scalpels.

Universal Precautions

This refers to those precautions taken to protect theatre staff from infection from every patient. They include:

- washing hands before and after contact with every patient and before putting on and after removing surgical gloves
- cover existing wounds and skin lesions
- avoid sharps use where possible
- avoid wearing open footwear
- clearing blood spillages promptly.

Special Precautions

These are used for all high-risk patients, e.g. hepatitis, HIV, or patients suspected of having these conditions:

- All personnel involved in patient care should be aware of the risk.
- Any patient considered a risk should be indicated as belonging to a high-risk category on the operating list (under no circumstances should the disease causing

the risk be placed on the operating list, for reasons of patient confidentiality).

- Arrangements should be made for contaminated fluid, dressings, etc., to be handled and disposed of correctly.
- Appropriate theatre techniques should be adopted:
  - minimize theatre staff: only essential personnel; no spectators
  - remove all but essential equipment
  - disposable drapes and gowns
  - double-gloving and use of 'indicator' glove systems
  - visors to prevent splashing in eyes
  - blunt suture needles
  - stapling devices rather than needles where possible
  - pass instruments in kidney dish
  - 'no-touch' technique
  - all disposable equipment should be removed in specifically marked containers
  - theatre should be thoroughly cleansed with dilute bleach solution at the end of the procedure.
- Recovery staff must also be aware of the risk.

These special precautions should also be used for other cases where spread of infection is possible, e.g. patients with MRSA.

Immunization

Immunization is available against hepatitis B but not hepatitis C or HIV.

Hepatitis B

Hepatitis B vaccine is offered to all high-risk staff, i.e. those performing exposure-prone procedures (EPPs). These include:

- surgeons
- theatre nurses and other operating department personnel
- pathology department staff
- A&E staff
- liver transplant unit staff
- GI unit staff
- workers in residential units for those with learning disabilities
- staff of infectious diseases units.

Dialysis units are often quoted as being 'high-risk' areas; however, following outbreaks of hepatitis B several years ago, all staff and patients of dialysis units are tested for HBsAg.

Management of Sharp Injuries

Immediately after the injury:

- let the site of injury bleed
- wash area with soap and water
- report the incident to supervisor/senior officer/occupational health **immediately**
- contact the occupational health department or nearest emergency department as soon as possible, according to local protocols.

Procedure at occupational health (OH) or emergency department:

- Take detailed information:
  - source patient risk factors for having a blood-borne virus (including IVDU, born in sub-Saharan Africa, etc.)
  - nature of the incident – type of injury and sharp involved (open-bore needle, probe, etc.)
  - HBV vaccination status of the exposed person
  - when the incident occurred.
- Explain transmission risks; risk is small.
- Depending on local protocol (your hospital will have its own), take serum/blood to store in case future testing required.
- If the source patient is known (i.e. the original use of the needle in needlestick injury), they should be asked to consent for testing for HIV, HBV and HCV. They should be counselled before the tests are done, by someone other than the person exposed.
- The person sustaining the 'sharps' injury should be advised about the risks of transmission until the test results are received. They should practise safe sex and not donate blood. They may continue operating and performing EPP. Follow-up testing **must** be performed as directed by the OH department, the timing of which will depend on the source patient's status. Generally, antibody tests to HBV, HCV and HIV are performed at 3 and 6 months, but additional testing for HCV RNA and/or HIV RNA may be required if the patient is known to be infectious.

Post-Exposure Prophylaxis

Hepatitis B

- OH or exposed person should be aware of their own HBV vaccine status, particularly if they have not responded to the initial immunization course ('non-responder').
- If the exposed person has responded to HB vaccine (documented anti-HBsAg >10 mIU/mL) then a booster dose may be given regardless of the source patient's status.
- If the exposed person has received two or more doses of HB vaccine, then the course is completed regardless of the source patient's status.
- If the exposed person has received one or no doses of HB vaccine or is a known 'non-responder' and a significant exposure from an HBsAg-positive source has occurred, then HB immunoglobulin will be required and an accelerated HB vaccine course may be initiated.
- Similar procedures should be followed when the source patient cannot be identified or refuses to be tested. Liaison with OH and a microbiology/virology consultant is mandatory.

Hepatitis C

- No vaccine or post-exposure prophylaxis is currently available.
- Risk of infection only if source patient is viraemic.

HIV

- Carry out tests after counselling at 3 months and 6 months.
- No vaccine available.
- Post-exposure prophylaxis (PEP) may be recommended depending on the nature of the injury and the risk of transmission (which is always low). Which drugs are used varies although commonly a combination of two NRTIs (nucleoside reverse transcriptase inhibitors, e.g. zidovudine, lamivudine) and a PI (protease inhibitor, e.g. lopinavir, ritonavir) are used.
- The decision on whether PEP is appropriate should be taken by someone experienced in HIV medicine as the drugs are always poorly tolerated, and specific counselling is needed. If the source patient has a drug-resistant virus (which is known about), then alternative agents may be used.

CJD and vCJD

- Two types of human prion protein (PrP) disease causing spongiform degeneration of the brain (transmissible spongiform encephalopathy).
- Creutzfeld–Jakob disease (CJD) is a progressive sporadic disease occurring over the age of 50.
- Variant CJD (vCJD) has been directly linked to BSE (bovine spongiform encephalopathy) in cattle and arises following the consumption of infected meat. It has a longer clinical course (years rather than months) and affects a younger age group (mean age is 25 years).
- No effective management exists and the conditions are usually fatal.
- Although no evidence exists for person-to-person spread by close contact, transmission may occur with specific surgical or medical treatment (iatrogenic).
- Hospitals have strict guidelines in place to prevent spread from those suspected or known to have the condition or from those with a greater than average risk, due either to their medical or family history, or from patients undergoing brain biopsy.
- Examples of precautions taken include:
  - including screening questions in preoperative checklists to determine risk
  - provision of single-use equipment for neurosurgical and endoscopic procedures
  - use of leucocyte-depleted blood in transfusions
  - appropriate disposal of waste and post-mortem material.

OSCE SCENARIOS

OSCE Scenario 21.1

A 37-year-old male attends A&E, complaining bitterly of pain in his left groin. On examination the skin appears red and cellulitic. He is in severe pain when it is touched, and he has a tachycardia of 133 beats/min and a temperature of 38.8°C.

1. Given the above information, what broad differential diagnoses are you considering?
2. What questions would you like to ask this patient to get a rapid idea of the diagnosis?
3. What investigations and management plan would you initiate?

The patient rapidly becomes haemodynamically unstable and a diagnosis of septic shock due to severe soft tissue infection is assumed. He is taken to theatre where extensive debridement of infected and necrotic tissue is performed along the fascial planes of his leg.

4. What are the diagnosis and prognosis, and which organisms are commonly associated with this condition?

OSCE Scenario 21.2

A 68-year-old male patient develops acute retention of urine after repair of a right inguinal hernia. An indwelling urethral catheter was inserted and he has now developed a urinary tract infection. He was started on appropriate broad-spectrum antibiotics and is now systemically much better. He has asked to speak to one of the surgical team as he is upset about developing a hospital-acquired infection (HAI).

1. Answer the patient's questions about HAI.

He is satisfied with your explanation and feels much happier now; however, he is worried about the possibility of getting an MRSA infection whilst he is in hospital, as he has read so much about it in the newspapers.

2. Explain what MRSA is, the different sources of infection and methods of spread.
3. Explain the methods employed in hospitals for prevention and control of HAI.

OSCE Scenario 21.3

A 31-year-old male patient who admits to regular intravenous drug use is admitted with cellulitis of his right groin, which began 48 h after repeated attempts to inject his femoral vessels. He saw his GP and was started on oral antibiotics but tells you the redness is increasing, although he is systemically well. On examination, the area is warm, pink and swollen but there is no evidence of abscess.

1. Which two bacterial species are the most likely to be the cause of this patient's infection?

Microbiology culture results of a wound swab taken by the patient's GP report that a resistant organism has been isolated.

2. Explain how organisms develop resistance to antimicrobials.

The antibiotics are changed, but as the erythema settles the patient develops a fluctuant area in the skin, consistent with an abscess. The patient is prepped for theatre.

3. What special considerations and precautions should be taken when operating on this patient?

OSCE Scenario 21.4

A 67-year-old male patient was admitted with perforated duodenal ulcer that necessitated laparotomy and repair. Postoperatively, he recovered on the high-dependency unit and was stepped down to the ward and deemed medically fit for discharge. He was commenced on *H. pylori* eradication therapy and was awaiting a social package. However, he developed severe diarrhoea a few days later along with abdominal pain and distension. He had T of 39.5°C, PR of 140/min, RR of 25/min and his blood tests showed WBC count of 35,000 106/dL. Abdominal X-ray showed very dilated colon.

1. What is the most likely diagnosis and responsible microorganism?
2. What are the predisposing risk factors for acquiring this infection in this context?
3. How do you confirm the diagnosis?
4. How do you manage this condition?
5. What are the precautions required to prevent this infection from occurring and spreading in hospitals?

OSCE Scenario 21.5

You attend the minor operation room to perform excision of skin lesions under local anaesthesia. Your consultant reminds you of using the pink disinfectant for skin preparation and performing the procedures under strict sterile measures using sterile instruments, gloves and gowns.

1. What disinfection agents are used on skin?
2. What is the difference between cleaning, disinfection, and sterilization?
3. What are the four main methods of sterilization?

Answers in Appendix pages 481–484

Please check your eBook at https://studentconsult.inkling.com/ for more self-assessment questions. See inside cover for registration details.

22

System-Specific Pathology

NERVOUS SYSTEM

Head Injury

In the UK, head injuries account for annual attendance rates at A&E of almost 1 million patients. Head injuries account for 9 deaths per 100 000 population and in young males, account for 15–20% of all deaths. Head injuries may be classified as follows:

- missile injury to the brain
- non-missile injury to the brain.

Missile Injury to the Brain

Typically caused by bullets. May result in:

- depressed injuries: missile causes depressed skull fracture with contusion, but does not enter brain
- penetrating injuries: where missile enters cranial cavity but does not exit, resulting in focal damage
- perforating injury: where missile enters and exits from cranial cavity, usually resulting in severe extensive haemorrhage around the track of the bullet.

Non-Missile Injury to Brain

- More common than missile injury.
- Range from relatively minor injuries to severe injuries, which may be fatal.
- Main damage to brain occurs as a result of acceleration/deceleration forces causing rotational and shearing forces acting on the mobile brain anchored within a rigid skull.

The types of brain damage occurring in non-missile injuries may be classified as:

- Primary brain injury:
    - immediate result of trauma
    - results in contusions, lacerations and diffuse brain damage
    - treatment cannot reverse primary brain injury.
- Secondary brain injury:
    - result of complications
    - prevention, recognition, and treatment is mainstay of management of patients with head injuries.

Primary Brain Damage

There are two main forms:

- Focal damage:
    - commonest type of focal damage is contusion
    - often occurs at site of impact, particularly if skull fracture
    - may be more severe on the side opposite the impact, i.e. contrecoup
    - large contusions may be associated with intracerebral haemorrhage
    - may be associated with tears of cranial nerves.
- Diffuse axonal injury:
    - results where there is shearing of axons as a result of acceleration/deceleration/torsional forces
    - changes are usually only detectable histologically
    - useful pointers to an occurrence are petechial haemorrhages in the corpus callosum and the cerebellar peduncles
    - patients who have sustained diffuse axonal injury and survive are generally severely disabled.

Secondary Brain Damage

- Results from complications developing after the moment of injury.
- Complications include:
    - intracranial haemorrhage
    - cerebral hypoxia
    - cerebral oedema
    - intracranial herniation
    - cerebral infection, e.g. meningitis.

Outcome of Non-Missile Head Injury

Complications include:

- Post-concussion syndrome resulting in:
    - headache
    - dizziness
    - fatigue
    - poor memory
    - labile emotional state.

- Post-traumatic epilepsy.
- Persistent vegetative state.
- Post-traumatic dementia.
- Brainstem death.

INTRACRANIAL HAEMORRHAGE

This may be:
- extracerebral: occurring in relation to the coverings of the brain
- intracerebral: occurring within the brain.

Extracerebral

Extracerebral intracranial haemorrhage may be divided into different types according to the anatomical space in which it occurs in relation to the meninges:
- extradural
- subdural
- subarachnoid.

Extradural Haemorrhage

- Bleeding into the extradural space, i.e. between skull and dura.
- Usually caused by trauma to the skull associated with a fracture tearing an artery or dural venous sinus.
- Particularly common with fractures of the temporal bone tearing the middle meningeal artery.
- Haematoma develops outside the dura, causing compression of the underlying brain, resulting in transtentorial herniation.
- Commonly fatal unless diagnosed early and treated by surgical evacuation.
- Clinical features include:
  - temporary concussion
  - recovery ('lucid interval')
  - decreased conscious level
  - coma
  - falling pulse rate
  - rising BP
  - dilated ipsilateral pupil
  - contralateral hemiparesis
  - focal fits
  - may be boggy swelling overlying the site of fracture as extradural blood tracks through the fracture into the subcutaneous tissues.

Subdural Haemorrhage

- Bleeding into the subdural space between dura and arachnoid.
- Caused by bleeding from veins which cross the subdural space.
- Divided into:
  - acute subdural haemorrhage: seen following head injury caused by falls or assaults
  - chronic subdural haemorrhage: usually seen in the elderly, where brain shrinkage makes the bridging veins between cortex and venous sinuses vulnerable; may result from trivial and forgotten head injury.
- Haematoma appears as a layer of gelatinous blood (acute type) or an organized layer of granulation tissue and clot (chronic type).
- Compression of underlying brain causes decline in conscious level.

Subarachnoid Haemorrhage

- Bleeding into the subarachnoid space, i.e. between arachnoid and pia.
- Causes include:
  - traumatic: in association with head injury
  - spontaneous:
    - rupture of berry aneurysm
    - rupture of vascular malformation
    - rupture of intracerebral haematoma into subarachnoid space.
- Pathologically there is a layer of blood over the cerebral surface in the subarachnoid space.
- Blood present in CSF.
- Presents with headache and signs of meningeal irritation.
- 60% of cases die immediately.
- One-third of survivors are permanently disabled as a consequence of hypoxic brain damage.
- Hydrocephalus can occur in survivors where fibrous obliteration of the subarachnoid space or arachnoid granulations may occur.

Intracerebral Haemorrhage

- An expansile haematoma within the brain substance.
- Causes include:
  - hypertensive vascular disease (most common cause)
  - trauma
  - bleeding into a tumour
  - vascular malformation
  - cerebral vasculitis
  - associated with coagulopathies.
- Commonest sites for intracerebral haematoma include basal ganglia, internal capsule, thalamus, cerebellum and pons.

Diffuse Petechial Haemorrhages

- Small pin-point haemorrhages scattered throughout brain.
- Result from disruption of wall of small cerebral blood vessels.

- Causes include:
  - vasculitis
  - acute hypertensive encephalopathy
  - fat embolism
  - head injury.

RAISED INTRACRANIAL PRESSURE

- Skull contains brain, CSF and blood.
- At normal intracranial pressures (10–15 mmHg or 12–18 cmH_2O), these three components are in volumetric equilibrium. If one component is elevated, intracranial pressure will increase unless the volume of the other two components decreases proportionately (Monro–Kellie doctrine) (see Ch. 22, Raised Intracranial Pressure section).
- Compensatory properties among the intracranial contents follow a pressure/volume exponential curve.
- Increased volume of any of three components can be balanced up to a certain level without any increase in intracranial pressure.
- Eventually a critical volume is reached where any further volume increase results in raised intracranial pressure.
- The effects of raised intracranial pressure include:
  - hydrocephalus
  - cerebral ischaemia
  - brain shift and herniation
  - systemic effects.

Hydrocephalus

- Common complication of space-occupying lesions of posterior cranial fossa, which compress cerebral aqueduct and fourth ventricle.

Cerebral Ischaemia

- Effects of raised intracranial pressure are exerted on vascular component and result in progressive reduction in cerebral perfusion pressure (cerebral perfusion pressure = blood pressure − intracranial pressure).

Brain Shift and Herniation

- Occurs following a critical increase in intracranial pressure.
- Lumbar puncture contraindicated as there is a risk of precipitating a potentially fatal brainstem herniation.
- Herniation may occur at the following sites:
  - transtentorial herniation (clinical manifestation shown in Box 22.1)
  - tonsillar herniation
  - herniation of cerebellar tonsils into foramen magnum, causing compression of medulla
  - medullary compression results in decerebrate posture, respiratory failure and death.

BOX 22.1 Clinical Manifestations of Tentorial Herniation

Affected (Compressed) Structure	Clinical Manifestation
Oculomotor nerve (cranial nerve III)	Ipsilateral pupillary dilatation
Ipsilateral cerebral peduncle	Contralateral hemiparesis
Contralateral cerebral peduncle	Ipsilateral hemiparesis
Posterior cerebral artery	Cortical blindness
Cerebral aqueduct	Headache and vomiting from hydrocephalus
Reticular formation	Coma
Midbrain	Decerebrate rigidity, death

Systemic Effects

These include:

- hypertension
- bradycardia
- slowing of respiration
- pulmonary oedema
- gastrointestinal ulceration (Cushing's ulcer).

Clinical Manifestations of Raised Intracranial Pressure

These include:

- headache, due to distortion and compression of pain receptors within the dura mater and around the cerebral vessels
- nausea and vomiting, due to pressure on the vomiting centre in the pons and medulla
- papilloedema, due to venous obstruction
- decrease in level of consciousness ranging from drowsiness to coma, depending upon the level of the intracranial pressure.

CEREBRAL ABSCESS

Cerebral abscesses usually develop following focal inflammation of the brain parenchyma. They usually occur as a result of:

- direct spread of infection from sepsis in the middle ear or paranasal sinuses
- septic cerebral sinus thrombosis, due to spread of infection from the mastoid or middle ear via the sigmoid sinus

- blood-borne infection, e.g. from infective endocarditis or bronchiectasis; in immunocompromised patients abscesses may be caused by fungal or protozoal organisms
- trauma, e.g. following open skull fractures.

Abscesses may occur at preferential sites according to their aetiology:

- temporal lobe or cerebellum from otitis media
- frontal lobe from paranasal sinuses
- parietal lobe from haematogenous spread.

Complications

Complications of cerebral abscesses include:

- meningitis
- intracranial herniation
- focal neurological deficit
- epilepsy.

TUMOURS OF THE NERVOUS SYSTEM

Classification of cerebral tumours is shown in Box 22.2.

Astrocytoma

- Peak incidence in early middle age.
- Vary in malignancy, some being slow growing and infiltrative.
- Most malignant astrocytomas are radioresistant and overall survival is usually less than 5 years.
- In children the tumour is often well differentiated and cystic and occurs in the cerebellum. This type is histologically benign and may often be completely excised with potential cure.

BOX 22.2 Classification of Cerebral Tumours

Primary
Glial (gliomas)
Astrocytomas
Glioblastoma multiforme
Medulloblastomas
Ependymomas
Oligodendrogliomas

Non-glial
Meningiomas
Acoustic neuromas
Pituitary tumours

Secondary
Lung
Breast
Kidney
Melanoma

Glioblastoma Multiforme

- Most malignant brain tumour.
- Grows rapidly.
- Occurs between 40 and 60 years old.
- Rarely removable surgically.
- Radioresistant.
- Most patients die within 1 year.

Medulloblastoma

- Commonest glioma of childhood.
- Occurs in first decade of life.
- Arises in roof of fourth ventricle and infiltrates into cerebellum.
- May cause obstructive hydrocephalus.
- Spreads by CSF and may seed on spinal cord.

Ependymomas

- Those arising from the choroid plexuses of the ventricles may be totally removable.
- Those arising from the ventricular walls are difficult to remove.
- Most are well differentiated.
- Malignant forms, however, may seed via the subarachnoid space.

Oligodendrogliomas

- Occur in the cerebral hemispheres.
- Slow growing.
- Usually ill-defined infiltrating neoplasms.
- Most patients die within 5 years of diagnosis.

Meningiomas

- Arise from arachnoid cells.
- Usually occur in females in the 40–60 age group.
- Compress cerebral cortex early in their growth and therefore fits may be an early sign.
- May cause osteoblastic change in overlying bone, giving rise to exostosis, producing a palpable lump over vault of skull.
- Most frequent sites are parasagittal region, sphenoidal wing, olfactory groove and foramen magnum.
- Usually slow growing; do not invade brain tissue but compress it.
- Small tumours are usually curable by excision.
- Even with subtotal excision for large tumours the prognosis is good.

Acoustic Neuroma

- Arises from Schwann cells of the nerve sheath of cranial nerve VIII at the internal auditory meatus.

- As tumour grows it expands the internal auditory meatus, extending into the cerebellopontine angle and compressing the pons, cerebellum and adjacent cranial nerves.
- May be a feature of von Recklinghausen's disease.
- Diagnosis should always be considered in patient with unilateral sensorineural deafness with tinnitus.
- Usually occurs in 30–60 age group.
- Facial weakness with unilateral taste loss is a later manifestation.
- Corneal reflexes are lost relatively early when trigeminal nerve is stretched by the tumour.
- Dysphagia, hoarseness and dysarthria may arise due to involvement of cranial nerves IX, X and XI.
- Unilateral cerebellar signs and features of raised intracranial pressure may occur.

Secondary Tumours

- CNS common site for metastases.
- Commonest neoplasms metastasizing to CNS are:
  - breast
  - bronchus
  - kidney
  - colon
  - malignant melanoma.

Clinical Features of CNS Tumours

CNS tumours may present clinically in two main ways:

- Local effects, including:
  - cranial nerve palsy
  - epilepsy
  - paraplegia with spinal cord tumour.
- Mass effects:
  - many tumours may present with non-specific signs of space-occupying lesions without any localizing signs; these symptoms include confusion, drowsiness, headache and vomiting
  - other features may relate to development of hydrocephalus and intracranial herniation.

Pituitary Tumours

These may cause symptoms because of:

- endocrine capacity
- effects on optic chiasma.

Secretory Tumours (e.g. Prolactinoma)

- Many tumours contain a mixture of secretory cells.
- Presentation is influenced by the hormonal production and size of the tumour.
- Secretory tumours are usually small.
- Secretory tumours may result in the following:
  - overproduction of growth hormone: before fusion of the epiphysis, this will result in gigantism; in adult life, acromegaly results
  - hyperprolactinaemia: this is characterized by amenorrhoea, infertility, galactorrhoea and impotence
  - Cushing's disease (see Chapter 12).

Non-Secretory Tumours

- Usually grow to a large size and present through local effects.
- Symptoms and signs depend upon whether tumour is due to endocrine capacity or local pressure effects.
- Bitemporal hemianopia results from compression of the optic chiasma.
- Compression of secretory cells by non-secretory tumours may result in hypopituitarism.
- Symptoms of hypopituitarism include:
  - reduced libido
  - infertility
  - amenorrhoea
  - myxoedema
  - depression
  - loss of sex characteristics
  - hypoadrenalism
  - in children, growth arrest may occur.

SPINAL CORD INJURIES

Two main groups of injury are recognized clinically:

- open injuries
- closed injuries.

Open Injuries

- Cause direct trauma to the spinal cord and nerve roots.
- Penetrating injuries may result in incomplete cord transection (see below).

Closed Injuries

- Account for most spinal injuries and are usually associated with fractures/dislocation of the vertebral column.
- Damage to the cord depends upon the extent of bony injury and may result in:
  - primary damage
  - contusion
  - nerve fibre transection
  - haemorrhagic necrosis
  - secondary damage
  - extradural haematoma
  - infarction
  - infection
  - oedema.

Complete Transection of Spinal Cord

- Total loss of voluntary movement distal to the level of transection; this loss is irreversible.
- Loss of all sensation from those areas which depend on ascending pathways crossing the site of injury.

Incomplete Spinal Cord Injury (see Fig. 6.10)

- Anterior cord syndrome:
  - associated with flexion/rotation injuries producing anterior dislocation; or compression fracture of vertebral body with bone encroaching on the vertebral canal
  - loss of power below level of lesion
  - loss of pain and temperature below the lesion
  - in addition to direct damage, the anterior spinal artery may be compressed
  - the dorsal columns remain intact and proprioception is not affected.
- Central cord syndrome:
  - occurs in syringomyelia and centrally placed tumours
  - initially involves decussating spinothalamic fibres so that pain and temperature are lost below the lesion
  - later the lateral corticospinal tract is involved, with the more centrally placed cervical tract supplying the arm being involved more than the peripheral tracts supplying the legs. Classically there is flaccid weakness of the arms, but because the distal leg and sacral motor and sensory fibres are spared, perianal sensation and some leg movement and sensation are preserved
  - proprioception and fine touch are preserved in the dorsal columns until late.
- Posterior cord syndrome:
  - seen in hyperextension injuries with fractures of the posterior elements of the vertebrae
  - loss of proprioception with profound ataxia and unsteady faltering gait
  - usually good power and pain and temperature sensation below the lesion.
- Brown-Séquard syndrome:
  - hemisection of the cord
  - stab injury; or damage to lateral mass of vertebra
  - paralysis on affected side below lesion (pyramidal tract)
  - loss of proprioception and fine discrimination (dorsal columns on affected side below lesion)
  - loss of pain and temperature on opposite side below lesion (normal on affected side because of decussation below level of hemisection)
  - therefore the *uninjured side* has good power but absent sensation to pin-prick and temperature.
- Cauda equina syndrome:
  - compression of lumbosacral nerve roots below the conus medullaris
  - caused by bony compression or disc protrusion in lumbosacral area
  - lower motor neuron lesion
  - bowel and bladder dysfunction, together with leg numbness and weakness.

PERIPHERAL NERVE INJURIES

Peripheral nerve injuries may be classified as follows:

- Neuropraxia:
  - a condition of transient physiological block without degeneration
  - continuity of axons and the myelin sheaths remain intact
  - function returns spontaneously in about 6 weeks.
- Axonotmesis:
  - usually the result of compression or traction injuries causing disruption of the axons with intact myelin sheaths
  - distal axons show degeneration, but since the myelin sheaths are intact return of function can be anticipated
  - axons regenerate at the rate of about 1 mm a day
  - return of function can be anticipated but may take many months.
- Neurotmesis:
  - division of nerve in whole or in part which occurs after incised or lacerated wounds, or may be the complication of a fracture
  - complete disruption of both axon and myelin sheath
  - surgical repair is required
  - residual neurological defect likely and neuroma may occur.

Wallerian Degeneration

- Damage to neuronal body, e.g. anterior horn cell, spinal nerve roots or nerve trunks, results in degeneration of the axon distal to the site of the injury.
- In myelinated fibres, this is accompanied by secondary breakdown of myelin around the degenerating axons.
- Regeneration commences 3–4 days following injury.
- Regenerating axonal sprouts grow at 1–2 mm/day.
- This is accompanied by central chromatolysis in the neuronal perikaryon.
- Remyelination occurs by Schwann cells.
- If regeneration and remyelination are successful, reinnervation of the target organ occurs.
- Reinnervation may be prevented by the following factors:

- ischaemia
- cytotoxic drugs
- disruption of perineurium
- haematoma
- scar tissue.

MUSCULOSKELETAL SYSTEM

Osteomyelitis

Acute Osteomyelitis

- Inflammatory lesion due to bacterial infection of bone.
- Disease of growing bones in children but may occur in immunosuppressed or diabetic adults.
- Is being seen increasingly in elderly patients.
- Usually due to *Staphylococcus aureus* and rarely due to streptococci, pneumococci, *Haemophilus* or *Salmonella*.
- The classical sequence of changes in osteomyelitis is as follows:
  - transient bacteraemia, e.g. *S. aureus*
  - focus of acute inflammation in the metaphysis of long bone
  - necrosis of bone fragments forming the sequestrum
  - new subperiosteal bone forms around the dead bone forming a shell (involucrum)
  - in untreated cases, sinuses form draining pus to the skin surface
  - rarely, pus may decompress into the joint, causing septic arthritis.

Chronic Osteomyelitis

- May follow acute osteomyelitis but is more common following surgery for a common fracture, especially when foreign material is implanted.
- It may be chronic from the outset, e.g. tuberculosis.
- Chronic osteomyelitis may occur as a result of tuberculosis, tertiary syphilis or mycotic infections; tuberculosis is the most common cause.
- Children with haemoglobinopathies, e.g. sickle cell disease, have an increased risk of osteomyelitis; unusual organisms such as *Salmonella* are sometimes responsible.

Septic Arthritis

Most cases of septic arthritis are a result of bacterial infection. Arthralgia may be associated with viral diseases.

- Septic arthritis is the result of blood-borne spread from a focus of infection elsewhere.
- The epiphyseal plate forms an effective barrier and it is unusual for an area of osteomyelitis in the metaphysis to spread and involve adjacent joints; this may occasionally occur in the hip joint where the metaphysis may lie within the joint capsule.
- Children are more commonly affected than adults.
- Organisms responsible include:
  - *S. aureus*
  - *Staphylococcus epidermidis* (prosthetic joints)
  - *Streptococcus pyogenes*
  - *Streptococcus pneumoniae*
  - *Neisseria gonorrhoeae*
  - *Haemophilus influenzae* (children)
  - Gram-negative organisms (drug addicts)
  - *Mycobacterium tuberculosis*
  - *Brucella abortus* (intervertebral discitis).
- Risk factors for septic arthritis include:
  - diabetes mellitus
  - rheumatoid arthritis
  - immunosuppression
  - intra-articular injections, e.g. corticosteroids.

Fractures

The healing of fractures has been considered in Chapter 14.

Complications of Fractures

These may be:

- immediate (at the time of fracture)
- early (during the period of initial treatment)
- late (after the period of initial treatment).

Immediate

- Haemorrhage: this may be internal or external. Internal haemorrhage can be considerable at the fracture site, i.e. up to 1.5 L with a fractured femoral shaft.
- Injury to nerves and vessels.
- Injury to underlying structures, e.g. brain damage with skull fractures, splenic rupture with left lower rib fractures, urethral trauma with pelvic fractures.

Early

These may be divided into:

- local
- general.

Local

- Gangrene due to vessel damage or tight plasters.
- Nerve palsies from tight plasters or involved in callus.
- Wound infection or wound dehiscence.
- Loss of position.
- Tetanus.
- Gas gangrene.

General

- DVT.
- Acute urinary retention.
- Fat embolism.
- Compartment syndrome.
- Crush syndrome.

Late
- Delayed union.
- Non-union.
- Mal-union.
- Reflex sympathetic osteodystrophy (Sudek's atrophy).
- Avascular necrosis of bone.
- Myositis ossificans.
- Osteoarthritis.

Delayed union
- Fracture does not heal in expected time.
- Absence of callus and mobility at the fracture are features.

Non-union
- Attempt at repair by normal body mechanisms have ceased and the fracture remains un-united.
- Persistent mobility of fracture site.
- Radiographs show no trabeculae across the fracture line.
- A pseudoarthrosis (false joint) may result.
- Causes of non-union include:
  - inadequate blood supply
  - infection
  - poor immobilization
  - excessive movement at fracture site
  - interposition of soft tissue between bone ends
  - pathological fracture.

Mal-union
- Healing has resulted in a deformed position.
- This may be shortening, overlap or angulation.
- Deformity may put strain on adjacent joints, resulting in osteoarthritis.

Complex regional pain syndrome (CRPS)
- Can be related, or unrelated, to a nerve injury.
- Can follow relatively mild hand trauma.
- Limb becomes painful, swollen and stiff with a reddened, smooth, shiny appearance to skin.
- The cause is unknown.

Avascular necrosis of bone
- Part of bone necroses when its blood supply is interrupted by the fracture.
- Common sites are:
  - the head of the femur in intracapsular fractures where the retinacular vessels supplying the femoral head are disrupted
  - the proximal part of the scaphoid bone in fractures across the body; the blood supply enters from the distal end.

Myositis ossificans
- Calcification with subsequent ossification occurs in a haematoma associated with stripping of the periosteum and release of osteoblasts into the surrounding muscle and tissue.
- Most common in injuries around the elbow and those involving quadriceps femoris.

Osteoarthritis
- Results from misaligned fractures putting strain on joints.
- After intra-articular fractures.

PATHOLOGICAL FRACTURES

A pathological fracture is one that occurs through a bone already weakened by an underlying disease. Causes of pathological fractures may be:
- general
- local.

General
- Osteoporosis.
- Metabolic conditions, e.g. rickets, osteomalacia.
- Adrenal overactivity or excessive steroid therapy.
- Hyperparathyroidism.
- Paget's disease of bone.
- Neuropathic conditions, e.g. syphilis, syringomyelia.
- Osteogenesis imperfecta.

Local
- Bony metastases from:
  - breast
  - prostate
  - thyroid
  - kidney
  - bronchus.
- Benign and malignant primary bone tumours.
- Simple bone cysts.
- Irradiation of bone.
- Bone atrophy, e.g. polio.

Compartment Syndrome
- Compartment syndrome is caused by increased tissue pressure in a closed fascial compartment, compromising circulation to the nerves and muscles within the involved compartment.
- The fascial compartments to the leg and forearm are most commonly involved.
- Causes include:
  - fracture with subsequent haemorrhage and oedema in the compartment
  - limb compression or crush
  - vigorous exercise.
- Ischaemia results from pressure on surrounding small arteries.

- Distal pulses may still be palpable and the diagnosis therefore missed.
- In the lower limb, the posterior compartment (flexors of the ankle), anterior compartment (extensors) or peroneal compartment (evertors) may be involved.
- Treatment is by prompt fasciotomy, which allows the muscle to expand and relieves pressure on the vessels.

ARTHRITIS

Osteoarthritis

- Common, painful, disabling, degenerative joint disease.
- Primarily affects cartilage of weight-bearing joints, e.g. hips, knees.
- Occurs spontaneously in older age groups and is increasingly common above the age of 60 years.
- Occurs in joints of younger persons following any form of previous mechanical damage, e.g. trauma, developmental dysplasia of hip, osteochondritis.
- Macroscopic features include:
  - erosive changes in cartilage (fibrillation)
  - exposed bone develops an ivory-like surface (eburnation)
  - thickening of the subchondral bone plate
  - subchondral bone pseudocyst may form, due to entry of synovium under pressure into the subchondral plate
  - at margins of the articular cartilage, bony outgrowths develop (osteophytes).
- Pain results from stimulation of nerve endings in joint capsule and synovium by inflammation or abnormal load-bearing/joint movement.
- Deformity results due to:
  - synovial inflammation
  - effusion into joint
  - erosion of articular surfaces
  - abnormal remodelling of subchondral bone
  - loss of alignment of joint surfaces by cartilage destruction and bone deformity.
- Restricted movement occurs because of:
  - synovial swelling
  - fibrosis
  - limitation by pain.

Rheumatoid Arthritis

- Common systemic chronic inflammatory disorder involving joints.
- Associated with rheumatoid factor – an autoantibody reactive with altered autologous immunoglobulin.
- Females affected more than males.
- Occurs in all age groups, e.g. Still's disease in children.
- Up to 75% of patients are HLA-DR4 positive.
- Multisystem disease characterized by chronic inflammatory granulomatous lesions (rheumatoid nodules).
- Affects many small joints, particularly those of the fingers, hands and wrists, but larger joints such as ankle, hip and knee are also affected.
- Joints are painful, swollen and tender.
- The synovial membrane is thickened with villus overgrowth, increased vascularity, and pannus, which grows over and replaces the articular cartilage.
- Extra-articular features of rheumatoid disease are:
  - subcutaneous rheumatoid nodules
  - anaemia
  - lymphadenopathy
  - splenomegaly
  - pericarditis
  - dry eyes and mouth (Sjögren's syndrome)
  - uveitis and scleritis
  - vasculitis, especially fingers and nail beds
  - pulmonary changes (nodules, interstitial fibrosis, obstructive airways disease)
  - amyloidosis.

Gout

- Painful, acute, inflammatory response to tissue deposition of urate crystals, e.g. subcutaneous tophi or in periarticular tissues.
- Usually occurs in middle-aged or elderly males, although females may be affected, especially when there is a family history of gout.
- The first metatarsophalangeal joint is the predominant site but many other joints including those of hands may be affected.
- Joint is swollen, red and shows white 'chalky' patches in the skin through which crystals can often be expressed.
- Serum uric levels are raised.
- May be associated with chronic renal failure.

Neuropathic Arthritis (Charcot's Joint)

- A degenerative joint disease which occurs due to loss of sensory nerve supply.
- Most frequently seen in knee or hip joints in tabes dorsalis, and shoulder or elbow joint in syringomyelia.
- Clinical features include:
  - recurrent swelling
  - degenerative changes in ligaments and tendons, resulting in subluxation of the joint.

BONE TUMOURS

These may be benign or malignant. Secondary tumours are much more common than primary. Primary malignant tumours are rare, but they have a bad prognosis and affect patients in a younger age group. Benign tumours include:

- osteoma ('ivory' osteoma)
- osteoid osteoma
- chondroma
- fibroma and fibrous dysplasia
- bone cysts.

Primary Malignant Tumours

These include:
- osteosarcoma (osteogenic sarcoma)
- osteoclastoma (giant cell tumour)
- Ewing's tumour
- chondrosarcoma
- fibrosarcoma
- myeloma.

Secondary Malignant Tumours

These occur from:
- lung
- thyroid
- breast
- prostate
- kidney.

Benign Tumours

Osteoma ('Ivory' Osteoma)

- Growth from surface of bone
- Common on the surface of the vault of the skull.
- A smooth, non-tender mound, rarely causing symptoms.
- If symptomatic, can be cured by excision.

Osteoid Osteoma

- Usually occurs in long bones in young males.
- Continuous, severe, boring pain, usually worse at night and relieved by aspirin.
- Probably not a true neoplasm.
- Radiographs show dense sclerosis surrounded by a central small lucent zone (osteoid).
- Treatment is by excision, which gives dramatic relief of pain.

Chondroma

- A cartilaginous tumour common in the phalanges and metacarpals.
- Enchondroma: a chondroma growing in the centre of a bone.
- Ecchondroma: a chondroma growing on the surface of a bone.
- Osteochondroma: a cartilage-capped bony outgrowth (commonest bone tumour; malignant potential; especially if >2 cm or multiple).
- Treatment consists of observation for malignant transformation or bony destruction, and removal only if the Chondroma is causing pain or fracture.
- Occasionally multiple enchondromatosis occurs in long bones (Ollier's disease).

Fibroma and Fibrous Dysplasia

- A spectrum of conditions with failure or partial failure of ossification replaced by fibrous tissue.
- Usually asymptomatic and often regress at puberty or after a fracture.

Bone Cysts

- Fluid- or blood-filled cavities.
- Vary from multiloculated cysts containing clear fluid in children and adolescence to large aneurysmal bone cysts which may cause 'bulging out' of one side of a bone.
- Pathological fractures common.
- Treatment is by excision and bone grafting.

Primary Malignant Tumours

Osteosarcoma (Osteogenic Sarcoma)

- Most common primary tumour of bone.
- More common in males.
- Occurs under the age of 30 years.
- Occurs in long bones.
- In the young it commonly affects the lower end of the femur or upper end of tibia, usually affecting the metaphysis.
- In older patients, may be associated with Paget's disease.
- Spread is via the bloodstream to the lungs.

Osteoclastoma (Giant Cell Tumour)

- Occurs in young adults.
- Occurs at end of long bones.
- Has low malignant potential but is locally recurrent.
- Metastases uncommon, occur late and are to the lungs.
- Pathological fractures may occur.

Ewing's Tumour

- Highly malignant.
- Arises from marrow.
- It is not confined to the ends of long bones and may occur in any bone.
- Affects children and young adults.
- Spreads rapidly via the bloodstream to lungs, liver and other bones.

Chondrosarcoma

- Slow-growing tumour arising from chondroblasts.
- Occurs between 30 and 50 years.
- May arise de novo or in a pre-existing osteochondroma.
- Occurs in long bones, pelvis and ribs.
- Metastases occur to lungs.
- Treatment is by wide excision or amputation.

Fibrosarcoma

- More common in soft tissues (malignant fibrous histiocytoma).
- Much less aggressive in bone.

Myeloma

- Common primary bone malignancy.
- It arises from marrow plasma cells.
- Rare before 50 years.
- Early dissemination with widespread marrow replacement (multiple myelomatosis).
- Clinically presents with:
    - anaemia
    - malaise
    - bone pain (backache)
    - pathological fracture.

Secondary Bone Malignancy

- Secondaries may occur from lung, thyroid, breast, prostate and kidney.
- Clinical features include:
    - past history of primary tumour
    - primary may not be apparent
    - bone pain
    - pathological fracture.

METABOLIC BONE DISEASE

Rickets and Osteomalacia

- Deficient mineralization of organic bone matrix.
- Rickets is the name given to osteomalacia affecting the growth of the skeleton in children.
- Rickets is characterized by bone deformities.
- Osteomalacia occurs in adults, causing susceptibility to fractures but few deformities.
- Causes of osteomalacia/rickets include:
    - dietary deficiency of vitamin D
    - deficiency of vitamin D metabolites
    - intestinal malabsorption
    - renal disease
    - liver disease.
- In children, classical deformities occur:
    - bowing of the femur and tibia
    - large head ('bossing' of the skull due to persistence of suture lines and fontanelles)
    - pronounced swelling of the costochondral junctions ('rickety rosary')
    - enlarged epiphyses
    - stunted growth
    - delayed dentition.
- Treatment is with vitamin D and calcium.

Osteoporosis

- Reduction in bone mass per unit volume.
- Common in the elderly, particularly females.
- May be complication of steroid therapy and Cushing's syndrome.
- Common predisposing cause of fractures, e.g. neck of femur, Colles' fracture, wedge fractures of vertebra.
- Occurs with any form of immobility.
- Associated with alcoholism, diabetes, liver disease and smoking.
- Localized osteoporosis is inevitable after immobilization of any part of the skeleton.

Hyperparathyroidism

See Chapter 12.

Paget's Disease of Bone

- Difficult disease to categorize, probably not metabolic.
- Aetiology unknown.
- Localized increase in bone turnover.
- May affect part of one bone, an entire bone or many bones.
- Disorderly bone resorption and replacement leads to softening, increased vascularity, painful enlargement and bowing of bones.
- Occurs in middle to old age and is more common in males.
- Skull, vertebra, pelvis and long bones are affected.
- Some cases are symptomless, being picked up on routine radiography.
- Complications include:
    - compressive symptoms due to skull enlargement, e.g. blindness, deafness, cranial nerve entrapment
    - paraplegia
    - pathological fractures
    - high-output cardiac failure, due to vascularity of bone
    - osteogenic sarcoma may develop after many years.

LUNG TUMOURS

Lung tumours may be primary or secondary. Both are common.

Primary Carcinoma of the Lung

- Most common primary malignant tumour worldwide.
- Largest cancer-causing death in UK: 35 000/year.
- 30% of all male cancer deaths.
- Male/female ratio 2:1 (was 7:1 but rise in incidence in women parallels increase in numbers of female smokers).

- Directly related to cigarette smoking.
- Associated with occupational exposure to carcinogens.
- Overall 5-year survival rate around 5%.

Aetiology

Major risk factors are:

- Cigarette smoking.
- Occupational hazards:
  - asbestos
  - haematite
  - radioactive gases, e.g. radon.
- Other factors:
  - nickel
  - chromates
  - mustard gas
  - arsenic
  - coal-tar distillates
  - fibrosis: peripheral lung cancers may arise in areas of previous scarring, e.g. old tuberculous foci or infarcts.

Classification of Lung Cancer

Four histological types are described:

- adenocarcinoma (30–45%)
- squamous cell carcinoma (35–40%)
- small cell (oat cell) carcinoma (15–25%)
- undifferentiated large cell carcinoma (rarest).

Clinical Features

Primary

- May be asymptomatic and seen on routine chest X-ray.
- Cough.
- Haemoptysis.
- Dyspnoea.
- Chest pain.
- Wheeze.
- Hoarseness.
- Recurrent chest infections.
- Dysphagia.

Complications

- Thoracic: pleural effusion, recurrent laryngeal nerve palsy (hoarseness).
- Superior vena cava obstruction, Horner's syndrome (ptosis, miosis, enophthalmos, anhidrosis), especially with Pancoast tumour (invasive cancer of apex of lung).
- Metastatic (cachexia, malaise), brain (headaches, fits, personality change), bone (pathological fractures), liver (jaundice), adrenal (Addison's disease).
- Non-metastatic, extrapulmonary, ADH, ACTH secretion, hypercalcaemia, myasthenic neuropathy, hypertrophic pulmonary osteoarthropathy, thrombophlebitis migrans, gynaecomastia, clubbing.

Prognosis

- Ultimately depends on cell type and stage of disease at time of diagnosis.
- Small cell carcinoma has the worst prognosis.

Other Primary Lung Tumours

Primary tumours other than carcinomas are rare. They may be classified as:

- benign, e.g. bronchial gland adenomas, benign mesenchymal tumours
- malignant, e.g. sarcomas, adenocystic carcinomas, lymphomas, carcinoid tumours.

Pneumothorax

This is air in the pleural cavity. The causes are as follows:

- Spontaneous:
  - primary: blebs on the pleural surface leak spontaneously or are triggered by a minor event, e.g. exertion; more common in young males; may be bilateral; may be familial
  - secondary: to lung disease that breaches pleura, e.g. COPD, bullous emphysema.
- Traumatic, e.g. following trauma to the chest, fractured ribs.
- Iatrogenic, e.g. following central lines for CVP, intravenous feeding or haemodialysis.

Pneumothorax may be further classified as follows:

- Open, e.g. following stabbing or shooting. Air is sucked into the pleural cavity during inspiration. This causes a to-and-fro movement of the mediastinum during respiration, leading to respiratory embarrassment.
- Closed: this is when the chest wall is intact, e.g. with rib fractures.
- Tension: occurs when there is a valve-like mechanism at the site of communication between the air and the pleural cavity, allowing air to enter the cavity in inspiration but not to escape in expiration. As pressure rises:
  - the lung collapses
  - mediastinal shift occurs to the opposite side with tracheal deviation to the opposite side
  - compression of the contralateral lung
  - compromise of venous return.

Tension pneumothorax is a life-threatening condition.

Pleural Effusions

- Haemothorax:
  - blood in the pleural cavity
  - due to chest injury, ruptured thoracic aortic aneurysm.
- Hydrothorax:
  - transudate (low-protein fluid) due to liver failure, cardiac failure, renal failure

  - exudate (high-protein fluid) due to tumours, infection, inflammation.
- Chylothorax:
  - lymph in the pleural cavity
  - due to neoplastic obstruction of the thoracic duct.
- Pyothorax (empyema):
  - pus in the pleural cavity
  - due to infection.

LUNG INFECTIONS

Respiratory infections are very common. The general factors predisposing to lung infections include:

- loss or suppression of cough reflex, e.g. anaesthesia, after surgery, coma, neuromuscular disorders
- ciliary defects, e.g. non-motile cilia or loss of ciliated cells with squamous metaplasia
- mucus disorders, e.g. cystic fibrosis, chronic bronchitis
- immunological defects, e.g. hypogammaglobulinaemia
- inhibition of macrophage function, e.g. smokers
- pulmonary oedema.

Mode of Infection

Pathogens may reach the lung via:

- inhalation from the environment, e.g. nebulizers
- aspiration of oropharyngeal flora
- colonization of diseased/abnormal lower respiratory tract, e.g. bronchiectasis
- blood spread: bacteraemia, septicaemia.

Predisposing Conditions

These include:

- chronic obstructive pulmonary disease
- mucus disorders, e.g. cystic fibrosis
- immunosuppressive disorders
- immunosuppressive drugs.

Bronchopneumonia

- Chiefly in old age and infancy.
- Occurs in patients with debilitating disease, e.g. cancer, cardiac failure, renal failure.
- Predisposing factors include COPD and cystic fibrosis.
- Occurs in early post-operative period due to failure to remove respiratory tract infections.
- Causative organisms include:
  - *S. pneumoniae*
  - *H. influenzae*
  - rarer causes include *S. aureus* and coliforms
  - *S. aureus* pneumonia seen in hospital patients, after influenza as a severe secondary bacterial pneumonia; intravenous drug abusers; in the immunocompromised. It may be fulminating and rapidly fatal
  - coliform bronchopneumonia is rare: may be encountered in hospital patients, the immunocompromised and those on ventilatory support in ITUs.
- Bronchopneumonia is of characteristically patchy distribution and tends to be basal and bilateral.
- Histological examination reveals inflammatory cells in the bronchi and bronchioles with alveoli filled with inflammatory exudate.

Lobar Pneumonia

- Rarely seen in surgical patients.
- May result in referred pain to the abdomen, particularly right lower lobar pneumonia; enters into the differential diagnosis of appendicitis, the intercostal nerves being irritated and pain being referred to the right iliac fossa.
- Commonly caused by *S. pneumoniae.*
- Part of post-splenectomy sepsis.
- Relatively uncommon in infancy and old age.
- Clinical features include:
  - cough
  - fever
  - 'rusty' sputum
  - rigors may occur
  - acute pleuritic chest pain
  - consolidation of a lobe or part of lobe results.
- Classically, four stages of the disease are recognized pathologically:
  - congestion: lasts about 24 h and is due to protein-rich exudate filling alveoli, with venous congestion
  - red 'hepatization': lasts a few days, with inflammatory cells and red cells in the alveolar spaces; fibrinous exudate on pleura; lung is red, solid, airless and bears a resemblance to the cut surface of fresh liver
  - grey 'hepatization': accumulation of fibrin with the destruction of white cells and red cells; lung appears grey and solid
  - resolution: occurs in 8–10 days; inflammatory cells and fibrin are re-absorbed and the underlying lung architecture is preserved.

The above is a classical pattern of lobar pneumonia. Most cases resolve as above, although the pattern may be modified by early and appropriate antibiotic therapy.

Aspiration Pneumonia

- Occurs when upper gastrointestinal contents are aspirated in lung.
- Results in consolidation and inflammation.
- Clinical situations in which this may occur include:
  - induction of anaesthesia
  - recovery from anaesthesia

  - sedation
  - coma
  - severe debility.
- Part of lung affected depends on the patient's posture.
- Abscess and empyema may result.
- Causative organisms are usually commensals of the upper respiratory tract, principally *S. pneumoniae*, although anaerobes are also involved in the majority of cases.

Atypical Pneumonia

- Main causative organisms are:
  - *Mycoplasma pneumoniae*
  - *Coxiella burnetii*
  - *Chlamydia psittaci*
  - *Chlamydia pneumoniae*.
- *Mycoplasma pneumoniae* is responsible for most cases of primary atypical pneumonia.
- School-aged children and young adults are the group most affected.
- Spread by droplet infection.
- Effective drugs include tetracycline and erythromycin.

Legionnaires' Disease

- Caused by *Legionella pneumophila*.
- Patients typically middle-aged smokers, often in poor general health.
- May also affect patients who are previously healthy.
- Spread by water droplets from contaminated air humidifiers or water storage tanks.
- Symptoms initially those of flu-like illness, which progresses to severe pneumonia and respiratory failure.
- Other features include:
  - headache
  - mental confusion
  - myalgia
  - nausea
  - vomiting
  - diarrhoea
  - acute renal failure.
- 10–20% of cases are fatal.
- Treatment usually with erythromycin, but those failing to respond may be treated with rifampicin or ciprofloxacin, either singly or in combination.

Chest Infections in the Immunocompromised

- These are opportunistic infections and include:
  - fungi, e.g. *Candida*, *Aspergillus fumigatus*, *Pneumocystis jirovecii* (formerly *carinii*)
  - viruses, e.g. cytomegalovirus (CMV).
- Characterized by:
  - fever
  - cough
  - shortness of breath
  - pulmonary infiltrates on chest X-ray.

Pneumocystis jirovecii (formerly carinii)

- Results from reactivation of latent infection.
- Common in patients with AIDS, and transplant patients.
- Diagnosis depends on identification of characteristic organisms in bronchial aspirates, bronchial lavage or lung biopsy.
- Treatment with intravenous co-trimoxazole.

Fungi

- Both *Candida* and *Aspergillus* can cause widespread areas of necrosis.
- Microabscesses containing characteristic fungal filaments may occur in the lungs.
- Treatment requires intravenous amphotericin B alone or in combination with 5-fluorocytosine.

New imidazoles, e.g. fluconazole, may be effective.

Viruses

- Cytomegalovirus causes diffuse alveolar damage.
- Characteristic intranuclear inclusions are seen with CMV infections.
- Treatment is with intravenous ganciclovir.

Bronchiectasis

- Abnormal and irreversible dilatation of bronchi.
- Now relatively uncommon in Western countries due to the decline in predisposing childhood infections, particularly whooping cough and measles.
- Condition may be congenital or acquired.
- Chief congenital cause is cystic fibrosis; may be seen in immunodeficiency syndromes.
- Chief acquired causes include:
  - whooping cough
  - measles
  - bronchial obstruction (enlarged lymph nodes from tuberculosis)
  - bronchial tumours.
- Recurrent infection and inflammation lead to further airway damage and destruction of lung tissue.
- Destruction of alveolar walls, fibrosis of lung parenchyma.
- Clinical features include:
  - production of large amounts of foul-smelling sputum
  - dyspnoea.
- Complications include:
  - pneumonia
  - lung abscess
  - empyema

  - septicaemia
  - amyloid formation
  - pulmonary fibrosis
  - cor pulmonale
  - remote abscesses, e.g. cerebral abscesses and meningitis.

EMPYEMA

This is pus within the pleural cavity. The causes include:

- pulmonary infection: complication of intrapulmonary infection, e.g. pneumonia, tuberculosis, lung abscess
- other infections: spread from subphrenic abscess, acute mediastinitis, distant infective foci
- surgery: as a complication of thoracic surgery
- penetrating chest wall injury.

Organisms

These include:

- Gram-positive organisms, e.g. *S. pneumoniae* or *S. aureus*, especially when empyema complicates pulmonary parenchymal infection
- empyema secondary to surgery, trauma or oesophageal disease may be due to Gram-negative organisms.

Complications

- Systemic sepsis.
- Lung collapse.
- Bronchopleural fistula.
- Pleural scarring.

Lung Abscess

- May be single or multiple.
- Usually occur in patients who are malnourished, cachectic or immunocompromised.
- Causes include:
  - aspiration pneumonia
  - bronchiectasis
  - carcinoma
  - inhaled foreign bodies
  - infected pulmonary infarcts
  - infection from drug abuse.
- Organisms include:
  - *S. pneumoniae*
  - *H. influenzae*
  - *S. aureus*
  - *Klebsiella*
  - *Entamoeba histolytica* (spreading from the liver via the diaphragm).

BREAST DISORDERS

Benign Tumours

Benign breast tumours comprise:

- fibroadenoma
- duct papilloma
- adenoma
- connective tissue tumours.

Fibroadenoma

- Commonest type of benign tumour, mainly in young women (15–35).
- Arises from connective tissue and epithelium.
- Clinically mobile on palpation (breast mouse).
- Firm rubbery masses that are well circumscribed. Rarely larger than 3 cm.
- Cut surface has a characteristic appearance which is greyish-white with a whorled appearance.
- May calcify with age.
- Juvenile fibroadenomas occurring in the breasts of young girls may grow quite rapidly and reach up to 10 cm in diameter; more frequent in Africans and West Indians than Caucasians.

Duct Papilloma

- More frequent in middle-aged females.
- Commonest cause of nipple discharge, often blood-stained.
- Consist of branching fibrovascular cores covered by epithelium, which is benign.
- Solitary duct papillomas are not premalignant.
- Multiple duct papillomas arising in smaller ducts at a younger age may be associated with an increased risk of malignancy.

Adenoma

- Rare.
- Tubuloadenomas are well-circumscribed tumours occurring mainly in women in their early 20s.
- Lactating adenomas are tubuloadenomas that undergo secretory changes during pregnancy.
- Nipple adenomas occur as nodules under the nipple; may occur at any age but most common between 30 and 50 years; overlying skin may ulcerate and there may be blood-stained discharge; nipple adenomas may be mistaken for Paget's disease.

Connective Tissue Tumours

- Lipomas and haemangiomas may occur but are rare.

Carcinoma of the Breast

This accounts for 20% of all cancers in women and is the commonest cause of death among women in 35–55 age group.

Risk Factors

These include:

- Female sex:
  - risk increases with age.

- Long interval between menarche and menopause:
  - early menarche and late menopause are each associated with an increased risk
  - thought to be related to prolonged exposure to oestrogen.
- Childbirth:
  - nulliparous women have a greater risk of developing breast carcinoma than parous women
  - in parous women, protection is related to early age for first full-term pregnancy
  - if first birth is delayed to mid- or late thirties, the woman is at greater risk of developing breast cancer than a nulliparous woman.
- Family history of breast cancer:
  - first-degree female relatives of breast cancer patients have an increased risk of developing breast cancer
  - inherited mutations of a gene on the long arm of chromosome 17 (BRCA1) are found in almost all families with susceptibility to female breast and ovarian cancer.
- Atypical hyperplasia in previous breast biopsy:
  - women with benign breast disease whose breast biopsies show atypical epithelial hyperplasia have a definite increased risk of developing breast cancer.
- Previous chest wall radiotherapy:
  - individuals who have undergone chest wall irradiation as a young adult, e.g. for lymphoma, have an increased risk of developing breast cancer.
- Geographic factors:
  - marked variation in breast cancer rates between different countries
  - highest rates are in North America, North-West Europe, Australia and New Zealand
  - lowest rates in South East Asia and Africa
  - this difference may be due to age at menarche, age at a full first-time pregnancy, age at menopause.
- Lifestyle factors:
  - some evidence to suggest that obesity and alcohol consumption can increase risks of breast cancer also, with weaker evidence for smoking and lack of exercise.

Aetiological Mechanisms

- Overexposure to oestrogen and underexposure to progesterone.
- Increased risk with hormone replacement therapy; debate over possibility of small risk with oral contraceptives.
- Some tumours contain oestrogen and progesterone receptors. Affected patients are more likely to respond to some form of hormone manipulation.

Non-Invasive Carcinomas

- Tumour confined to ducts (ductal carcinoma in situ) or acini (lobular carcinoma in situ).
- Ductal carcinoma in situ is unilateral, occurs in pre- and post-menopausal women, has several forms and may become invasive.
- Lobular carcinoma in situ occurs in premenopausal women, has no clinical features (i.e. does not present as a palpable lump and is usually found in biopsies removed for other reasons), is often bilateral, can be multifocal, and is a risk factor for invasive carcinoma.

Invasive Carcinomas

- Occur in pre- and post-menopausal women.
- Most are infiltrating ductal carcinomas of no special type.
- Infiltrating lobular carcinomas can be multifocal.
- Less common types include mucinous, medullary, papillary and tubular carcinomas.

Gross Features

Macroscopic appearances depend upon the amount of stroma within the carcinoma.

- Scirrhous: implies prominent fibrous tissue reaction resulting in the carcinoma having a dense, white appearance which grates when cut (like the surface of an unripe pear).
- Medullary (encephaloid): like substance of brain, tumour feels much softer; cellular with little stroma.
- Mucinous carcinomas: predominance of mucin or jelly-like material.

Paget's disease of the nipple

- Erosion of the nipple, clinically resembling eczema.
- Associated with underlying ductal carcinoma in situ or invasive carcinoma.
- Eventually destroys the nipple.
- Differentiated from eczema in that eczema is usually bilateral, does not destroy the nipple and is not associated with an underlying lump.

Spread of Breast Carcinoma

- Directly into skin and muscle:
  - tethering to skin
  - skin dimpling
  - ulceration
  - fungation
  - fixity to pectoral muscles.
- Via lymphatics to axillary, cervical and internal mammary nodes.
- Via bloodstream to lungs, bone, liver and brain:

- lungs: pleural effusion, lymphangitic carcinomatosa
- bone: pathological fractures, hypercalcaemia
- liver: jaundice
- brain: confusion, fits.
- May be considerable delay before metastases occur.

Prognostic Factors

- Presence of invasion: non-invasive tumours are curable if all lesions are resected; multicentricity may require mastectomy.
- Tumour size: the smaller the tumour, the higher the survival.
- Tumour type: tubular, medullary, mucinous and papillary are associated with more favourable prognosis.
- Staging: outcome depends upon involvement of lymph nodes and distant metastases.
- Degree of differentiation.
- Expression of hormone receptors – an indication of likely response to anti-oestrogens.
- Overexpression of products of proto-oncogene C-*erb* B-2/HER-2.

Phylloides Tumour

- Can occur at any age, but mean age of presentation is 45.
- Can become very large (not to be confused with giant fibroadenoma).
- Should be excised with wide margin of normal breast tissue.
- Recurrence is a major problem.
- Risk of recurrence is less if tumours are small with low mitotic rate and minimal cellular atypia, and have a rounded rather than an infiltrative edge.
- Chance of metastases increases with recurrence.
- Metastases occur in about 10% of cases of recurrence.

Inflammatory Conditions

These include:

- acute pyogenic mastitis
- tuberculosis
- actinomycosis
- mammary duct ectasia
- fat necrosis.

Acute Pyogenic Mastitis

- Painful, acute inflammatory condition due to *S. aureus*.
- Occurs in the first few weeks after delivery, during breastfeeding.
- Usually associated with cracked nipple, although blockage of a duct may be a factor.
- Results in localized swelling and erythema.
- Responds to flucloxacillin, but if fluctuation has occurred indicating abscess, incision and drainage will be required.

Tuberculosis

- Rare.
- Due to haematogenous spread.
- Caseous mass with marked fibrous reaction, mimicking carcinoma.

Actinomycosis

- Rare.
- May be due to spread of infection from the lung through the thoracic wall, or occur as primary infection.
- Usually presents with hard lump beneath the nipple, which may be painful.
- Results in abscess formation with pus containing typical 'sulfur granules'.

Mammary Duct Ectasia

- Usually affects ducts behind nipple.
- Usually occurs in fifth decade.
- Thick, creamy nipple discharge, which may occasionally be blood-stained.
- Fibrosis around ducts may cause nipple retraction, thus mimicking carcinoma.
- Ducts are dilated and are filled with inspissated material.
- Condition sometimes known as periductal mastitis or plasma cell mastitis because of the prevalence of plasma cells on histological examination.

Fat Necrosis

- Caused by trauma, e.g. seat-belt injury, partner's teeth.
- Presents with hard lump that may mimic carcinoma.
- Macroscopically, yellow tissue with haemorrhagic areas of calcification.
- Occurs more frequently in the obese.

Proliferative Conditions of the Breast

- Known by a variety of names including cystic mastitis, fibrocystic disease and chronic mastitis.
- Causes severe discomfort in the breast before period.
- One component, i.e. epithelial hyperplasia, is associated with an increased risk of cancer.
- Causes palpable lumps, mimicking breast cancer.
- Cysts occur in the breast and may require aspiration.
- Histological features are numerous and include:
  - adenosis
  - sclerosing adenosis
  - epithelial hyperplasia
  - cysts
  - fibrous.

Gynaecomastia

Breast tissue in men contains only ductular structures with no evidence of acini. Gynaecomastia is the benign enlargement of male breast tissue. It occurs most commonly in adolescent and older age groups.

Causes are shown in Box 22.3.

Breast Cancer in Men

- Rare: accounts for 1% of all breast carcinomas.
- Increased risk in patients with Klinefelter's syndrome.
- Usually presents as a lump, but there can be nipple discharge or retraction.
- Prognosis affected by such factors as lymph node status and size.

BOX 22.3 Causes of Gynaecomastia

Physiological
Neonates
Puberty
Old age

Pathological
Drugs
Oestrogens
Cyproterone
Spironolactone
Cimetidine
Digitalis
Griseofulvin
Amphetamines
Tricyclic antidepressants
Cannabis
Anabolic steroid abuse

Carcinoma of the male breast
Liver failure
Renal failure
Hyperthyroidism
Hypogonadism
Klinefelter's syndrome
Agenesis

Testicular tumours
Other tumours
Bronchial carcinoma (inappropriate secretion of hormones)
Pituitary tumours (e.g. prolactinoma)

Malnutrition
Idiopathic

CARDIOVASCULAR SYSTEM

Atherosclerosis

Atherosclerosis is by far the most common disorder leading to death and serious morbidity throughout the developed world. It is responsible for more deaths than all forms of cancer.

Lesions of Atherosclerosis

Fatty streaks

- First visible lesion.
- Seen in young, even infants, and consist of intracellular lipid deposits.
- Appear as raised subendothelial yellow streaks.

Gelatinous plaques

- Small, soft, blister-like elevations.
- Occur more commonly in aorta and large vessels.
- May be precursors of mature plaques.

Fibrolipid plaques (Fig. 22.1)

- Characteristic lesions of atherosclerosis.
- Most commonly, have a lipid-rich core with overlying fibrous cap on the luminal surfaces.
- Great variations from the basal accumulation of lipid, being very large with only a thin overlying cap to the opposite extreme, where the cellular and connective tissue elements predominate.
- Plaques tend to be found at certain sites, but especially the lower abdominal aorta, coronary arteries, renal arteries, distal superficial femoral and popliteal arteries, descending thoracic aorta, internal carotid and circle of Willis. Arteries of the upper limb tend to be spared.
- Microscopically, plaques have three components:
  - cells: mainly vascular smooth muscle cells, macrophages and lymphocytes
  - connective tissue fibres of collagen, elastin and proteoglycans
  - lipids, mainly cholesterol and oxidized cholesterol in the form of low density lipoproteins. These are quite irritant and have been shown to cause severe inflammatory reactions in connective tissue; may result in periarterial inflammation, fibrosis and lymphocyte infiltration.

Complicated plaques

Typical fibrolipid plaques may undergo several complications, as follows:

- Rupturing or ulceration of the luminal surface may occur. This may result in fat in the fatty part discharging into the bloodstream as so-called 'cholesterol emboli'.
- Thrombosis may occur over ulcerated plaques, which may extend, leading to arterial occlusion, particularly in the coronary circulation.

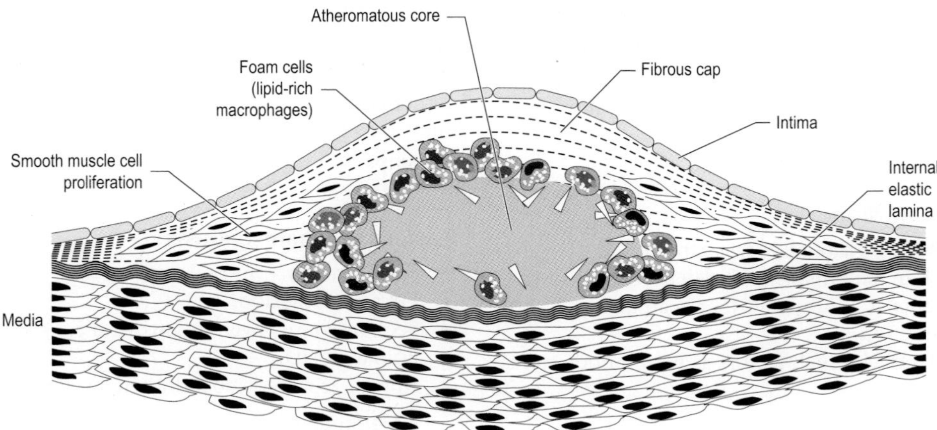

Fig. 22.1 Typical fibrolipid atheromatous plaque.

- Haemorrhage may occur into a plaque because of breakdown of the overlying fibrous cap. This may balloon the plaque, narrowing the lumen, or lead to its rupture.
- Calcification frequently occurs.
- Extensive necrosis of the plaque may occur, which may cause embolism of plaque material, leaving large areas of ulceration.
- May be thinning and weakening of media, which may result in aneurysmal dilatation.

Risk Factors

Predisposing factors to atherosclerosis include:

- increasing age
- male sex
- race
- smoking
- diabetes mellitus
- obesity
- systemic hypertension
- hyperlipidaemia
- family history.

Pathogenesis

Pathogenesis must account for:

- focal nature of the lesion
- the place of risk factors in causation, especially hyperlipidaemia
- the presence of lipids in most lesions
- smooth muscle proliferation, which is an early and characteristic feature.

The various theories of pathogenesis are as follows:

- response to injury, e.g. chemicals from cigarette smoke, cholesterol, hypertension
- increased permeability to lipids
- raised lipids: increased lipid absorption more likely in hyperlipidaemia, and the low density lipoprotein is likely to be oxidized by free radicals at the site of injury where they are absorbed into the intima
- oxidized low density lipoprotein itself is toxic to endothelial cells, and attracts monocytes and macrophages
- smooth muscle proliferation: proliferates under the influence of PGDF
- thrombogenic theory: plaques arise from mural thrombi formed at sites of endothelial injury with subsequent organization.

ISCHAEMIC HEART DISEASE

Ischaemic heart disease (IHD) is the term used for several closely related conditions where the supply of oxygenated blood to the heart is inadequate. Atherosclerotic narrowing is the main cause, but may be aggravated by:

- increased demand due to ventricular hypertrophy
- increased demand due to impaired oxygen transport, e.g. severe anaemia, advanced lung disease, carbon monoxide poisoning.

Four ischaemic syndromes may result, depending on the severity and speed of onset:

- stable angina
- acute coronary syndromes (unstable angina and acute myocardial infarction)
- sudden cardiac death
- ischaemic cardiomyopathy.

Angina of Effort

- Characterized by central chest pain, which may radiate down the left arm, up and into the jaw.

- Caused by a shortage of oxygenated blood supplying the heart muscle, due to increased demand during exercise in the presence of narrowed coronary arteries.

Acute Coronary Syndrome (Unstable Angina and Acute Myocardial Infarction)

Myocardial infarction may be:
- subendocardial
- transmural.

Subendocardial (partial thickness or non-Q-wave infarct)

- Inner third of heart muscle is least well perfused and therefore more vulnerable to reduced coronary flow.
- In subendocardial infarct, although there is usually diffuse coronary arteriosclerosis, there is less commonly superimposed thrombosis.
- Frequently S/T-wave changes but no Q-wave.

Transmural infarction (full thickness or Q-wave infarct)

- More common.
- More serious and usually involves left ventricle.
- May follow disruption of arteriosclerotic plaque with superimposed thrombosis.
- Platelet activation and aggregation responsible for this may be reduced if the patient is on antiplatelet drugs.
- Normally Q-waves on ECG.

Pathological consequences of acute transmural infarct

These are:
- arrhythmia
- acute heart failure
- papillary muscle infarct, leading to rupture with acute mitral regurgitation
- pericarditis
- mural thrombus: may result in peripheral arterial embolus, causing stroke, acutely ischaemic limb or mesenteric ischaemia
- scarring of heart muscle with subsequent ventricular aneurysm
- myocardial rupture, causing intraventricular septal defect, bleeding into the pericardium with tamponade, depending on site of rupture.

Sudden Cardiac Death

- Defined as unexpected death from cardiac cause within an hour of onset of acute symptoms.
- Majority of cases are due to ischaemic heart disease.
- In a small percentage of cases, no cause is found.
- Final cause of death is almost always a lethal arrhythmia.

Ischaemic Cardiomyopathy

- Tends to occur in the elderly.
- Insidious and gradually deteriorating congestive cardiac failure with ECG changes.
- Often a history of angina or myocardial infarction.
- May be due to multiple small infarcts or chronic myocardial ischaemia or a combination of both.
- Histologically the main finding is diffuse myocardial atrophy and interstitial fibrosis.

ANEURYSMS

An aneurysm is abnormal dilatation of an artery. Aneurysms may be classified as:
- true: where the wall is formed totally by the three normal elements of the arterial wall, i.e. intima, media and adventitia
- false: a pulsating haematoma, the cavity of which is in direct continuity with the lumen of an artery, i.e. where the wall is formed by connective tissue which is not part of the vessel wall.

The types of aneurysm are shown in Fig. 22.2.

True Aneurysms

These may be:
- fusiform: dilatation due to a segment of the vessel wall being affected around the whole circumference
- saccular: where only part of the circumference is involved.

Congenital Aneurysms

'Berry' Aneurysms

- Due to congenital defect in media at junction of vessels around the circle of Willis.
- Most common cause of subarachnoid haemorrhage.
- Commonest age of presentation is around 50 years.
- Increased incidence in patients with hypertension.
- Increased incidence in patients with adult polycystic kidney disease.

Acquired Aneurysms

These may be:
- atheromatous
- mycotic
- syphilitic
- dissecting (acute aortic dissection)
- false
- arteriovenous aneurysms (aneurysmal varices).

Atheromatous Aneurysms

These are most common at:
- abdominal aorta
- popliteal artery
- femoral artery.

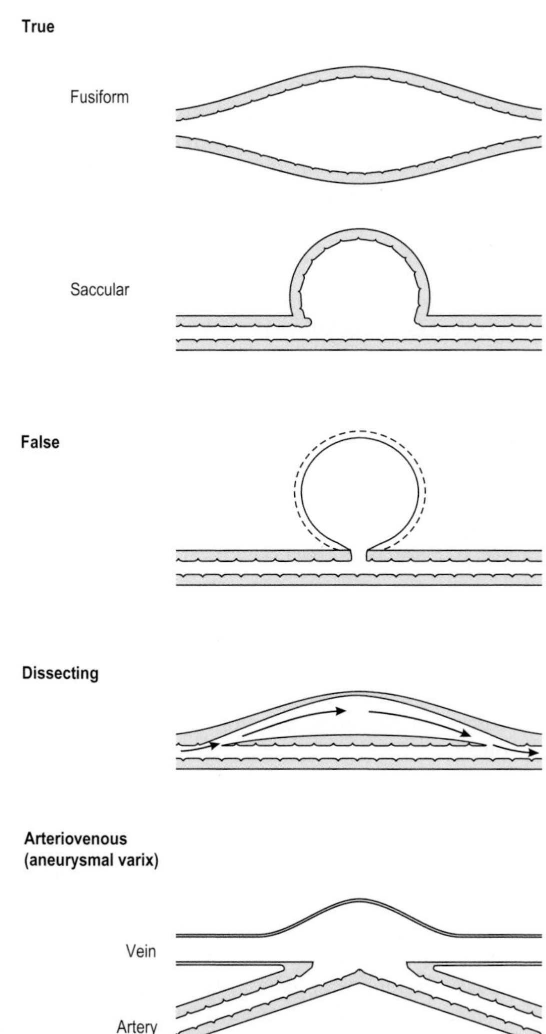

Fig. 22.2 Types of aneurysm.

Abdominal aortic aneurysm

- Incidence is rising.
- Risk factors include smoking and hypertension.
- Main complication is rupture, which may be intraperitoneal, accompanied by rapid death, or retroperitoneal.
- May be a familial tendency.
- May be associated aneurysms of common iliac arteries.
- May also be increased incidence of femoral and popliteal artery aneurysms.

Mycotic Aneurysms

- Commonly associated with subacute infective endocarditis.
- May be due to any form of bacteraemia, e.g. *Salmonella*.
- Usually saccular.

Syphilitic Aneurysms

- Common many years ago but now rare.
- Tend to involve the thoracic aorta, especially the arch.
- Due to endarteritis of vasa vasorum with inflammatory process extending into the media and causing ischaemic damage of the vessel wall.

Dissecting Aneurysm (Acute Aortic Dissection)

- Most common in thoracic aorta.
- Blood enters the diseased media, which splits into two layers.
- Associated with Marfan's syndrome.
- Associated with hypertension.
- Blood enters false lumen and then ruptures, either back into the main lumen of the artery distally, in which case the patient may survive for some time; or externally, with sudden death.
- If it involves the ascending aorta, it may dissect across a coronary ostium, leading to myocardial infarction; or across the aortic valve, causing aortic regurgitation.

False Aneurysm (Pulsating Haematoma)

- Results from a small tear in an artery which is followed by haematoma, the wall of which becomes organized and holds the aneurysm in check for some time before it ruptures.
- May follow stab wounds, intra-arterial injections or intra-arterial radiological procedures.
- Repaired by controlling artery above and below, closing the small defect and evacuating the haematoma.

Arteriovenous Aneurysms

- Sometimes known as aneurysmal varices.
- May be traumatic, but more commonly follow formation of an AV fistula for dialysis.

General Complications of Aneurysms

- Rupture.
- Thrombosis with occlusion, e.g. in popliteal artery aneurysms.
- Distal emboli from mural thrombus.
- Pressure on adjacent structure, e.g. abdominal aortic aneurysm eroding vertebral bodies; femoral aneurysms pressing on femoral nerve; popliteal artery aneurysm compressing popliteal vein leading to DVT.

ENDOCRINE SYSTEM

See also Chapter 12.

Thyroid Disease

Goitre

This is an enlargement of the thyroid gland. Causes range from the physiological, when the gland increases in size as result of increased demand for thyroid hormone, e.g. at puberty, to frank malignant disease. The causes of goitres are shown in Box 22.4.

Hyperthyroidism

Hyperthyroidism (thyrotoxicosis) is a clinical syndrome resulting from the effects of excess circulating T_3 and T_4. Hyperthyroidism results from three main pathological lesions:

- Graves' disease
- functioning adenoma
- toxic nodular goitre.

Clinical features of thyrotoxicosis

- Anxiety.
- Nervousness.
- Irritability.
- Sweating.
- Heat intolerance.
- Insomnia.
- Hair loss.
- Palpitations.
- Menorrhagia.
- Diarrhoea.
- Tremor.
- Eye signs: exophthalmos lid retraction, lid lag.
- Tachycardia.
- Atrial fibrillation.
- Proximal myopathy.
- Pretibial myxoedema.
- Warm, moist palms.
- Hyper-reflexia.
- Osteoporosis.

BOX 22.4 Causes of Goitres

Simple (non-toxic) goitre
Simple hyperplastic goitre
Multinodular goitre

Toxic goitre
Diffuse goitre (Graves' disease)
Toxic nodule
Toxic multinodular goitre

Neoplastic goitre
Benign
Adenoma

Malignant
Papillary
Follicular
Anaplastic
Medullary

Inflammatory
De Quervain's thyroiditis
Riedel's thyroiditis

Autoimmune
Hashimoto's thyroiditis

Hypothyroidism

Hypothyroidism (myxoedema) is the clinical syndrome resulting from inadequate levels of circulating T_3 and T_4. Causes include:

- Hashimoto's thyroiditis
- Iatrogenic:
  - surgical removal of thyroid tissue
  - drugs, e.g. sulfonylureas, lithium, amiodarone.

Clinical Features of Myxoedema

- Slowness of thought, speech and movement.
- Weight gain.
- Cold intolerance.
- Tiredness.
- Lethargy.
- Constipation.
- Loss of hair.
- Menstrual irregularities.
- Dry hair.
- Puffy, swollen face.
- Loss of outer third of eyebrows.
- Ischaemic heart disease.
- Bradycardia.
- Carpal tunnel syndrome.
- Muscle weakness.

Hashimoto's Thyroiditis

- Commonest cause of hypothyroidism.
- Disease of middle age occurring more often in females.
- Association with human leucocyte antigen (HLA), DR5.
- Autoimmune.
- Microscopically, gland is infiltrated by lymphocytes and plasma cells.
- Presents with goitre; patient is usually euthyroid.
- Later, atrophy and fibrosis of gland with development of myxoedema.

Carcinoma of the Thyroid Gland

Carcinoma of the thyroid gland is uncommon, accounting for less than 1% of all cancer deaths. It is associated with:

- radiation exposure, e.g. neck X-rays, or as a result of nuclear fallout
- family history of multiple endocrine neoplasia syndromes IIa and IIb.

There are four types of thyroid carcinoma, which are summarized in Table 22.1.

Clinical presentation

This includes:

- goitre
- dysphagia
- signs of local invasion, e.g. Horner's syndrome, hoarseness
- cervical lymphadenopathy
- pathological fractures due to bone secondaries
- cough due to lung metastases
- rarely, thyrotoxicosis.

Adrenal Disorders

Medulla

Commonest adrenal medullary tumour is a phaeochromocytoma.

- Peak incidence at 30–50 years.
- Male/female ratio is 1 : 1.
- Derived from adrenal medullary chromaffin cells.
- 10–20% of cases are familial and associated with other conditions:
  - MEN IIa
  - MEN IIb
  - neurofibromatosis
  - Von Hippel–Lindau syndrome
  - tuberous sclerosis
  - Sturge–Weber syndrome.
- 10% are extra-adrenal associated with paraganglia.
- Clinical features include:
  - hypertension (occasionally intermittent)
  - pallor
  - headaches
  - sweating and nervousness
  - palpitations
  - abdominal pain.
- Occasionally malignant.
- Curable cause of secondary hypertension.
- Laboratory diagnosis depends on elevated 24 h urine vanillylmandelic acid (VMA) estimation.

Cortex

The adrenal cortex produces the following steroid hormones:

- glucocorticoids (zona fasciculata)
- mineralocorticoids (zona glomerulosa)
- sex steroids (zona reticularis).

Hyperfunction of the Adrenal Cortex

Hyperfunction of the adrenal cortex produces generalized effects, the nature of which depends on whether it is glucocorticoids, mineralocorticoids or sex steroids that are produced in excess.

Cushing's syndrome

- Due to excess glucocorticoids.
- Causes include:
  - iatrogenic: therapeutic administration of glucocorticoids
  - excess ACTH secretion from the pituitary gland
  - adrenal cortical neoplasms
  - ectopic ACTH secretion.

TABLE 22.1 Types of Thyroid Carcinoma

Type	Proportion of all Cases (%)	Age (Years)	Spread	Prognosis
Papillary	65	16–40	Lymphatic Local nodes	Excellent
Follicular	20	40–60	Blood Especially bone	Good
Anaplastic	10	Old age	Locally aggressive Lymph nodes	Very poor
Medullary	5	Over 40 Younger in familial cases	Local, lymph nodes, blood	Variable: poor if bone metastases; more aggressive in familial cases

Systemic features of Cushing's syndrome:

- Moon face.
- Buffalo hump.
- Central obesity.
- Avascular necrosis of bone.
- Stunted growth.
- Proximal myopathy.
- Hypertension.
- Peptic ulceration.
- Hyperglycaemia.
- Menstrual disturbances.
- Stria on the abdomen.
- Acne.
- Cataracts.
- Osteoporosis: pathological fractures.
- Predisposition to infection.
- Thinning of the hair.
- Thinning of the skin.
- Psychosis.

Hyperaldosteronism

Conn's syndrome (primary hyperaldosteronism)

- Due to autonomous secretion of excess aldosterone.
- Usually caused by an adenoma of the zona glomerulosa.
- Increased renal retention of sodium and water leads to hypertension.
- Potassium loss leads to muscular weakness and cardiac arrhythmias.
- Hypokalaemia associated with metabolic alkalosis causing tetany and paraesthesia.
- Diagnosis rests on raised plasma aldosterone while renin is low.

Secondary hyperaldosteronism

- Reduction in renal glomerular perfusion activates the renin–angiotensin system.
- This stimulates aldosterone secretion in an attempt to correct renal glomerular perfusion.
- This is the commonest type of hyperaldosteronism.
- Aldosterone levels raised but are appropriate response to high renin levels.

Hypersecretion of Sex Steroids

- Some adrenal cortical adenomas secrete sex steroids, most commonly androgens.

Hypofunction of the Adrenal Cortex

Adrenocortical hypofunction can be primary, due to lesions within the adrenal gland, or secondary, due to failure of ACTH secretion by the pituitary gland. Causes of chronic primary insufficiency include:

- tuberculosis
- autoimmune disease
- amyloidosis
- haemochromatosis
- metastatic tumours
- atrophy due to prolonged steroid therapy.

Acute insufficiency

- Waterhouse–Friderichsen syndrome: acute haemorrhagic necrosis of the adrenals associated with meningococcal septicaemia.
- Other acute septicaemias, e.g. Gram-negative septicaemia, may cause similar effects.
- May be due to disseminated intravascular coagulation within the adrenal gland.

Chronic insufficiency (Addison's disease)

- Effects of chronic adrenal insufficiency include:
  - anorexia, weight loss, vomiting
  - weakness
  - lethargy
  - hypertension
  - skin pigmentation
  - hyponatraemia with hyperkalaemia
  - chronic dehydration
  - sexual dysfunction.
- During acute illnesses patients may undergo an acute Addisonian crisis with vomiting, dehydration, electrolyte disturbances and circulatory collapse.
- Plasma cortisol levels are low.
- Estimation of ACTH levels enables a distinction to be made between primary adrenocortical insufficiency (ACTH raised) and secondary insufficiency (ACTH low).

Tumours of the Adrenal Cortex

These are:

- adenoma
- carcinoma.

Adenoma

- 'Functioning' adenomas cause Cushing's syndrome or Conn's syndrome.
- Clinically unsuspected 'non-functioning' adenomas may be found in about 2% of adult autopsies or picked up incidentally on CT scans for other conditions.

Carcinoma

- Rare.
- Usually hormone-secreting with a tendency to produce androgens.
- May be extremely large and exhibit invasive growth.

GENITOURINARY SYSTEM

Gynaecological Causes of Acute Abdominal Pain

These include:

- ruptured ectopic pregnancy

- torsion of ovarian cyst
- ruptured ovarian cyst
- salpingitis
- severe dysmenorrhoea
- mittelschmerz
- endometriosis
- torsion or degeneration of a fibroid.

Pelvic Inflammatory Disease

Infection of the fallopian tubes usually involves the ovaries and peritoneum, and the combined infection is called pelvic inflammatory disease (PID).

- Results from ascending infection of organisms from vagina or cervix.
- Most episodes are associated with traditional sexually transmitted disease pathogens, i.e. *Chlamydia* and gonorrhoea.
- Predominantly disease of young, sexually active women.
- Secondary invasion with anaerobes is common, so that a combination of antibiotics is required to cover the spectrum of likely pathogens.
- Associated with tubule damage, leading to ectopic pregnancy or infertility.
- Partner notification is important in management.

Acute Pelvic Inflammatory Disease

Causes are:

- Primary:
  - sexually transmitted diseases
  - *Escherichia coli*, *Bacteroides* or other gut organisms
  - iatrogenic, e.g. following D&C, termination of pregnancy, insertion of an intrauterine contraceptive device
  - after delivery or miscarriage.
- Secondary:
  - direct spread from nearby pelvic organs, e.g. appendicitis or schistosomiasis.
- Pathological consequences of acute pelvic inflammatory disease include:
  - salpingitis
  - pyosalpinx
  - hydrosalpinx
  - acute pelvic peritonitis
  - salpingo-oophoritis
  - tubo-ovarian abscess
  - adhesions.

Sequelae

These include:

- chronic pelvic pain
- subfertility
- ectopic pregnancy
- recurrent PID with:
  - heavy periods
  - dysmenorrhoea
  - dyspareunia
  - chronic pelvic pain due to adhesions
  - infertility.

Chronic Pelvic Inflammatory Disease

This may be due to:

- inadequately treated, recurrent, acute pelvic inflammatory disease
- tuberculosis (rare).

Ovarian Disease

Ovarian lesions present either with pain, due to inflammation, or swelling of the organ. Rarely do they present with the remote effects of endocrine secretion.

Ovarian Cysts

- Both normal follicles and corpus luteum are cystic.
- Retention cysts form frequently and by definition must be >2 cm.
- Luteal cysts may rupture with slight haemorrhage into the peritoneal cavity.
- Follicular cysts have an inner layer of granulosa cells and contain clear fluid; they may be multiple.
- 'Chocolate' cysts of the ovary are a feature of endometriosis.
- Ovarian cysts cause symptoms by either rupture or torsion.

Ovarian Tumours

Ovarian tumours may be divided into five main categories:

- epithelial
- germ cell
- sex-cord stromal
- metastatic
- miscellaneous.

Epithelial tumours

- Majority of ovarian tumours are derived from surface epithelium.
- Several varieties, which depend upon embryonic differentiation.
- Mucinous type may be benign or malignant.
- Benign mucinous cystadenoma may grow to be a very large size, filling the peritoneal cavity, and may be mistaken for ascites.
- Benign tumours may rupture, releasing tumour cells which seed onto the peritoneum and continue to produce mucus (pseudomyxoma peritonei).
- Some tumours are borderline between cystadenoma and cystadenocarcinoma.

- The commonest malignant ovarian tumour is the serous carcinoma:
  - occurs most frequently between 40 and 60 years
  - may be largely cystic (25%), semi-solid (65%) or entirely solid (10%)
  - poor prognosis: 15% 5-year survival.

Germ cell tumours

- May be either benign or malignant.
- Commonest is the benign cystic teratoma (dermoid cyst).
- Dermoid cysts may present at any age, although usually in younger patients.
- Dermoid cysts characteristically contain hair, sebaceous material and teeth, the latter often being apparent on a plain abdominal X-ray.
- May undergo torsion.
- Malignant transformation is rare.

Sex-cord stromal tumours

- About 5% of all ovarian tumours.
- Fibromas comprise about half of that 5%.
- Ovarian fibromas are not associated with steroid hormone production.
- Other sex-cord stromal tumours are associated with steroid hormone production, e.g. thecoma, granulosa cell tumour, Sertoli–Leydig tumours.
- Meigs' syndrome occurs in approximately 1% of patients with ovarian fibromas and includes ascites and pleural effusions which disappear following removal of the ovarian fibroma.

Metastatic tumours

These arise from:

- stomach (Krukenberg tumours)
- large intestine
- breast.

Clinical presentation of ovarian tumours

- Pain.
- Rupture or torsion of a cyst.
- Abdominal mass.
- Ascites: peritoneal seedlings, pseudomyxoma peritonei, Meigs' syndrome.
- Excess hormone production: abnormal uterine bleeding with oestrogen production; virilization due to androgen production.
- Pleural effusion: Meigs' syndrome, lung secondaries, symptoms of other distant metastases.

Ectopic Pregnancy

- Incidence of 10–12 per 1000 pregnancies.
- Risk of recurrence after one ectopic pregnancy is 10–20%.
- Fallopian tube is commonest site.
- May be associated with chronic inflammatory disease in the tubes or intrauterine contraceptive devices (controversial).
- Pain occurs as ectopic pregnancy expands tube.
- Pain and haemorrhage on rupture.
- Pregnancy-associated changes seen in endometrium.

Endometriosis

Endometriosis is the presence of endometrial glands and stroma in sites other than the body of the uterus. Endometriosis may be responsible for:

- pelvic inflammation
- infertility
- pain.

Sites include:

- ovaries (80%)
- round ligaments
- fallopian tubes
- pelvic peritoneum
- intestinal wall
- umbilicus
- laparotomy scars
- lymph nodes (rare)
- lung and pleura (rare)
- synovium (rare).

Clinical features

- Retrograde menstruation may be important in the aetiology of endometriosis in the peritoneal cavity, but cannot explain spread to distant sites.
- Endometrial tissue retains its sensitivity to hormones, and bleeding occurs into the lesions at the time of menstruation.
- Fibrosis may occur at the site of the lesion; in the peritoneal cavity, this may lead to adhesion formation with subsequent obstruction.

Fibroids

Fibroleiomyoma

- Common tumours of smooth muscle origin.
- Grow during reproductive years; regress after the menopause but do not completely disappear.
- Firm, white, whorled, well-circumscribed lesions, which may be submucous, subserosal or intramural.
- Subserosal ones may be pedunculated.
- Aetiology unknown.
- Clinically they may present as follows:
  - abdominal mass
  - abnormal uterine bleeding
  - urinary problems due to pressure on the bladder
  - pain due to complications, e.g. red degeneration, torsion of the pedicle of a pedunculated fibroid.

Complications

- Cystic degeneration.
- Necrosis with haemorrhagic infarction (red degeneration).
- Dystrophic calcification (calcified fibroids may be seen on a plain abdominal X-ray).
- Sarcomatous change extremely rare.

Endometrial Carcinoma

Two types are recognized:

- First type occurs in young women with polycystic ovary syndrome or in perimenopausal women.
- It may complicate post-menopausal oestrogen replacement therapy.
- This type is associated with a good prognosis.
- Second type affects elderly post-menopausal women and is not oestrogen-related.
- It is poorly differentiated with deep myometrial invasion.
- Poor prognosis.

Aetiological factors for endometrial carcinoma include:

- obesity
- hypertension
- diabetes mellitus
- nulliparity
- long-term tamoxifen therapy.

Spread

This occurs:

- by direct extension into pelvis and adjacent viscera
- to the iliac and para-aortic nodes
- via the bloodstream to the liver and lungs.

Urinary Tract Calculi

Urinary calculi occur in 1–5% of the population in the UK. Stones may form in the kidney or bladder. Ureteric calculi are in transit from the kidney to bladder. 90% of calculi are radio-opaque.

Types of Calculi

Calculi are classified according to their composition. The types are:

- Calcium oxalate (75%):
  - ‘mulberry’ stones covered with sharp projections
  - occur in alkaline urine
  - cause bleeding and are often black owing to altered blood on their surface
  - because of their sharp surface they give symptoms when comparatively small.
- Magnesium ammonium phosphate (struvite) stones (15%):
  - smooth and dirty white
  - may enlarge rapidly and fill the calyces, taking on their shape, i.e. staghorn calculus
  - occur in strongly alkaline urine.
- Urate (5%):
  - arise in acid urine
  - hard, smooth, faceted and light brown in colour
  - radiolucent.
- Cystine (2%):
  - usually multiple
  - arise in acid urine
  - are of metabolic origin, owing to decreased reabsorption of cystine from the renal tubules
  - white and translucent
  - radio-opaque because of their sulfur content.
- Xanthine and pyruvate stones:
  - rare
  - due to inborn error of metabolism.

Precipitating Factors

These include:

- diet
- dehydration
- stasis
- infection
- hyperparathyroidism
- idiopathic hypercalciuria
- milk-alkali syndrome
- hypervitaminosis D
- cystinuria
- inborn errors of purine metabolism
- gout
- chemotherapy (excess uric acid following treatment of leukaemia or polycythaemia).

Sites

Renal pelvis

- Solitary or multiple.
- Unilateral or bilateral.
- Small stones are commonest, but large-branched ‘staghorn’ calculi may occur and completely fill the pelvis and calyces.

Bladder

- Bladder stones may originate in the kidney with subsequent enlargement in the bladder due to phosphate encrustation.
- Formed primarily in the bladder, usually of phosphates.

Ureteric and urethral stones

- Ureteric stones in transit from kidney to bladder.
- Urethral stones in transit from bladder to outside.

Clinical Effects

These are:

- Obstruction:
  - at the pelviureteric junction
  - in the ureter

- at the bladder neck
  - rarely at the external urethral meatus.
- Ulceration:
  - of calyces, pelvic mucosa or bladder, causing haematuria.
- Chronic infection, e.g. pyelonephritis, pyonephrosis.

Urinary Tract Infections (UTIs)

These may be divided into those affecting the kidney (pyelonephritis) and those affecting the bladder (cystitis). UTIs are more common in women and the majority of women will have had a UTI at some time during their life. Risk factors include:

- pregnancy
- urinary tract malformations
- urinary tract obstruction
- calculi
- prostatic obstruction
- bladder diverticulum
- spinal injury
- trauma
- urinary tract tumour
- diabetes mellitus
- immunosuppression.

Acute Pyelonephritis

Infection of the kidney by pyogenic organisms.

Pathogenesis

- Haematogenous spread.
- Retrograde ureteric spread.
- Organisms include *E. coli*, *Proteus*, *Enterobacter*, *Klebsiella*, *Pseudomonas* and faecal streptococci.

Clinical features

These include:

- malaise
- fever
- dysuria
- urgency of micturition
- pain and tenderness in the loin.

Complications

These include:

- renal papillary necrosis
- pyonephrosis
- perinephric abscess.

Chronic Pyelonephritis

Chronic pyelonephritis occurs in association with:

- vesicoureteric reflux, either due to congenital lesions or occurring in early life
- obstruction developing during childhood.

Clinical features

- Vesicoureteric reflux is associated with abnormal entry of the ureter into the bladder.
- Reflux of urine into the kidney during micturition raises intrapelvic and intracalyceal pressure.
- The presence of infection accelerates scarring, due to reflux.
- End result is scarring of the kidney with interstitial fibrosis.
- Atrophic and dilated tubules containing eosinophilic casts, giving the appearance of 'thyroidization' of the kidney.
- Unless vesicoureteric reflux is successfully corrected, the condition may proceed to chronic renal failure and need for dialysis and transplantation.

Cystitis

Inflammation of the bladder (cystitis) is a common occurrence as part of a urinary tract infection.

Aetiology

- Causative organism usually derived from patient's faecal flora, e.g. *E. coli*, *Proteus* and *Klebsiella*.
- Mostly due to retrograde spread of the organisms along urethra.
- 20–30% of women will have bacterial cystitis at some time during their lives.
- Predisposing factors in females:
  - short urethra
  - urethral trauma during sexual intercourse
  - pregnancy.
- Instrumentation of the urinary tract in both sexes increases both the incidence and variety of infecting organisms.
- Other organisms include *Candida* in immunosuppressed patients or patients on prolonged antibiotic therapy; tuberculous cystitis always reflects tuberculosis elsewhere in the urinary tract.
- Irradiation, trauma due to instrumentation and drugs (e.g. cyclophosphamide) may cause cystitis, which is often sterile.

Clinical features

These include:

- frequency
- lower abdominal pain
- dysuria
- occasionally haematuria
- general malaise and pyrexia in some patients.

Sterile Pyuria

Pus cells are apparent on microscopy but there is no growth on culture. Causes include:

- inadequately treated UTI

- tuberculosis
- tumour
- stone
- prostatitis
- polycystic kidneys
- appendicitis (appendix adheres to and 'irritates' the bladder)
- diverticulitis (adheres to bladder)
- analgesic abuse.

Urinary Tract Tuberculosis

This has shown a decline in the past 30 years but remains a problem in the Third World and in immigrant populations in the UK. Features include:

- always secondary to TB elsewhere
- urinary tract is involved by haematogenous spread
- kidney is affected most frequently
- lower urinary tract secondarily infected by descending infection, giving rise to cystitis or infection of the epididymis or seminal vesicles.

Clinical features

- Often silent.
- Repeated UTIs with frequency, dysuria, haematuria.
- Occasionally dull loin pain.
- Weight loss, fever, night sweats.
- Symptoms of uraemia.
- Epididymitis.
- Scrotal sinuses.

Tumours of the Urinary Tract

Kidney

Tumours of the kidney include:

- benign:
  - adenoma
  - angiomyolipoma
- malignant:
  - Wilms' tumour (nephroblastoma)
  - renal cell carcinoma (hypernephroma)
  - transitional cell carcinoma of renal pelvis.

Benign Neoplasms

Cortical adenoma

- Commonest benign tumour of kidney.
- Usually small, <2 cm in diameter.
- Distinction from well-differentiated adenocarcinoma not easy.
- Lesions <3 cm are classified as adenoma.
- Those >3 cm are classified as carcinoma.
- Malignancy may develop in cortical adenomas.

Angiomyolipoma

- Intrarenal mass composed of mixture of blood vessels, muscle and mature fat.
- Best regarded as hamartoma.
- 40% associated with tuberous sclerosis.
- May be painful if there is intralesional haemorrhage.

Malignant Renal Tumours

Wilms' tumour

- Commonest renal tumour of childhood.
- Peak incidence 1–4 years.
- Commonest clinical presentation is with an abdominal mass.
- Other presentations include haematuria, hypertension, abdominal pain and intestinal obstruction.
- Aggressive tumour – rapidly growing, spread to lungs often present at time of diagnosis.
- Spread occurs as follows:
  - into renal parenchyma and perinephric tissues
  - lymphatic to regional lymph nodes
  - blood: commonly to lung, less frequently to liver, peritoneum, and rarely to bone.
- Prognosis: over 90% survival due to aggressive therapy involving radiotherapy, chemotherapy and surgery.

Renal cell carcinoma (hypernephroma, Grawitz tumour)

This is the commonest primary kidney tumour in adults.

Aetiology

- Smoking
- Genetic predisposition in von Hippel–Lindau disease.

Clinical presentation

This includes:

- Haematuria.
- Loin pain.
- Loin mass.
- Paraneoplastic manifestations:
  - pyrexia of unknown origin
  - polycythaemia from erythropoietin production
  - hypercalcaemia
  - hypertension.
- Left-sided tumour may present with varicocele due to invasion of the left renal vein with tumour and obstruction of the left testicular vein.

Spread

- Direct into renal parenchyma, renal pelvis and perinephric tissues.
- Lymphatic: 30% have tumour in para-aortic nodes at presentation.
- Blood: lungs (cannon-ball metastases), bone.

Prognosis

- Depends on staging and differentiation.
- If tumour is localized to kidney, nephrectomy offers a 5-year survival rate of 70%.

Transitional cell carcinoma of renal pelvis

These form 5–10% of renal tumours and arise from the urothelium of the renal pelvis.

Aetiology

- Analgesic abuse.
- Exposure to aniline dyes used in the dye, rubber, plastics and gas industries.

Clinicopathological features

- May present with:
  - haematuria
  - infection secondary to hydronephrosis
  - ureteric colic due to obstruction or clot.
- In presence of pelvic stones, urothelium may undergo squamous metaplasia. Squamous cell carcinoma may subsequently develop, and is known to be associated with calculi and chronic infection.
- Tumours may seed down the ureter and involve the bladder.

Bladder Tumours

Epithelial tumours of the bladder are common. The majority are transitional cell carcinomas but a small proportion are squamous. Adenocarcinoma of the bladder is uncommon.

Aetiology

- Chemical substances – seen particularly in aniline dye and synthetic rubber workers; chemical substances implicated include β-naphthylamine and benzadine; dyes used in textiles, printing, rubber, and cable and plastic industries.
- Smoking.
- Schistosomiasis.
- Leucoplakia: associated with squamous cell carcinoma.
- Bladder diverticulum: tumour complicates about 2% of diverticulae.
- Ectopia vesicae: adenocarcinoma may complicate this condition.

Transitional Cell Carcinoma

Transitional cell carcinomas arise from the urothelium and are frequently multiple. Carcinoma is often preceded by dysplasia.

Clinical features

- Painless haematuria commonest presenting feature.
- Dysuria.
- Frequency and urgency.
- Obstruction with unilateral pyelonephritis or hydronephrosis if tumour obstructs ureteric orifice.
- Urethral obstruction: retention of urine.
- Extension to other organs: fistula formation; vesicocolic fistula with pneumaturia; vesico-vaginal fistula with incontinence.

Staging and grading

- Transitional cell carcinomas are graded I–III according to degree of cytological atypia.
- Grading is a guide to prognosis.
- TNM staging is also used to judge prognosis.
- Good correlation between grade and stage.
- Majority of papillary growth are grade I and non-invasive.
- Grade III lesions are usually flat, ulcerated, invasive and carry a poor prognosis.

Squamous Cell Carcinoma

These arise from metaplastic squamous epithelium. Metaplasia occurs most often in association with:

- calculi
- schistosomiasis.

Clinicopathological features

- Solid invasive tumours.
- Prognosis is not as good as for transitional carcinoma.

Conditions of the Urethra

Urethral obstruction

- Extrinsic compression by prostate gland enlargement.
- Intrinsic lesions include:
  - congenital valves
  - rupture
  - stricture.

Urethritis

May be associated with:

- More proximal infection in the urinary tract.
- Adjacent to a local urethral lesion, e.g. calculus.
- Indwelling urinary catheter.
- Sexually transmitted infection:
  - gonococcal urethritis
  - non-gonococcal (non-specific) urethritis.

Gonococcal urethritis

- A purulent infection due to *Neisseria gonorrhoeae*.
- Bacteria multiply on urethral mucosa and invade periurethral glands in male and endocervix and Bartholin's glands in female.
- Yellow, purulent discharge 3–8 days after initial infection.
- Organisms may be seen as Gram-negative intracellular diplococci in Gram stain of smears.

Course and complications

- May resolve in 2–4 weeks, either spontaneously or following treatment.
- May progress to chronic infection with abscesses and fibrosis, leading to urethral stricture in males.
- Important cause of pelvic inflammatory disease in females.
- Systemic spread is rare, but may produce suppurative arthritis, tenosynovitis, skin rashes and endocarditis.

Non-gonococcal (non-specific urethritis)

- Commonest sexually transmitted disease.
- Mucopurulent urethral discharge and dysuria develop within a few days of infection in males.
- Discharge contains pus cells but gonococci cannot be identified.
- Commonest organisms are *Chlamydia*, *Trachomatosis* and *Ureaplasma urealyticum*.

Tumours

Tumours of the urethra include:

- viral condyloma
- transitional cell carcinoma.

Viral condyloma

- Viral warts in penile urethra.
- Caused by human papillomavirus.
- Relation to neoplasia uncertain.

Transitional cell carcinoma

- Papillary transitional cell carcinoma may rarely develop in urethra.
- Often in association with similar tumour in bladder.
- May develop as a result of tumour implantation in the urethra following instrumentation of the bladder.

Conditions of the Penis

These include:

- congenital malformations
- tumours
- infections.

Congenital Lesions

These include:

- hypospadias
- epispadias.

Hypospadias

- Due to failure of fusion of urethral folds over urogenital sinus.
- Urethra does not reach tip of penis but opens on inferior aspect.
- Commonest site of meatus is on inferior aspect of glans.

Epispadias

- Much less common than hypospadias.
- Urethra opens onto dorsum of penis.
- Results in urinary incontinence and infections.
- Sometimes associated with extrophy of the bladder.

Inflammation and Infections

Balanoposthitis

- Inflammation of the prepuce is posthitis.
- Inflammation of the glans is balanitis.
- Balanoposthitis often associated with tight prepuce (phimosis).
- Bacteria include staphylococci, coliforms or gonococci.
- In diabetic and immunosuppressed patients, *Candida* infection is a further risk.
- Redness and swelling of prepuce and glans associated with purulent exudate.
- Scarring may occur with formation of preputial adhesions or severe phimosis.

Phimosis

- Prepuce cannot be retracted over glans penis.
- In most cases it is an acquired lesion as a late sequel of ammoniacal preputial dermatitis in infancy.
- Prepuce may 'balloon' on micturition.
- Indication for circumcision.

Paraphimosis

- Tight prepuce retracted behind glans may not be reducible, and causes obstruction of venous return from glans and prepuce.
- Oedematous swelling of glans and prepuce.
- Requires circumcision.

Balanitis xerotica obliterans

- Affects 30–50-year age group.
- Uncommon.
- Thickened white plaques and fissures on glans and prepuce.
- Non-retractile prepuce or preputial discharge.
- Requires circumcision.

Genital herpes

- Acute infectious disease caused by herpes simplex virus (HSV).
- Usually HSV type II as sexually transmitted disease.
- Acute vesicular eruption on glans penis or in coronal sulcus.
- Vesicles produce shallow, painful ulcers.

Genital warts

- Prevalence increasing.
- Caused by human papillomavirus (HPV6, HPV11).
- Warts (condylomata acuminata) occur usually on glans but may occur in urethra, penile shaft, perineum and around anus.
- Clinical diagnosis is usually obvious.
- High incidence of recurrence.

Tumours of the Penis

These include:

- Intraepidermal carcinoma:
  - Bowen's disease on the foreskin
  - erythroplasia of Queyrat (on the glans).
- Invasive squamous carcinoma.

Invasive squamous carcinoma

- Rare in UK.
- Only occurs in uncircumcised men.
- May follow premalignant conditions described above.
- Presents clinically as an indurated nodule or plaque which later ulcerates.
- May be hidden under the foreskin and eventually produces an offensive purulent discharge.
- Spread:
  - direct: through prepuce and proximally along shaft of penis
  - lymphatic: to inguinal nodes
  - blood spread is uncommon.
- Prognosis:
  - if lymph nodes free of tumour, 80–90% 5-year survival occurs following amputation
  - prognosis poor with node involvement.

Conditions of the Prostate

Prostatitis

This may be:

- acute suppurative prostatitis: caused by coliforms, gonococcus, *Staphylococcus*
- chronic non-specific prostatitis
- granulomatous prostatitis: idiopathic, tuberculous; following transurethral resection.

Acute suppurative prostatitis

- Usually from spread of infection along prostatic ducts secondary to urethritis or cystitis.
- Common causative organisms include coliforms, staphylococci and gonococci.
- May follow urethral catheterization or endoscopy.
- May be blood-borne.
- Clinically characterized by fever, rigors, low back pain, dysuria, perineal pain. Prostate palpably enlarged, often tender.
- Prostatic abscess may occur with discharge into urethra.

Chronic non-specific prostatitis

- May develop from recurrent episodes of acute infective prostatitis. Organisms include *E. coli*, *Chlamydia* and *Ureaplasma*.
- Clinical features include:
  - symptoms of UTI, dull perineal ache, normal or indurated irregular prostate
  - bacterial infections can be diagnosed by culture of urine following prostatic massage.

Benign prostatic hypertrophy

- A common non-neoplastic lesion of the prostate.
- Involves periurethral zone.
- Nodular hyperplasia of glands and stroma.
- Not premalignant.
- Affects most men over the age of 50, but only 10% present with symptoms.
- Severity of symptoms depends on degree of encroachment on prostatic urethra.
- Clinical features include:
  - cardinal symptoms are difficulty in starting micturition and a poor stream of urine
  - nocturia
  - frequency
  - dribbling
  - incontinence
  - acute retention
  - haematuria from ruptured dilated bladder neck veins
  - occasionally, palpable bladder.
- Examination reveals smooth enlarged prostate, midline sulcus, enlarged lateral lobes.

Complications

These include:

- hypertrophy of bladder muscle with trabeculation
- hydroureter with reflux of urine
- hydronephrosis
- pyonephrosis
- pyelonephritis and impaired renal function.

Carcinoma of the Prostate

This is one of the commonest forms of malignant disease and is the second leading cause of male deaths from malignancy in Europe and the USA. The tumour is rare below the age of 50 years, the peak incidence being between 60 and 85 years.

Aetiology

- Largely unknown.
- Possibly related to changes in circulating androgen levels.
- Family history: 2- to 3-fold risk of tumour developing in men with first-degree relatives in whom prostatic carcinoma was diagnosed under the age of 50 years.
- Rare in eunuchs.

Clinicopathological types

Two clinicopathological types are recognized, which differ in their behaviour:

- clinical (symptomatic) carcinoma
- latent (incidental) carcinoma.

Clinical (symptomatic) carcinoma

- Arises in posterior subcapsular area of gland.
- Adenocarcinoma.

- Invades stroma.
- Asymmetrical, hard, irregular enlargement of prostate palpable per rectum.
- Metastasizes, especially to bone.

Latent (incidental) carcinoma

- Microscopic focus of tumour found incidentally, e.g. at histological examination of prostatectomy specimens removed for benign hyperplasia or at autopsy.
- Common; incidence high in old age.
- Dormant lesions; metastases in 30% after 10 years.

Spread

Spread of prostatic carcinoma may be:

- direct: stromal invasion through the prostatic capsule, urethra, bladder base, seminal vesicles
- via lymphatics to sacral, iliac and para-aortic nodes
- via blood to bone (pelvis, lumbosacral spine, femur), lungs, liver.

Clinical presentation and features

Clinical presentation and features of prostatic carcinoma include:

- urinary symptoms: dysuria, haematuria, hesitancy, dribbling, retention, incontinence
- bone metastases: pain, pathological fractures, anaemia
- rectal examination revealing hard, craggy prostate.

Prognosis

- Variable.
- Dependent on stage at presentation.
- Patients with clinically localized tumours treated radically may expect normal life expectancy.
- Those with metastatic disease at presentation have a median 3-year survival.

GASTROINTESTINAL SYSTEM

Carcinoma of the Oesophagus

Carcinoma of the oesophagus accounts for about 2% of all malignant disease in the UK. Incidence is increasing worldwide. There is considerable geographical variation in its incidence, being 300 times higher around the Caspian Sea than in the UK.

Causes

These include:

- High dietary intake of tannic acid, e.g. in strong tea.
- Dietary deficiency of vitamin A.
- Dietary deficiency of riboflavin.
- Dietary deficiency of zinc.
- Fungal contamination of food.
- Opium ingestion.
- Thermal injury.
- Possible association with cigarette smoking and drinking spirits.
- Higher incidence in patients with Barrett's oesophagus.
- Oesophageal stasis may increase risk of carcinoma:
    - 22-fold increase with lye strictures
    - 9-fold increase with oesophageal webs
    - 7-fold increase in achalasia
    - 6-fold increase with peptic strictures
    - post-cricoid carcinoma usually occurs in females and is part of the Plummer–Vinson syndrome.

Types

- Most are squamous cell carcinomas.
- In the lower third, adenocarcinomas are the predominant type.
- Squamous cell carcinoma usually commences as an ulcer, spreading to become annular and constricting, causing dysphagia.
- Dysplasia usually precedes malignant change.

Spread

- Lymphatic spread occurs within submucosa beyond the recognizable margins of the tumour viewed endoscopically.
- Lymphatic metastases occur early to local lymph nodes.
- Local spread within the mediastinum may result in tracheo-oesophageal fistula, pleural effusion, superior vena caval obstruction.
- Haematogenous spread occurs to lung and liver.

Prognosis

- At time of presentation, spread has usually occurred to adjacent organs.
- Surgical resection possible in only 30–40%.
- Prognosis extremely poor: most patients survive less than 6 months.
- 5-year survival only 5%.

Peptic Ulcer Disease

A peptic ulcer is a breach of the epithelial surface of the gastrointestinal tract due to attack by acid and pepsin. Peptic ulcers may occur in the:

- stomach (common on lesser curve)
- duodenum (anterior or posterior aspect of first part of duodenum)
- lower oesophagus
- gastrojejunal anastomosis, following past surgery for duodenal ulcer
- Meckel's diverticulum (containing gastric mucosa).

Peptic ulcers may be acute or chronic.

Acute Peptic Ulceration

- Part of acute gastritis as a response to severe stress.

- Due to severe hyperacidity such as Zollinger–Ellison syndrome.
- Acute ulcers arising following acute gastritis are usually a consequence of:
  - steroids
  - non-steroidal anti-inflammatory drugs
  - alcohol.
- Stress-induced ulcers may follow:
  - severe sepsis
  - acute pancreatitis
  - major trauma
  - head injury (Cushing's ulcer)
  - burns (Curling's ulcer).

Chronic Peptic Ulceration

Chronic peptic ulceration occurs when the action of acid and pepsin is not opposed by adequate mucosal protection mechanisms. The mucosal defences against acid attack consist of a mucus–bicarbonate barrier and the surface epithelium. Several factors show an association with peptic ulceration:

- acid hypersecretion
- *Helicobacter*-associated gastroduodenitis
- non-steroidal anti-inflammatory drugs
- steroids
- smoking
- alcohol
- diet
- stress.

An increased incidence of peptic ulceration, especially duodenal ulceration, has been associated with:

- uraemia
- hyperparathyroidism
- hypercalcaemia
- chronic obstructive pulmonary disease
- alcoholic cirrhosis.

Complications of peptic ulcer

These include:

- perforation, resulting in peritonitis
- bleeding, due to erosion of vessel in the base of an ulcer
- penetration into underlying structures, e.g. pancreas, liver
- scarring: this may result in pyloric stenosis
- malignant change: this may occur rarely in gastric ulcers but never in duodenal ulcers.

Carcinoma of the Stomach

Gastric cancer is the second most common fatal malignancy (after lung cancer) in the world. There is a high incidence in Japan, China, Colombia and Finland, but in these countries as elsewhere in the world, the incidence of carcinoma of the stomach is declining.

Aetiology

- Nitrosamines: possible relationship between high levels of nitrates in the diet and carcinoma. Nitrates converted to nitrites, which ultimately lead to potential carcinogenic *N*-nitroso compounds.
- High-salt diet.
- High vegetable content in diet: vegetables contain antioxidants such as vitamin C and vitamin E.
- High intake of animal fat and proteins.
- High intake of refined carbohydrate.
- Cigarette smoking.
- Blood group A.
- Only 4% of patients with gastric cancers have a family history of the disease.

Conditions associated with an increased risk of gastric cancer are:

- Achlorhydria
  - due to chronic gastritis
  - autoimmune
  - *Helicobacter*-associated.
- Following partial gastrectomy, risk is increased 3- to 6-fold, with peak 20–30 years after surgery.
- Intestinal metaplasia.
- Epithelial dysplasia.
- Ménétrier's disease.

Pathogenesis

Gastric cancer is believed to develop by a sequence of pathological changes:

Normal mucosa → chronic gastritis → intestinal metaplasia → dysplasia → intramucosal carcinoma → invasive gastric carcinoma

Classification

Gastric cancers are classified on the basis of their direct spread through the stomach wall as:

- early
- advanced.

Early

- Confined to either mucosa or submucosa.
- Increased diagnosis at this stage due to routine endoscopies and introduction of screening, e.g. in Japan, where the number of early cases has increased from 4% to 30%.
- Early gastric cancer has a 5-year survival of 80–100%.

Advanced

- Cancer extending beyond muscularis propria.
- More than 80% of gastric cancers in the UK are in this category.
- Mainly in prepyloric region, pyloric antrum and lesser curve.

- Macroscopically, three types are recognized:
  - ulcerating
  - nodular or fungating
  - infiltrating.
- Spread:
  - direct to adjacent organs, e.g. pancreas
  - lymphatic: initially to local lymph nodes along the right and left gastric artery, then to coeliac glands; retrograde spread to nodes at the porta hepatis (obstructive jaundice); distal nodes, e.g. to left supraclavicular fossa (Virchow's node, Troisier's sign)
  - blood: usually via portal vein to liver
  - transcoelomic, e.g. to ovaries (Krukenberg tumours).

  Prognosis: overall 5-year survival 10%.

Hepatobiliary Disorders

Jaundice

Jaundice is yellow discoloration of the tissues, noticed especially in the skin and sclera due to the accumulation of bilirubin. Jaundice is clinically apparent when the circulating level of bilirubin is in excess of 35 μmol/L. Jaundice may be:

- prehepatic (due to haemolysis)
- hepatic (due to intrinsic liver disease)
- cholestatic (due to either intrahepatic cholestasis or posthepatic biliary obstruction). The causes of jaundice are shown in Box 22.5.

BOX 22.5 Causes of jaundice

Prehepatic (unconjugated hyperbilirubinaemia)
Congenital defects
Gilbert's disease
Crigler–Najjar syndrome

Haemolysis
Congenital red cell defects
Hereditary spherocytosis (congenital acholuric jaundice)
Sickle cell disease
G6PD deficiency
Thalassaemia

Acquired red cell defects
Malaria
Incompatible blood transfusion
Autoimmune
Haemolytic disease of the newborn
Absorbing large haematoma
Hypersplenism

Hepatic
Acute hepatocellular disease
Viral hepatitis
Hepatitis A, B, C
Epstein–Barr virus
CMV

Other infections
Leptospirosis
Drugs, e.g. paracetamol, halothane
Toxins, e.g. carbon tetrachloride
Autoimmune
Chronic hepatocellular disease
Chronic viral hepatitis
Chronic autoimmune hepatitis
End-stage liver disease
Alcohol
Cirrhosis
Haemochromatosis
Wilson's disease

Cholestatic
Intrahepatic
Drugs, e.g. chlorpromazine
Total parenteral nutrition (TPN)
Primary biliary cirrhosis
Viral hepatitis
Pregnancy

Extrahepatic (obstructive)
In the lumen
Gallstones
Infestation: clonorchiasis (liver fluke); schistosomiasis

In the wall
Congenital biliary atresia
Cholangiocarcinoma
Stricture, e.g. inflammatory, post-operative
Cholangitis
Sclerosing cholangitis
Choledochal cyst

Outside the wall
Carcinoma of the head of the pancreas
Carcinoma of the ampulla of Vater
Malignant nodes in the porta hepatis
Chronic pancreatitis
Mirizzi syndrome

Gall Bladder

Gallstones (cholelithiasis)

Gallstones are common, found in 10–15% of patients.

Aetiology

Predisposing factors include:

- sex: more common in females; multiple pregnancies may also increase predisposition
- age: incidence increases with age
- diet/obesity: possibly related to increased cholesterol secretion from liver
- gastrointestinal disease: affecting terminal ileum, which interferes with enterohepatic circulation of bile salts – Crohn's disease; intestinal resection
- drugs: clofibrate and oestrogens
- geographical: high incidence in developed countries, e.g. Europe, North America
- haemolytic disease: increased incidence of pigment stones – sickle cell disease, thalassaemia, hereditary spherocytosis.

Types of stone

- Mixed:
  - 80% are mixed
  - predominantly cholesterol with small amounts of calcium and bile pigments
  - characteristically multiple with faceted surface and laminated on cross-section.
- Pure cholesterol stones:
  - 10% of stones
  - usually solitary
  - up to 5 cm in diameter
  - radial arrangement of crystals on cross-section
  - usually form in bile, which is supersaturated with cholesterol.
- Pigment stones:
  - 10% of stones
  - composed of calcium bilirubinate
  - usually multiple, small and black in colour.

Pathological consequences of gallstones

These are:

- inflammation of gall bladder: acute cholecystitis, chronic cholecystitis, acute-on-chronic cholecystitis
- obstructive jaundice due to impaction of a stone at the lower end of the common bile duct; secondary biliary cirrhosis may result
- ascending cholangitis
- empyema of the gall bladder
- mucocoele
- gallstone ileus: a fistula occurs between the gall bladder and duodenum, and a large stone enters the small bowel, causing obstruction usually at the terminal ileum
- acute pancreatitis, usually associated with multiple small stones
- carcinoma of the gall bladder
- perforation of the gall bladder.

Acute cholecystitis

- Usually associated with stones.
- Occasionally occurs without stones, i.e. acalculous cholecystitis.
- Acalculous cholecystitis may be due to infection with *E. coli*, clostridia or rarely *Salmonella typhi*.
- Acalculous cholecystitis may occur after prolonged starvation or TPN; stasis is probably a contributing factor.
- Gall bladder becomes oedematous with mucosal ulceration and fibropurulent exudate.
- Cystic artery may thrombose but gangrene is rare, as gall bladder gains a second blood supply from the liver directly via the gall bladder.
- Occasionally gangrene does occur with perforation.
- Suppuration may occur with formation of empyema.
- Occasionally gall bladder may fistulate into second part of duodenum.

Chronic cholecystitis

- Invariably associated with gallstones.
- May develop after several episodes of acute cholecystitis.
- More often develops insidiously without any preceding clinically evident acute attacks.
- Gall bladder wall becomes thickened, fibrotic and relatively indistensible.
- Glandular outpouchings are formed by the lining of the mucosa and are known as Rokitansky–Aschoff sinuses.
- Obstructive jaundice may occur if stone impacts in common bile duct.
- Gall bladder does not usually distend as the wall is relatively rigid due to fibrosis consequent on chronic cholecystitis.

Mucocoele

- Due to impaction of stone in neck of gall bladder or cystic duct without super-added infection.
- Bile absorbed from gall bladder and mucus is secreted into it from mucus-secreting cells of epithelium.
- Lack of inflammation in wall allows gall bladder to distend to several times its normal size.

Empyema

- Due to impaction of stone in neck of gall bladder or cystic duct with super-added infection.
- Gall bladder full of pus.
- In 50% of cases organisms cannot be cultured from the pus.
- May result from:

- acute cholecystitis
- infection of mucocoele.

Cholesterolosis

- Lipid-laden macrophages accumulate in gall bladder wall, producing yellowish flecks in red mucosa – 'strawberry' gall bladder.
- Often asymptomatic but may accompany or predispose to cholesterol stones.

Pancreatitis

Acute pancreatitis

Acute pancreatitis is an acute inflammatory process caused by the effects of enzymes released from the pancreatic acini. Aetiological factors include:

- gallstone disease
- chronic alcoholism
- infection, e.g. mumps, Coxsackie virus, typhoid
- hypercalcaemia, e.g. hyperparathyroidism
- trauma
- post-operative, e.g. after upper GI operations where pancreas is handled
- hyperlipidaemia
- drugs: corticosteroids, oestrogen-containing contraceptives, azathioprine, thiazide diuretics
- hypothermia
- vascular insufficiency, e.g. shock, polyarteritis nodosa
- scorpion bites
- iatrogenic, e.g. after ERCP.

Pathogenesis

- Duct obstruction: may lead to reflux of bile into the pancreatic ducts causing injury; increased intraductal pressure may damage pancreatic acini, leading to leakage of pancreatic enzymes with further damage to pancreas.
- Direct acinar damage: due to viruses, bacteria, drugs or trauma.
- Protease release causes widespread destruction of pancreas and increases further enzyme release with consequent further damage.
- Lipase causes fat necrosis, resulting in characteristic yellowish-white flecks on the pancreas, mesentery and omentum, often with calcium deposition (fat necrosis).
- Elastase destroys blood vessels, leading to haemorrhage within the pancreas and haemorrhagic exudate into the peritoneum.
- Haemorrhage may be extensive, leading to acute haemorrhagic pancreatitis.

Biochemical changes

- Increased serum amylase: released from damaged acini into bloodstream.
- Hypocalcaemia: arises because of deposition of calcium in areas of fat necrosis.
- Hyperglycaemia: occurs because of associated damage to pancreatic islets.
- Abnormal liver function tests, especially raised bilirubin and alkaline phosphatase, due to mild obstruction of bile ducts by oedema.

Complications

These include:

- pancreatic pseudocyst: localized collection of fluid in lesser sac of peritoneum
- pancreatic abscess
- stress-induced gastric erosions with haematemesis or melaena
- acute renal failure
- toxic psychosis
- multiple organ failure
- chronic pancreatitis.

Prognosis

- Overall mortality 10–20%.
- Severe haemorrhagic pancreatitis has mortality rate of 50%.
- Usual cause of mortality is multiple organ failure.

Chronic pancreatitis

Chronic pancreatitis is a relapsing disorder which may arise insidiously or follow repeated attacks of acute pancreatitis. Aetiological factors include:

- Chronic alcoholism (70–85%).
- Biliary tract disease.
- Cystic fibrosis.
- Rare familial pancreatitis inherited as an autosomal dominant.
- Pathological changes include parenchymal destruction, fibrosis, loss of acini and duct stenosis with dilatation behind the stenosis.
- Calcification may be seen on plain abdominal X-ray.
- Clinical effects include:
  - abdominal pain
  - malabsorption resulting in steatorrhoea, hypoalbuminaemia and weight loss
  - diabetes mellitus
  - jaundice
  - pancreatic calcification.

Carcinoma of the Pancreas

Pancreatic cancer is increasing in incidence in many countries. It accounts for about 5% of deaths from cancer in the UK.

Aetiology

Factors include:

- cigarette smoking
- high-fat diet
- diabetes mellitus
- familial pancreatitis.

Clinical features

- About two-thirds arise in the head of the pancreas.
- Carcinomas of the head of the pancreas may present with obstructive jaundice.
- Carcinomas at other sites may be symptomless until they invade local organs, e.g. vertebral column, stomach, colon.
- Weight loss.
- Thrombophlebitis migrans, i.e. Trousseau's sign.

Prognosis

- Poor: 5-year survival 2%.

Portal Hypertension

Cirrhosis is the commonest cause of portal hypertension in the UK. Worldwide, schistosomiasis is the commonest cause. The causes of portal hypertension are shown in Box 22.6.

Intestinal Fistulae

Small bowel fistulae

Fistulae involving the small bowel may be external, where the fistula opens onto the skin; or internal, between two pieces of bowel. The result of a fistula is:

- loss of absorptive surface
- loss of nutrients
- loss of water
- loss of electrolytes.

Fistulae may have high output or low output, depending on the site:

- high-output fistulae: upper small bowel, e.g. duodenal fistula
- low-output fistulae: ileum.

High-output fistulae

- Approximately 3–4 L of fluid lost per day.
- Derived from gastric juice, bile, pancreatic juice or duodenal secretions.
- Depletion of intravascular and interstitial volume; requires replacement with isotonic saline.
- Loss of alkaline pancreatic juice and bile gives rise to a metabolic acidosis.
- Skin protection required with external fistula because of activated pancreatic trypsin digesting the keratin of the skin, causing excoriation.
- Treatment requires:
  - intravenous administration of water and electrolytes commensurate with losses
  - total parenteral nutrition until fistula closes or is surgically closed.

Low-output fistulae

- May put out initially up to 1.5 L per day.
- Low-output small bowel fistula similar to ileostomy.
- Proximal ileum can gradually adapt to loss of any colonic surface distal to it, and more fluid and electrolytes are absorbed.
- Fluid loss less in low-output fistulae because there is still a large proximal surface for absorption.
- Loss of nutrients less, because most have already been absorbed in the proximal small bowel.
- In initial stages, fluid and electrolyte management is important, but nutrition may be maintained by elemental diets.

Disorders of Colon and Rectum

Polyps

These are a heterogeneous group of protuberant growths into the bowel lumen. They may be:

- sessile or pedunculated
- benign or malignant.

Polyposis is a term reserved for hundreds of polyps occurring in the large bowel. The most common forms of polyps are shown in Box 22.7.

Adenomas

- Tubular, tubulovillous or villous.
- May give rise to adenocarcinoma.
- Malignant potential of an adenoma depends on:

BOX 22.6 Causes of portal hypertension

Prehepatic (obstruction of portal vein)
Congenital atresia or stenosis
Portal vein thrombosis
Extrinsic compression, e.g. tumour

Hepatic (obstruction to portal flow within liver)
Cirrhosis
Hepatoportal sclerosis
Schistosomiasis
Sarcoidosis

Post-hepatic
Budd–Chiari syndrome
Idiopathic hepatic venous thrombosis, e.g. due to polycythaemia, contraceptive pill, congenital obliteration, tumour invasion of hepatic veins
Constrictive pericarditis

BOX 22.7 Polyps of the large intestine

Type	Histology
Neoplastic	Benign
	Adenoma
	Tubular
	Tubulovillous
	Villous
	Malignant
	Polypoid adenocarcinomas
	Carcinoid polyps
Inflammatory	Pseudopolyp (ulcerative colitis)
Hamartomatous	Peutz–Jegher's polyp
	Juvenile polyp
Unclassified	Metaplastic (hyperplastic)
Others	Mesenchymal in origin
	Benign
	Lipoma
	Fibroma
	Leiomyoma
	Haemangiomas
	Malignant
	Sarcomas
	Lymphomatous polyps

  - size
  - growth pattern
  - degree of epithelial dysplasia.
- Malignant change is found in:
  - 1% of adenomas <1 cm in diameter
  - 10% of adenomas 1–2 cm in diameter
  - up to 40% >2 cm in diameter.
- Malignant potential depends upon type of adenoma: 5% of tubular adenomas, 20% of tubulovillous adenomas and 40% of villous adenomas become malignant.
- Sessile lesions are more likely to become malignant than pedunculated ones.

Inflammatory polyps (pseudopolyps)

- Associated with ulcerative colitis; result from mucosal ulceration.

Hamartomas

- Rare.
- May be solitary, e.g. juvenile polyps.
- May be present throughout the gastrointestinal tract, e.g. Peutz–Jegher's syndrome.

Metaplastic polyps

- Not neoplastic, therefore no malignant potential.
- Origin unknown.

Malignant epithelial polyps

- Vast majority arise within pre-existing adenomas.
- Small number may be carcinoid tumours of low malignant potential.
- Complete local excision is usually curative.

Familial adenomatous polyposis (FAP) – (aka familial polyposis coli)

- Rare condition inherited as autosomal dominant.
- Equal sex incidence.
- Hundreds of polyps carpet colon and rectum.
- Cancer develops before age of 40 years in almost all patients.
- Gene responsible for FAP is on the long arm of chromosome 5.

Gardner's syndrome

- FAP-associated.
- Desmoid tumours, osteomas of the mandible, sebaceous cysts.

Rectal Cancer

In Western countries, colorectal cancer ranks second only to lung cancer in incidence and mortality rates. Multiple synchronous colonic cancers, i.e. two more carcinomas occurring simultaneously, are found in 5% of patients. Metachronous cancer is a new primary lesion in a patient who has had a previous resection for cancer. The risk of metachronous tumours reaches 25% after 20 years of follow-up.

Progression of adenoma to carcinoma (see Fig. 18.1)

There is considerable evidence that most colorectal cancers develop from adenomas:

- colorectal cancers develop in familial adenomatous polyposis
- adenomas and carcinomas frequently occur together in the resected specimen of bowel; such patients have an increased risk of developing a metachronous cancer compared with those having carcinoma alone in the resected specimen
- marked geographical variation in the prevalence of adenomas: there is a strong correlation with the incidence of colorectal cancer in the same geographical areas.

Aetiology

- Inherited genetic factors:
  - familial adenomatous polyposis
  - autosomal dominant hereditary non-polyposis colorectal cancer (HNPCC). There are two types:
    - cancer family syndrome (CFS: Lynch syndrome 2; early onset – age 20–30 years) and associated

with other adenocarcinomas, especially endometrial carcinoma
  - hereditary site-specific colon cancer (HSSCC: Lynch syndrome 1): shows same characteristics except for extracolonic carcinomas; in the absence of the above syndromes, first-degree relatives of patients with colorectal cancer have 2- to 3-fold increased risk of the disease.
- Environmental factors:
  - low-fibre/high-fat diets: high fat leads to an increase in bile acid production; bile acids are promoters of carcinogenesis. Dietary fibre contains plant lignans, which are converted to human lignans by bacterial action in the colon; lignans may protect against cancer.
- Inflammatory bowel disease: greater risk in ulcerative colitis than Crohn's disease.
- Colorectal polyps.
- Schistosomal colitis.
- Exposure to radiation.
- Presence of a ureterocolostomy – this operation is rarely performed nowadays.

Molecular basis for development of colorectal cancer

- Activation of *ras* oncogene:
  - *c-Ki-ras* is affected in 80% of cases.
- Abnormalities of long arm of chromosome 5:
  - 5q deletion (FAP gene).
- Deletions on long arm of chromosome 18:
  - 18q deletion
  - seen in 70% of carcinomas and 50% of large adenomas.
- Deletions on short arm of chromosome 17:
  - inactivation of p53 in 75% of colorectal cancers.

Site

See Fig. 22.3.

Spread

- Direct:
  - encircles bowel lumen
  - longitudinal submucosal spread occurs, but rarely more than 2 cm from edge of tumour
  - to bowel wall and into neighbouring structures, e.g. liver, greater curvature of stomach, duodenum, small bowel, pancreas, kidneys, bladder, ureters or vagina. Carcinoma of the rectum may invade the bladder, prostate or sacrum.
- Lymphatic: regional nodes along vessels are involved but not necessarily in a progressive or orderly fashion. Positive nodes may be found at some distance from the primary intervening nodes, which are normal.
- Blood:
  - liver
  - lungs.
- Transcoelomic: seedlings on serosal surface with ascites.

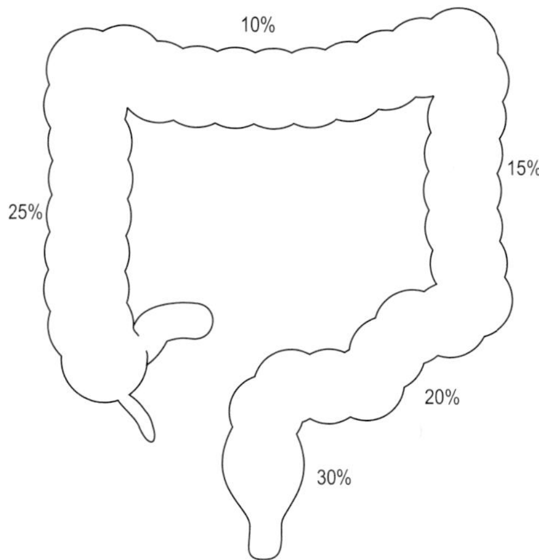

Fig. 22.3 The distribution of colorectal cancer.

Complications

These include:

- obstruction
- perforation
- perforation of the caecum in closed loop obstruction with competent ileocaecal valve
- perforation into an adjacent organ with fistula formation, e.g. colovesical, ileocolic, colovaginal
- symptoms relating to direct extension.

Prognosis

This depends on:

- degree of differentiation of tumour
- completeness of excision degree of spread
- examination of resection margins (proximal, distal and circumferential needed to assess completeness of excision)
- extent of spread is given by Dukes' classification, which also relates to prognosis (Table 22.2).

Carcinoid Tumours

- Arise from enterochromaffin cells throughout the gut.
- May be associated with multiple endocrine neoplasia (MEN type I and type II).
- Commonest in the midgut, the appendix being the most common site.
- Firm, yellowish, subcutaneous nodules.
- In the appendix they are often an incidental finding at appendicectomy.
- Approximately 30% of small bowel carcinoids cause symptoms such as obstruction, pain, bleeding or carcinoid syndrome.

Carcinoid syndrome

- Extensive metastases, particularly in the liver, result in carcinoid syndrome.

TABLE 22.2 Staging of Colorectal Carcinoma Based on Dukes' Classification, With Survival Rates after Surgery

Dukes' Grade	Spread	5-Year Survival (%)
A	Confined to the bowel wall	90
B	Spread through the bowel wall	70
C	Spread to lymph nodes	30

Stage D was added to Dukes' classification later, based on clinical rather than pathological evidence. Stage D implies distant metastases.

- Syndrome consists of cutaneous flushing, diarrhoea, bronchoconstriction with wheezing and right-sided cardiac valvular disease (usually pulmonary stenosis) due to collagen deposition.
- Principal cause of symptoms and signs is 5-hydroxytryptamine (5-HT, serotonin).
- 5-HT in circulation is degraded to 5-hydroxyindoleacetic acid (5-HIAA), which is measured in the urine as a diagnostic marker.

Inflammatory Bowel Disease

Crohn's Disease

Crohn's disease is a chronic inflammatory granulomatous disorder that may occur anywhere in the alimentary canal from the mouth to the anus. It is most common in temperate climates and among those of European origin.

Aetiology

The aetiology is largely unknown. Hypotheses include:

- infection, e.g. mycobacteria and viruses
- abnormal immune mechanisms
- environmental factors, e.g. cigarette smoking and intake of refined sugars
- family history of disease in 15–20% of patients.

Appearances

Macroscopic

- Classically segmental with areas of normal bowel separating areas of involved bowel – 'skip' lesions.
- Thickening of wall, which becomes firm and rigid.
- Encroachment on mesenteric fat.
- Linear mucosal ulceration.
- A 'cobble-stone' pattern of islands of surviving mucosa.
- Deep linear ulceration.

Microscopic

- Transmural inflammation from mucosa to serosa.
- Marked oedema of submucosa.
- Lymphoid aggregates.
- Patchy mucosal ulceration and fissuring.
- Presence of non-caseating granulomas (found in only 60% of cases).

Complications

- Intestinal obstruction.
- Fistula formation.
- Abscess formation.
- Malabsorption syndrome.
- Malignancy (increased risk of adenocarcinoma).
- Toxic dilatation.
- Haemorrhage.
- Perianal complications.
- Gallstones (reduction of enterohepatic circulation of bile in terminal ileum).

Extragastrointestinal manifestations

- Eyes: conjunctivitis, episcleritis, uveitis.
- Joints: sacroiliitis, arthritis, ankylosing spondylitis.
- Skin: erythema nodosum, pyoderma gangrenosum.
- Liver: sclerosing cholangitis (rare).

Ulcerative Colitis

Ulcerative colitis is a chronic inflammatory disease that involves the whole or part of the colon. Inflammation is initially confined to the mucosa and nearly always involves the rectum, extending to involve the distal or whole colon.

Aetiology

- Abnormal immune response to gut micro-organisms.
- Autoimmunity against colonic epithelial cells.
- Genetic factors:
  - familial clustering occurs
  - association with HLA-DR2
  - higher concordance rate in monozygotic twins.
- Geographic factors: much commoner in Western countries than in developing world.

Appearances

Macroscopic

There may be:

- Proctitis: inflammation limited to rectum.
- Varying extent of colitis extending for a variable distance proximally from the rectum.
- Total colitis with or without backwash ileitis.
- Affected mucosa red, inflamed, with contact bleeding on sigmoidoscopy.
- Fistulae do *not* occur.

Microscopic

- Diffuse, mixed inflammatory cell infiltrate.
- Crypt abscess formation.
- Distortion of glandular architecture.
- Mucosal ulceration.

Complications

- Toxic dilatation.

- Perforation.
- Increased risk of colorectal cancer.
- Electrolyte disturbances with severe diarrhoea.

Extragastrointestinal manifestations

- Eye: iritis, uveitis, episcleritis.
- Joint: ankylosing spondylitis, arthritis.
- Skin: pigmentation, erythema nodosum, pyoderma gangrenosum.
- Liver: fatty change, pericholangitis, sclerosing cholangitis, cirrhosis, hepatitis.

Diverticular Disease

A diverticulum is an outpouching of the colonic mucosa through a defect in the muscular wall of the colon. This occurs where blood vessels pierce the wall of the colon. Diverticular disease is common in Western civilization and is attributed to a low-fibre diet.

Pathogenesis

- Formed due to increased intraluminal pressure, forcing the mucosa to herniate through weaknesses in the muscle wall (pulsion diverticulum).
- 90% occur in the sigmoid colon, but the whole colon may be affected.
- The term diverticular disease covers the whole spectrum, i.e. diverticulosis (presence of diverticulae but no inflammation); diverticulitis (inflammation of diverticulae).

Complications

- Diverticulitis.
- Perforation:
  - into local tissues, where it becomes walled off as a paracolic abscess
  - into the general peritoneal cavity, giving rise to faecal peritonitis
  - into an adjacent viscus, e.g. colovesical fistula (bladder), vaginocolic fistula (vagina), ileocolic fistula (ileum).
- Bleeding: due to erosion into adjacent vessel.
- Intestinal obstruction: due to repeated attacks of diverticulitis causing fibrosis and consequent narrowing of bowel lumen.

OSCE SCENARIOS

OSCE Scenario 22.1

A 28-year-old right-handed female attends A&E with a wound on the radial and volar border of her right index finger, just proximal to the Proximal Interphalangeal Joint. She explains that she cut it last night with a knife whilst washing dishes, and complains of radial numbness distal to the wound.

1. Outline how you would examine the patient's finger to establish what structures have been injured other than the digital nerve.
2. Explain to the examiners what would happen pathologically and clinically if the nerve injury was left untreated.
3. Explain your management plan to the patient and answer any questions she may have.

OSCE Scenario 22.2

A 19-year-old male attends your outpatient clinic with a 3-month history of right knee pain and swelling. The pain and swelling are worsening, waking him at night, and he now walks with a limp. He denies any traumatic injury, is otherwise fit and well and on no medications. An X-ray arranged by his GP whilst waiting for his referral is shown in the figure (Fig. 22.2Q).

1. Describe the pathological signs on the X-ray.
2. What is the likely diagnosis, given the history and the X-ray?

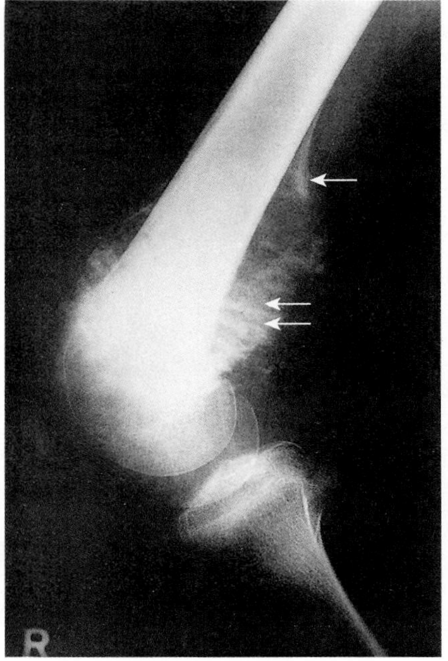

Fig. 22.2Q X-ray of the patient's right knee.

3. What other investigations could you arrange?
4. What are the management options?

OSCE Scenario 22.3

A 45-year-old female has presented in A&E after falling down some steps. She is alert and her pulse and blood pressure are normal, though her oxygen saturations are only 80% on high-flow oxygen. She is complaining bitterly of pain down her right chest wall, though only grazes are present.

1. How will you approach the assessment of this patient?
2. Her chest X-ray is shown below (Fig. 22.3Q). What is the condition shown? What is the likely cause?
3. How would you treat this condition?
4. Explain to the examiners the classification of causes and types of this condition, and how you would have treated the patient if she had presented with tracheal deviation and haemodynamic instability.

OSCE Scenario 22.4

A 14-year-old boy attends your clinic with his mother, who is concerned that her son seems to be developing breasts. The boy is overweight, with a BMI of 29, but both he and his mother state that he has lost weight recently and his breasts are still enlarging. His examination reveals enlarged nipples with small firm breast bud development.

1. What is the likely diagnosis? What questions would you like to ask to confirm this?
2. Explain the diagnosis and its causes in layman's terms, and outline the options for investigation and management.

OSCE Scenario 22.5

A 62-year-old male attends A&E with acute onset of severe abdominal pain radiating to the back. He is pale and sweaty with a tense, distended, tender abdomen. A CT of his abdomen is shown below (Fig. 22.5Q).

1. What pathology is shown? The patient is still in the radiology department and his blood pressure is stable at 90 mmHg systolic.
2. Outline the management of this patient.
3. What risk factors exist for this condition?
4. What is the operative mortality risk for this condition?
5. Explain to the examiners the different types of this condition, their classification and their aetiology.

OSCE Scenario 22.6

A 37-year-old female attends your clinic having been referred by her GP with excessive sweating, diarrhoea and neck swelling.

1. Ask this patient about her symptoms and give the examiners your differential diagnosis.
2. What physical signs may you expect to see on examination?
3. What investigations might you arrange? The results of your investigations suggest a benign toxic goitre with a dominant nodule.
4. What treatment options are available?

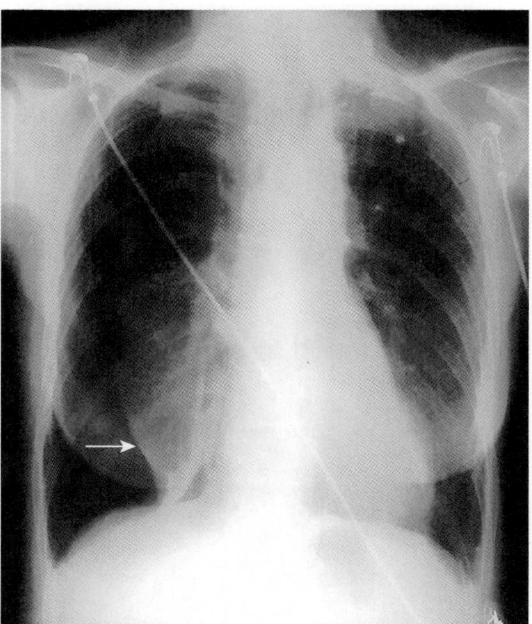

Fig. 22.3Q The patient's chest X-ray.

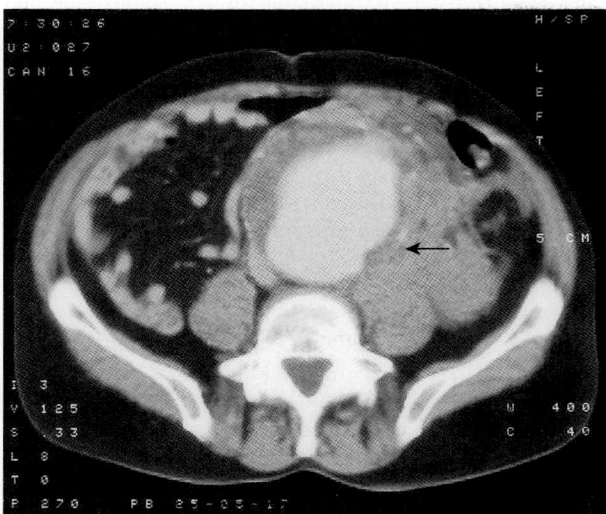

Fig. 22.5Q CT scan of the patient's abdomen.

5. If the patient opts for surgery, which nerves are at risk of intra-operative damage?

OSCE Scenario 22.7

The blood results displayed below are those taken from a 49-year-old male ex-alcoholic, feeling generally unwell with vague abdominal pain, whose GP has referred him to your clinic.

Bilirubin 57 μmol/L
Albumin 22 g/L
Total protein 64 g/L
Alkaline phosphatase (ALP) 152 IU/L
Alanine aminotransferase (ALT) 188 IU/L
Aspartate aminotransferase (AST) 220 IU/L
Gamma glutamyltransferase (GGT) 129 IU/L

1. What biochemical abnormalities are shown?
2. Explain to the examiners the different types of jaundice and give examples of the causes of each type.
3. Which type is this patient's likely to be from the blood results?
4. Closer questioning reveals that the patient has developed abnormal stools which are pale, float and are difficult to flush away. What other condition is the patient likely to have developed?

OSCE Scenario 22.8

An 82-year-old male is brought into the emergency department with an acutely painful right leg. The symptoms include the leg feeling cold, looking very pale and pins and needles. The patient's ECG is shown below (Fig. 22.8Q).

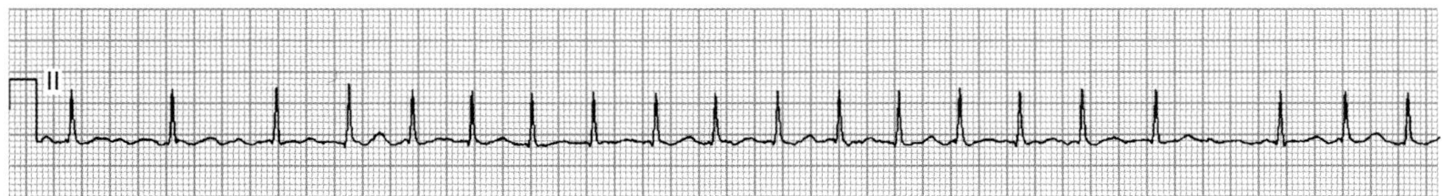

Fig. 22.8Q ECG from an 82-year-old patient.

1. What is the likely diagnosis?
2. What are the causes?
3. What other symptoms can occur and which are the most clinically important?
4. What investigations would you perform?
5. Are you aware of any classification systems for this condition?
6. If the patient had a paralysed and insensate leg with a purple discolouration which did not blanch under pressure, what would be the likely management plan?

OSCE Scenario 22.9

A 56-year-old male is admitted with severe dehydration and vomiting, his urea and creatinine are raised at 15 mmol/L and creatinine at 215 μmol/L. A blood gas shows the following abnormalities: pH 7.55, PO_2 10.9 kPa, CO_2 6.9 kPa and HCO_3 is 21.

1. What type of metabolic abnormality is this patient displaying?
2. How has it occurred?
3. The patient has a 'sucsussion splash' on examination – what is the diagnosis?
4. How would you manage this condition?

OSCE Scenario 22.10

A 62-year-old male is in the A&E department and is complaining of epigastric pain. This feels like his normal heartburn but has not been relieved by antacids. In addition he is sweating and has a bradycardia. An ECG is performed and shows raised ST segments.

1. From the history, what type of myocardial infarction is the patient having and in what leads would you expect to see the ST segment rises?
2. Which coronary artery is involved?
3. Why is it common to see a bradycardia?

Answers in Appendix pages 484–489

Please check your eBook at https://studentconsult.inkling.com/ for more self-assessment questions. See inside cover for registration details.

SECTION IV

Appendix

OSCE Scenario Answers

OSCE SCENARIO ANSWER 1.1

A 19-year-old male is admitted with a right-sided spontaneous pneumothorax. He has a past history of a treated coarctation of the aorta. He requires a chest drain.

1. ***Describe the anatomy of a typical intercostal space.***
   - A typical intercostal space contains three muscles comparable to those of the abdominal wall:
     - the external intercostal muscle passes downwards and forwards from the rib above to the rib below. It is deficient in front where the anterior intercostal membrane replaces it
     - the internal intercostal muscle passes downwards and backwards. It is deficient behind where it is replaced by the posterior intercostal membrane
     - the innermost intercostal muscle may cover more than one intercostal space.
   - The neurovascular bundle lies between the internal and innermost intercostals and consists of (from above down) the vein, artery and nerve, the vein lying directly in the groove on the undersurface of the corresponding rib.
2. ***Why is this knowledge important in your technique of insertion of an intercostal drain?***

Insertion of a chest drain should be close to the upper border of the rib below the intercostal space to avoid the neurovascular bundle.

3. ***What is the 'triangle of safety' when inserting a chest drain?***
   - The 'triangle of safety' is defined by the anterior border of latissimus dorsi, the lateral border of pectoralis major and a horizontal line lateral at the level of the nipple with an apex below the axilla. This corresponds to the 5th intercostal space.
   - This basically corresponds to an insertion of a drain between the anterior axillary line and the mid-axillary line at the level of the nipple. Insertion of a drain at a lower level risks damage to abdominal contents.
4. ***Explain the anatomical basis for notching of the lower border of a rib seen on a chest X-ray of a patient with coarctation of the aorta.***
   - In coarctation of the aorta, collaterals develop between vessels above and below the narrowing. Blood reaches the aorta beyond the narrowing via branches of the subclavian artery, which arise above the aortic narrowing. This results in extreme vascularity of the whole thoracic wall owing to the many arteries which arise indirectly from the aorta above its obliterated portion, anastomosing with vessels connecting with the aorta below the obliteration and the connecting channels become greatly enlarged.
   - On the anterior chest wall, the thoraco-acromial, lateral thoracic and subscapular arteries from the axillary artery, the suprascapular from the subclavian artery, and the 1st and 2nd posterior intercostal arteries from the costocervical trunk anastomose with the 3rd and lower posterior intercostal arteries, whilst the internal thoracic artery and its terminal branches anastomose with the lower posterior intercostal arteries and the inferior epigastric arteries. The anterior and intercostal branches of the internal thoracic artery pass blood by a reverse flow to the lower posterior intercostal with which they anastomose and hence into the descending aorta. As a consequence, the intercostal arteries dilate and become more tortuous because of the increased blood flow, eroding the lower border of the ribs and hence giving rise to notching of the ribs, which can be seen on chest X-ray.

OSCE SCENARIO ANSWER 1.2

A 35-year-old male sustains a crushing upper abdominal injury in a road traffic accident. On admission to A&E he has a tachycardia of 120 beats/min and a systolic blood pressure of 90 mmHg. He is complaining of abdominal and bilateral shoulder tip pain. Urgent CT scan reveals liver and splenic trauma as well as a ruptured left hemidiaphragm.

1. ***Describe the three origins of the muscular part of the diaphragm.***
   - A vertebral part arising from the crura and the arcuate ligaments.
   - A costal part arising from the inner aspect of the lower six ribs and costal cartilages.
   - A sternal portion arising by two slips from the deep surface of the xiphisternum.
2. ***At what vertebral levels do the oesophagus and the IVC pass through the diaphragm?***

The oesophagus passes through the right crus at the level of T10 whilst the IVC passes through the central tendon of the diaphragm at the level of T8.

3. ***What is the nerve supply of the diaphragm?***

The diaphragm receives its entire motor supply from the phrenic nerve (C3, 4, 5). The sensory nerves from the central part of the diaphragm run in the phrenic nerve, whilst the peripheral part of the diaphragm receives sensory fibres from the lower six intercostal nerves.

4. ***Explain why in some cases irritation of the diaphragm may result in referred pain to the shoulder, while in others it may result in referred pain to the abdomen.***

The sensory nerve supply of the parietal pleura and peritoneum on the upper and lower surfaces of the diaphragm, respectively, is as follows:

- Serous membranes related to the central part of the diaphragm are innervated by the phrenic nerve, while those related to the peripheral regions of the diaphragm are supplied by the lower six intercostal nerves.
- This double sensory innervation explains the different distribution of referred pain that may be felt in cases of infection or inflammation of the diaphragm such as may occur in pleurisy or pneumonia, affecting its upper surface, or in peritonitis, affecting its lower surface. For example, if it is more the central part of the diaphragm that becomes inflamed in cases of acute peritonitis, the patient may complain of pain referred to the area of the cutaneous distribution of C4, i.e. the shoulder.
- On the other hand, if the periphery of the diaphragm becomes involved in a patient with pleurisy or pneumonia, the patient may complain of pain in the area of distribution of the cutaneous branches of the lower intercostal nerves and the pain is referred into the abdomen.
- This partly explains why right lower lobar pneumonia in a child results in pain referred to the right lower quadrant, which may be mistaken for acute appendicitis.

OSCE SCENARIO ANSWER 1.3

A 60-year-old female undergoes a right open nephrectomy via a loin approach through the bed of the 12th rib. A post-operative chest X-ray shows a small right pneumothorax.

1. ***Describe the surface anatomy of the pleura.***
   - The cervical pleura extends above the sternal end of the 1st rib. It follows a curved line drawn from the sternoclavicular joint to the junction of the inner one-third and outer two-thirds of the clavicle, the apex arising 2.5 cm above the clavicle.
   - A line of pleural reflection passes behind the sternoclavicular joint on each side to meet in the midline at the angle of Louis (2nd costal cartilage level). The right pleural edge passes vertically down to the level of the 6th costal cartilage and crosses:
     - 8th rib in the mid-clavicular line
     - 10th rib in the mid-axillary line
     - 12th rib at the lateral border of erector spinae.
   - The left pleural edge arches laterally at the 4th costal cartilage and descends lateral to the border of the sternum, where it follows a path similar to the right side. The medial end of the 4th and 5th left intercostal spaces are therefore not covered by pleura.
   - The pleura descends below the 12th rib at its medial extremity.
2. ***Why has this patient developed a right pneumothorax?***

The pleura descends below the medial extremity of the 12th rib and therefore may be inadvertently opened in the loin approach to the kidney.

3. ***At which other site, other than surgery on the thorax, may surgery or trauma result in a pneumothorax?***

The pleura arises above the clavicle in the neck. It may be injured at surgery in the lower part of the neck, by a stab wound, or during insertion of an internal jugular line.

OSCE SCENARIO ANSWER 1.4

A 22-year-old male is brought to A&E with a penetrating injury in the left third intercostal space, anterior to the mid-axillary line. His blood pressure is 80/40, pulse rate 140 beats/min and has muffled hear sounds and distended neck veins. A diagnosis of cardiac tamponade is established.

1. ***Describe the surface anatomy of the heart.***

Distance in cm is from sternal border. Red is superior border, blue is right border, black is left border and green is inferior border (Fig. 1.4A).

2. ***Why does cardiac tamponade result in drop in blood pressure and clinical shock?***

The pericardium is formed by a fixed fibrous layer that is lined by a parietal layer of serous pericardium. While the

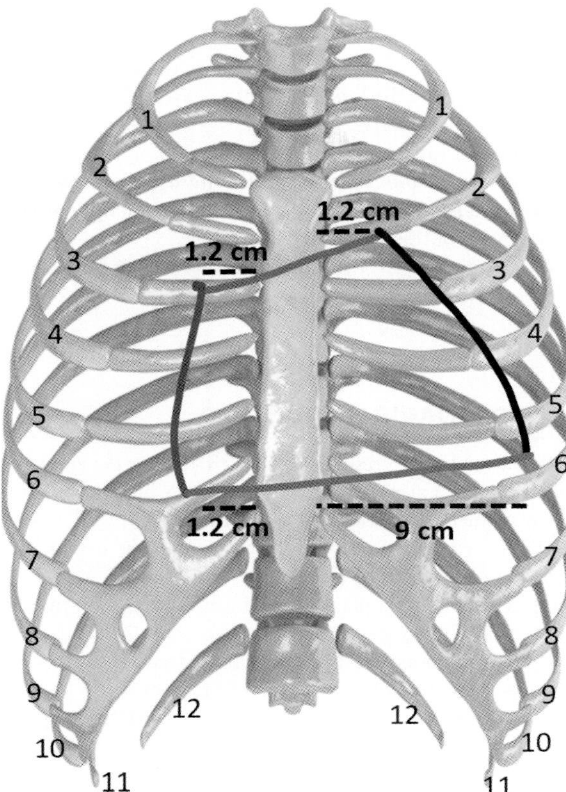

Fig. 1.4A Surface anatomy of the heart.

fibrous pericardium can stretch gradually if there is enlargement of the heart, a sudden increase in the pericardial content (as in a sudden bleed) can result in cardiac malfunction due to inability of the fibrous pericardium to stretch. A relatively small amount of blood can restrict cardiac activity and interfere with cardiac filling, resulting in shock.

3. Describe how you would treat a cardiac tamponade.
When cardiac tamponade is diagnosed, the most recent edition of the ATLS® manual recommends emergency thoracotomy or sternotomy by a qualified surgeon as soon as possible. Administration of intravenous fluid will raise the patient's venous pressure and improve cardiac output transiently while preparations are made for surgery. If surgical intervention is not possible, pericardiocentesis can be therapeutic, but it does not constitute definitive treatment for cardiac tamponade. Subxiphoid pericardiocentesis can be performed by cleaning the skin and performing a puncture to the left of the xiphisternum using a 16–18 gauge 15 cm cannula. Aim at a 45° angle towards the tip of the left scapula. Aspirate continuously; blood in the syringe confirms the correct position. Push the needle too far and the ECG will show ST changes (injury pattern) and should be withdrawn immediately. After the removal of blood (it doesn't need to be much) the blood pressure should improve. Remove the needle leaving the cannula and attach a three-way tap. If symptoms return the three-way tap can be opened and re-aspirated. Because complications are common with blind insertion techniques, pericardiocentesis should represent a lifesaving measure of last resort in a setting where no qualified surgeon is available to perform a thoracotomy or sternotomy. Ultrasound guidance can facilitate accurate insertion.

OSCE SCENARIO ANSWER 1.5

An 18-month-old girl developed sudden-onset bouts of cough and wheezes. A bowl of peanuts was found nearby while she was playing unwitnessed. She was rushed to A&E and found to be conscious but distressed, tachypnoeic and wheezy. A chest X-ray revealed a collapsed lung.

1. In which main bronchus is a foreign body more likely to be dislodged and why?
The right main bronchus is wider and more vertical; hence, foreign bodies are more likely to be aspirated into this bronchus

2. In relation to the surface anatomy, where does the trachea commence and terminate?
The trachea extends from lower border of cricoid cartilage (level of the sixth cervical vertebra) to terminate into the right and left main bronchi at the level of the sternal angle (level of fifth thoracic vertebra).

3. Describe briefly how you would treat the patient.
The treatment would involve taking the child to theatre and performing a GA – a bronchoscope can then be passed to retrieve the foreign body. A rigid bronchoscope is usually used as it allows better visualization of the airways and manipulation of the foreign body. Once visualized, grasping forceps or a fogarty catheter can be used to remove the foreign body.

OSCE SCENARIO ANSWER 2.1

A 19-year-old male presents with a history of vague central abdominal pain of 8 h duration. He has now developed a sharp pain in the right iliac fossa which is exacerbated by moving and coughing. He has a temperature of 37.4°C and a white cell count of 15 × 10^9/L. He is tender with rebound in the right iliac fossa. A provisional diagnosis is made of acute appendicitis and he elects for an open appendicectomy.

1. Explain the anatomical basis for the two types of pain he has experienced.

Initial pain

- The initial pain in the central abdomen at the level of the umbilicus is referred pain. Referred pain occurs due to nerve fibres in areas that have a high level of

sensory input, e.g. skin, and nerve fibres from areas that have low levels of sensory input, e.g. internal organs, coming together in the same area of the spinal cord.
- Afferent pain-conducting fibres from the viscera combine with afferent pain-conducting fibres from the skin on one central neuron of the spinothalamic tract. Impulses from the viscera travel in the same central pathway as pain impulses from the skin to reach the same final sensory neuron in the brain.
- The final sensory neuron projects pain sensation to the skin in the place from which it usually receives pain signals.
- The appendix is a derivative of the mid-gut. The mid-gut relates to the T10 segment, which is the periumbilical area of the central abdomen, and therefore pain referred from a mid-gut structure is experienced in the central abdomen in the periumbilical area.
- In the case of an inflamed appendix, which causes spasm of muscle in its wall, the pain is appreciated as periumbilical abdominal colic, although the inflamed appendix lies in the right lower quadrant. The appendix localizes as mid-gut pain to T10 through its autonomic nerve supply.

Localized pain
- As inflammation of the appendix proceeds, the inflamed serosal peritoneum abuts against the parietal peritoneum of the right lower quadrant, which has somatic innervation. The pain is now well localized to the right iliac fossa. Pain is then experienced at the site of inflammation near the classic site of McBurney's point.
- The pains therefore are two separate pains: one a visceral pain, due to either distension of the appendicular lumen or muscle spasm in the wall of the appendix; and the other a sharp somatic pain, due to inflammation of the parietal peritoneum. It is incorrect to say that the pain moves; it is a different pain that develops in the right iliac fossa.

2. ***Describe the structures encountered in a gridiron incision for appendicectomy.***

The incision is centred on McBurney's point (two-thirds of the way along a line drawn from the umbilicus to the anterior superior iliac spine). Structures encountered include:
- Skin.
- Camper's fascia.
- Scarpa's fascia at the lower medial end of the incision.
- The external oblique aponeurosis and muscle is then encountered, which is split in the line of its fibres, exposing the internal oblique muscle.
- The internal oblique muscle is also split in the line of its fibres.
- Transversus abdominis muscle is then exposed and also split in the line of its fibres; extraperitoneal fat is then encountered.
- The peritoneum is then incised.

3. ***What variations in position of the appendix may be encountered when attempting to locate the appendix?***

The position of the appendix is variable:
- 75% lie behind the caecum or colon, i.e. retrocaecal or retrocolic
- 20% are pelvic
- 5% are either pre-ileal or retroileal.

OSCE SCENARIO ANSWER 2.2

A 40-year-old male presents with severe pain in the right loin radiating into the right groin. A diagnosis of right ureteric colic is made and a plain abdominal radiograph is requested.

1. ***Where would you look for the course of the ureter projected onto the bony skeleton?***

A ureteric stone on a plain radiograph may be seen in relation to the following structures:
- running along the tips of the lumbar transverse processes
- crossing in front of the sacroiliac joint
- swinging out onto the pelvic wall and crossing the ischial spine
- passing medially to the bladder.

2. ***At which points along the course of the ureter is a stone likely to impact?***

The narrowest parts of the ureter where a stone is likely to impact are:
- pelvi-ureteric junction
- at the brim of the pelvis
- at the entry to the bladder.

3. ***How would you identify the ureter during an extraperitoneal approach?***

The ureter may be identified at operation as it strips up with the peritoneum and worm-like movements (vermiculation) may be noticed in its wall, particularly if it is stimulated by the tip of a pair of forceps.

4. ***What is the blood supply of the ureter and why, when removing a kidney for transplantation, is it important to leave abundant connective tissue around the ureter?***
   - The ureter receives a segmental blood supply from the following vessels:
     - renal arteries, from which it may receive a considerable contribution
     - lower polar artery
     - testicular or ovarian artery
     - internal iliac artery
     - inferior vesical arteries.

- There is a rich anastomosis between these vessels in the peri-ureteral connective tissue. When a kidney is removed for transplantation, the blood supply of the ureter depends solely on the renal artery. Blood flow down the length of the ureter is now via collaterals, which are in the peri-ureteral connective tissue. If this tissue is stripped up, there is a risk of ureteric necrosis following transplantation.

OSCE SCENARIO ANSWER 2.3

A 40-year-old female has had two attacks of acute cholecystitis and has recently had an attack of biliary colic. She has been admitted for laparoscopic cholecystectomy.

1. ***Describe biliary colic. What causes it?***
   - Sudden onset of severe pain across the epigastrium (it is not confined to the right upper quadrant [RUQ]). There are severe spasms of colic against a background of continuous severe pain. The patient rolls around in agony and cannot get into a comfortable position.
   - It is caused by a stone impacted in the neck of the gallbladder or in the cystic duct. The stone may fall back into the gallbladder or pass through the cystic duct into the common bile duct, when the pain abates suddenly.
2. ***What is Calot's triangle?***

Calot's triangle is formed by the liver, the cystic duct and the common hepatic duct. It must be exposed carefully to define the anatomy of the area, as variations of the anatomy are not uncommon. The cystic artery (usually a branch of the right hepatic artery) lies within Calot's triangle, where it is exposed and ligated/clipped.

3. ***Why is a knowledge of the structures in the free edge of the lesser omentum important while*** performing ***gallbladder surgery?***

The hepatic artery and the portal vein lie in the free edge of the lesser omentum. If haemorrhage occurs during cholecystectomy, bleeding can be controlled by compressing the hepatic artery and portal vein between the finger and thumb in the free edge of the lesser omentum (Pringle's manoeuvre).

4. ***What may result from the close relationship between the fundus of the gallbladder and the duodenum?***

The close relationship between the fundus of the gallbladder and the duodenum may result in an inflamed gallbladder adhering to, and ulcerating into, the duodenum, causing a cholecystoduodenal fistula and subsequent gallstone 'ileus'.

5. ***Gangrene of the gallbladder with perforation is rare, even if the cystic artery has thrombosed. Why?***

Gangrene of the gallbladder is rare because, even if the cystic artery thromboses, it gets a second blood supply directly from the liver bed.

OSCE SCENARIO ANSWER 2.4

A 78-year-old male is brought into the Accident and Emergency department with a history of a sizeable fresh blood haematemesis. He has a history of peptic ulcer disease. He is hypotensive and tachycardic.

1. ***Describe your initial management of this patient?***

The initial management of the patient would be along the lines of ABC. He will need supplemental oxygen and large-bore i.v. access to allow rapid fluid resuscitation. Bloods should be sent for full blood count, clotting profile, urea and electrolytes (U&Es), liver function tests and blood for cross matching. Clotting should be normalized in patients on warfarin using either fresh frozen plasma (FFP) or prothrombin complex concentrate (i.e. Beriplex). Platelet count is not associated with bleeding risk or mortality but if platelet dysfunction is present should be $>100 \times 10^9$/L. Consideration should be given to high-dose i.v. proton pump inhibitor (PPI); these allow clot stabilization and allow platelet aggregation. Giving erythromycin as a prokinetic has been associated with a reduced need for repeat endoscopy and can be considered in some cases. A nasogastric tube can be placed to allow old blood to be removed prior to endoscopy and in stable patients give an indication of early re-bleeding. The mainstay of treatment in these patients is early endoscopy.

2. ***What are the potential options for treating bleeding duodenal ulcers?***

There are a number of ways in which bleeding duodenal ulcers can be treated. The main stay is endoscopy; there are a number of methods available. These can be divided into the following:

- Injection agents – these include epinephrine (vasoconstriction and tamponade), tissue adhesives, thrombin and fibrin (vessel sealing and tamponade) and sclerosing agents (thrombosis of vessels by tissue injury).
- Mechanical therapy – endoscopic ligation clips and banding.
- Thermal therapy – these include electrocautery (diathermy), heater probes and argon plasma coagulators. These work by pressure of the device stopping bleeding and heat coagulating the vessel
- Haemostatic powders – a number of topical powders to induce coagulation have shown promise.

If a patient re-bleeds following endoscopy then a further endoscopic attempt can be made to stop the bleeding. If this fails again the options are then limited to laparotomy and opening the duodenum and oversewing the bleeding vessel, or angiography and identification of the bleeding vessel and selective embolization. The vast majority of bleeds are treated successfully with endoscopy.

3. *Which vessel is most commonly involved in bleeding duodenal ulcers – describe its anatomy?*

The vessel most commonly involved in a bleeding duodenal ulcer is the gastroduodenal artery (GDA); it is a branch of the hepatic artery, and it descends behind the first part of the duodenum and divides into the right gastroepiploic artery and the superior pancreaticoduodenal artery.

4. *Name three other causes of upper GI bleeding.*

The common causes of upper GI bleeding (other than peptic ulcers) include gastric erosions, oesophageal varices, oesophagitis, Mallory-Weiss tears and gastric cancers.

OSCE SCENARIO ANSWER 2.5

A 62-year-old male presents to his GP with weight loss, abdominal pain, jaundice and a palpable gallbladder. He has dark urine and pale stools.

1. *What are three potential causes for his jaundice?*

Jaundice can be divided into pre-hepatic, hepatic or post-hepatic. This patient clearly has post-hepatic or obstructive jaundice due to the dark urine and pale stools. Causes of this can be divided into those in the lumen of the bile duct, in the wall of the bile duct or outside the wall of the bile duct.

- In the lumen – gallstones, parasites, blood clots
- In the wall – congenital atresia, traumatic stricture, sclerosing cholangitis, cholangiocarcinoma, choledochal cysts.
- Outside the wall – carcinoma (pancreas, ampulla of Vater, malignant nodes), Mirrizi's syndrome.

2. *What is Courvoisier's Law?*

This law states that in the presence of jaundice and a palpable gallbladder the cause is not gallstones. The theory being that gallstones tend to lead to chronic inflammation, meaning the gallbladder becomes scarred and fibrotic and so unable to distend with obstruction.

3. *What would you expect to see on the liver function tests?*

The blood tests will obviously show a raised bilirubin (conjugated – as it has already passed through the liver). There will also be a dramatically raised alkaline phosphatase. Liver enzymes can be mildly elevated but not in comparison to levels seen in hepatitis.

OSCE SCENARIO ANSWER 3.1

A patient attempts suicide by slashing the flexor aspect of his wrists in a radial to ulnar direction.

1. *Which tendons are likely to be divided and how would you test their integrity?*

- Tendons which may be cut include:
  - palmaris longus
  - flexor digitorum superficialis
  - flexor carpi radialis
  - flexor carpi ulnaris.
- It is unlikely that flexor digitorum profundus will be damaged. To test whether flexor digitorum superficialis tendons have been damaged, the patient should be asked to flex the fingers at the proximal interphalangeal joints against resistance while the distal interphalangeal joints are held extended (to prevent the action of flexor digitorum profundus).
- Damage to the tendons of flexor carpi radialis and flexor carpi ulnaris will result in weakness of flexion of the wrist against resistance. If the flexor carpi ulnaris tendon alone is damaged, an attempt at flexion of the wrist will result in radial deviation. If the flexor carpi radialis tendon alone is damaged, an attempt at flexion of the wrist will result in ulnar deviation.

2. *Which nerves are likely to be affected?*

Median and ulnar nerves.

3. *How would you test the integrity of these nerves?*

The median nerve lies just deep to palmaris longus, and the ulnar nerve lies between the ulnar artery and pisiform bone.

- To test the ulnar nerve, the hand is placed palm downwards and the fingers straightened then abducted and adducted against resistance. Alternatively, a sheet of paper can be held between the adducted fingers and an attempt made to dislodge it. There would also be loss of sensation over the medial 1½ fingers.
- To test the median nerve, the patient is asked to abduct his thumb against resistance. This involves bringing the thumb forward at right angles to the plane of the palm against resistance and feeling the muscle contracting. With a median nerve lesion this would not be possible. There would also be loss of sensation over the lateral 3½ digits.

OSCE SCENARIO ANSWER 3.2

A patient with chronic renal failure is being assessed for construction of a radiocephalic arteriovenous fistula on the left wrist.

1. *Where would you palpate the radial and ulnar pulses to assess their integrity?*

- Pulsation of the radial artery is felt lateral to the tendon of flexor carpi radialis at the wrist.
- Pulsation of the ulnar artery is felt lateral to the tendon of flexor carpi ulnaris at the wrist.

2. *The ulnar pulse is not readily palpable. What test would you use to assess the integrity of the circulation to the hand and how would you perform it?*

- It is important to check the integrity of the palmar arch before performing a radio-cephalic fistula as there is a small risk of radial artery thrombosis. If the ulnar artery is not patent then the hand will be rendered ischaemic.

- The Allen test is performed. The patient is asked to repeatedly clench the fist while the radial artery and ulnar artery are occluded by pressure at the wrist. The patient is then asked to extend the fingers, palm up, which should demonstrate blanching of the hand. Pressure on the ulnar artery at the wrist is removed. If the hand flushes rapidly (within 5 s) then the ulnar flow is satisfactory. The test may be repeated, keeping the ulnar artery occluded and releasing the radial artery to inflow.

OSCE SCENARIO ANSWER 3.3

A 30-year-old male is taken to A&E, having fallen from a horse and landed on the point of his right shoulder. On examination, any attempt to move the shoulder is painful.

1. ***Describe the anatomy of the upper end of the humerus.***
   - The head of the humerus forms one-third of a sphere and faces medially, upwards and backwards.
   - The head is separated from the greater and lesser tuberosities by the anatomical neck.
   - The tuberosities are separated from one another by the bicipital groove, which contains the tendon of the long head of biceps.
   - The upper end and shaft meet at the surgical neck.
2. ***X-ray shows a fracture of the surgical neck of the humerus. Which nerve is likely to have been*** damaged?

The axillary nerve may be damaged by fractures of the surgical neck of the humerus.

3. ***Describe the distribution of the nerve and how you would test for damage to the nerve.***
   - The axillary nerve arises from the posterior cord of the brachial plexus. It passes through the quadrangular space accompanied by the posterior circumflex humeral artery. It ends by dividing into an anterior and posterior branch.
   - The anterior branch accompanied by the posterior circumflex humeral artery winds round the surgical neck of the humerus deep to deltoid, which it supplies, giving off a few small cutaneous branches to the skin covering the insertion of the deltoid.
   - The posterior branch supplies teres minor and is continued as the upper lateral cutaneous nerve of the arm, which supplies the skin over the lower part of the deltoid.
   - Paralysis of the deltoid results in loss of abduction of the arm from 15° to 90°. This is difficult to test because of pain on any movement of the shoulder. It is therefore more appropriate to test for loss of sensation in the skin over the lower part of the insertion of deltoid (the 'badge' area).

OSCE SCENARIO ANSWER 3.4

A 30-year-old motorcyclist is brought to the Accident and Emergency department after a road traffic accident. Following application of the ATLS protocol, secondary survey revealed significant soft tissue injury to the right shoulder and axillary areas. He was unable to abduct his arm and you suspect he has shoulder dislocation with tear to the rotator cuff muscles and possible injury to the brachial plexus.

1. ***What muscles make up the rotator cuff?***

The rotator cuff comprises the subscapularis, supraspinatus, infraspinatus, and teres minor.

2. ***What muscles are involved in abduction of shoulder joint?***

The supraspinatus initiates the movement of abduction. Then, the deltoid is responsible for further abducting the arm. The scapula then rotates, bringing the glenoid upwards. This is performed by the trapezius and serratus anterior. The lateral rotation of humerus is achieved by infraspinatus and teres minor.

3. ***The patient is noted to have his arm hanging adducted by his side, medially rotated while the elbow is extended and pronated. Which part of the brachial plexus is affected and what is this injury called?***

This position (waiter's tip hand) is caused by upper brachial plexus injury (Erb's palsy), which is the commonest injury of the brachial plexus. It affects roots C5 and 6 and results in loss of abduction (deltoid and supraspinatus paralysis) and lateral rotation movements (infraspinatus and teres minor paralysis) of the arm and flexion (biceps, brachialis and brachioradialis paralysis) and supination of forearm (biceps and supinator paralysis).

4. ***Where does the long thoracic nerve originate from? What muscle does it supply? How can you test for potential injury to it after axillary dissection?***

The long thoracic nerve originates from the anterior rami of C5, 6 and 7. It supplies serratus anterior muscle. Injury to this nerve can occur secondary to axillary surgery and results in winging of the scapula. To assess that, you ask the patient to stand up facing a wall. The patient then is asked to push firmly with both hands against the wall. The examiner observes for winging of the scapula from behind.

OSCE SCENARIO ANSWER 3.5

A 63-year-old female attends breast clinic after feeling a left breast lump. On examination, she had a 3×3 cm palpable hard lump in the upper outer quadrant, and you noticed skin puckering with arm elevation. Axillary examination demonstrated palpable enlarged lymph nodes.

1. ***What is the blood supply to the breast?***

The blood supply of the breast arises from:

- The axillary artery via its lateral thoracic and acromiothoracic branches.
- The internal mammary artery via its perforating branches.
- The intercostal arteries via the lateral perforating branches.

2. ***What is the lymph drainage to the breast?***

Most of the breast tissue drains into the axillary lymph nodes, while the medial part drains into internal mammary lymph nodes. Occasionally there may be drainage along the intercostal vessels, and lymphatic channels exist from one breast to the other; therefore, drainage is possible across the chest wall. Rarely there may be direct drainage to the supraclavicular nodes; these should not be missed out on breast examination.

3. ***How do you classify axillary lymph nodes anatomically and surgically?***

Axillary lymph nodes are classified anatomically into five areas: anterior, posterior, lateral, central and apical, while in surgery, the term 'axillary clearance' refers to axillary lymph node dissections which can be at level I, II or III. Level I dissection involves removing nodes in the axillary tail (if present) and clearing the lymph nodes inferior to the inferolateral border of the pectoralis minor. Level II includes nodes posterior to the pectoralis minor and Level III clears nodes superior to the muscle and up to the apex of the axilla.

OSCE SCENARIO ANSWER 4.1

An 85-year-old female trips over the edge of a carpet at home. She cannot get up from the floor. On arrival at hospital she complains of pain in the right groin. On examination the right leg is externally rotated, shortened and adducted.

1. ***Classify fractures of the neck of the femur.***

These fractures may be classified as either:

- intracapsular (subcapital, transcervical)
- extracapsular (basal, intertrochanteric).

2. ***Explain the anatomical basis for external rotation, shortening and adduction.***
   - Shortening of the fractured femur is due to the strength of the longitudinally lying muscles, especially the quadriceps and hamstrings, as well as the adductor group, which combine to pull the limb superior and medially.
   - In external (lateral) rotation, the femoral head normally rotates about a vertical axis, passing through the centre of the head of the femur and medial condyle. The femoral neck swings about this axis. Due to the angle between the neck and the shaft, this axis of rotation does not pass through the shaft of the femur. When the neck of the femur is fractured, rotation takes place about an axis passing through the shaft of the femur. Iliopsoas can now externally rotate the femur, leaving it in the characteristic position of fractured neck of femur, i.e. externally rotated.
3. ***What is the blood supply of the head of the femur?***
   - This comes from three sources:
     - vessels from the hip capsule, where this is reflected onto the neck in longitudinal bands or retinacula (retinacular vessels)
     - vessels travelling up the diaphysis
     - an artery in the ligamentum teres, which is a negligible source in the adult.
   - The chief source is from the retinacular vessels.
4. ***Explain why some fractures require a dynamic hip screw while others require a hemiarthroplasty.***
   - Fractures of the femoral neck completely interrupt the blood supply from the diaphysis. If the retinacular vessels are torn, avascular necrosis of the femoral head will occur. Avascular necrosis of the femoral head is much more likely to occur with intracapsular fractures than extracapsular fractures because intracapsular fractures are more likely to disrupt the retinacular flow.
   - Therefore, with extracapsular fractures a dynamic hip screw will be satisfactory, while with intracapsular fractures there is a danger of avascular necrosis of the femoral head and a hemiarthroplasty is more appropriate.

OSCE SCENARIO ANSWER 4.2

You are asked to examine the pulses in a patient's lower limb.

1. ***Describe the anatomical landmarks you would use to locate the peripheral pulses in the lower limb.***
   - The femoral artery is located at the mid-inguinal point, which is midway between the anterior superior iliac spine and the pubic symphysis.
   - The popliteal artery is located in the midline of the popliteal fossa behind the knee. It should be palpated in the lower half of the popliteal fossa where it can be compressed against the flat posterior surface of the tibia. The knee should be flexed to about 130° in order to relax the muscles and fascia to facilitate palpation.
   - The posterior tibial artery is located posterior to the medial malleolus, midway between the latter and the medial border of the tendo calcaneus.
   - The dorsalis pedis artery may be palpated on the dorsum of the foot against the navicular and medial cuneiform bones. It lies lateral to the tendon of extensor hallucis longus and medial to the tendon of extensor digitorum longus to the 2nd toe.

OSCE SCENARIO ANSWER 4.3

A 60-year-old female presents with a swelling in the right groin.

1. ***What are the boundaries of the femoral triangle?***

The boundaries are:

- above is the inguinal ligament
- medially is the medial border of adductor longus
- laterally is the medial border of sartorius.

2. ***On examination, the lump is below the inguinal ligament. Based on your knowledge of the contents of the femoral triangle, with the exception of lymphadenopathy, what pathological conditions may arise from the contents of the triangle?***

Possible conditions are femoral hernia (coming down the femoral canal), aneurysm of the femoral artery, saphena varix at the sapheno-femoral junction, neuroma of the femoral nerve.

3. ***On examination, you believe that the lump is a lymph node. Which structures drain to the inguinal lymph nodes?***

The following structures drain to the inguinal lymph modes:

- the skin of the leg
- the skin of the buttock as far up as the iliac crest
- the skin of the lower abdominal wall up to and including the umbilicus
- the skin of the labia
- the lower one-third of the vagina
- the lower half of the anal canal
- the fundus of the uterus (lymphatics accompanying the round ligament to the groin).

OSCE SCENARIO ANSWER 4.4

A 27-year-old male is impaled on a metal pole after falling from some scaffolding. It has entered his right buttock. You are asked to see him on the ward several days after recovering from surgery. The nurse looking after him is concerned he has a nerve injury.

1. ***What is the likely nerve to be injured in a penetrating injury to the buttock?***

The most likely nerve to be injured in the buttock is the sciatic nerve. If the nerve injury is not complete it may present as a common peroneal nerve injury as the fibres to this nerve lie uppermost in the sciatic nerve.

2. ***What are the roots of this nerve?***

The roots of the sciatic nerve are L4–5 and S1–3.

3. ***If he has a nerve injury what are the likely clinical signs and why?***

The sciatic nerve has both motor and sensory components. The motor signs would be difficulty in flexing the knee, although some is possible via the sartorius (femoral nerve) and gracilis (obturator nerve). There will be plantar flexion or foot drop and all the muscles below the knee are paralysed (loss of tibial and common peroneal nerve). Sensation in the thigh is preserved but is lost below the knee apart from some sensation along the medial aspect of the leg and foot from the saphenous nerve (femoral nerve).

OSCE SCENARIO ANSWER 4.5

A 52-year-old male has been hit by a car on the outside of his left leg as he crossed the road. It is obvious he has a nasty fracture of his lower leg. The plain X-ray has shown a nasty comminuted proximal fibular fracture and a tibial fracture.

1. ***What is the likely nerve to have been injured and what would be the examination findings?***

The common peroneal nerve leaves the popliteal fossa and winds round the neck of the fibula where it is easily injured from fractures of the fibula. Injury leads to paralysis of the muscles of the anterior and lateral compartments of the calf. The patient will experience foot drop (foot is plantar flexed and pulled inwards (equinovarus). Sensory loss is the anterior and lateral sides of the leg, dorsum of the foot and toes, and the medial side of the hallux.

2. ***What other nerves are injured in fractures/dislocations?***

Examples include:

- The axillary nerve can be injured by fractures of the humerus and anterior dislocations of the shoulder.
- The radial nerve can be injured by fractures/dislocations of the humerus, fractures of the spiral groove of the humerus and fracture/dislocations of the radial head.
- The ulnar nerve can be injured by fractures/dislocations of the elbow.
- The median nerve is at risk of injury with supra-condylar fractures.
- The sciatic nerve can be injured with fractures of the pelvis.
- The obturator nerve can be injured by anterior dislocations of the hip.

3. ***He is placed in a plaster-cast but just after midnight the nurse on the ward calls to tell you he is in tremendous pain and his leg feels 'odd'. What is the likely diagnosis and what would be the treatment?***

Pain of this magnitude following a severe lower limb fracture is likely to be compartment syndrome. Swelling of the muscles of the lower limb compress the neurovascular structures in the calf, causing tingling and numbness, pain on passive movement of the calf, and eventually vascular compromise. It is a clinical diagnosis – the old adage is 'if you think its compartment syndrome then treat it as compartment syndrome'. The treatment of this is a surgical fasciotomy in which the four compartments of the calf have their fascia opened via two incisions. A medial incision to open the superficial and deep posterior compartments and a lateral incision for the lateral and anterior compartments.

OSCE SCENARIO ANSWER 5.1

A 55-year-old female undergoes a right superficial parotidectomy for a pleomorphic adenoma of the parotid gland.

1. ***What is the order of structures traversing the gland from without in?***

From without in the structures are:

- the facial nerve
- the retromandibular vein, formed by the junction of the superficial temporal and maxillary veins
- the external carotid artery, dividing at the level of the neck of the mandible into its superficial temporal and maxillary branches.

2. ***Name the divisions of the facial nerve within the gland.***

These are from above downwards:

- temporal
- zygomatic
- buccal
- mandibular
- cervical.

3. ***How would you test the integrity of the individual branches of the facial nerve in the postoperative period to exclude intraoperative damage?***
   - The temporal branch supplies frontalis. Ask the patient to wrinkle the forehead by raising the eyebrows.
   - The zygomatic branch supplies orbicularis oculi. Ask the patient to close the eyes tightly and attempt to open them against resistance.
   - The buccal branch supplies buccinator and part of orbicularis oris. Buccinator compresses the cheek, as in the act of blowing, and allows the cheek to cave in, as in the act of sucking. Test this by asking the patient to whistle. Inability to whistle suggests damage to the buccal branch.
   - The marginal mandibular branch supplies the muscles around the mouth, including orbicularis oris. There will be drooping of the mouth on the affected side and inability to smile. Ask the patient to smile – the lips do not separate on the affected side. This branch is the thinnest and has the longest course through the parotid, and therefore is most likely to be injured.
   - The cervical branch supplies platysma. Ask the patient to pull down the corners of the mouth. The patient will be unable to do this on the affected side.
4. ***What is Frey's syndrome? Explain its anatomical basis.***
   - Frey's syndrome (gustatory sweating) is redness and sweating on the face adjacent to the parotid gland precipitated by eating (or anything else which precipitates salivation).
   - It is caused by damage to the auriculotemporal nerve at the time of surgery. The auriculotemporal nerve provides both parasympathetic innervation to the parotid gland and sympathetic innervation to the sweat glands and subcutaneous vessels. Damage to the auriculotemporal nerve results in aberrant regeneration of parasympathetic secretomotor fibres, which grow along the cut sympathetic nerve fibres to the skin, blood vessels and sweat glands. When the patient eats, activation of the parasympathetic nerve fibres produces sweating and flushing.

OSCE SCENARIO ANSWER 5.2

A 50-year-old male presents to a general surgery clinic with a lump in the right side of his neck.

1. ***What are the boundaries of the anterior and posterior triangles of the neck?***
   - The boundaries of the anterior triangle of the neck are:
     - the midline anteriorly
     - the anterior border of sternocleidomastoid posteriorly
     - the lower margin of the mandible superiorly.
   - The boundaries of the posterior triangle are:
     - the posterior border of sternocleidomastoid anteriorly
     - the anterior border of trapezius posteriorly
     - the middle third of the clavicle inferiorly.

Examination reveals that the lump is in the right posterior triangle.

2. ***What are the possible differential diagnoses?***

Possible differential diagnoses are:

- sebaceous cyst
- lipoma
- abscess
- lymph node
- cervical rib
- subclavian artery aneurysm.

On further examination you suspect lymphoma and discuss the case with a haematologist. The haematologist requests an excision biopsy. The lump lies centrally in the posterior triangle.

3. ***What structure do you need to avoid at surgery and what is the effect of injury to this structure?***
   - The spinal accessory nerve enters the posterior triangle of the neck from behind the posterior border of sternocleidomastoid at the junction of the upper

third and lower two-thirds. It runs downwards and laterally across the triangle on levator scapulae muscle and passes deep to the anterior border of trapezius at the junction of the upper two-thirds and lower third.

- Injury to the spinal accessory nerve in the right posterior triangle of the neck will result in inability to shrug the shoulder on that side due to paralysis of trapezius.

OSCE SCENARIO ANSWER 5.3

A 40-year-old female is to undergo a subtotal thyroidectomy for a multinodular goitre.

1. Describe the gross anatomy of the thyroid gland.

The gland is composed of two lateral lobes connected by an isthmus. The lateral lobes extend from the lateral aspect of the thyroid cartilage to the level of the 6th tracheal ring. The isthmus overlies the 2nd and 3rd tracheal rings. An inconstant pyramidal lobe extends up from the isthmus.

2. When exposing the gland at surgery, which structures are encountered?

Skin, platysma, deep investing fascia (which is opened longitudinally between the strap muscles and between the anterior jugular veins) and pretracheal fascia. The strap muscles are overlapped by the sternocleidomastoid muscles in the lateral part of the incision.

3. Describe the arterial blood supply of the thyroid gland.

The arterial supply comes mainly from two arteries.

- The superior thyroid artery arises from the external carotid artery and passes to the upper pole.
- The inferior thyroid artery arises from the thyrocervical trunk of the first part of the subclavian artery.
- A small inconstant artery, the thyroidea ima, arises from the aortic arch.

4. Where are the nerves situated in relation to the gland and when are they in danger of damage?

- The external branch of the superior laryngeal nerve is close to the superior pole of the gland and is in danger when ligating the superior thyroid artery, which must be ligated close to the upper pole of the gland.
- The recurrent laryngeal nerve lies in the groove between the trachea and oesophagus close to the inferior thyroid artery, which must be ligated far away from the gland.

OSCE SCENARIO ANSWER 5.4

A 35-year-old female is referred to the ENT clinic after recurrent episodes of nasal congestion, nasal discharge, fever, headache, tiredness, and facial pain in the right cheek. COVID-19 swabs were negative on several occasions and the GP is seeking advice for management of possible chronic sinusitis and is concerned that the symptoms are unilateral.

1. What are the paranasal sinuses and where are they located?

The paranasal air sinuses are four, paired, complex air-filled cavities that open into the nasal cavity and are lined by columnar ciliated epithelium. These are:

- The frontal sinuses are in the frontal bone and are separated by a bony septum.
- The maxillary sinuses are located within the maxilla at the lateral margin of the nasal cavity.
- The ethmoid sinuses are a group of 8–10 air-containing cavities within the lateral mass of the ethmoid bone, in between the upper nasal cavity and the orbit.
- The sphenoid sinuses lie within the body of the sphenoid bone.

2. Where do they drain into?

- The maxillary sinus: opens into the hiatus semilunaris in middle meatus. The opening of the sinus lies high on the medial wall just below the floor of the orbit. As the ostium is high on the wall, drainage depends on ciliary action and not gravity.
- The anterior and middle ethmoidal sinuses: drain into the middle meatus.
- The posterior ethmoidal sinus: drains into the superior meatus.
- The sphenoidal sinus: drains into the sphenoethmoidal recess.

3. How would you go about draining the maxillary sinus surgically?

The maxillary sinus is the largest paranasal sinus and washout can be performed through a cannula insertion via the inferior meatus of the nasal cavity, most commonly performed endoscopically, while antral drainage through the gingivolabial fold (known as the Caldwell Luc procedure) traditionally involved removing part of the anterior bony wall of the maxillary sinus.

4. How can carcinoma of the maxillary sinus present?

This depends on which surrounding structures it invades.

- Invading the floor of the sinus causes dental problems.
- Invading the medial wall may block the nasolacrimal duct causing epiphora or it may invade the nasal cavity causing nasal blockage or epistaxis
- Invading superiorly can cause proptosis
- Invading the posterior wall may involve the palatine nerves and produce severe pain referred to the teeth of the upper jaw.

The GP is right to be concerned that the symptoms are unilateral.

OSCE SCENARIO ANSWER 5.5

A 29-year-old male presented to Accident and Emergency with mandibular pain and inability to occlude the teeth following a bout of excessive laughter while watching a comic movie in the cinema. Examination of the temporomandibular joint (TMJ) revealed prominent mandibular head anteriorly.

1. ***What is the likely diagnosis and what other events can cause it?***

The likely diagnosis is a dislocation of the jaw or temporomandibular joint. Causes range from yawning, laughing, prolonged dental procedures, trauma or seizures.

2. ***What would you find on examination?***

The most common symptom is an inability to close the mouth. Pain is often present on the affected side. The patient may find it difficult to talk and swallow saliva. Palpation over the pre-auricular area may reveal an emptiness in the joint space (it may just feel different to the other side).

3. ***What type of joint is TMJ?***

Formed by articulation of the head of the mandible with mandibular fossa and articular eminence of temporal bone, the TMJ is atypical synovial joint consisting of a fibro-cartilaginous disc and fibrocartilage on the bony surfaces.

4. ***How would you treat the patient?***

This patient has suffered from an anterior dislocation which is the most common type that affects this joint and can be reduced by pressing down the mandible on the molar teeth to stretch the masseter and temporalis which are in spasm then pulling up the chin to lever the condyle back into the mandibular fossa (essentially downwards and backwards). This can be done using an auriculotemporal nerve block or local anaesthetic infiltration into the joint or under general anaesthesia.

OSCE SCENARIO ANSWER 6.1

An 18-year-old male is assaulted at a party. He is struck on the left temporal region with a bottle. He briefly loses consciousness. He is taken to hospital where on examination his GCS (Glasgow Coma Scale) is 15. Four hours following admission, he suddenly deteriorates with a GCS of 8 and his left pupil dilates.

1. ***What is the most likely diagnosis?***

Extradural haematoma.

2. ***What is the explanation for the 'lucid' interval?***

The lucid interval occurs after the patient comes round from the concussion caused by the force of the initial trauma and before lapsing into unconsciousness again due to bleeding into the cranial cavity, which gives rise to increased intracranial pressure with resulting brain damage.

3. ***What is the anatomical basis for the left pupillary dilatation?***

The haematoma pushes the most medial part of the temporal lobe, the uncus, across the tentorial hiatus, compressing the ipsilateral 3rd (oculomotor) nerve. This paralyses the constrictor pupillae, allowing unopposed action of the sympathetic nerves which supply the dilator papillae.

4. ***Where would you locate the middle meningeal artery for the purpose of making a burr hole?***
   - The anterior branch of the middle meningeal artery lies in the region of the pterion and is the usual source of extradural haemorrhage.
   - The middle meningeal artery enters the skull at a point level with the midpoint of the zygomatic arch and divides 2 cm above it.
   - The pterion, a point important for making a burr hole, is 4 cm above the zygomatic arch and 3.5 cm behind the lateral angle of the eye.
5. ***What layers of the scalp would you encounter in your incision?***

The layers are:
- skin
- subcutaneous tissue
- aponeurosis
- loose areolar tissue
- temporalis muscle
- periosteum (pericranium).

OSCE SCENARIO ANSWER 6.2

A 55-year-old male presents with low back pain, bilateral sciatica, numbness over the buttock area and weakness in the lower limbs. He has also developed difficulty in passing urine. Examination reveals reduced lower limb reflexes and loss of anal tone and sensation.

1. ***What is the most likely diagnosis?***

Cauda equina syndrome.

2. ***At what level does the spinal cord end in the adult?***

At the level of the disc between the 1st and 2nd lumbar vertebrae.

3. ***Describe the level and type of disc lesion that is likely to cause the symptoms.***

It is likely to be caused by a central disc lesion at L4–5 or L5–S1 level.

4. ***Describe the anatomy of an intervertebral disc.***

Each intervertebral disc consists of:
- Peripheral annulus fibrosus, which is adherent to the thin, cartilaginous plate on the vertebral body above and below.
- Nucleus pulposus, which is a gelatinous fluid surrounded by the annulus fibrosus.

- The posterior part of the annulus fibrosus is relatively thin and prone to rupture due to degenerational injury. The nucleus pulposus protrudes into the vertebral canal through intervertebral foramen.
- In the case of cauda equina syndrome, the disc lesion is directed posteriorly or central.

5. ***Explain the anatomical basis of bladder and bowel dysfunction.***
   - S2, 3, 4 give off nerve fibres (pelvic splanchnic nerves) which are distributed to the pelvic organs.
   - The sacral parasympathetic fibres supply motor fibres to the bladder and inhibitory fibres to the internal vesical sphincter. Damage to these nerves leads to flaccid paralysis of the bladder and internal sphincter dysfunction.
   - The parasympathetic system also supplies motor fibres to the muscles of the rectum and inhibitory fibres to the internal anal sphincter. Damage results in bowel dysfunction.
6. ***What investigation would you carry out to confirm the diagnosis and what action would you take if the diagnosis was confirmed?***
   - Urgent MRI.
   - If the diagnosis is confirmed, urgent referral is required for surgical decompression.

OSCE SCENARIO ANSWER 6.3

A 55-year-old insulin-dependent diabetic develops a boil on the right upper lip. She does not seek treatment. A few days later she develops a severe headache and redness and swelling around the right orbit. A diagnosis of cavernous sinus thrombosis is made.

1. ***Describe the anatomy of the cavernous sinus.***
   - The cavernous sinuses lie one on either side of the body of the sphenoid bone against the wall of the pituitary fossa. They extend from the superior orbital fissure to the apex of the petrous temporal bone. They communicate with one another via the intercavernous sinuses. The internal carotid artery and abducent nerve (VI) pass through it.
   - On the lateral wall from above down are:
     - ocular motor nerve (III)
     - trochlear nerve (IV)
     - ophthalmic nerve (V1)
     - maxillary nerve (V2).
   - The ophthalmic veins drain into the anterior part of the sinus.
   - Emissary veins pass through foramina of the middle cranial fossa connecting the cavernous sinus to the pterygoid plexus and facial veins.
   - The optic tract and the internal carotid artery lie above the sinus, the latter piercing the roof of the sinus then doubling back to lie against it.
2. ***Why does cavernous sinus thrombosis develop following an infection on the upper lip?***

Cavernous sinus thrombosis may develop as a result of the spread of infections from the lips and part of the cheek via the anterior facial and ophthalmic veins, or from deep infections via pterygoid venous plexus, all of which drain into the sinus. Diabetics and immunosuppressed patients are particularly at risk of cavernous sinus thrombosis following infections on the upper lips and cheek.

3. ***Describe the characteristic clinical picture of cavernous sinus thrombosis.***

The characteristic clinical picture consists of:

- oedema of the conjunctiva (chemosis) and eyelids
- exophthalmos with transmitted pulsations from the internal carotid artery (pulsating exophthalmos)
- ophthalmoplegia due to pressure on the contained cranial nerves
- papilloedema, venous engorgement and retinal haemorrhages are seen on ophthalmoscopy.

OSCE SCENARIO ANSWER 6.4

A 75-year-old male has been referred to you by the Accident and Emergency department for a possible stroke. His main symptom is left arm and leg weakness.

1. ***Which hemisphere has suffered a stroke?***

When describing carotid symptoms following a TIA it can be quite confusing; the symptoms are left sided but this would mean the right carotid is the symptomatic side, so we would refer to this as a right hemispheric event.

2. ***If the patient had suffered left sided amaurosis fugax which hemisphere would have been affected?***

Amaurosis fugax is a sensation of a curtain closing over ones eye. It happens when a clot passes through the retinal artery. Unlike weakness, which is the contralateral carotid, the side affected by amaurosis is the same as the symptomatic carotid, i.e. a left amaurosis fugax is caused by a left carotid artery stenosis.

3. ***The patient is right-handed and has had dysphasia only. Which hemisphere is the most likely to have been affected and why?***

Dysphasia is difficulty finding words and is not an uncommon symptom; indeed it may well be the only presenting complaint. In 90% of right-handed people the speech area lies in the left hemisphere. In left-handed people it is not quite so simple and can be in the left hemisphere in 50% of people. In the above example one could be confident the patient had a symptomatic left carotid lesion, as he is right-handed.

OSCE SCENARIO ANSWER 6.5

A 70-year-old non-smoking female presents with a hoarse voice. A CT angiogram is shown below Fig. 6.5Q.

1. What is the diagnosis?

The patient has a thoracic aortic aneurysm.

2. What are the treatment options?

The options, as with any condition, can be divided into conservative, medical or surgical. Clearly there are no medical treatment options but conservative management may be appropriate for patients who do not wish to have treatment or are not fit enough. Surgical treatment can be divided into open or endovascular. In the majority of conditions the preferred treatment would be an endovascular repair using a thoracic stent graft (TEVAR – thoracic endovascular aneurysm repair). Surgery may be preferred in the very young or those with congenital conditions affecting the aorta, such as Marfans or Ehlers-Danlos syndrome.

3. What is the anatomical explanation for the hoarse voice?

The left recurrent laryngeal nerve branches off the vagus nerve as it crosses the aortic arch. The nerve then passes underneath the aortic arch behind the ligamentum arteriosum and passes superiorly into the neck. As thoracic aneurysms grow, the nerve is compressed against the ligamentum arteriosum causing nerve palsy (see Fig. 6.5A). The left recurrent laryngeal nerve supplies all the intrinsic muscles of the larynx except the cricothyroid muscles.

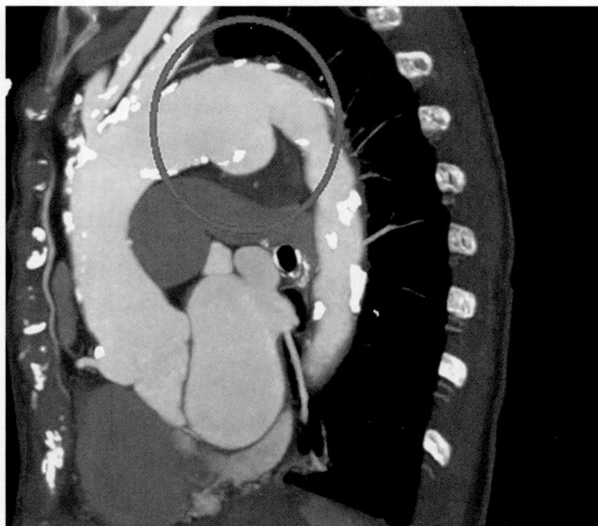

Fig. 6.5A CT angiogram of the Thoracic Aorta showing a large aneurysm (circled).

OSCE SCENARIO ANSWER 7.1

A 64-year-old male is admitted for a right hemicolectomy and is found to have a serum sodium of 120 mmol/L.

1. What are the possible causes of hyponatraemia in this patient?

Hyponatraemia has a number of causes, which may be defined by asking two questions:

- What is the volume status of the patient: is he hypovolaemic, hypervolaemic or normovolaemic?
- Is the sodium in the urine >20 mmol/L or <20 mmol/L?
  - Hypovolaemia + urine Na >20 mmol/L = excessive renal loss (diuretics and salt losing renal disease), mineralocorticoid deficiency.
  - Hypovolaemia + urine Na <20 mmol/L = extrarenal losses or sequestration.
  - Hypervolaemia + urine Na >20 mmol/L = renal failure.
  - Hypervolaemia + urine Na <20 mmol/L = cirrhosis, cardiac failure, nephritic syndrome.
  - Normovolaemia + urine Na >20 mmol/L = glucocorticoid deficiency, hypothyroidism, SIADH (syndrome of inappropriate ADH secretion).

2. Describe what investigations you would carry out in order to identify the cause of the hyponatraemia.

The investigations are:

- U&Es
- TFTs
- LFTs
- serum and urine osmolality
- urine sodium
- serum cortisol
- serum ADH
- Synacthen test (identifies adrenal failure).

3. How would you correct it?

The treatment depends on the cause. If hypervolaemic, then volume restriction is appropriate. If the patient is volume depleted, then intravenous normal saline is required. Hyponatraemia should not be rapidly corrected, as this may lead to central pontine myelinolysis.

OSCE SCENARIO ANSWER 7.2

An 82-year-old male is transferred to ITU following a Hartmann's procedure for perforated diverticular disease. He has been anuric for 3 h. A number of fluid challenges have been given, achieving a BP of 120/90 mmHg, pulse of 87 beats/min and a CVP of 10 mmHg. ABG analysis shows a pH of 7.2 and U&Es reveal serum potassium of 7.1 mmol/L.

1. What are the possible causes of hyperkalaemia in this patient?

The possible causes of hyperkalaemia include:

- acute renal failure
- metabolic acidosis
- excess administration of potassium
- adrenal insufficiency (rare).

2. ***What are the ECG changes associated with hyperkalaemia?***

The ECG changes associated with hyperkalaemia are:

- peaked T-waves
- loss of P-waves
- widened QRS complexes.

3. ***What would be your possible treatment options for this patient? Explain how each works to lower the serum potassium.***

The treatment options for hyperkalaemia include:

- 10 mL of 10% calcium gluconate intravenously. It stabilizes cardiac myocytes, decreasing the risk of arrhythmia. It has no effect on the serum potassium level and the effect is short lived.
- Insulin and dextrose infusion (10 units of Actrapid in 50 mL of 50% glucose). Insulin promotes K^+ and glucose influx into cells via stimulation of the Na/K ATPase pump. Dextrose prevents the development of hypoglycaemia.
- Salbutamol (can be given by nebulizer). Stimulates β_2 receptors, leading to increased cellular uptake of K^+.
- Oral or rectal calcium resonium. This is an ion exchange resin, calcium being exchanged for potassium, which is then lost in the faeces. It takes 24 h to work and is therefore inappropriate in the emergency situation.

OSCE SCENARIO ANSWER 7.3

A 56-year-old male is admitted with severe dehydration and vomiting. His urea and creatinine are raised at 15 mmol/L and 215 µmol/L, respectively. A blood gas analysis shows the following abnormalities – pH 7.55, PO_2 10.9 kPa, PCO_2 6.9 kPa and HCO_3^- is 21 mmol/L.

1. ***What type of metabolic abnormality is this patient displaying?***

The patient has a metabolic alkalosis – this is indicated by the pH showing alkalosis. The fact that it is metabolic in nature is indicated by the raised CO_2 (compensatory hypoventilation) and the low HCO_3^- (compensatory loss by the kidneys). The fact that the HCO_3^- is low would suggest the cause of the alkalosis is loss of H+ ions rather than excess HCO_3^-.

2. ***How has it occurred?***

Vomiting results in a loss of H^+ ions and thus a metabolic alkalosis.

3. ***The patient has a 'succussion splash' on examination. What is the diagnosis?***

A 'succussion splash' is a characteristic finding in gastric outlet obstruction which leads to severe vomiting.

4. ***How would you manage this condition?***

The management of this condition would fall into:

- Resuscitation and correction of electrolyte abnormalities.
- Investigation as to the cause – OGD and/or CT scan.
- Management of the cause – the commonest causes are peptic ulcer disease or malignancy. If due to malignancy, then surgical resection of the tumour or palliative gastro-jejunostomy would be appropriate. If due to peptic ulcer disease, then initial medical management with i.v. PPI is appropriate for 48–72 h. If there is no improvement, then surgical resection may be deemed appropriate.

OSCE SCENARIO ANSWER 7.4

A 35-year-old female patient with weight of 70 kg underwent uncomplicated appendicectomy. As she arrives back to the ward, the nurses ask you to prescribe her intravenous fluids for the next 24 h as she is unable to eat and drink due to nausea.

1. ***What are the volumes of the fluid compartments of the body?***

For a 70-kg man there would be approximately:

- 25 L of intracellular water
- 19 L of extracellular water, comprising:
  - 3 L plasma
  - 15 L interstitial fluid
  - 1 L transcellular fluid, e.g. CSF, peritoneal fluid, intraocular fluid.

2. ***In general, what are the average daily fluid and electrolyte requirements?***
   - Approximately 40 mL/kg/day of fluid
   - Sodium: 1–2 mmol/kg/day
   - Potassium: 0.5–1 mmol/kg/day
3. ***What intravenous fluids would you prescribe for the next 24 h?***
   - For uncomplicated patient, postoperative intravenous fluid prescription should include 2.5–3 L of fluid containing 150 mmol of Na+ and 60 mmol of K+ per day.
   - A suitable fluid regimen for 24 h would therefore be as follows:
     - 1000 mL 0.9% sodium chloride + 40 mmol KCL
     - 1000 mL 5% dextrose
     - 1000 mL 5% dextrose + 20 mmol KCl.

   Each bag to of fluid is given over 8 h.

OSCE SCENARIO ANSWER 7.5

A 65-year-old male patient is bought to the Accident & Emergency department with acute abdominal pain. He looks very unwell and is in obvious pain and is very confused. He is wearing a medical alert bracelet informing you he is diabetic. He has a temperature of 39°C and his blood pressure is 90/50 with a heart rate of 110. He has a rather strange smell of acetone or 'pear drop' sweets.

1. ***What is the diagnosis?***

The clue is in the medic alert bracelet and the characteristic 'pear drop' smell. This patient likely has diabetic ketoacidosis. This is often triggered by an infection, so he quite likely has an acute abdominal infection that has led to the ketoacidosis. The characteristic smell is ketones in the breath.

2. ***What would you expect his blood gases to show and why?***

The blood gas will show severe acidosis, the pH will be less than 7.3 (in severe cases may fall below 7) and the bicarbonate will also be low (around 10 mmol/L) as excess acid is neutralized. In addition the anion gap will be >10. This is due to the metabolism of fat (lipolysis) and resulting production of free fatty acids. The fatty acids are metabolized and produce acetyl CoA, the citric acid cycle (that breaks down the acetyl CoA) is overwhelmed and acetyl CoA gets converted to ketoacids. These are excreted in the urine (ketonuria) and the breath (hence the characteristic smell). The anion gap is a measure of acid–base balance and is a balance of cations (base) and anions (acids). The anion gap represents the difference in these. In acidosis the anion gap may be high, normal or low. As the acid in ketoacidosis is from an abnormal source, the anion gap will rise (i.e. more anions than cation).

3. ***How would you manage this patient, explaining which electrolyte needs specific management?***

The management of patients with diabetic ketoacidosis (DKA) can be divided into four parts: (1) fluid resuscitation, (2) administration of insulin, (3) correction of electrolyte abnormalities and (4) treatment of any precipitating cause. There are numerous protocols and regimes for DKA but the basics will involve giving insulin to lower the glucose levels and monitoring/giving adequate potassium. Potassium may be elevated at presentation but as insulin is given, it will cause potassium to be taken back into cells and lead to dangerous hypokalaemia and thus added potassium will be needed.

OSCE SCENARIO ANSWER 8.1

A 59-year-old male with severe acute gallstone pancreatitis has been on the ward for 5 days. He is complaining of acute shortness of breath with a respiratory rate of 32 and an SpO_2 of 88% despite oxygen by facemask. The junior doctor has obtained arterial blood gases (ABGs), the results of which are shown below:

pH 7.25
PaO_2 7.7 kPa
$PaCO_2$ 7 kPa
Base excess −9 mmol/L
HCO_3^- 18 mmol/L.

1. ***What are the possible differential diagnoses for the shortness of breath?***

The possible causes of shortness of breath in this patient include:

- ARDS
- pleural effusion (secondary to acute pancreatitis, usually left sided)
- aspiration pneumonitis
- hospital-acquired pneumonia.

2. ***How is respiratory failure classified?***

Respiratory failure is said to exist when PaO_2 <8 kPa. It is then divided into type I and type II:

- Type I occurs when the $PaCO_2$ is low or normal and is termed hypoxaemic respiratory failure.
- Type II occurs when the $PaCO_2$ is elevated and is termed ventilatory failure.

3. ***What is adult respiratory distress syndrome (ARDS)?***

ARDS is the pulmonary component of the systemic inflammatory response syndrome and may be caused by direct lung injury, e.g. aspiration, or indirect injury such as burns or pancreatitis.

4. ***How is ARDS diagnosed?***

There are a number of criteria for the diagnosis of ARDS:

- Known cause.
- Acute onset of symptoms.
- Hypoxia unresponsive to O_2 therapy.
- New bilateral 'fluffy' infiltrates on CXR.
- No cardiac failure or fluid overload (defined as PAWP) (pulmonary artery wedge pressure <18 mmHg).

5. ***How is ARDS managed?***

Management involves:

- Treating the precipitating cause.
- Preventing multi-organ failure (MOF) with judicious fluids and inotropes as needed.
- Respiratory support to maintain reasonable levels of oxygenation while minimizing further lung injury.

There are a number of ventilator strategies used in ARDS:

- Lung protective ventilator strategies with lower tidal volumes and peak airway pressures and allowing hypercapnia as long as pH <7.1.
- Prone ventilation.
- High-frequency jet ventilation.

- Inverse ratio ventilation (inspiration/expiration ratio prolonged, allowing a longer time for inspiration).
- ECMO (extra-corporeal membranous ventilation).

OSCE SCENARIO ANSWER 8.2

A 52-year-old male, 7 days post-right total knee replacement, has become acutely short of breath. He has severe chest pain on inspiration.

1. ***What is the differential diagnosis?***

Differential diagnosis includes:

- pulmonary embolism (PE)
- cardiac-related chest pain
- pneumothorax
- pneumonia.

2. ***What changes on ECG would support a diagnosis of pulmonary embolism (PE)?***

The following changes on ECG would support a diagnosis of PE:

- sinus tachycardia
- right bundle branch block (RBBB)
- T-wave inversion in V1–V3
- S1Q3T3 (S-wave in lead I, and Q-wave and inverted T-wave in lead III).

3. ***What is the treatment of PE?***
    - The management of PE depends on whether it is a non-massive PE or massive PE.
    - In patients with non-massive PE, management involves confirming the diagnosis and definitive treatment. In patients with a high degree of suspicion of PE, then treatment should be instituted immediately (see following).
    - Many hospitals have flow-chart protocols to assess the probability of PE from a list of clinical points and a raised D-dimer blood test. The imaging modality of choice is CT pulmonary angiography (CTPA).
    - Management of non-massive PE involves anticoagulation, initially with heparin (either unfractionated or low molecular weight), followed by oral anticoagulation with warfarin (maintaining the INR between 2 and 3) for a period of 6 months.
    - Patients with a massive PE will be acutely unwell and require immediate resuscitation according to ABC guidelines. They will need ITU support with inotropes for cardiovascular collapse while the diagnosis is confirmed. Options for massive PE include thrombolysis (treatment of choice) and surgical embolectomy (uncommon).
4. ***Describe the physiological changes that lead to hypoxia and hypotension, which occur in PE.***

Hypoxia is caused by two mechanisms:

- Firstly, there is an increase in dead space due to blockage of pulmonary arteries by thrombus (this leads to areas of lung that are ventilated but not perfused).
- After 24–48 h, the affected area of lung loses surfactant, leading to atelectasis; this may cause further hypoxaemia.

Hypotension, seen only in large PEs, is essentially due to right heart failure (cor pulmonale) due to obstruction of pulmonary arteries. This leads to a reduction in right ventricular output and thus left ventricular preload and therefore hypotension.

OSCE SCENARIO ANSWER 8.3

A 19-year-old male is involved in a fight. He has been stabbed in the left side of the chest. He is brought into A&E very pale and struggling to breathe.

1. ***What possible chest injury could he have?***

The possible chest injuries may include pneumothorax, tension pneumothorax, haemothorax or cardiac tamponade.

2. ***What would be the examination findings in each?***

These would depend on the injury:

- *Pneumothorax* – the patient will be short of breath with tachypnoea. There may be some mediastinal shift with large pneumothorax. The patient will have decreased breath sounds and hyper-resonant percussion.
- Tension pneumothorax – the patient will be in severe respiratory distress and shock. He will have mediastinal shift away from the injured side, have decreased breath sounds and will be hyper-resonant to percussion on the injured side.
- Haemothorax – the clinical signs will depend on the size of the haemothorax. With a small bleed, there may be very few clinical signs. With a large haemothorax, the patient will show signs of shock and respiratory distress. He will have absent breath sounds and be dull to percussion on the affected side.
- Cardiac tamponade – the patient will be in shock and may exhibit signs of respiratory distress. He will not have mediastinal shift or the lungs signs of a tension pneumothorax which may have a similar clinical presentation. Beck's triad includes hypotension, raised JVP and muffled heart sounds. ECG may show reduced complexes. Other signs, such as pulsus paradoxus and Kussmaul's sign, are more related to tamponade caused by chronic pericardial effusion and demonstrating them is not appropriate in a trauma scenario.

3. ***How would you manage this patient?***

The treatment of all conditions would initially be in line with ATLS protocols. Each of these chest injuries would be diagnosed and managed in the primary survey.

- Pneumothorax – chest drain
- Tension pneumothorax – initial needle decompression followed by chest drain.
- Haemothorax – i.v. fluid/blood resuscitation and chest drain. Depending on the amount of blood drained, the patient may require urgent thoracotomy.
- Cardiac tamponade – needle thoracocentesis followed by urgent thoracotomy.

OSCE SCENARIO ANSWER 8.4

A 56-year-old male has recently had major knee surgery and you are called to the ward as he has difficulty breathing. He also has pleuritic chest pain. You suspect a pulmonary embolus (PE).

1. ***What other signs may be associated with a PE?***

Clinical signs associated with PE – along with shortness of breath and pleuritic chest pain – may include haemoptysis, pyrexia, hypotension and a raised JVP. With massive PE the first presentation may be cardiac arrest. Remember that DVTs that cause PEs are rarely occlusive (i.e. free floating and more likely to embolize) and thus only 10% or so of patients with PE will also have symptoms of a DVT. ECG may also show a number of changes, which can include:

- Sinus tachycardia is most common
- Classic sign is S1Q3T3 – this is a prominent S wave in lead I, Q wave and T wave inversion in lead III – this indicates right heart strain and is not diagnostic of a PE.
- Atrial fibrillation or flutter.
- Right bundle branch block.
- Right deviation of the QRS complex.

2. ***What would you expect to see on ABGS and why would you see these changes?***

The changes on an arterial blood gas (ABG) are again not diagnostic but one would expect to see low oxygen (hypoxaemia) due to a V/Q mismatch from the blocked pulmonary vessels – i.e. alveoli have air but no perfusion. There is hypocapnea as a result of hyperventilation. This would be termed a respiratory alkalosis. In massive PE, there also maybe an element of metabolic acidosis due to low blood pressure and systemic hypoperfusion.

3. ***How would you investigate and treat this patient?***

Investigations would include CXR, VQ scanning and CT pulmonary angiography (CTPA). A CXR is usually taken at the acute episode that the patient became symptomatic, mainly to rule out other causes and is rarely diagnostic. VQ scanning uses radioisotopes to show the difference between ventilated and perfused lung but is rarely if ever used today, except in pregnancy. The mainstay investigation is with CTPA, which is very sensitive at showing clots within the pulmonary veins. Direct pulmonary angiography is performed prior to commencing endovascular treatment but is not used as a standard investigation.

The first stage in treatment must always be ABC; further treatment and investigation will depend on the stability of the patient – stable or unstable. Remember, treatment can always be divided into conservative, medical or surgical. Conservative treatment has no role unless a massive PE occurs in a very poorly patient not expected to survive. In the stable patient, the treatment is medical – this would include oxygen, fluids to support BP and anticoagulation with i.v. or LMW heparin and ensure the patient is wearing TED stockings if appropriate. Investigation with CTPA can then be performed when appropriate. Anticoagulation should be commenced if a high degree of suspicion before a CT confirms a PE. In the unstable patient then treatment involves stabilizing the blood pressure using inotropes before either systemic or catheter-directed thrombolysis. Clots can also be sucked out using special catheters. In some centres facilities maybe available to perform median sternotomy and pulmonary embolectomy.

OSCE SCENARIO ANSWER 8.5

A 26-year-old male has been shot in the chest with a shotgun and has a sizeable chest injury. He is very short of breath. Bubbles are coming from the wound.

1. ***What type of chest injury is this and how would you treat it?***

This patient has what is called an open pneumothorax or 'sucking' chest wound. This is when a defect in the chest wall allows intra-thoracic pressure and atmospheric pressure to equalize. If the defect is >2/3 the diameter of the trachea, air will preferentially enter the wound and not take part in gas exchange and thus cause hypoxia. The visible bubbles are from damaged lung surface. The first aid treatment is the placement of a dressing over the wound sealed on three sides to allow air out but prevent air going into the chest – this is a flutter valve. In hospital a sealed dressing can be placed over the wound and a chest drain distant from the site of injury.

2. ***He has hypoxia and hypoxaemia – which type of hypoxia and hypoxaemia does he have?***

Hypoxia is a deficiency of oxygen in the tissues – this patient will be suffering from hypoxic hypoxia due to low arterial oxygen levels. Hypoxaemia is low level of oxygen in the blood and will result from a ventilation perfusion mismatch.

3. ***What other types of chest injury can you describe?***

There are a number of other types of chest injury and these can be divided into immediately life-threatening and potentially life-threatening. A useful pneumonic is 'ATOM

FC' for immediate and 'ATOM PD' for potentially life threatening injuries.

Immediately Life-Threatening	Potentially Life-Threatening
Airway obstruction	**A**ortic disruption
Tension pneumothorax	**T**racheobronchial injury
Open pneumothorax	**O**esophageal injury
Massive haemothorax	**M**yocardial contusion
Flail chest	**P**ulmonary contusion and pneumothorax
Cardiac tamponade	**D**iaphragmatic rupture

OSCE SCENARIO ANSWER 9.1

An 80-year-old male is 5 days post-repair of abdominal aortic aneurysm. He has suddenly developed a tachycardia and become hypotensive. His ECG shows atrial fibrillation with a rate of 140.

1. What are the causes of atrial fibrillation?

The causes of atrial fibrillation can be divided into cardiac causes and non-cardiac causes.

- Cardiac causes include:
  - ischaemic heart disease
  - cardiomyopathy
  - left ventricular hypertrophy
  - hypertension
  - valvular heart disease.
- Non-cardiac causes include:
  - hyperthyroidism
  - PE
  - alcohol excess
  - sepsis (especially pneumonia)
  - hypoxia
  - biochemical derangements (e.g. low calcium, potassium and magnesium).

2. What are the physiological mechanisms which explain the hypotension seen in fast atrial fibrillation?

There are three physiological mechanisms to explain the hypotension in atrial fibrillation:

- Loss of atrial contraction leads to poor ventricular filling and thus reduced stroke volume and hypotension.
- Increased heart rate leads to reduced time for ventricular filling and thus reduced stroke volume and consequent hypotension.
- The increased heart rate leads to reduced time in diastole (coronary artery filling occurs mainly in diastole), leading to cardiac ischaemia and reduced strength of contraction.

3. How would you diagnose atrial fibrillation?

The two ways to diagnose AF are:

- irregular heart rate (both clinically and on ECG)
- absence of P-waves on ECG.

4. Describe your initial management of the patient.

Initial management involves:

- Airway, Breathing and Circulation
- confirmation of diagnosis:
- ECG
- FBC
- U&E
- cardiac markers
- calcium
- magnesium
- CXR
- ABG.

The further management of AF relates to control of the heart rate. This varies depending on a number of factors:

- If the patient is haemodynamically unstable, commence i.v. heparin and arrange urgent DC cardioversion.
- If the patient is not unstable, then treatment differs depending on whether the AF is of new onset or not:
  - new-onset AF: electrical or pharmacological cardioversion (amiodarone)
  - previous AF: pharmacological rate control (beta-blockers, calcium antagonists or amiodarone).

OSCE SCENARIO ANSWER 9.2

An 89-year-old male is 8 days post-laparotomy for repair of a perforated duodenal ulcer. He has developed a severe post-operative chest infection and is pyrexial and hypotensive.

1. Describe your initial management of this patient.

Assessment of any critically ill patient requires initial assessment and resuscitation (Airway, Breathing and Circulation) followed by appropriate investigations and treatment.

- ABC:
  - Airway: patient may require intubation if in respiratory failure.
  - Breathing: patient should be given high-flow oxygen.
  - Circulation: rapid intravenous access should be gained and a fluid bolus of colloid or crystalloid given; further management will depend on the response to the fluid. If the patient responds to a simple fluid bolus then investigation into the cause can be initiated. If the patient has been given adequate fluid resuscitation (which in septic patients can be several litres) then further invasive monitoring (arterial line and CVP line) should be used to guide treatment, e.g. inotropes.
- Diagnosis: screening for sepsis (sputum, wound swab, blood culture), FBC, CRP, CXR.

- Treatment: empirical broad-spectrum antibiotics should be commenced against the most likely source as soon as possible; respiratory support either as high-flow oxygen, non-invasive ventilation or intubation; and intensive management of hypotension with invasive monitoring guiding further fluid management and inotropic support.

2. ***Why does sepsis lead to hypotension?***

Sepsis leads to hypotension in three ways:

- Profound vasodilatation, leading to pooling of blood in the venous system.
- Third space losses due to inflammatory exudate.
- Poor cardiac contractility secondary to bacterial toxins and inflammatory mediators.

3. ***Which inotrope is commonly used in sepsis and what is its mode of action?***
   - The most commonly used inotrope is noradrenaline. This is given after adequate fluid resuscitation.
   - Noradrenaline (via alpha receptors) leads to vasoconstriction and thus an increase in blood pressure.
4. ***What is Starling's law of the heart and how do inotropes affect it?***
   - Starling's law states that the contraction of cardiac muscle is dependent on the degree of stretch: the greater the stretch, the greater the degree of contraction and thus the stroke volume. There is a finite limit to which the heart muscle can be stretched, after which point the heart will begin to fail.
   - Inotropes reset the contraction of the heart to a higher level, and for a given end diastolic volume will lead to a greater stroke volume.

OSCE SCENARIO ANSWER 9.3

A 58-year-old male is admitted with severe inter-scapular back pain. He is hypertensive with a BP of 200/140 mmHg. A CT angiogram shows a type B aortic dissection.

1. ***What is the difference between a type A and B dissection?***

Type A dissection refers to an aortic dissection which begins in the ascending aorta. A type B dissection is where the tear is located in the descending aorta – usually close to the origin of the left subclavian artery. Both type A and B dissections may involve the length of the aorta.

2. ***How is a type A dissection managed?***

Type A is a surgical emergency. Without operation the mortality is extremely high. Urgent transfer to a cardiothoracic centre is required. Surgery basically involves resection of the ascending aorta and replacement with a Dacron graft under cardiopulmonary bypass. The distal anastomosis often involves a combination of pledgeted sutures and glue to obliterate the false lumen.

3. ***How is an uncomplicated type B dissection managed?***

Type B dissections are managed medically unless there are signs of complications such as:

- end-organ ischaemia (renal, bowel or limb)
- rupture
- high BP resistant to treatment
- unremitting pain
- aneurysmal expansion.

Medical management consists of transfer to HDU/ITU and invasive BP management with a variety of medications. The most commonly used drug is labetolol – a rapidly acting beta-blocker that lowers BP and heart rate and thus applies less 'pressure' to the dissection flap and thus limits its propagation. In complicated dissection the management is similar but will involve the placement of an endovascular thoracic graft (TEVAR).

OSCE SCENARIO ANSWER 9.4

A 72-year-old male patient underwent elective open abdominal aortic aneurysm repair. An infra-renal aortic cross clamp was required.

1. ***What are the physiological and cardiovascular changes that result from aortic cross clamping?***

The main effect of aortic cross clamping is increasing the afterload which manifests as hypertension. An increase in afterload results in increased cardiac work and therefore oxygen consumption. Therefore in susceptible patients (i.e. those with a history of ischaemic heart disease) it can predispose the patient to myocardial ischaemia, arrhythmias, and left ventricular failure.

2. ***What techniques would the anaesthetists use to reduce these effects?***

Several techniques can be utilized to reduce afterload, such as increasing volatile anaesthetic agent and using beta-blockers or vasodilators such as glyceryl trinitrate (GTN). Vasodilatation leads to reduction of peripheral vascular resistance and the afterload, resulting in less stress on the heart.

3. ***What are the physiological and cardiovascular changes that result from releasing aortic cross clamp?***

This can be more significant than the initial cross clamping as it results in sudden reduction in the afterload and reperfusion of the ischaemic tissues. The impact is hypotension, release of vasodilatory metabolites from the pelvis and legs, an increase in potassium, lactate and CO_2, which can result in a degree of acidosis, and resultant myocardial ischaemia or arrhythmias.

4. ***What techniques would the anaesthetists use to reduce these effects?***

The anaesthetists ensure that patients are adequately prefilled prior to the release of cross clamping. Vasodilators are stopped if they have been commenced. The vascular surgeons can also gradually release cross clamping over several minutes by keeping the flow partially clamped, press on the femoral artery to perfuse the pelvis first prior to perfusing the leg and release one leg at a time.

OSCE SCENARIO ANSWER 9.5

A 75-year-old female patient underwent difficult open anterior resection. She has past medical history of hypertension, ischaemic heart disease and transient ischaemic attack (TIA). The procedure was complicated with significant blood loss that necessitated intraoperative blood transfusion. Postoperatively, she was admitted to the high-dependency unit as she required vasopressors support.

1. ***What methods can be utilised to monitor the cardiovascular system?***
   - ECG
   - blood pressure measurement (via cuff or arterial line)
   - central venous pressure
   - pulmonary wedge pressure (pulmonary artery occlusion pressure) via a Swann-Ganz catheter
   - pulse oximetry
   - cardiac output
   - urine output
   - echocardiogram
   - echo Doppler.
2. ***What is the best indicator to assess adequate fluid balance?***

Urine output remains the best indicator to assess adequate fluid balance. Normal urine output is 0.5–1 mL/kg/h. Assessment of the central venous pressure can be also a useful guide to fluid replacement in hypovolaemic patients.

3. ***How does the pulse oximetry work?***

It relies on the measurement of the different absorption of oxyhaemoglobin and deoxyhaemoglobin at different wavelengths. The pulse oximeter uses two different light emitting diodes at two wavelengths: 660 nm (red light) and 960 nm (infrared light)

4. ***What are the problems and pitfalls that can occur when reading pulse oximetry?***
   - delay: calculations are made from several pulses and there is a 20s delay between actual and displayed values
   - irregular pulse: atrial fibrillation
   - venous pulsation (tricuspid incompetence)
   - hypotension
   - vasoconstriction
   - abnormal Hb (carboxy-), and methaemoglobin
   - bilirubin
   - methylene blue dye
   - other factors: electrical interference (diathermy), flickering lights, patient movement, shivering, nail varnish (coloured or not).
5. ***What is a vasopressor? Give some examples used in common clinical practice.***

Vasopressors are drugs that constrict blood vessels through α-effect. Metaraminol and noradrenaline are commonly used vasopressors. Adrenaline has both vasopressor (α-effect) and inotropic (β-effect) mechanisms of action, depending on the dose given.

OSCE SCENARIO ANSWER 10.1

A 40-year-old male presents with recurrent attacks of right upper quadrant pain exacerbated by fatty food. His only significant past medical history is a right hemicolectomy 5 years previously for acute regional ileitis (Crohn's disease). Investigations reveal normal liver function tests but FBC reveals anaemia with a raised MCV. Abdominal ultrasound scan demonstrates gallstones.

1. ***Explain the pathophysiology underlying the development of gallstones in this patient.***
   - The terminal ileum is the site of bile salt absorption. Because the terminal ileum has been removed during the right hemicolectomy for terminal ileal Crohn's disease, the absorption of bile salts is reduced and they are lost in the faeces.
   - Due to the loss of enterohepatic circulation, there is a decrease in the bile salt pool. There is therefore not enough bile salt to keep cholesterol dissolved and thus cholesterol gallstones form.
2. ***What is the cause of the patient's anaemia?***

The terminal ileum is the site of absorption of vitamin B_{12}. Intrinsic factor (secreted in the stomach) binds to its specific receptor. The intrinsic factor–vitamin B_{12} complex is then taken up into the cell. Absence of the terminal ileum results in lack of B_{12} absorption and consequently B_{12} deficiency, leading to a megaloblastic anaemia (i.e. the cells are large), thus explaining the raised MCV.

3. ***What would be the effects of failing to treat the anaemia?***
   - Body stores of vitamin B_{12} far exceed requirements and deficiency may take years to develop.
   - Apart from the general symptoms of anaemia, paraesthesia and peripheral neuropathy may be present.
   - Less commonly spasticity, unsteadiness and altered gait may occur due to subacute combined degeneration of the spinal cord (damage to the posterior and lateral columns).
   - Visual disturbances (due to optic atrophy), dementia and weight loss (due to effects of the vitamin deficiency on intestinal mucosal cells) can also occur.
   - Cardiomyopathy may occur.
4. ***How would you treat the anaemia?***

Megaloblastic anaemia due to vitamin B_{12} deficiency is treated by replacement with intramuscular injections of 1 mg of hydroxocobalamin. Initially this is performed 3 times per week for 2 weeks. The maintenance dose is 1 mg every 3 months continued for life.

OSCE SCENARIO ANSWER 10.2

A 32-year-old female is admitted with jaundice and right upper quadrant pain. Liver function tests reveal a bilirubin of 112 μmol/L, a markedly raised alkaline phosphatase and gamma GT. Liver enzymes are normal.

1. *What is jaundice?*

Jaundice is a yellow discoloration of the tissues noticed especially in skin and sclera due to the accumulation of bilirubin.

2. *At what level of bilirubin is jaundice clinically apparent?*

For jaundice to be clinically apparent, the circulating bilirubin levels should be in excess of 35 μmol/L.

3. *Classify the types of jaundice.*

Jaundice may be:

- pre-hepatic (due to haemolysis)
- hepatic (due to intrinsic liver disease)
- post-hepatic/cholestatic (due to either intrahepatic cholestasis or post-hepatic biliary tract obstruction).

4. *What is the most likely cause in this case?*

Given the markedly elevated levels of alkaline phosphatase and gamma GT and the fact that the liver enzymes are normal, this would suggest a cholestatic cause.

5. *Describe the different types of gallstone.*

There are three types of gallstone:

- Mixed (80%): these are predominantly cholesterol with small amounts of calcium and bile pigment.
- Cholesterol stones (10%): these are usually solitary and can be up to 5 cm in diameter. They are usually formed in bile which is supersaturated with cholesterol.
- Pigment stones (10%): these are usually multiple, small and black in colour. They result most commonly due to haemolytic anaemia.

6. *List the complications of gallstones.*

The complications of gallstones are:

- cholecystitis (acute, chronic, acute-on-chronic)
- obstructive jaundice
- mucocoele of the gall bladder
- empyema of the gall bladder
- perforated gall bladder
- ascending cholangitis
- acute pancreatitis
- gallstone ileus
- carcinoma of the gall bladder.

OSCE SCENARIO ANSWER 10.3

A 63-year-old male is admitted with central abdominal pain radiating through to his back. He is hypotensive with a BP of 90/60 mmHg and tachycardic. The results of blood investigations are shown below:

WBC 19 × 10⁹/L
Glucose 8 mmol/L
AST 390 U/L
LDH 500 U/L
Amylase 2235 U/L.

1. *The raised amylase suggests acute pancreatitis. What are the common causes of acute pancreatitis?*

The commonest causes of acute pancreatitis are gallstones (40%) and alcohol excess (35%). Other causes include hyperlipidaemia, hypercalcaemia, viral infections (mumps and Coxsackie virus), hypothermia, trauma, drugs, hereditary/autoimmune disorders, scorpion bites, post Endoscopic Retrograde Cholangiopancreatography (ERCP) and pancreatic cancer.

2. *What is the patient's initial Ranson score?*

On admission, Ranson's criteria are

- WBC > 16 × 10^9/L
- Age >55 years
- Glucose >10 mmol/L
- AST >250 U/L
- LDH >350 U/L.

This patient thus scores 4. Amylase has no prognostic value.

3. *What are the criteria measured at 48 h for the Ranson score?*

At 48 h post-admission the following criteria are examined:

- Haematocrit drop >10% from admission
- Urea increase >5 mg/dL from admission
- Calcium <2 mmol/L
- Arterial PaO_2 < 8 kPa
- Base deficit <4
- 6 L fluids within 48 h.

The more factors present, the higher the predicted mortality.

4. *What pancreas-related complications can occur with acute pancreatitis?*

Complications of acute pancreatitis include:

- pancreatic necrosis
- pancreatic abscess
- pancreatic pseudocyst formation
- chronic pancreatitis
- diabetes.

OSCE SCENARIO ANSWER 10.4

A 50-year-old male patient presented to Accident and Emergency with epigastric pain after starting a course of NSAIDs 2 weeks ago for a flare-up of arthritis. His pain was getting worse over the last 24 h. Abdominal examination revealed peritonism with guarding. His HR was 130/min, temperature 38.5°C and BP 130/70. You suspect perforated peptic ulcer.

1. *What is the volume of daily gastric secretion? And what is its content?*

The stomach secretes 2-3 L/day; it contains

- Hydrochloric acid: helps to break down tissue, converts pepsinogen to active pepsin, and provides immunity against microorganisms.

- Pepsinogen: when activated to pepsin, it hydrolyses peptide bonds in proteins.
- Mucus: helps neutralize gastric acid to protect the stomach from digestion.
- Intrinsic factor: binds to vitamin B12 which is then absorbed as a complex in the ileum.
- Salt and water.

2. ***What are the classes of medications that are used to treat peptic ulcers and what are their mechanisms of action?***

Medical treatment of peptic ulcers frequently involves antibiotic therapy to eradicate *H. pylori* and drugs that reduce the gastric acid secretion or produce mucosal protection.

- Drugs that reduce gastric secretion can be divided into three groups:
  - histamine (H2-receptor) antagonists, e.g. cimetidine and ranitidine: these drugs act by blocking H2-receptors on parietal cells which prevents the intracellular increase in cAMP, and thus acid production
  - muscarinic antagonists are historic and not in clinical use.
  - proton pump inhibitors (PPI), e.g. omeprazole: activated at stomach low pH; these block the proton pump (H^{+}/K^{+} ATPase).
- Drugs that produce mucosal protection can be divided into three types:
  - sucralfate: forms a sticky layer that adheres to the base of the ulcer
  - bismuth chelate: acts the same; in addition, it helps eradicate *H. pylori*
  - misoprostol: stimulates secretion of mucus and bicarbonate and increases the mucosal blood flow.

3. ***The patient undergoes emergency laparotomy, and a large friable perforated duodenal ulcer is found that could not be closed with a patch. The surgeon decides to perform distal gastrectomy with Roux-en-Y gastrojejunostomy. What are the potential complications of gastrectomy?***
   - malnutrition
   - iron deficiency anaemia
   - vitamin B12 deficiency
   - dumping syndrome
   - diarrhoea
   - bilious vomiting
   - infection
   - carcinoma
   - risk of vagotomy.
4. ***Why does dumping syndrome develop?***
   - Early dumping (30–45 min after eating): due to the rapid gastric emptying of a hyperosmolar meal into the small bowel, resulting in fluid moving into the small bowel by osmosis (third space loss), and results in dizziness, weakness, and palpitations.
   - Late dumping (1–3 hours after eating): due to the rapid swings in insulin secretion in response to the glucose load in the small bowel, this leads to rebound hypoglycaemia.

OSCE SCENARIO ANSWER 10.5

A 65-year-old female patient with background of smoking and hypertension presents with chronic postprandial pain (sitophobia), weight loss and loose stools. She is found to be cachexic due to food fear and admission is for urgent investigations and addressing nutritional problems with total parenteral nutrition (TPN).

1. ***A CT abdomen is arranged (see** Fig. 10.5Q**). What is the main finding on this CT scan? What is the diagnosis?***

The CT scan clearly shows that there is occlusion of the superior mesenteric artery (SMA) from its origin (see arrow, Fig. 10.5A). The SMA is the main artery that supplies the small intestine and right colon; however, rich anastomoses take place between the SMA and the celiac artery and inferior mesenteric artery (IMA) via their terminal branches; hence, significant ischaemia usually occurs when more than one mesenteric artery is affected. This is called chronic mesenteric ischaemia. The CT scan also shows that the patient is cachexic.

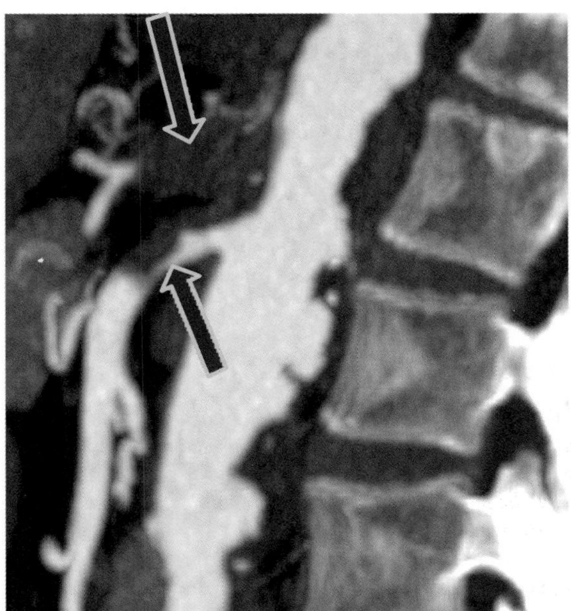

Fig. 10.5A CT angiogram showing occlusion of the Coeliac artery (top arrow) and tight stenosis of the superior mesenteric artery (SMA).

2. ***What are the pros and cons of enteral and parenteral feeding?***

Enteral feeding should be always preferred to maintain mucosal integrity of bowels. It is also associated with lower cost and infective complications than TPN. However, it can be difficult to adopt in cases of poor abruption/ileus, it can cause diarrhoea and increases risk of ventilator-associated pneumonia and sinusitis in ITU patients. TPN, on the other hand, does not depend on bowel integrity and function and provides easy route for full energy requirements. However, it is associated with risk of infection, liver dysfunction and metabolic complications such as mineral or trace element deficiency.

3. ***How would you treat this condition?***

As the patient is symptomatic and continues to lose weight, revascularization of the SMA would be indicated; however, before that, the patient's nutritional status should be optimized by referring the patient to the dietician; occasionally TPN is indicated. In addition, the patient should be on the best medical therapy for atherosclerotic disease in the form of antiplatelet therapy and statin. In addition, lifestyle modification, including smoking cessation and control of other risk factors such as diabetes, hypertension and hyperlipidaemia, should be addressed. Revascularization of the SMA can be via the endovascular route such as stent insertion or through open surgery such as endarterectomy of aorto- (or ilio)-mesenteric bypass.

4. ***Five days after her admission, the patient is found to have low levels of K, Mg and PO4. What is this condition called? And why does it develop?***

This is called refeeding syndrome. This metabolic disturbance is important to consider prior to feeding malnourished patients. The body adapts to a state of starvation and refeeding can cause insulin levels to rise in response to glycaemia, resulting in cellular uptake of K, PO_4 and Mg and causing their catastrophic depletion. Hypophosphataemia can reduce ATP and 2,3-DPG, causing cellular dysfunction that can cause respiratory and cardiac failure. It is also important to replenish thiamine, particularly in alcoholics.

OSCE SCENARIO ANSWER 11.1

A 70-year-old male is 2 days post-repair of a ruptured abdominal aortic aneurysm. Urine output has been poor, the last 4 h having been 20 mL, 10 mL, 5 mL and 5 mL per hour, respectively. The patient has been haemodynamically unstable.

1. ***How would you define oliguria?***

   Oliguria is a urine output of <0.5 mL/kg/h.

A specimen of urine is sent for examination and reveals the following results:

Specific gravity >1020
Urine osmolality >500 mOsm/kg
Urine sodium <20 mmol/L
Fractional sodium excretion <1.

2. ***What is the likely cause of the oliguria?***

This is physiological (pre-renal) oliguria. Likely causes are either dehydration, hypovolaemia or impaired cardiac function.

3. ***What action would you take based on these results?***
   - Fluid challenge with a bolus of 250–500 mL of fluid. CVP monitoring is often required in these patients. Fluid should be given until there is a sustained rise in the CVP, indicating that the patient is well filled.
   - If fluid challenges do not produce a diuresis, the next step is to ensure adequate renal perfusion pressure using inotropes such as noradrenaline. Furosemide rarely has a place in the acute management of poor urine output as it results in depletion of intravascular volume, although it may increase urine output; and dopamine has never been shown to improve outcome from acute renal failure, even though it may increase urine output.

Appropriate measures fail to produce a diuresis. Serum creatinine is now 350 mmol/L and urine analysis reveals the following:

Specific gravity <1010
Urine osmolality 290 mOsm/kg
Urine sodium >40 mmol/L
Fractional sodium excretion >2

4. ***What is now the cause of the patient's renal dysfunction?***

The patient is developing acute tubular necrosis.

5. ***What techniques are available for renal replacement therapy in this patient?***
   - The available techniques are:
     - haemodialysis
     - haemofiltration
     - haemodiafiltration.
   - Peritoneal dialysis is inappropriate in this patient as he has recently undergone major abdominal surgery and a prosthesis has been inserted (risk of infection).

6. ***What are the absolute indications for renal replacement therapy?***

The absolute indications for renal replacement therapy are:

- hyperkalaemia (>6.5 mmol/L)
- severe metabolic acidosis (HCO_3^- <10 mmol/L)
- fluid overload with pulmonary oedema
- symptoms of severe uraemia, e.g. fits, pericarditis.

7. ***Which mode of renal replacement therapy will be the most appropriate in this patient?***
   - Haemofiltration is the most appropriate.
   - Haemodialysis involves movement of large volumes between body compartments, and risk of gross hypotension and cardiac arrhythmias in the haemodynamically unstable patient. With haemofiltration,

fluid removal can be achieved gradually over a period of time.

- It is highly efficient, giving good ECF volume control, and can be used in the hypotensive patient.
- With continuous veno-venous haemofiltration, almost any quantity of fluid can be removed in a 24 h period, allowing administration of other fluids, e.g. parenteral nutrition.

OSCE SCENARIO ANSWER 11.2

A 19-year-old male is admitted to A&E having been stabbed in the abdomen. On examination he is pale, sweating, with a tachycardia of 120 and a systolic blood pressure of 80 mmHg.

1. What are the grades of haemorrhagic shock?

Haemorrhagic shock can be classified from 1 to 4 and allows a rough clinical assessment of the amount of blood lost.

- Class 1: 15% blood loss or <750 mL, pulse is <100, BP is normal, pulse pressure is normal and there may be a mild increase in respiratory rate. Urine output is normal. Clinically this occurs when donating blood.
- Class 2: 15–30% blood loss or >750 mL and <1500 mL, the pulse is elevated, the BP is normal but the pulse pressure has narrowed due to an increase in diastolic pressure owing to the release of natural vasoconstrictors. The patient has a mild tachypnoea (20–30 breaths/min) and urine output may fall (20–30 mL/h).
- Class 3: 30–40% blood loss or >1500 to <2000 mL, the patient looks in shock from the end of the bed, and is anxious or confused, pale and tachypnoeic. The pulse rate is above 120, the systolic blood pressure is <100 mmHg and urine output is markedly reduced (<10 mL/h).
- Class 4: >40% or >2000 mL blood loss, the patient is in extremis and is white, barely rousable and will die very soon if haemorrhage is not arrested. Pulse rate is >140, blood pressure may be unrecordable (or sometimes only systolic) and the urine output is negligible.

2. What is renal blood flow autoregulation and how is it affected by shock?

- Autoregulation is the physiological ability of the kidney to maintain perfusion at a constant level across a range of perfusion pressures. Autoregulation occurs between 80 mmHg and 180 mmHg. The main site of autoregulation in the kidney is the afferent glomerular arteriole. Two main factors affect vascular tone in the afferent arteriole:
  - myogenic: with an increase in transmural pressure the arterioles are distended, thus stretching the muscle in the wall, resulting in vasoconstriction, an increase in vascular resistance and decrease in renal blood flow
  - tubulo-glomerular feedback via the juxtaglomerular apparatus: complex signals pass from the macula densa to the afferent arteriole, regulating its tone.
- These mechanisms fail below around 80 mmHg, i.e. in a state of severe shock, and other mechanisms, namely hormonal, will attempt to compensate, e.g. antidiuretic hormone (ADH), aldosterone and the renin–angiotensin system (RAS).

3. Describe the hormonal response to shock with specific reference to ADH, aldosterone and the renin–angiotensin system.

The effect of ADH, aldosterone and the RAS all aim both to increase blood pressure (and thus perfusion pressure) and to maintain intravascular volume. They have the following effects:

- ADH: leads to an increase in the permeability of the distal tubule and collecting ducts to water and thus increases absorption and increases intravascular volume. It is also a potent vasoconstrictor.
- Aldosterone: leads to an increased absorption of sodium in the distal convoluted tubules and thus acts to increase plasma volume and blood pressure.
- RAS: renin leads to the conversion of angiotensinogen to angiotensin II. This is a powerful vasoconstrictor (thus increasing blood pressure) and also stimulates the release of both ADH and aldosterone.

OSCE SCENARIO ANSWER 11.3

A 75-year-old male with a known lung malignancy is admitted in an acute confusional state. He is found to have a sodium level of 117 mmol/L. He is not dehydrated and has no signs of sepsis.

1. What possible explanation is there for the electrolyte abnormality?

The lung malignancy and hyponatraemia in the presence of normovolaemia would suggest SIADH (syndrome of inappropriate antidiuretic hormone secretion).

2. What other tests would help confirm it?

Measuring the urine sodium content and urine/plasma osmolality. In the face of hyponatraemia the urine will have sodium level >40 mmol/L and urine osmolality will be >100 mOsm/kg and the plasma osmolality is <280 mOsm/kg.

3. Which type of lung cancer most commonly causes it?

Small cell lung cancer is the commonest cause of SIADH.

4. How would you treat it?

An endocrinologist should be consulted. Treatment in the acute setting consists of:

- 3% hypertonic saline
- water restriction 0.5–1.5 L per day
- loop diuretics to excrete free water
- vasopressin receptor antagonists (e.g. tolvaptan); these block the AVP V2 receptors.

OSCE SCENARIO ANSWER 11.4

A 40-year-old male who was a restrained driver in a motor vehicle crash was found to be paraplegic at the level of T10. After primary and secondary survey, he was admitted to the high-dependency unit and abdominal examination revealed palpable bladder.

1. ***What is the normal innervation to the urinary bladder?***
    - L1–2: sympathetic outflow via the hypogastric plexus that acts to inhibit micturition by suppressing detrusor contraction and stimulating internal sphincter contraction.
    - S2–4: parasympathetic outflow via the pelvic splanchnic and pudendal nerves which stimulate micturition by stimulating the detrusor muscle and suppressing the internal sphincter contraction.
    - Efferent sensory fibres enter the spinal cord at L1–2 and S2–4.
2. ***What are the three bladder abnormalities that can occur following spinal injury?***
    - Atonic bladder: or flaccid bladder, refers to a bladder whose muscles do not fully contract. Hence, the patient might sense that they need to urinate, but they are unable to because their bladder muscles will not contract. As a result, the bladder can overflow with urine, causing leakage and discomfort.
    - Automatic reflex bladder: with a reflex bladder, the nerve impulses (known as the reflex arc) between the bladder and spinal cord remain intact but messages no longer reach the brain. A reflex bladder allows automatic, involuntary control of the bladder so when the bladder fills above a certain level it contracts and urine flows out automatically. However, the reflex bladder may not empty completely due to the sphincter not relaxing fully. This can leave a pool of urine in the bladder which increases the risk of infection and back pressure on the kidneys.
    - Autonomous bladder: with autonomous bladder, there is interruption in both the afferent and efferent limbs of the reflex arcs. Bladder sensation is absent; dribbling is constant; residual urine amount is large.
3. ***Describe the bladder function following the initial phase of spinal injury.***

Atonic bladder occurs during the initial phase of spinal shock and may last for several weeks; the following abnormalities are seen:

- Bladder wall muscle is relaxed.
- Sphincter vesicae is contracted.
- Sphincter urethra is relaxed.
- Bladder becomes distended and eventually empties by overflow. If the level of injury is above L1–2 then the patient becomes unaware of the bladder distension; if the injury is below L1–2 then the patient is aware of the distended bladder.

OSCE SCENARIO ANSWER 11.5

A 70-year-old male is admitted to the emergency surgical unit with suprapubic pain and inability to pass urine for 12 h. He reported recent history of hesitancy, weak stream and nocturia. Abdominal examination revealed a palpable distended bladder. His creatinine is found to be 220 μmol/L and GFR of 32 mL/min/1.73 m², while his baseline test 2 months ago showed GFR of 60 mL/min/1.73 m² and Cr of 87 μmol/L.

1. ***What volume in the bladder normally triggers the urge to urinate?***

The intravesical pressure is normally around 3 cmH_2O and the pressure does not change much until the intravesical volume reaches 200–300 mL, at which point the desire to pass urine is felt. As the volume increases further, the intravesical pressure rises steeply.

2. ***What is the differential diagnosis?***

The clinical scenario suggests acute on chronic bladder urinary retention with a background of symptoms of benign prostatic disease. The commonest cause is benign prostate hypertrophy. Other causes include prostate cancer, severe constipation, urethral stricture, urinary tract infection, drugs, general anaesthesia and a mass or cancer in the pelvis.

3. ***What is the likely cause of his renal function deterioration?***

Causes of acute kidney injury can be classified into prerenal, renal, or post-renal. In this case, the cause is postrenal due to obstructive uropathy and inability to void, which results in tubulointerstitial injury. This tends to be reversible if urinary retention is treated promptly.

4. ***The patient was found to have been recently commenced on tamsulosin by his GP. How does tamsulosin work?***

Tamsulosin is a drug that inhibits α1 sympathetic receptors located in the prostate smooth muscles which in turn relax the bladder neck and relieve some of the symptoms associated with benign prostatic disease.

OSCE SCENARIO ANSWER 12.1

A 32-year-old female is admitted with suspected acute appendicitis. She is sweating, agitated, confused and complaining of palpitations. Her symptoms do not fit with a straightforward diagnosis of acute appendicitis. Examination reveals a temperature of 40°C and a tachycardia of 140 with an irregularly irregular pulse. You check her thyroid function, which reveals an elevated T_3 and T_4 with suppressed TSH.

1. ***What is the most likely diagnosis?***

The symptoms and signs suggest a thyroid storm (crisis).

2. ***What may precipitate the condition?***

Thyroid storm is an uncommon condition but has a mortality rate >50%. It is a hypermetabolic state that occurs in undiagnosed patients with hyperthyroidism and also in inadequately treated patients with hyperthyroidism. It is commonly precipitated by infection, trauma or surgery.

3. ***How is the condition managed?***

Immediate recognition of the condition is the key to managing patients with a thyroid storm (crisis). Thyroid storm (crisis) is manifest by hyperpyrexia, tachycardia, hypertension, severe tremor, agitation, confusion and high output cardiac failure. Confirmation of the diagnosis is with urgent thyroid function tests. Medical management consists of:

- ABC: high-flow oxygen i.v. access and fluids
- if infection is suspected, treat empirically with antibiotics
- high-dose propylthiouracil: prevents the production of more T_4 and T_3 and blocks the peripheral conversion of T_4 to T_3
- 1 h after administration of propylthiouracil, administer Lugol's iodine. This blocks the release of stored T_4 and T_3. If it is given before the propylthiouracil works, it will increase the release of thyroid hormone
- hydrocortisone: blocks the peripheral conversion of T_4 to T_3
- beta-blocker: used to treat tachycardia, tremor and agitation.

OSCE SCENARIO ANSWER 12.2

A 40-year-old male presents to his GP with intermittent headaches, palpitations, sweating, anxiety and intermittent chest pains. Examination reveals a blood pressure of 180/110 mmHg.

1. ***What endocrine condition do you need to consider? Explain the condition.***
   - A diagnosis of phaeochromocytoma must be considered in this case.
   - Phaeochromocytomas are tumours of the chromaffin cells. Around 90% arise in the adrenal glands. Phaeochromocytomas are known as the '10%' tumour as 10% are bilateral, extra-adrenal, multiple or familial (especially MEN IIa and IIb) and malignant.
2. ***How could you confirm the diagnosis?***

The diagnosis is confirmed by:

- Biochemical diagnosis: 24 h acidified urine sample for VMA (vanillylmandelic acid), which is a breakdown product of catecholamines.
- Imaging diagnosis: CT and MRI are accurate in the majority of cases. MRI is preferred as it is more accurate in identifying extra-adrenal tumours. Radioisotope MIBG scans (^{131}I-metaiodobenzylguanidine) may be used for extra-adrenal tumours and metastases in cases of malignancy.

3. ***What measures would you take to prepare the patient for surgery?***

Two main forms of medication are required:

- Alpha-adrenergic blockade with phenoxybenzamine. Treatment should be given prior to surgery until nasal stuffiness and postural hypotension occur. High dosage may need to be gradually introduced to block the adrenergic effects of the tumour.
- Beta-blockade with propanolol should be used only when alpha-blockade is complete. If used before, it may precipitate a hypertensive crisis.

OSCE SCENARIO ANSWER 12.3

A 64-year-old female is admitted for major gastrointestinal surgery. She is taking 5 mg prednisolone and has been doing so for 6 months.

1. ***What are the risks of failing to replace steroids pre-operatively?***

Steroids will cause adrenal suppression. At the time of major surgery the body needs increased steroids as a part of the acute phase response. If this is not met due to the adrenal suppression, then an Addisonian crisis may occur. This presents as low BP, hypoglycaemia, confusion, hyponatraemia, hyperkalaemia and hypercalcaemia.

2. ***How would you manage her steroid administration prior to major surgery?***

For major surgery the patient takes the usual pre-operative steroid dose. She should have 25 mg of hydrocortisone i.v. on induction and then 100 mg i.v. daily for 48–72 h unless there are post-operative complications.

3. ***How long after stopping steroids would a patient not require pre-operative replacement?***

If the patient has stopped taking steroids, a period of stress may still cause an Addisonian crisis. This is a potential risk up to 3 months from the time of stopping steroids. After 3 months, steroid replacement is not required.

OSCE SCENARIO ANSWER 12.4

A 46-year-old female has undergone a total thyroidectomy – you are called to the ward as the patient is suffering from severe cramps and numb peripheries.

1. ***What are Chovstek's and Trousseau's signs?***

Chovstek's sign is a contraction of the facial muscles when you tap the facial nerve just in front of the external auditory meatus. Trousseau's sign is a spasm of the hand when a blood pressure cuff is inflated.

2. ***What is causing the above symptoms and why? What would you expect to see on an ECG and how would you treat it?***

The above symptoms are due to hypocalcaemia. The likely cause for this in this patient is either ischaemia or inadvertent removal of all parathyroid glands. An ECG would typically show a prolonged QT interval. Treatment is with a combination of i.v. calcium gluconate acutely and a combination of oral calcium and vitamin D.

3. ***Why has the hypocalcaemia happened and what will be the long-term treatment?***

The parathyroid glands are intimately related to the thyroid gland and may be removed or damaged during surgery. In addition, ligation of the inferior thyroid artery may render them ischaemic. Preservation during surgery is the mainstay of preventing this complication. If the gland is removed accidentally it can be diced and then placed in an intra-muscular pocket in the sternomastoid where it will eventually be revascularized. Even if this is not done, parathyroid function will eventually return to normal as ectopic islands will grow or retained parathyroid tissue will revascularize. In the short term, the hypocalcaemia may need to be managed with i.v. calcium gluconate acutely or vitamin D and oral calcium in the long term if symptoms persist.

OSCE SCENARIO ANSWER 12.5

A 45-year-old male attends a GP surgery with some strange symptoms – he describes episodes of sweating, palpitations, being confused and forgetting things, and also abdominal pain and diarrhoea. A friend thought it might be diabetes and measures his blood sugar during an episode and found it to be 3 mmol/L.

1. ***What is the diagnosis and what is the classic triad associated with this condition?***

There are a number of possibilities but the symptoms would be highly suggestive of an insulinoma. Symptoms are either due to a lack of glucose, i.e. weakness, sweating, lack of cerebral glucose (confusion, forgetfulness or odd behaviour) or from GI tract problems, such as hunger or diarrhoea. The classic triad is Whipple's triad, which is symptoms due to hypoglycaemia, a diagnosis of low glucose at the time of the symptoms and having glucose relieves the symptoms.

2. ***What cells does the disorder arise from?***

Insulin is produced in β-cells so insulinomas arise from pancreatic β-cells.

3. ***What percentages are benign or malignant?***

Malignancy is not common and only around 10% are malignant.

4. ***What syndrome are they associated with?***

Insulinomas can be related to a group of conditions known as multiple endocrine neoplasia; this is an autosomal dominant condition and there are three types. Most typically insulinomas are associated with MEN I. MEN I is associated with hyperparathyroidism, pancreatic/duodenal tumours and pituitary tumours. MEN IIA is associated with medullary thyroid carcinoma, phaeochromocytoma and hyperparathyroidism. MEN IIB is associated with same as IIa but patients have multiple ganglioneuromas and a marfanoid appearance.

OSCE SCENARIO ANSWER 13.1

An 18-year-old male is admitted to A&E following an assault. He has severe head injuries. His GCS is 6.

1. ***How is brain injury classified?***

Brain injury is classified as primary or secondary.

- Primary: this is the damage caused as an immediate result of trauma. It results in contusions, lacerations and diffuse brain damage. There are two mains types: focal damage or diffuse axonal injury. Treatment cannot reverse primary brain injury.
- Secondary: this develops as a result of complications. Complications include intracranial haemorrhage, cerebral hypoxia, cerebral oedema, intracranial herniation and cerebral infection, e.g. meningitis. The prevention, recognition and treatment of these secondary complications are the mainstay of treatment of the patient with head injuries.

2. ***Describe the mechanism of compensation for an acute rise in intracranial pressure.***

- The skull, which is a rigid container, contains the brain, CSF and blood. The volume of the brain is static and cannot alter. Compensation occurs following head injury as the swelling/haematoma pushes CSF and blood out of the skull vault. This will compensate for a mass of approximately 100–150 mL. After this point the ICP sharply increases as compensation can no longer occur.
- This is referred to as the Monro–Kellie hypothesis, which states that the ICP will increase if the volume of one component is increased. The increase in ICP

can only be compensated for by a decrease in one or both of the other components.

The patient is transferred to ITU and you are called because the intracranial pressure (ICP) has risen acutely.

3. ***Describe the possible management options.***

As with any critically ill patient, the initial management should be according to ABC principles. In an isolated head injury, ICP should be kept below 20 mmHg. In a patient with an ICP above this, options for management include:

- Position the patient head up 30° to improve venous drainage (removing a spinal collar can only help if safe to do so).
- Sedate the patient: this decreases cerebral metabolism and can be achieved with propofol or thiopental.
- Hyperventilation: normally a patient should be normocarbic but in instances of sudden increase in ICP, a period of hyperventilation may buy time.
- Treat with i.v. mannitol, an osmotic diuretic that reduces brain water and thus volume.
- Inducing hypothermia may be protective.
- Contact the neurosurgical team. They may advise re-scanning of the patient to identify a reason for deterioration. Surgical options include CSF drainage, evacuation of haematoma, craniectomy and lobectomy.

OSCE SCENARIO ANSWER 13.2

A 55-year-old male presents to a pain clinic with a long history of lumbar back pain that has become more severe recently. There is no history of sciatica and there is no neurological deficit on examination. Paracetamol has been of no benefit.

1. ***Why is paracetamol unlikely to have been of benefit?***
   - Paracetamol is an effective analgesic and anti-pyretic. It is believed to inhibit COX-3 (cyclo-oxygenase-3) in the spinal cord and brain, and this results in analgesia. It has little effect on COX-1 and 2, thus explaining its poor anti-inflammatory action.
   - This patient is likely to have a significant inflammatory component to his pain and this explains the lack of benefit from paracetamol.

He is commenced on ibuprofen.

2. ***Why is this more likely to be of benefit than paracetamol?***

Ibuprofen is an inhibitor of COX-1 and COX-2 enzymes, leading to inhibition of a number of prostaglandins involved in pain transmission (thus explaining the analgesic effect). It also inhibits prostaglandins involved in inflammation.

Treatment with ibuprofen brings about little improvement and he is treated with a TENS machine.

3. ***What is the mechanism of action of TENS?***
   - TENS is thought to work by closing the gate on pain, i.e. preventing onward transmission of pain signals from the dorsal horn of the spinal cord to the ascending sensory nerves (spinothalamic tract) which connect to the pain centres in the brain.
   - TENS signals arrive at the dorsal horn by large sensory A-fibres at the same time as pain signals arriving via small sensory C-fibres. If the large A-fibre input is significantly strong, the C-fibre input is inhibited, producing pain relief.

TENS provides initial improvement but the benefit is slowly lost. He is treated by facet joint injections with local anaesthetic and steroid.

4. ***What is the purpose of the local anaesthetic injection and what is the mechanism of action of local anaesthetics?***
   - The combination of steroid and local anaesthetic injections produces a combination of the short-lived pain relief given by local anaesthetic followed by the longer-term relief provided by the anti-inflammatory action of the steroids.
   - Local anaesthetics reversibly block nerve conduction by inactivating sodium channels. This preferentially affects smaller nerve endings that transmit sharp pain.

Facet joint injections with steroid fail to give lasting relief and he is commenced on Oramorph (morphine).

5. ***What is the mechanism of action of Oramorph and what side effects might be expected?***
   - Oramorph is a liquid form of morphine, a member of a group of drugs known as opiates. Opioid painkillers work by mimicking the action of naturally occurring pain-reducing chemicals called endorphins. Endorphins are found in the brain and spinal cord and reduce pain by combining with opioid receptors.
   - Oramorph interacts predominantly with the opioid mu receptor in the brain (posterior amygdala, thalamus, caudate nucleus and putamen) and spinal cord (substantia gelatinosa).
   - Side-effects of opiates include dependence, respiratory depression, sedation, itching, nausea and constipation.

OSCE SCENARIO ANSWER 13.3

A 24-year-old male is in a critical condition on ITU following a road traffic accident. He has severe head injuries. The ITU consultant has discussed his poor prognosis with the family and they ask about organ donation. Answer the following questions regarding testing for brainstem death.

1. ***What are the preconditions required before diagnosing brainstem death?***

There are four preconditions for diagnosing brainstem death:

- patient must be in a coma
- known cause for coma
- cause is irreversible
- patient dependent on ventilator.

2. ***What are the exclusion criteria?***

There are three exclusion criteria prior to carrying out brainstem death tests:

- no residual effects from drugs: e.g. narcotics, hypnotics, tranquilizers, muscle relaxants, alcohol or illicit drugs
- core body temperature >35°C
- no reversible causes that may contribute coma (circulatory, endocrine or metabolic).

3. ***Which cranial nerves are involved in the following tests:***

Corneal reflex
Gag reflex
Cough reflex
Vestibulocochlear reflex

The cranial nerves involved in each test are as follows:

- Corneal reflex – V and VI
- Gag reflex – IX and X
- Cough reflex – IX and X
- Vestibulocochlear reflex – III, VI and VIII.

OSCE SCENARIO ANSWER 13.4

A 75-year-old male patient is found confused during a night shift, 5 days following left hemicolectomy. He has past medical history of TIA, IHD and BPH. On examination, his GCS is 13/15, he appears combative and hallucinating, his temperature is 38.9°C, RR is 25/min, PR is 120/min and irregular and blood pressure is 115/65. His chest examination shows possible reduced air entry on the left side, he is diffusely tender in the abdomen, and he has a urinary catheter with urine output averaging 20/h over the last 3 h. Bedside ECG shows new fast AF. You are the night surgical SPR and asked to review the patient.

1. ***How would you manage this patient?***

This patient is suffering from acute onset postoperative confusion and management should be along the guidance of the care of critically ill surgical patients' course (CCrISP) with assessment of ABCDE, etc. In summary, oxygen therapy and commencement of intravenous fluid resuscitation should be followed by history and examination, including a review of his medical notes, drug chart, vital signs, fluid balance charts and recent lab results. In addition to bedside ECG, up-to-date blood tests including FBC, U&E, LFT, glucose and ABGs should be sought. As the patient has signs of sepsis, it is important to look for a source and initial assessment with blood cultures, chest X-ray, sputum culture (if applicable), midstream urine and wound swabs should be sent. Assessment should include examination for infected lines and early commencement of broad-spectrum intravenous antibiotics. While the patient is very confused and has fast AF, these are secondary signs to sepsis and addressing the acute presentation with sedation, e.g. haloperidol, and medical control of fast AF, e.g. digoxin, might be required at certain points in his management but should not be the sole management plan.

2. ***What is the differential diagnosis?***

The presence of fever in this scenario suggests infection as the underlying cause; however, other causes should be ruled out with a detailed assessment. Other causes can be:

- dehydration
- electrolyte abnormalities
- hypoxia
- drugs
- uraemia
- hypoglycaemia
- pre-existing psychiatric disorder or dementia
- alcohol and drug withdrawal
- urinary retention
- pain and anxiety
- cerebrovascular accident (CVA)
- head injury (especially trauma patients)
- sleep deprivation
- ITU syndrome: pain, fear and sleep deprivation can lead to visual and auditory hallucinations and inability to differentiate reality from fantasy.

3. ***What is the most likely cause?***

The clinical scenario suggests infection as the underlying cause of confusion and the patient has mainly abdominal signs. In the context of recent colonic surgery, the possibility of anastomotic leak or intra-abdominal infected collection should be considered, and CT abdomen and pelvis would be indicated.

4. ***Who would you inform at this stage?***

In addition to the surgical consultant on call, it would be relevant to inform the on-call radiologist regarding the urgency of the CT scan; the critical team outreach as the patient might need perioperative admission to critical care; the on-call anaesthetic and theatre team as he might need emergency laparotomy and patient's next of kin to inform them of his progress.

OSCE SCENARIO ANSWER 13.5

A 65-year-old male patient has been stepped down from the high-dependency unit to the ward on day 2 following open *repair of abdominal aortic aneurysm. As you review him on the ward round, you notice that he is comfortable in bed; however, his blood pressure is low at 95/60 and pulse rate is 58/min. He is apyrexial and his RR is 16/min and his oxygen saturation is 98% on room air. His abdominal examination is unremarkable, and his pain is well controlled, having epidural catheter in situ. The night FY1 gave him intravenous fluid challenge 2h earlier, which improved his BP reading slightly, and arranged for blood tests. His Hb is 12.5g/dL, WBC 11.2 × 10^6/dL, while the rest of his blood tests are unremarkable.*

1. ***What are the possible causes of his low blood pressure?***

The most common cause of postoperative hypotension remains hypovolaemia which can be either due to dehydration, third space fluid loss or bleeding. Other causes can be cardiogenic, such as myocardial infarction, pulmonary embolism, sepsis or anaphylaxis. However, the clinical scenario did not raise suspicion of any of these possibilities, which raises the possibility of the epidural infusion being the cause of hypotension and bradycardia.

2. ***What drugs are usually infused in epidural catheters?***

Most commonly the infusion would consist of:

- Local anaesthetic agents which block sensory afferent nerve roots and reduce transmission of pain.
- Opioids (e.g. fentanyl): diffuse through the dura into CSF and bind to spinal cord opioid receptors.

3. ***How does epidural infusion cause hypotension?***

It can cause a degree of blockage to the sympathetic nervous system (runs from T1–L2) which results in vasodilatation and hypotension.

4. ***Why is postoperative analgesia important for surgical patients?***

In addition to alleviating the unpleasant sensation of pain and associated psychological stress, postoperative analgesia is important to prevent complications including respiratory (e.g. atelectasis and pneumonia), cardiovascular (e.g. myocardial strain), thromboembolism due to immobilization, GI (e.g. ileus, stress ulcers) and urinary retention.

5. ***What are the side effects and complications of epidural catheters?***

These can be classified into those related to:

- Side effects of the drugs used such as nausea and vomiting, pruritus, sedation, reduced sensation of needing to urinate (hence, the need for urinary catheter), respiratory centre depression and hypotension.
- Complications of insertion such as haematoma, infection, dural puncture and headache and failure to achieve adequate block.

6. ***How would you treat hypotension related to epidural catheters?***

Anaesthetic review to consider reduction in rate, intravenous fluids and, in severe compromise, vasoconstrictor can be administered to reverse the effect of vasodilatation.

OSCE SCENARIO ANSWER 14.1

A 77-year-old female presents to your clinic with a suspicious-looking lesion on her temple.

1. ***Outline your history, examination, investigations and management plan.***

History

Salient points in the history should include:

- Length of time lesion has been present.
- How it has changed over this time, and how rapidly, specifically changes in or presence of:
  - size
  - shape
  - colour
  - borders
  - crusting/bleeding
  - itching
  - trauma.
- Any history of skin neoplasms or previous similar lesions.
- History of significant sun exposure or episodes of blistering sunburn.
- Any pre-malignant skin conditions (i.e. giant hairy naevus or xeroderma pigmentosum).
- Any family history of skin neoplasms.
- Systemic review to exclude cutaneous metastatic deposits of other malignancies (rare).
- Quick review of any past medical conditions, allergies, previous local anaesthetics and drugs (particularly warfarin/aspirin/clopidogrel).

Examination

Examination should include:

- Search for other scars of excised lesions or similar lesions.
- Measurement of the lesion (not approximated guesses).
- Assessment of pigmentation, borders, edges.
- Mention any ulceration, telangectasia, satellite lesions, etc.
- Check for regional lymphadenopathy.

Investigations

Investigations are:

- Clotting screen if on anticoagulants.
- Imaging/FNA of any nodes.

Management

A suspicious lesion that is small and can be closed directly should be managed by excision biopsy in the first instance.

2. ***Draw around the lesion on the diagram** (Fig. 14.1Q) **to indicate your surgical margins and direction of incision.***

See Fig. 14.1A.

The pathology report of the lesion indicates an incompletely excised poorly differentiated squamous cell carcinoma with ulceration. A multi-disciplinary skin cancer meeting suggests re-excision of the scar with a 1 cm margin.

3. ***Outline your options for closing this defect.***

Direct closure is unlikely to be an option. Options for closure of the defect would include:

- skin graft (split or full thickness)
- local flap (advancement/transposition/rotation are all acceptable choices).

4. ***Explain the pathological findings and management plan to the patient including her follow-up.***

Salient points would include (in layman's terms):

- Tell the patient she did have a form of skin cancer.
- Explain the incomplete excision and need to take further tissue to reduce risks of it returning.
- Explain that direct closure is not an option, and outline the process of either a local flap (moving tissue near to the area to close the skin) or a skin graft and the donor site of either choice.
- The patient should be aware that she will have a larger scar if a local flap is used and a donor scar if a graft is used.
- The patient should be counselled about the possibility of needing further tissue excised and the possibility of flap or graft failure.

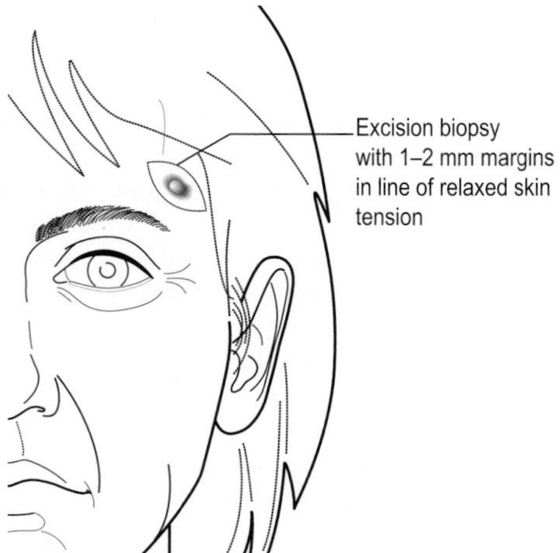

Fig. 14.1A Excision margins (2 mm) in lines of relaxed skin tension.

- The patient should know that her flap/graft will need to be checked in approximately 1 week and she will be seen in 4–6 weeks with the pathology results. She should also know that she will be followed up every few months to check the lesion has not returned or spread.

OSCE SCENARIO ANSWER 14.2

You are the A&E doctor in a district general hospital at 3 a.m. A 33-year-old male has been trapped in a fire in his home, and had to be rescued from the house by the fire brigade, who think the fire started at around 1 a.m. He has superficial non-blistering burns to his face with soot around his nose, and blistering burns to the whole of his left leg and arm, including his hand. He appears confused and the ambulance crew think he may be intoxicated.

1. ***Approximately what percentage is this man's burn? What features would you use to assess the depth of the blistered burn?***

This man has burnt the whole of one arm (9%) and leg (18%) = approximately 27% burns. You are told that the facial burns are non-blistering; therefore these are not included in the burns estimation. Features that you would use to assess the depth of the blistered burn would include:

- colour (pink/red/white/black)
- presence/absence of pain/sensation
- presence/absence of capillary refill.

2. ***Assuming that his facial burns are epidermal and his arm/leg burns are full-thickness, calculate this man's fluid resuscitation requirements and detail how this should be administered.***

- This man weighs 65 kg and has 27% burns. Using the Parkland formula: 4 (mL) × 65 (kg) × 27 (% TBSA) = 7020 mL of Hartmann's solution over 24 h.
- The estimation of time of burn is given at 1 a.m.; therefore, as it is now 3 a.m., the first half of this volume (3510 mL) needs to be given over 6 h, not 8 h, as we are 2 h post-burn.
- Therefore in the next 6 h this man needs 3510/6 = 585 mL/h of fluid.
- After this initial 8 h post-burn, he requires the second half of the resuscitation volume to be given over 16 h = 3510 mL/16 = 220 mL/h.

3. ***What acute injuries and pathology specific to burns would this man be at risk of from the above description?***

- Inhalational injury: you are told that the man was in a house fire (enclosed space) and had to be removed by the fire brigade, indicating that he may have been in a smoke-filled area for some time.
- Compromised limb vascularity: as this man's entire left arm and leg have sustained full-thickness burns,

it is very possible that to avoid vascular compromise he will require escharotomy to release swelling compartments from the inelastic burn eschar.
- Carbon monoxide poisoning: you are told that the man appears confused, possibly intoxicated. It is very dangerous to assume that his confusion is due to intoxication, and carbon monoxide poisoning must always be excluded.

4. Which allied medical staff would you like to involve?

Given your above suspicions, it would be reasonable to initially involve the following:
- anaesthetist (possible early intubation)
- surgeon (possible escharotomies)
- intensivist (possible ITU admission)
- paramedics (possible transfer if no burns service at the hospital)
- A&E nurses (repeat observations/catheter/fluids).

Later, the following would also be important to patient care:
- physiotherapist (splints, exercises, walking aids)
- dietician (enteral or parenteral nutritional support)
- occupational therapist (pressure garments, home assessments)
- psychosocial support (counselling, treatment for depression/anxiety/post-traumatic stress).

OSCE SCENARIO ANSWER 14.3

You see a 63-year-old male in clinic who describes a 2-year history of an ulcer on his leg. He has been self-managing the wound with dressings from the pharmacy, but recently it has become malodorous and his children encouraged him to seek medical advice.

1. What salient features from this man's history would you like to know?

Salient points in the history should include:
- Symptoms of the ulcer: e.g. pain, purulence, itch, bleeding.
- How has it changed over the past 2 years?
- Any history of similar ulcers in the past.
- Past medical history of peripheral vascular disease, diabetes, varicose veins, cardiac disease, skin cancers, autoimmune diseases, previous fractures in the limb.
- Review of medications and allergies.

2. What is your differential diagnosis?
- Venous ulcer.
- Ischaemic/arterial ulcer.
- Neuropathic ulcer.
- Skin neoplasm.

3. Describe the factors affecting wound healing.

Factors affecting wound healing can be classified into local and systemic:
- Local factors include:
  - inadequate blood supply
  - infection
  - foreign material
  - irradiation
  - neuropathy.
- Systemic factors include:
  - advanced age
  - poor nutrition
  - immunosuppression
  - neoplasia.
- Systemic disease, e.g. jaundice, uraemia.

On further questioning the patient tells you he has previously had radiotherapy to this limb for a 'kind of skin cancer'.

4. What effects does radiotherapy have on the body? How does this change your differential diagnosis?

Radiotherapy effects may be classified into acute and chronic, local and systemic:
- Acute: cell death, inflammation.
- Chronic: vascular damage and insufficiency, tissue atrophy and fibrosis, neoplasia.
- Local: skin burns/irritation, hyperpigmentation, telangectasia, alopecia, local discomfort.
- Systemic: fatigue, marrow suppression, diarrhoea, strictures, fibrosis, sterility.

The differential diagnosis should now have neoplastic ulcers and radiation-induced ulcers at the top of the list.

OSCE SCENARIO ANSWER 14.4

A 79-year-old diabetic has neglected a foot infection and is admitted extremely unwell. The whole forefoot is black, wet and malodorous.

1. What type of necrosis has occurred in the foot?

This type of necrosis is known as gangrenous necrosis. The necrotic tissue provides an excellent anaerobic environment for bacteria to proliferate and produce toxins that cause local tissue damage but also damage the microcirculation, leading to more extensive tissue damage.

2. What clinical term is used for this type of tissue loss?

This would be referred to as wet gangrene. It is a life-threatening infection and will continue to progress and lead to systemic illness. It is easy to spot as the wound will characteristically smell bad and the black tissue is wet and friable. If gangrene does not get secondarily infected it will eventually dry out and the body will try to demarcate healthy and dead tissue. Indeed for toes it may auto-amputate and drop off. This is known as dry gangrene.

3. What would be the clinical management of this patient?

The patient may be very unwell so ABC should be the initial management with particular attention to C as they may be septic and hypotensive. It is imperative to give broad-spectrum antibiotics early. Cultures and swabs should be taken but not at the expense of giving antibiotics. Early surgery to debride the dead tissue or amputate an unsalvageable limb is required when the patient is stabilized.

OSCE SCENARIO ANSWER 14.5

A 53-year-old female is in the breast cancer clinic following surgery for a right-sided breast tumour. As you are taking a history she tells you she has also had ovarian cancer and that a close relative had a brain tumour and a rare muscle tumour.

1. ***Do you know of any inherited condition that relates to all these tumours?***

Li Fraumeni syndrome would link all these conditions. This syndrome has an inherited abnormality in the *p53* gene and leads characteristically to breast and ovarian carcinomas, astrocytomas and sarcomas.

2. ***What does p53 normally do and how does it lead to neoplasia when genetic abnormalities occur?***

p53 is a tumour-suppressor gene – these are a group of genes that either repair DNA damage (caretaker) or ensure cells with damaged DNA cannot replicate (gatekeeper). *p53* is a gatekeeper gene and is a very common abnormality in a number of cancers. *p53* is involved in repair of DNA by halting the cell cycle until repair is carried out. If DNA cannot be repaired then it will initiate cell death (apoptosis) – if abnormal then cells will continue to have cells with DNA damage and eventually this will lead to further mutations that will give rise to cancerous cells.

OSCE SCENARIO ANSWER 15.1

A 66-year-old male is admitted through A&E with painless red bleeding per rectum. He has no past medical history and a subsequent colonoscopy shows multiple benign-looking polyps only, which have been biopsied. He is anxious and worried about his condition and has asked to speak to a doctor.

1. ***Answer the patient's questions about polyps and rectal bleeding. Explain the different types of polyps and the need for the biopsy, avoiding medical jargon.***
   - Polyps can be found all over the body including in the bowel, nose and uterus.
   - Most polyps are benign but some are cancerous or have the potential to cause cancer if left without treatment.
   - They can cause different symptoms as they can differ in size and shape. Some can bleed; some can twist on themselves or become inflamed and cause pain.
   - It is important that we find out what type of polyp you have, although the surgeon did say that they didn't look like cancerous polyps when he saw them with the camera.
   - The only way to be sure is to take a sample and see what it shows under the microscope.
   - Some people are more prone to developing polyps and this can mean that we need to keep checking them to make sure the polyps aren't turning cancerous. This would involve camera tests every few years.

The patient then explains that several members of his family have had 'camera tests' in their bowel, and you notice some small dark dots on his lower lip.

2. ***Name the most likely condition causing this patient's polyps.***

Peutz–Jeghers syndrome.

3. ***Explain to the examiners the type of polyps caused by this condition, any risks from the polyps and any screening procedures that need to be in place.***
   - Peutz–Jeghers syndrome results in multiple hamartomatous polyps throughout the gastrointestinal system.
   - A hamartoma is a benign tumour-like lesion which contains two or more mature cell lines from the parent organ from which it developed.
   - Debate exists whether the polyps have a malignant potential, but evidence suggests that Peutz–Jeghers individuals have a higher risks of GI, GU and breast malignancies overall. Therefore, current recommendations suggest baseline gastroscopy and colonoscopy as a child, repeated 3-yearly until age 50 if polyps found at this stage, or to start at age 18 if no polyps found. Colonoscopy should continue after 50 years of age at 2-yearly intervals.

OSCE SCENARIO ANSWER 15.2

A 40-year-old-male presents to your orthopaedic outpatient clinic having been referred by his GP for 'tingling' sensations in his hands. He complains of the symptoms progressing over the last 9 months. He is a carpenter by trade and is starting to drop things due to weakness in his grip. He has no past medical history and takes no medications. He is concerned about his hands, as being self-employed his inability to work is impacting upon him financially.

1. ***Take a brief history regarding this patient's symptoms and examine his hands.***

History

- Location of symptoms.
- Frequency.
- Timing and onset.
- Character: tingling or burning? Pain? Numbness?

- Severity.
- Constancy.
- Radiation.
- Association with any change in shape of the hands?

Examination

- Flattening of thenar eminence?
- Test sensation in areas of median/ulnar and radial nerves.
- Test motor power and function for median/ulnar and radial nerves.
- To reproduce symptoms, could try Phalen's wrist flexion test, Tinel's test and the carpal compression test.

2. What is the diagnosis?

Bilateral carpal tunnel syndrome.

The patient then explains that he has seen his GP for headaches recently, which he feels are stress-related due to his worry about his job.

3. In view of this new information and your previous diagnosis, what condition are you now concerned about?

Acromegaly.

4. Explain to the examiners the other symptoms and signs you would now check for in this patient, and briefly outline the investigations and management.

Features

- Visual field defects due to optic chiasma compression.
- Facial changes (frontal bossing, prognathism, macroglossia).
- Skin changes (thickened, oily skin; skin tags).
- Soft tissue/extremity swelling.
- Excess sweating.
- Glucose intolerance.
- Hormonal changes: increased prolactin levels and decreased glucocorticoids, sex steroids and thyroid hormone.

Investigations

- IGF-1 levels.
- Glucose tolerance test and GH levels.
- TSH, FSH, LH, ACTH, prolactin.
- MRI head.

Management

- Surgical hypophysectomy.
- Medical treatment (somatostatin analogues, dopamine agonists, GH receptor antagonists).
- Carpal tunnel symptoms should resolve with treatment of the cause, though may require surgery if median nerve function is threatened.

OSCE SCENARIO ANSWER 15.3

A nurse in your clinic asks you to see a very distressed 50-year-old male regarding the result of a biopsy performed on his cheek 2 weeks ago. He attended the outpatient clinic earlier today, and was informed by a different doctor that he had 'dysplasia', 'but it was completely removed and nothing to worry about', and was told to come back in 3 months. He has spent the last 2h near to tears in the hospital canteen, tells you 'he didn't understand any of it' and is terrified he has cancer.

1. Explain the diagnosis of dysplasia to this man, being sensitive to his heightened emotional state.

- Start by ensuring a good environment for this consultation, such as a private room with yourself and the nurse present, some tissues if required, the notes available for you to review with any results you need to check.
- Acknowledge the patient's distress and explain you are sorry that he has been so upset after his earlier consultation and that you will go through it with him now.
- After confirming all the details in the notes and with no medical jargon, explain in broad terms that:
  - The biopsy had shown some cells that were changing, but were not cancerous.
  - The changing cells have been completely removed by the biopsy, meaning that they cannot progress to cancer cells now.
  - The follow-up appointment in 3 months was to check the wound and make sure no more changing cells are seen.

2. Tell the examiners what known risk factors exist for oral cavity tumours and the names of any pre-malignant conditions you know of.

Risk factors include:

- Smoking.
- Alcohol.
- Infections (HPV virus/HIV virus).
- Betel nut.
- Previous irradiation.
- Previous oral tumour.

Pre-malignant conditions:

- Leukoplakia.
- Erythroplakia.
- Oral submucous fibrosis.

3. How would you draw this consultation to a close and ensure the patient felt supported?

- Repeat the main points of the consultation:
  - not cancer
  - areas have been removed
  - follow-up in 3 months.
- Check patient understanding – ask him to repeat the main points back to you.
- Ask him if he would like to discuss ways in which he could reduce his risk of more changing cells – offer information leaflets if possible.
- Ensure he has had all his questions answered.
- Offer yourself as a point of contact if further information is requested.

OSCE SCENARIO ANSWER 15.4

A 35-year-old male with a long-standing history of gastro-oesophageal reflux undergoes endoscopy which reveals suspicion of Barrett's oesophagus. Biopsy confirms the diagnosis, and the patient attends outpatient clinic to discuss the results.

1. Describe to the patient the diagnosis and pathogenesis.

The oesophagus (food pipe) is normally lined by certain type of cells called stratified squamous epithelium. The oesophagus continues into the stomach at a junction between the chest and abdomen. The lower part of the oesophagus is normally protected from the acidity of the stomach's secretion by a mechanism of high pressure at the lower end of the oesophagus that acts as a sphincter. However, if this is deficient, as is the case with hiatus hernia, the lining of the oesophagus becomes exposed to the acid secretions and can undergo reversible transformation (termed metaplasia) to another type of lining called columnar epithelium to adapt. Hence, the lower part of the oesophagus becomes abnormal and is termed Barrett's oesophagus.

2. What is the significance of Barrett's oesophagus?

It is a premalignant condition and requires regular endoscopic surveillance to detect the development of adenocarcinoma.

3. The patient does not attend any further medical appointments and after 15 years presents with history of dysphagia and weight loss. Investigations reveal advanced lower oesophageal cancer. Palliative chemotherapy is advocated. Describe the phases of cell cycle and the relationship to chemotherapy.

The cell cycle is the progressive steps a cell moves through to proliferate by undergoing mitosis. It is made up of the following phases:

- G0: resting phase.
- M phase: mitosis (nuclear division) and cytokinesis (cytoplasmic division).
- G1: first gap phase. Duration varies between cell types; hence it is the main determinant of the cell cycle.
- S phase: DNA synthesis.
- G2 phase: gap 2 phase.
- Cells can leave the cell cycle temporarily and re-enter, this is called the Go phase.

Various chemotherapy agents act on the different phases of the cell cycle and attack rapidly dividing cells. For example, anti-metabolites such as 5-flourouracil (a chemotherapy agent for oesophageal cancer) act by preventing DNA synthesis within the S phase. Other examples of chemotherapy agents and their relationship to the cell cycle phases are summarized in Fig. 15.4A.

4. As you discuss potential side effects of chemotherapy, explain to the patient the reason for the likelihood of hair loss, developing anaemia and the susceptibility to infection and bleeding.

As chemotherapy agents cannot differentiate between cells sometimes, they can attack normal rapidly dividing cells, such as skin, bone marrow and lymphoid tissue, resulting

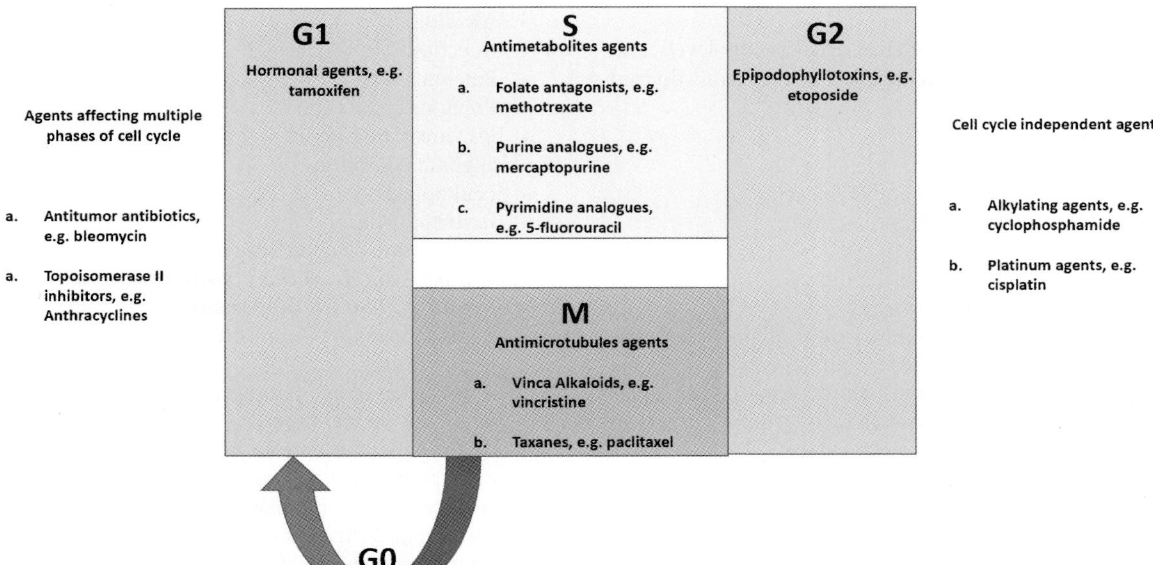

Fig. 15.4A Actions of antineoplastic agents within the cell cycle.

in side effects such as hair loss, anaemia, thrombocytopenia (low platelet count) and immunosuppression.

OSCE SCENARIO ANSWER 15.5

A 15-year-old boy attends the outpatient clinic with his parents after getting concerned regarding bilateral breast enlargement over the past year. This is causing embarrassment and he would like to understand its aetiology. Following assessment, you conclude that the findings are consistent with physiologic changes during puberty.

1. ***Explain to the patient and his family the underlying pathogenesis.***

This condition is called gynaecomastia, which can be due to the physiologic changes that occur at puberty when one or both breasts appear enlarged. This is due to hyperplasia, which is an increase in the size of the organ due to an increase in the cell number.

2. ***Give other examples of organs that can undergo physiologic changes during early adulthood.***
    - Thyroid hyperplasia due to the increased metabolic demands that can occur at puberty.
    - Thymus atrophy typically occurs in early adulthood. Atrophy is a decrease in the size due to loss of cells or a reduction in the size of individual cells.
3. ***What are the other causes of gynaecomastia that you need to be exclude?***
    - Drugs:
        - recreational drugs: marijuana, amphetamines, diazepam
        - gastrointestinal drugs: cimetidine, ranitidine
        - cardiovascular drugs: digoxin, ACE inhibitors, spironolactone, nifedipine, verapamil
        - antibiotics: metronidazole, isoniazid, ketoconazole.
    - Endocrine disorders:
        - hypo- or hyperthyroidism
        - hypogonadism
        - Klinefelter's syndrome
        - acromegaly.
    - Malignancy:
        - testicular tumours
        - lymphoma.
    - Chronic liver disease.

OSCE SCENARIO ANSWER 16.1

A 16-year-old male presents to your clinic with a 6-month history of weight loss and vague abdominal pain with intermittent rectal bleeding.

1. ***Outline your history, examination and investigations.***

History

- Pain history:
    - location
    - frequency
    - timing and onset
    - character/severity
    - constancy
    - radiation
    - association with movement, food, defecation, vomiting.
- Bowel habit:
    - associated diarrhoea/constipation
    - bleeding: colour, clots, frequency, painful
    - presence of mucus or pus
    - tenesmus
    - character/severity.
- Any past medical history of trauma, abdominal operations, abdominal pain.
- Any allergies or medications.
- Any family history of bowel pathology.
- Systemic review to elicit presence of any weight loss, mouth ulcers, skin conditions, jaundice, urinary symptoms, musculoskeletal complaints, etc.

Examination

Examination should include:

- Search for systemic signs of disease, e.g. clubbing, jaundice, oral ulceration, rashes, lymphadenopathy.
- Look for abdominal scars, distension, masses, external haemorrhoids, or anal ulcers or fissures.
- Palpate the abdomen, feeling (whilst watching the patient's face for pain) for tenderness, masses and organomegaly.
- Auscultate for bowel sounds.
- Perform a per rectal examination.

Investigations

- FBC/ESR/U&E/LFT/amylase.
- AXR/CXR if suspecting perforation or obstruction.
- Colonoscopy +/− biopsy.
- Barium study/small bowel enema.
- CT/MRI scan.

2. ***What is your differential diagnosis?***

Differential diagnoses would include (in descending order of likelihood):

- inflammatory bowel disease (Crohn's disease or ulcerative colitis)
- polyps
- fissure-in-ano
- gastric/duodenal ulcer
- carcinoma
- diverticular disease.

The colonic mucosal biopsy shows chronic inflammation with focal colitis and granulomas. The patient is currently well but is worried as he does not know what this means.

3. ***Explain the findings and diagnosis to the patient.***
   - The results of your biopsy have shown that there are parts of your bowel which are inflamed. This means that something is irritating your bowel lining, which is why you have had some diarrhoea and bleeding.
   - The type of inflammation on your biopsy suggests that you have a condition called Crohn's disease, which can affect any part of the gut, from the mouth to the anus. This may explain why you have had a lot of mouth ulcers recently and may have lost some weight.
   - The cause of Crohn's disease is largely unknown, but we know that it can run in families.
   - The treatment for Crohn's is mainly medical, using tablets to control the inflammation to allow the bowel to function normally, but sometimes people need surgery if parts of the bowel are very affected.
   - We'd like to arrange a meeting with you and the medical doctors who help us treat this condition, and also some nurses and dieticians so we can plan your treatment together.

OSCE SCENARIO ANSWER 16.2

A 19-year-old male is admitted with a history of central abdominal pain localizing to the right iliac fossa after 12 h. It is now 5 days since the onset of symptoms. On admission to A&E he has a temperature of 38.5°C with a tachycardia of 120, and abdominal examination reveals a tender mass in the right iliac fossa. A clinical diagnosis of appendix abscess is made and this is confirmed by CT scan.

1. ***What is suppuration? Why in some cases does acute appendicitis perforate and cause peritonitis while in others abscess formation occurs?***
   - Suppuration is the formation of pus. Pus is a mixture of living, dead and dying bacteria and neutrophils with cellular debris and liquefied tissue.
   - An abscess (a localized collection of pus) forms and becomes surrounded by a pyogenic membrane, i.e. capillaries, neutrophils and occasional fibroblasts. In some cases the appendix perforates into the general peritoneal cavity. In other cases adhesions (particularly from the omentum and surrounding viscera) form around the appendix and wall off the inflammation, resulting in the formation of an appendix mass. The appendix may then perforate within the mass, giving rise to an abscess walled off by adhesions.
2. ***Why do abscesses require drainage?***

Bacteria within abscess cavities are relatively inaccessible to antibiotics and antibodies: hence the need to drain pus. Prolonged treatment with antibiotics may halt expansion of an abscess and even sterilize the pus, resulting in a sterile abscess known as an 'antibioma', which will ultimately cause symptoms and require drainage.

3. ***What organisms are likely to be cultured from the pus?***

These are usually a mixture of aerobic and anaerobic organisms. The organisms most commonly isolated are *E. coli* and *Bacteroides fragilis*.

4. ***What sequelae other than suppuration may follow acute inflammation?***

Other sequelae include:
- resolution
- organization
- chronic inflammation.

The patient is re-admitted to hospital 1 year later with vomiting, central abdominal colicky pain, abdominal distension and constipation. Plain abdominal X-ray shows dilated loops of small bowel and a diagnosis of small bowel obstruction is made.

5. ***Why is this likely to have occurred? Explain the pathology of the condition.***
   - The patient has small bowel obstruction due to adhesions. This is a result of organization occurring at the time of the appendix abscess.
   - Organization is replacement of tissue by granulation tissue. Factors favouring organization include excessive fibrin with swamping of the fibrinolytic system; a substantial volume of necrotic tissue; and exudate and debris, which cannot be removed or discharged. Capillaries grow into the inflammatory tissue, bringing fibroblasts that proliferate under the influence of TGF-β, resulting in fibrosis.
   - The bowel in relation to the appendix abscess is covered by fibrinous exudate, which causes loops of bowel to stick to the abscess and to one another. Failure of removal of this fibrinous exudate by the fibrinolytic system results in its invasion by capillaries accompanied by fibroblasts, which lay down collagen, resulting in permanent fibrous adhesions. Small bowel loops then twist or kink around the adhesions.

OSCE SCENARIO ANSWER 16.3

You see an 8-year-old girl, along with her mother, in A&E, who fell over earlier today and banged her arm, which is slightly pink and swollen. The child is happy and playing with her arm in a sling, with normal observations and no evidence of serious injury or infection. The girl's mother explains that the nurse practitioner performed an X-ray, which showed no fracture, but that she doesn't understand why it is red and sore if it isn't infected or broken. She asks if her daughter needs antibiotics.

1. ***Explain to this worried parent the difference between inflammation, fractures and infection and answer her question regarding antibiotics.***

Explain in general terms, avoiding jargon that:

- There is no broken bone, but that doesn't mean that the soft tissues around the bone have not sustained an injury – this is causing the redness and swelling.
- The redness and tenderness is due to inflammation – a normal response of the body to injury.
- Acknowledge her worry but explain that infection is just one of the causes of inflammation, and though it is sometimes difficult to tell them apart, certain features help – such as there being no wound, only a few hours since the injury, normal vital signs, etc.
- Reassure her that most inflammation settles within a few days and that if it was not settling down, or the redness and discomfort were increasing, then you would be happy to review her again.
- Explain that you would not prescribe antibiotics.

2. ***Explain to the examiners the stages of acute inflammation, what clinical features these processes produce and the key chemical mediators involved.***

Three key stages:

- Vascular phase:
  - change in vessel calibre
  - increase in vascular permeability
  - formation of fluid exudates.
- Exudative cellular phase:
  - adhesion of neutrophils
  - neutrophil migration
  - diapedesis
  - neutrophil chemotaxis.
- Outcome:
  - resolution
  - suppuration
  - organization
  - chronic inflammation.

The combination of the above mechanisms produces the clinical picture of a red (increased vessel dilatation), warm (increased blood flow to the skin), swollen (tissue oedema from fluid egress), painful (stretch of tissues, chemical mediators of pain such as prostaglandins and bradykinin) area which may exhibit loss of function (restricted by pain, swelling or protective reflexes): these are also known by their Latin descriptions as: rubor, calor, tumour, dolor, functio laesa, respectively.

Key chemical mediators include:

- Histamine – vasodilates, increases vascular permeability.
- Lysosomal compounds – increase vascular permeability and activate complement.
- Prostaglandins – increase vascular permeability, affect platelet aggregation.
- Leukotrienes – increase vascular permeability, chemotaxis.
- Cytokines – chemotaxis.
- Nitric oxide – bactericidal, vasodilates.

3. ***Explain to the examiners what factors in the presentation of a child to A&E would make you think of non-accidental injury (NAI)?***

All clinicians have a duty to look for features of NAI in any child they assess with an injury. Some features that would increase the index of suspicion of NAI include:

- Delay in presentation.
- Changing history.
- Different history from different parents/caregivers.
- Injuries inconsistent with description of trauma.
- Injuries incompatible with child's developmental stage, i.e. newborn 'rolling over' or 4-month-old 'crawling to the stove'.
- Child brought to A&E by someone other than primary caregiver.
- Red-flag injuries – i.e. glove-and-stocking burns (indicating being held in hot water), cigarette burns, multiple injuries of different ages, e.g. bruises of different colours.

OSCE SCENARIO ANSWER 16.4

A 44-year-old female is brought in unwell with severe central abdominal pain radiating through to her back with nauseas and vomiting. Her amylase is 3400 U/L.

1. ***What is the diagnosis?***

The most likely diagnosis with an amylase in this range and her symptoms is pancreatitis but other causes of raised amylase can include pancreatic cancer, mesenteric ischaemia, mumps and trauma.

2. ***Five days later she has clinically deteriorated and is hypotensive and anaemic. A CT scan has shown considerable bleeding in and around the pancreas. What is this type of inflammation called and why does it occur?***

This is likely to be haemorrhagic pancreatitis, a specific type of inflammation seen in the pancreas. The inflammation that occurs in pancreatitis is due to the release of proteolytic enzymes released from the pancreas. Normally this is responsible for causing the swelling and inflammation in and around the pancreas; however, in severe cases it can digest blood vessel walls and lead to haemorrhage. It indicates a very severe type of pancreatitis and the prognosis can be poor.

3. ***Do you know any common causes of pancreatitis?***

There are many causes of acute pancreatitis, the two commonest of which are gallstones and alcohol excess, but a useful mnemonic for all causes is 'I GET SMASHED':

- I = idiopathic
- G = gallstones
- E = ethanol (Alcohol excess)
- T = trauma
- S = steroids
- M = mumps
- A = autoimmune
- S = scorpion bites
- H = hyperlipidaemia/hypercalcaemia
- E = ERCP
- D = drugs.

OSCE SCENARIO ANSWER 16.5

A 48-year-old male has accidentally been given i.v. penicillin – he is known to have a severe allergy to all penicillin-based antibiotics. He is very unwell and has collapsed on the ward, he is struggling to breathe, his arm is swollen and he is profoundly hypotensive.

1. ***What type of shock does he have?***

This is called anaphylactic shock or anaphylaxis, and is triggered by an allergic response to certain drugs, foods and insect stings. It is a type 1 hypersensitivity reaction caused by the over production of IgE on mast cells and basophils.

2. ***Explain why he is having difficulty breathing and is hypotensive?***

The binding of IgE antibodies leads to the degranulation of mast cells and the release of a number of different mediators that have a profound effect on the body. The difficulty in breathing is due to the release of a number of substances that lead to intense bronchospasm, including histamine, leukotrienes, prostaglandins, and PAF (platelet activating factor). These and other substances, such as those in the complement system, lead to increased vascular permeability (loss of intravascular volume and swelling) and vasodilation (leading to low blood pressure), both of which lead to profound hypotension.

3. ***How would you treat this patient?***

The initial treatment would be along the lines of ABCDE – first aid measures can include laying the patient flat or raising the legs. The airway should be secured (anaphylaxis can cause significant airway swelling). Give high flow oxygen and secure vascular access so a fluid challenge can be given and drugs administered. Adrenaline should be given as soon as possible, 0.5 mL 1:1000 adrenaline or 500 µg; this can be repeated every 5 min. In addition to this, 10 mg chlorpheniramine and 200 mg hydrocortisone should be given.

OSCE SCENARIO ANSWER 17.1

A 42-year-old female on your ward develops a painful calf 5 days after having a mastectomy and free flap reconstruction for breast cancer. She has a body mass index BMI of 25, is otherwise fit and well, and takes no medications.

1. ***Take a brief history from this patient.***

Salient points in the history should include:

- Speed of onset of pain: immediately post-op or slowly developed?
- Character of pain: dull throbbing or sharp stabbing?
- Any change in the size of the calf or ankle swelling.
- Any trauma to the leg since the operation.
- Previous history of DVT/PE.
- Previous history of leg/calf pain.
- Family history of thrombotic disease.
- Drug history, particularly any oestrogen analogues, e.g. oral contraceptives.
- Screen for PE symptoms: breathlessness, malaise, cough or haemoptysis.

2. ***What is your diagnosis?***

Deep vein thrombosis.

3. ***What specific risk factors does this patient have for a DVT?***
   - Operating time >90 min.
   - Active cancer.
4. ***What venous thromboembolism prophylaxis measures would you check that she had received?***
   - Compression stockings from admission.
   - Prophylactic low-molecular-weight heparin from admission.
   - Pneumatic calf-compression devices intra-operatively.
5. ***Outline your assessment and any investigations you would perform.***

Examination

- Inspect for swelling and ankle oedema.
- Feel for tenderness and warmth.
- Measure calf circumferences.
- Perform a chest examination.

Investigations

- Vital signs: pulse, blood pressure, temperature, oxygen saturation.
- Bloods: FBC, U&Es, clotting screen (D-dimer test alone is not accurate enough in the early detection of DVT because plasma D-dimer levels can be influenced by such conditions as cancer, infection and surgery).
- Duplex Doppler scan of calf.

The vital signs and blood tests were all unremarkable; however, the duplex Doppler reveals a DVT in the popliteal vein of the affected calf.

6. ***Outline your management plan.***
   - Explain the diagnosis to the patient.
   - Start treatment dose of low-molecular-weight heparin.
   - Start warfarin and arrange anticoagulation clinic follow-up for INR checks post-discharge.

- Explain to the patient that the heparin injections will continue until the warfarin levels are stabilized and that warfarin treatment will usually continue for 3–6 months.

OSCE SCENARIO ANSWER 17.2

A 69-year-old male presents to A&E an hour after developing acute pain in his left buttock, thigh and calf. He has a history of angina and hypertension, and admits to episodes over several months of cramp-like pain in the left buttock, thigh and calf when walking uphill. On examination his left leg is paler, cooler and the patient complains of a 'pins and needles' sensation in it.

1. ***What is the likely diagnosis?***

Acute-on-chronic peripheral artery occlusion due to thrombus/embolus. Given the location of the symptoms (buttock/thigh), the left common iliac artery is likely to be involved.

2. ***An arteriogram is carried out** (Fig. 17.2Q). **What abnormalities are shown? Is there evidence that this is acute-on-chronic rather than simply acute?***

Complete occlusion of the left common iliac artery. Multiple collaterals exist, suggesting that this is acute-on-chronic. The chronic ischaemia has led to the development of collaterals. Additionally, the right external iliac and the right internal iliac artery have stenotic lesions at their origins (Fig. 17.2A).

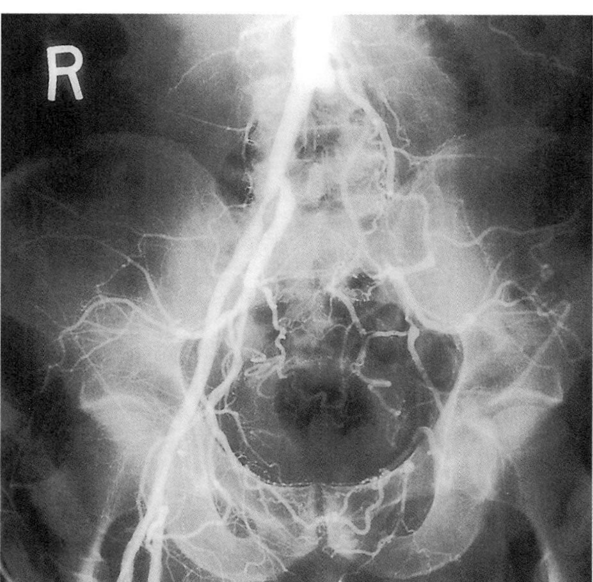

Fig. 17.2A The patient's arteriogram showing complete occlusion of the left common iliac and external iliac arteries.

3. ***Outline your immediate management plan to the examiners.***
   - Explain your findings and suspected diagnosis to the patient.
   - Explain the need for urgency: ideally surgery needs to be performed within 6–8 h of symptom onset.
   - Explain the investigations you would like to perform and why: FBC/U&Es/clotting/cross-match/CXR/ECG/arteriogram (performed, but should not delay a threatened limb from proceeding directly to theatre).
   - Give the patient 100% oxygen.
   - Proceed to theatre for emergency thrombectomy/embolectomy or intra-arterial thrombolysis +/− angioplasty or bypass graft.
   - Fasciotomies may need to be performed to prevent compartment syndrome and post-operative anticoagulation with heparin.

OSCE SCENARIO ANSWER 17.3

You are asked to see a 60-year-old male in ICU who has been intubated and ventilated for 2 days after a cardiac arrest – attributed to a myocardial infarction. He had approximately 45 min of CPR before a heartbeat was restored. The intensivists are concerned as he has a rising serum lactate and acidosis despite good cardiac output and no obvious evidence of infection. He has reduced bowel sounds, although no abdominal distension exists. He has a temperature of 38.1°C. His WCC is 14.2 $\times 10^9$/L and his lactate 5.6 mmol/L.

1. ***What is your differential diagnosis?***
   - Ischaemic colitis.
   - Infective colitis.
   - Bowel obstruction.
   - Appendicitis.
   - Diverticulitis.
2. ***A plain AXR is non-contributory and a CT scan is carried out and is shown below** (Fig. 17.3Q). **Explain to the examiners what the CT scan shows and the most likely diagnosis.***
   - The patient's CT scan (an axial image through the upper descending colon) shows thickening of the bowel wall at the splenic flexure (large arrow) and descending colon (small arrow). The low attenuation of the submucosa represents submucosal oedema related to ischaemia (Fig. 17.3A).
   - The most likely diagnosis is ischaemic colitis. A CT scan of the abdomen will be accurate in 85–90% of patients with ischaemic colitis.

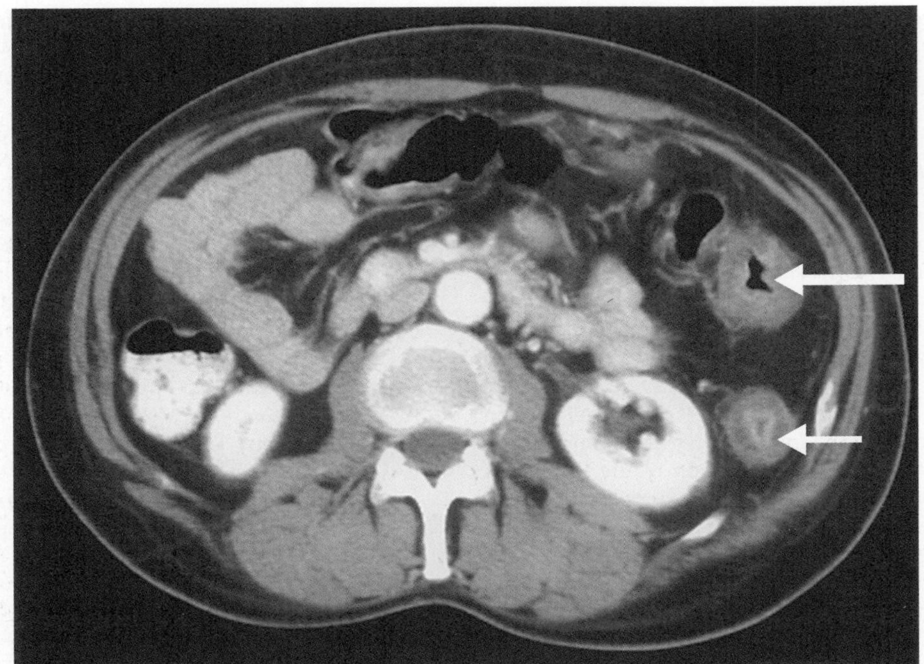

Fig. 17.3A The patient's CT scan showing thickened bowel wall loops (arrows). From Pretoris ES, Solomon JA. Radiology Secrets Plus, 3rd edition, Mosby, 2011, with permission.

3. ***What other investigation could be carried out to establish the diagnosis?***
    - Colonoscopy – early changes include petechial haemorrhages and pale, oedematous mucosa, whilst late changes include segmental erythema, mucosal bleeding, ulceration and necrosis.
4. ***Outline your management plan.***
    - Immediate management would include:
        - Preparation for immediate exploratory laparotomy with likelihood of bowel resection – check for cross-matched blood and inform anaesthetic colleagues.
        - Discussion with the patient's next of kin regarding the serious and potentially life-threatening nature of the suspected diagnosis, need for surgery and probable need for a stoma.
        - Consent form to be completed with another senior colleague for a patient who is unable to give consent (highlighting that this is an emergency situation).
5. ***Explain to the examiners the likely cause of this patient's pathology.***

This man has likely suffered a 'watershed' infarction of the colon at the splenic flexure, which sits between the territories supplied by the superior mesenteric artery and the inferior mesenteric artery and is therefore vulnerable to ischaemic insult. This ischaemia was likely the result of prolonged downtime at his recent coronary event, leading to under-perfusion of the bowel, infarction and ischaemic colitis.

OSCE SCENARIO ANSWER 17.4

A 65-year-old smoker is referred to you due to episodes of unsteadiness, blurred vision in the left eye and a numb left arm. During your history you find out he is a painter and these symptoms occur only when he is painting or using his arm for other physical tasks. He is left-handed.

1. ***What is the potential diagnosis?***

The diagnosis is likely to be subclavian steal syndrome, given that the symptoms occur when the arm is exercising. In addition, he is a smoker and this will obviously increase his risk of arterial disease.

2. ***Would you expect to find a difference in the blood pressure of each arm, and why? Are there any other significant examination findings?***

There will almost certainly be a difference in blood pressure, with the left arm having a lower blood pressure (at least >20 mmHg to be significant) due to the stenosis in the left subclavian artery. In addition, you may find weak wrist pulses and a bruit over the left shoulder region. In severe cases of subclavian artery stenosis there may be ischaemic lesions on the fingers and they may be pale and cold.

3. *Can you explain his symptoms given the diagnosis?*

The subclavian artery is divided into three parts. The first part lies medial to the scalene anterior, the second part lies behind and the third part lies from the lateral edge of scalene anterior the edge of the first rib where it becomes the axillary artery. The common positon for subclavian stenotic disease is at its origin from the aortic arch. The vertebral artery is a branch of the first part of the subclavian artery and is usually proximal to the stenosis. When a patient exercises or uses the arm, the arm will need more blood flow for muscles to work. Due to the stenosis this is not possible, so blood is drawn from (or stolen) from the cerebral circulation in a reverse direction via the vertebral artery to supply blood to the arm. This explains why symptoms occur only when the arm is used. The blood is preferentially drawn from the posterior part of the brain and leads to symptoms such as vertigo, diplopia, dysarthria, visual loss and syncope (all posterior cerebral symptoms). The patient may also suffer arm claudication.

4. *You order a duplex ultrasound scan; can you describe the findings you would expect to see?*

The diagnosis can be confirmed anatomically by CT or MR angiogram to show the subclavian stenosis but a duplex ultrasound is diagnostically more useful as it can confirm the direction of vertebral artery blood flow. A positive diagnosis will demonstrate retrograde flow on the vertebral artery (i.e. flowing the wrong way).

OSCE SCENARIO ANSWER 17.5

A 29-year-old male is involved in a road traffic accident and has a badly fractured right femur, a splenic haematoma and broken right wrist. He is taken to theatre early the next morning and has had his femur nailed to fix the fracture. You are called by the nurse caring for him to tell you he is very confused – he is pulling away when the nurse has tried to take a blood gas, he is making noises and opens his eyes when you speak. In addition, his SpO_2 is 88% and his chest is covered in a petechial rash.

1. *What is the likely diagnosis and what is the cause? What differential diagnosis should you consider?*

The likely diagnosis given the symptoms is fat embolism syndrome but given the cause of his injury any other serious chest injuries or a head injury is essential to diagnose.

2. *What tests would you order?*

The tests are very much to confirm the absence of other injuries causing the symptoms. Blood tests are non-specific as is a chest X-ray. An arterial blood gas will confirm the degree of hypoxia. A CT scan of the head and chest will rule out any traumatic chest or head injuries as a cause of his symptoms. The diagnosis is usually clinical with a collection of symptoms in a patient at risk, i.e. hypoxia, petechial rash and confusion in a patient with a long bone fracture or post fixation of a fracture (manipulation of the bone marrow cavity and nailing increases the risk of developing fat embolism).

3. *How would you treat this patient?*

The management is supportive and essentially involves ruling out other treatable diagnoses and treating hypoxia or hypotension. The disease is usually self-limiting although can be life threatening.

4. *What is his GCS score?*

His GCS is 9 to 10: he is withdrawing from pain (5; could also be 4 flexing away), opens his eyes to speech (3) and is making noises only (2).

OSCE SCENARIO ANSWER 18.1

A 32-year-old female attends your clinic after triple assessment has shown her breast lump to be a benign cyst. She remains very anxious. Although she has no family history of breast cancer, her sister-in-law has just been diagnosed with ductal carcinoma in situ (DCIS) and is due to have a mastectomy. She wishes to know about the screening programme for breast cancer and to discuss any risk factors she has.

1. *Answer this patient's questions about cancer and carcinoma in situ.*

Explain the difference between cancer and carcinoma in situ in layman's terms. For example:

- A tumour can be benign (it doesn't spread but may cause problems as it grows locally) or malignant (often causes problems locally and can spread to other parts of the body and be fatal).
- Cancer can develop at different speeds, and sometimes there are features in body tissues which we can pick up using tests if the risk of developing cancer is increased.
- Carcinoma in situ is a condition that has not spread into the deeper tissues of the organ and therefore at this stage does not have the potential to metastasize.

2. *Answer her questions about risk factors for cancer, in particular breast cancer.*

The chances of getting cancer can be altered with various risk factors, some of which are possible to change (such as smoking, diet, sun exposure, etc.) and some of which are not (e.g. sex, increased age, race and inherited risks). Known risk factors for breast cancer include:

- Increasing age.
- Oestrogen exposure (starting periods early, not having children, having your first baby later in life, menopause at an older age).
- Use of oral contraceptives (small risk).
- Use of hormone replacement therapy.

- Close family member with breast cancer (though 85% of these women do not develop breast cancer and 85% of breast cancer patients have no relatives with breast cancer).
- Genetic breast cancer genes (BRCA 1&2, Li–Fraumeni syndrome, Cowen's syndrome, etc.).
- Alcohol consumption.
- Obesity.
- Radiation exposure (e.g. radiotherapy).

3. ***Explain the breast screening programme to her.***
   - Breast screening is a way to detect breast cancer at an early stage using mammograms (X-rays of the breasts).
   - It is not a test for cancer, and there are small numbers of women who have a 'positive' test result who do not have cancer, and those who have a 'negative' test result who do have cancer.
   - Currently women between the ages of 50 and 70 years old are invited to attend every 3 years, though this range is increasing over the next 2 years to between 47 and 73 years old.
   - Women below this age are not invited unless they have particular risk factors such as genetic predisposition, and as their breasts are more dense, they may need other tests such as scans (ultrasound or magnetic resonance imaging).
   - If the screening mammogram is unclear or shows anything that looks abnormal, the patient is asked to come back to have more tests, which can include a physical examination, more X-rays or scans, or taking a sample of some cells or tissue from the breast to check it for cancer.

OSCE SCENARIO ANSWER 18.2

A 58-year-old female with known breast cancer is admitted with pain in the back and ribs which has been present for several weeks but has suddenly become much worse. She is in obvious pain but has no neurological symptoms. A bone scan had been carried out 1 week previously (Fig. 18.2Q).

1. ***What is your suspected diagnosis? What does the bone scan show?***

Metastatic breast cancer. The bone scan shows secondary deposits (hot spots) in the bony skeleton, especially the ribs and spine (Fig. 18.2A).

The patient is admitted for pain relief. A CT scan shows liver and bone metastases. She has completed her surgery and chemotherapy and understands that her disease has spread. She wishes to go home as soon as possible as her eldest daughter is getting married in 3 weeks.

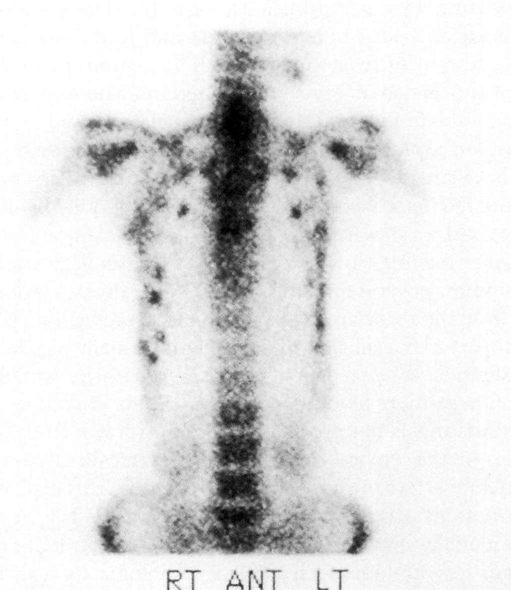

Fig. 18.2A The patient's bone scan.

2. ***After ruling out any fractures, what multidisciplinary treatment plan may be appropriate for her now? What specific treatment may help her back pain?***
   - Palliative care team: involvement of specialist nurses, dieticians and pain teams to control her symptoms. This may involve morphine sulphate with breakthrough top-ups, antiemetics and dietary supplementation. Consider involving the Macmillan nurses or equivalent for when the patient goes home. Offer the support of the counselling or pastoral care teams.
   - Therapeutic radiation to the spinal bony metastases may be an effective way to control her symptoms whilst allowing her to be at home.
3. ***How does therapeutic radiotherapy work? On which tissues does it work best?***
   - Ionizing radiation induces the formation of reactive free radicals or oxygen species, which can damage cellular structures and DNA.
   - Depending on the dose of radiotherapy, this results in either cell death, permanent cell genome change or cell repair and recovery.
   - Cells that are most radiosensitive are those which renew themselves frequently, e.g. bone marrow, blood, skin, intestines.

4. ***What side-effects can radiotherapy have in the short and long term?***

Obviously depends on the area irradiated, but general side effects include:

- Acute:
  - skin: ranges from hair loss with mild erythema to severe irritation and breakdown
  - bowel: diarrhoea
  - bone marrow: anaemia and neutropenia
  - gonads: sterility.
- Chronic:
  - skin: permanent redness, pigmentation and telangiectasia
  - bowel: fibrosis and stricture formation
  - bone marrow: risk of aplastic anaemia and leukaemia
  - gonads: sterility
  - lung: pulmonary fibrosis
  - kidney: renal failure.

OSCE SCENARIO ANSWER 18.3

A 22-year-old male attends your clinic after referral by his GP for testicular discomfort. He describes a vague history of trauma during football several weeks ago. Examination reveals a firm, painless mass near the superior pole of the testis but no other clinical abnormalities.

1. ***What is your differential diagnosis?***
   - Testicular cancer.
   - Epididymal cyst.
   - Intermittent torsion.
   - Epididymo-orchitis.
   - Haematoma.

Any mass within the testicle must be considered cancer until proven otherwise.

2. ***What other clinical features would you look for on examination?***
   - Cough/shortness of breath.
   - Supraclavicular lymphadenopathy.
   - Gynaecomastia.

3.. ***Explain to the examiners some known risk factors for testicular cancer and the most common pathological types.***

Some known risk factors include:

- Cryptorchidism, even after orchidopexy.
- Klinefelter's syndrome (46XXY).
- Family history (first-degree relative).
- Infertility.

95% of testicular tumours are germ-cell tumours. Five types of testicular germ cell tumour exist:

- Seminomas.
- Embryonal carcinomas.
- Teratomas.
- Yolk sac tumours (most common in infants/small children).
- Choriocarcinomas.

Broadly divided into seminomas (most common pure germ-cell tumour), non-seminomas and mixed germ-cell tumours, which contain more than one histological pattern.

4. ***How should this man be investigated? How are these tumours staged?***
   - Blood tests:
     - β-hCG
     - LDH
     - AFP (elevated in non-seminomas only).
   - Imaging:
     - testicular USS (ultrasound scan) by experienced clinician
     - chest X-ray
     - CT abdomen and pelvis +/− chest.

Suspicious lesions should proceed to an inguinal orchidectomy (some units perform intra-operative frozen-section histology). Biopsies and scrotal orchidectomy are not recommended due to risk of tumour seeding and recurrence. Testicular tumours are staged using the TNM system.

OSCE SCENARIO ANSWER 18.4

A 70-year-old smoker has had a cough for the last 6 months and has been losing weight due to a poor appetite. The GP does some baseline blood tests and sends the patient for a chest X-ray. The blood tests come back before the chest X-ray and show a sodium of 120 mmol/L.

1. ***What are you concerned about?***

As the patient is a smoker, I would be concerned about lung cancer, particularly with the cough and weight loss. The low sodium may represent syndrome of inappropriate ADH secretion (SIADH).

2. ***What further tests would you need to do to secure the diagnosis?***

The patient should have plasma and urine osmolality measured, urinary sodium, thyroid function tests and a short Synacthen test (a test to diagnose adrenal insufficiency). The plasma sodium should be <135 mmol/L, the plasma osmolality should be <280 mOsm/kg, the urine osmolality should be >100 mOsm/kg and the patient should be euvolaemic. Diuretic use and adrenal or thyroid dysfunction should also be excluded.

3. ***What type of lung condition is it most often associated with?***

It can be seen with TB or lung abscess, but lung cancer is the commonest lung cause, particularly small cell carcinoma.

4. ***What is this type of condition called and can you name any others?***

SIADH is known as a paraneoplastic disorder. This is a group of wide ranging conditions that are caused by a tumour but not as a result of the tumour itself or its metastasis. They may be humoral, e.g. secretion of ACTH and SIADH; immunological, e.g. dermatomyositis; metabolic, e.g. insulin from an insulinoma. There are others disorders that do not fit into these three categories, such as cachexia, hypertrophic pulmonary osteoarthropathy and thrombophlebitis migrans.

OSCE SCENARIO ANSWER 18.5

A 30-year-old male is seen in the general surgery clinic with a history of rectal bleeding and abdominal pain. In the process of your history-taking you discover his father died from bowel cancer at a young age. At colonoscopy you find hundreds of colorectal polyps.

1. ***What is the diagnosis?***

The likely diagnosis is familial adenomatous polyposis (FAP); this is a condition characterized by hundreds of colorectal polyps that present at a young age. It is also associated with duodenal polyps and extra-intestinal conditions such as osteomas, dental cysts and desmoid tumours.

2. ***What gene is abnormal and what group of genes is it part of? Describe how these genes cause cancer when they are abnormal.***

The gene involved in FAP is the adenomatous polyposis coli gene or APC. It is an autosomal dominantly inherited condition. The APC gene is known as a tumour suppressor gene; these are a group of genes that help to prevent cancer by repairing damaged DNA or preventing cells with damaged DNA to proliferate. In their absence, damaged DNA in cells goes unchecked and leads to cancerous cells. The risk of cancer developing in FAP is 100%.

3. ***Can you name another group of genes involved with cancer and describe how abnormalities in these genes can give rise to cancers? Give some examples.***

The other group of genes involved in cancers are known as oncogenes. These genes are normally involved in producing proteins that signal cells to divide. When abnormal, oncogenes produce excessive amounts of protein and lead to uncontrolled cell growth and division. Examples include sis gene and platelet derived growth factor (PDGF) and ras gene and G-proteins – both are involved in sarcomas.

OSCE SCENARIO ANSWER 19.1

A 17-year-old female presents to your trauma service with an infected dog bite to her right arm, with associated lymphangitis. Whilst on the ward awaiting theatre for washout and debridement, she is started on intravenous penicillin. Shortly after, the staff nurse in the patient's bay calls for help, and you find that the patient is flushed, anxious and you can hear a slight wheeze when she is breathing.

1. ***What is the most likely diagnosis?***

Anaphylactic reaction to penicillin.

2. ***What type of immune reaction is this?***

Type I hypersensitivity reaction.

3. ***What other signs/symptoms may be present in this type of reaction?***

Symptoms

- Dizziness.
- Itching.
- Palpitations.
- Nausea/vomiting.
- Abdominal cramp/diarrhoea.

Signs

- Swelling of eyes/lips/extremities.
- Urticaria-type rash.
- Hoarse voice/stridor.
- Tachycardia.
- Loss of consciousness/low blood pressure.
- Cardiac arrest.

4. ***Briefly outline your immediate management.***

Should be managed in an ABC approach as per ATLS guidance:

- STOP THE ANTIBIOTIC INFUSION.
- Ask staff nurse to put out an arrest call immediately.
- Administer 100% oxygen via a non-rebreather bag.
- Lay the patient flat/elevate legs.
- Administer 500 µg (0.5 mL) of 1 : 1000 adrenaline i.m.
- Secure i.v. access and give 500–1000 mL of i.v. fluid as a bolus.
- Give 10 mg chlorpheniramine i.v. and 200 mg hydrocortisone i.v.
- Consider inhaled/i.v. salbutamol.

5. ***Before the patient is discharged, what actions would you ensure had been taken?***
   - Make sure the patient understands she had a very severe anaphylactic reaction to penicillin and must avoid this drug in the future.
   - Check that details of the anaphylactic reaction to penicillin were recorded in the patient's case notes and ensure clear labelling of allergen as per local guidelines (e.g. red sticker on front of notes).
   - Ensure the patient's GP has been informed of the reaction and its trigger.
   - Refer the patient to an allergy specialist.

OSCE SCENARIO ANSWER 19.2

A 20-year-old male undergoes a first renal transplant from a well-matched deceased donor. He has no preformed cytotoxic antibodies.

1. ***What immunosuppressive regime would you commence in the post-operative period?***

This patient is at a low risk of rejection, having a well-matched kidney with no preformed antibodies. He should be commenced on steroid (prednisolone), an anti-proliferative agent (azathioprine) and a calcineurin inhibitor (ciclosporin).

The serum creatinine falls to 130 μmol/L by the 6th post-operative day. On the 8th post-operative day there is reduced urine output and the creatinine has risen to 200 μmol/L. The ciclosporin level in the blood is within therapeutic limits.

2. **What are the possible diagnoses?**
   - Acute rejection.
   - Ureteric obstruction.
3. **Name two investigations which you would perform to confirm the diagnosis. In which order would you perform them?**
   - Ultrasound scan to exclude ureteric obstruction.
   - If this is normal, then a core biopsy.
4. **What histological features suggest the diagnosis of acute rejection?**
   - In cell-mediated rejection there would be infiltration of the tubules and interstitium by cytotoxic T-cells.
   - In antibody-mediated rejection there would be intimal arteritis with thrombosis of the blood vessels and deposition of C4d in the peritubular capillaries.
5. **If cell-mediated rejection is confirmed, how would you treat it?**

Pulsed doses of methylprednisolone i.v. daily for 3 consecutive days.

6. **If the kidney fails to respond to planned treatment, what further treatment would you institute?**

The patient has steroid-resistant rejection and a course of ATG would be administered.

OSCE SCENARIO ANSWER 19.3

You have recently incised and drained an abscess on the neck of a 48-year-old male, which did not exhibit the usual features of an inflamed abscess. The microbiologist reports seeing acid- and alcohol-fast bacilli (AAFBs) on the Gram stain.

1. ***What infection does this suggest?***

AAFBs suggest infection with mycobacteria. Examples would include:

- Mycobacterium tuberculosis.
- Mycobacterium bovis.
- Mycobacterium leprae.

When you see the patient in clinic he tells you he has recently had a cough and shortness of breath. An X-ray and sputum culture performed by his GP has revealed a Pneumocystis pneumonia.

2. ***What possible underlying condition do you now suspect? How can you classify it?***

Infection with Mycobacterium (possible tuberculous) and a Pneumocystis pneumonia suggests an underlying immunodeficiency. This can be classified as:

- Specific deficiencies (in the immune system itself).
- Non-specific deficiencies (in neutrophils or complement).

Specific deficiencies in the immune system can be further subclassified into:

- Primary – present from birth and relatively uncommon
  - severe combined immune deficiency
  - di George syndrome.
- Secondary:
  - infection (HIV/CMV/viral hepatitis)
  - neoplasia (leukaemia/lymphoma/myeloma)
  - iatrogenic (medications such as steroids/cytotoxics, splenectomy)
  - advanced age
  - malnutrition.

3. ***Summarize the immune response.***
   - Antigen is presented to lymphocytes by antigen presenting cells (APCs).
   - Antigen is processed and presented to T-cells with MHC class II antigen.
   - B-lymphocytes produce antibodies with a unique antigen-binding site.
   - T-helper cells produce cytokines:
     - TH1 cells secrete TNF and IFN-γ and mediate cellular immunity.
     - TH2 cells secrete IL-4, IL-5, IL-10 and IL-13 and stimulate antibody production by B-cells (clonal expansion).
   - T-lymphocytes directly kill infected cells and release cytokines to increase inflammation.
4. ***Explain to the examiners the difference between the humoral and cell-mediated immune systems.***

Humoral immunity

- Involves production of antibodies (produced by B-lymphocytes differentiated into plasma cells) which causes:
  - bacterial lysis
  - toxin neutralization
  - opsonization (surface coating of foreign material by complement to promote engulfment by phagocytes)
  - promotion of antibody-dependent cell-mediated cytotoxicity.

Cell-mediated immunity

- Involves T-lymphocytes, of which there are two main types:

- helper T-cells (CD4+), which produce cytokines that activate other T-cells, B-cells and macrophages
- cytotoxic T-cells (CD8+), which destroy infected target cells.

5. ***What is complement?***

Complement is a complex, step-wise enzymatic cascade of proteins, activated by antigen–antibody complexes (the classical pathway) or by bacterial cell surfaces (the alternative pathway) to produce a membrane attack complex. This results in target cell death by membrane lysis, opsonization (and phagocytosis), removal of immune complexes and mediation of inflammation.

OSCE SCENARIO ANSWER 19.4

A 42-year-old male is having a blood transfusion following a major colorectal procedure; the nurse looking after him comes to tell you that the patient has just finished the first bag of blood but he has a temperature of 38°C and is very flushed and complaining of back and flank pain.

1. ***What is the possible diagnosis?***

The likely diagnosis given the symptoms and that he is receiving a blood transfusion is a significant reaction to the blood – given the early onset, it is likely a haemolytic transfusion reaction to preformed antibodies in the blood, i.e. ABO and Rhesus antibodies.

2. ***Explain how it occurs and what type of immune reaction it is.***

A blood transfusion reaction as acute as this would be due to a preformed antibody reacting with the transfused blood. It is a Type II hypersensitivity reaction in which antibodies are directed towards antigens on the surface of cells. There are three types of antibody-dependent mechanisms, which are complement mediated, antibody mediated cell mediated cytotoxicity (ADCC) and antibody mediated cellular dysfunction. In this case it is due to complement mediated cell destruction in which IgM and IgG antibodies attach to the antibodies on blood cells and lead to destruction by either the formation of the membrane attack complex (MAC) or increased risk of phagocytosis (complement or antibody binds to the cell – opsonisation – and triggers phagocytosis).

3. ***What is a Coombs test? Which will be the most relevant in this case?***

A Coombs test is used to look for antibodies that may cause a transfusion reaction. There is a direct and indirect test. In this case the direct test will be useful as a direct Coombs test uses antibodies to the human globulin fraction. It binds to antibodies attached to red cells and causes them to stick together (agglutinate). In a transfusion reaction, preformed antibodies will be attached to the transfused cells and thus the test will be positive. An indirect Coombs tests the serum of a patient for the presence of antibodies prior to giving a transfusion.

OSCE SCENARIO ANSWER 19.5

A 27-year-old female visits you in the transplant clinic; she is very upset regarding some unwanted facial hair growth, acne and excess growth of her gums. She had a cadaveric renal transplant 4 months ago and it has been functioning very well.

1. ***Which immunosuppressant drug has these side effects?***

The immunosuppressant drug with these side effects would be cyclosporine (ciclosporin) – hirsutism and ginigival hyperplasia are common side effects. Other common side effects are high blood pressure, numbness of fingers and toes, tremors and increased risk of infections. At high doses it is nephrotoxic, so dosing is controlled by measuring blood levels.

2. ***Explain how this drug works to prevent graft rejection.***

Hyperacute rejection is rare and should be avoided by correct cross-matching. Immunosuppressant drugs are mainly aimed at reducing episodes of acute rejection. T lymphocytes are key in mediating the cell mediated rejection. Following antigen presentation, intracellular signalling leads to the production of IL-2 (interleukin-2), this leads to cytotoxic T-cell proliferation. Cyclosporine is a calcineurin inhibitor. Calcineurin is an enzyme involved in the dephosphorylation of a nuclear protein which signals upregulation of IL-2. By blocking this pathway, rejection can be prevented/reduced due to the prevention of T cells proliferating.

3. ***Another patient attends who has had a working transplant for over 15 years. They are complaining of fevers, night sweats and palpable lumps in the right side of their neck. What is the likely diagnosis and how has the drug mentioned in question 1 led to this complication?***

This sounds like lymphoma – night sweats and fever are classic symptoms. In transplant patients immunosuppressant drugs can lead to a condition known as post-transplant lymphoproliferative disorder (PTLD). In immunocompetent patients B cells are controlled by immune-surveillance T cells. When T cells are reduced as with immunosuppressants like cyclosporine (ciclosporin), this allows abnormal B cells to proliferate and leads to lymphoma.

OSCE SCENARIO ANSWER 20.1

A 73-year-old female is seen in pre-assessment clinic as she is due to have a hip replacement in 4 weeks' time. Her bloods show a haemoglobin of 6.7 g/dL and an MCV of 69 fL with a normal clotting screen.

1. ***What type of anaemia is shown in the test results?***
Microcytic anaemia.
2. ***What are the common causes of this type of anaemia? Which is most likely in this case?***
   - The common causes of microcytic anaemia are:
     - iron deficiency: can be due to chronic blood loss, dietary insufficiency or malabsorption
     - thalassaemia
     - anaemia of chronic disease.
   - Iron deficiency anaemia is most likely and chronic blood loss needs to be ruled out.

You discuss the case with the operating surgeon, who asks you to take a full history and arrange any investigations required.

3. ***Ask the patient relevant questions about her health status, and explain what the next investigations you would suggest will involve. You should also introduce the possibility of her hip operation needing to be delayed.***

Questions
Important things to elicit would include:
- Recent feelings of tiredness, shortness of breath or chest pain.
- Change in bowel habit.
- Bleeding p.r. or dark stools.
- Vomiting and any presence of 'coffee ground' appearance.
- History of any GI malignancy or ulcers.
- History of any inflammatory bowel disease or coeliac disease.
- Weight loss, anorexia.
- Change in diet.
- Past medical history and drug history.
- Family history, particularly of GI pathology or bleeding disorders.

Investigations
- Repeat FBC and blood film.
- Serum iron and TIBC.
- Serum ferritin.

Possible further investigations
- Faecal occult blood sample.
- Colonoscopy.
- Gastroscopy.

OSCE SCENARIO ANSWER 20.2

You are fast-bleeped to a surgical ward by the nursing staff as a 68-year-old male patient has become pyrexial, short of breath and hypotensive. The staff nurse informs you that the patient is normally fit and well, on no medications, and had an uncomplicated hip replacement yesterday. This morning he was prescribed two units of blood as his haemoglobin was 6.9 g/dL and his transfusion was commenced about 5 min before the onset of these symptoms. The patient cannot answer your questions due to his dyspnoea.

1. ***What is your differential diagnosis?***
Major transfusion reaction due to:
   - haemolysis, e.g. ABO incompatibility
   - anaphylaxis
   - transfusion-related acute lung injury (TRALI)
   - allergic reaction to blood constituents/other source.

The nurse in charge shows you that the first name and date of birth on the detail label on the partially transfused bag of blood do not match those on the patient's wristband.

2. ***Outline your immediate actions.***
Immediately STOP THE TRANSFUSION and proceed in an ATLS fashion:
   - Give the patient 100% oxygen.
   - Commence rapid i.v. crystalloid fluids to maintain blood pressure and urine output.
   - As the patient may require inotropes to maintain blood pressure, ensure anaesthetic/intensivist colleagues are contacted.
   - Perform ABO and rhesus re-typing of the patient and send the discontinued transfusion bag of blood to blood bank intact.
   - Take blood for coagulation screen/U&Es/FBC and an arterial blood gas.
   - Test patient's urine for haemoglobinuria.
   - Request direct (anti-globulin) Coombs test.
   - Be aware of the possibility of renal failure and disseminated intravascular coagulation (DIC) and discuss with renal physician/haematologist.
   - Inform your consultant and the transfusion team regarding the situation and fill in a critical incident form.
   - With a senior member of the team, you should explain to the patient/family what has occurred and the next steps in management and investigation.

OSCE SCENARIO ANSWER 20.3

A 19-year-old female patient is admitted with a femoral fracture after a road traffic accident. When preparing her for theatre she tells you that she is a Jehovah's Witness and does not want blood under any circumstances, even if it would mean her death, and informs you she has a valid Advanced Decision recorded in her medical notes and wallet stating the same. You assess her as having full capacity, confirmed by a senior colleague.

1. ***If this patient required a life-saving transfusion during her operation, should you administer it? What is capacity?***
No. Administering blood to a patient who has the capacity to refuse it, even if it means they will die, can result in a criminal charge of assault. It is, however, worth establishing

with the patient whether they refuse all blood products (FFP, albumin, etc.) or only packed red cells. Patients' autonomy and religious beliefs must be respected, though doctors must assess the capacity of the patient making the decision.

Capacity is the ability to:

- Understand and retain relevant information.
- Use this information as part of the process to arrive at a decision.
- Communicate that decision by any means.

Capacity must be presumed until incapacity is established.

2. ***What if she was unconscious?***

No. An advance decision is made for this exact scenario. If the patient is brought in without capacity (e.g. unconscious), then a valid advanced decision should be respected.

3. ***What if she was 3 years old?***

If a child (under 16 years of age), who cannot give consent or is assessed as being too young to have capacity, has a life-threatening requirement for blood transfusion, then irrespective of parental wishes, the treating clinician can transfuse the child. This is performed by getting a special court order, which is available 24 hours a day. However, it must be stressed that every effort to avoid transfusion in these cases should be made.

4. ***What methods can be employed to reduce the need for transfusion?***
   - Pre-donation (in the non-urgent case) – blood taken from the patient at weekly intervals prior to elective surgery and that can be transfused back into the patient if required.
   - Normovolaemic dilution – collect blood immediately prior to surgery and replace with colloid. Thus any blood lost in surgery has fewer red cells and clotting factors in it and the patient's blood can be returned if required.
   - Intra-operative blood salvage – spilled blood is collected, processed, filtered and returned to the patient (aka 'cell saver').

OSCE SCENARIO ANSWER 20.4

A 38-year-old male has been involved in a high-speed motorbike accident. He has multiple injuries and has been in theatre for some time, having received 12 units of blood. He has returned to the ITU following surgery.

1. ***One of the nurses on ITU calls you an hour later and says that every time the blood pressure cuff goes up the hand of the patient spasms. What do you think this might be due to and what is the cause?***

This patient has had a massive blood transfusion – this is defined as transfusion of a patient's blood volume or greater in <24 h. The patient is demonstrating Trousseaus sign – a spasm of the hand on inflation of a blood pressure cuff. It is due to hypocalcaemia. This occurs due to binding of calcium by citrate. Citrate is used in transfused blood as an anticoagulant and normally it is broken down rapidly by the liver, but a massive transfusion may overwhelm this process, leading to hypocalcaemia.

2. ***While you are examining the patient you notice the ECG looks odd and the T waves are very high and peaked. What is the cause of this and what would be the urgent treatment?***

This sounds like hyperkalaemia – the peak T waves are a classic ECG finding. Transfused blood has high potassium content as stored blood has a low ATP content and thus potassium is not pumped back into cells. With a massive transfusion it can become dangerously high. If >7 mmol/L it is an emergency. Treatment involves a glucose and insulin infusion to push the potassium back into the cells. Typically calcium gluconate is also given at the same time to stabilize the heart.

3. ***Unfortunately, despite managing the above problems, after 3–4 h the patient starts to ooze from his nose, operative wounds and various different cannula sites. What could be the potential causes of this and how could you prevent it?***

Patients who have had a massive transfusion are at risk of coagulopathy of major trauma; in addition, patients who have suffered major trauma may have disseminated intravascular coagulation. In this patient you may have noticed that despite receiving 12 units of blood he has not had any clotting factors. Most hospitals will have a protocol for massive transfusions, for example transfusing a unit of FFP and platelets for every unit of blood transfused. Other reasons for a coagulopathy with massive transfusion include:

- Stored blood is low in platelets as they tend to clump together.
- Dilutional thrombocytopenia.
- Stored blood is cold and leads to hypothermia which causes platelet dysfunction.
- Hypotension leads to acidosis, which interferes with the clotting mechanism.
- Stored blood also loses clotting factors when stored – particularly factor V and VIII.

This could have been prevented by maintaining a good blood pressure, warming of blood and administering FFP and platelets along with the blood. The aim should be to maintain platelets >50,000 mm^3, PT <16 s and fibrinogen >100 mg/dL.

OSCE SCENARIO ANSWER 20.5

A 78-year-old male is seen in clinic for potential total hip replacement; he tells you he is on warfarin for a prosthetic heart valve – it is metallic.

1. ***Describe how you will manage this patient's warfarin prior to surgery.***

With elective surgery the best option is to stop the warfarin; after 3–5 days the INR should be below 2 and therapeutic low-molecular-weight heparin (LMWH) can be given instead. On the night before surgery a DVT prophylaxis dose can be given. Following the operation, full anticoagulation can be commenced when clinically safe to do so (i.e. risk of post-op bleeding). An alternative is using i.v. heparin; the anticoagulant effect will be gone after stopping the infusion after 60–90 min. The patient would need to be in hospital, however, receiving the infusion.

2. ***On the evening before the operation the INR has come back as 1.9; you tell your consultant who says it must be below 1.5 and asks if you will kindly sort this out. Describe what you can do to lower the INR and why it will work given the method of action of warfarin.***

The patient could be given vitamin K – a dose of 2 mg i.v. would likely be satisfactory but could be repeated. Warfarin acts as a vitamin K antagonist and interferes with the production by the liver of vitamin K dependent clotting factors II, VII, IX and X. It is important not to give too high a dose of vitamin K as you may find it difficult to re-warfarinize the patient post-op.

3. ***Imagine the patient has presented with an INR of 6 and has small bowel obstruction and needs urgent surgery; describe what options you have to reverse the action of warfarin.***

In an emergency it is not appropriate to wait for the INR to fall by omitting warfarin; vitamin K takes several hours to take effect and may need several doses. A patient can be given FFP, which is rich in all clotting factors, or a prothrombin concentrate complex can be used (e.g. Beriplex), which will reverse the effects of warfarin in under 30 min.

OSCE SCENARIO ANSWER 21.1

A 37-year-old male attends A&E, complaining bitterly of pain in his left groin. On examination the skin appears red and cellulitic. He is in severe pain when it is touched, and he has a tachycardia of 133 beats/min and a temperature of 38.8°C.

1. ***Given the above information, what broad differential diagnoses are you considering?***
   - Likely:
     - necrotizing fasciitis
     - cellulitis
     - infected femoral injection site +/− pseudo-aneurysm.
   - Less likely:
     - strangulated inguinal/femoral hernia.
2. ***What questions would you like to ask this patient to get a rapid idea of the diagnosis? Important points to elicit would include:***
   - history of trauma, particularly intravenous drug abuse
   - course of illness and spread of erythema
   - loss of sensation of skin over groin
   - systemic illness, e.g. anorexia, rigors
   - predisposing factors, e.g. diabetes, immunological compromise.
3. ***What investigations and management plan would you initiate?***

Investigations

- Blood tests: FBC/U&Es/LFT/CRP/ESR/blood cultures.
- Arterial blood gas.
- Wound swabs.
- If time permits, X-rays may show gas in tissues.

Management

- Surgical debridement is urgently needed as a life-saving measure.
- Prepare for theatre immediately.
- Resuscitate using i.v. fluids.
- Start high-dose i.v. antibiotics after discussion with a senior microbiologist regarding the antibiotic protocol in your hospital for suspected necrotizing infections.
- Contact senior anaesthetist and request help with lines/monitoring, etc.
- Send multiple tissue cultures for microbiology at time of surgery.

The patient rapidly becomes haemodynamically unstable and a diagnosis of septic shock due to severe soft tissue infection is assumed. He is taken to theatre where extensive debridement of infected and necrotic tissue is performed along the fascial planes of his leg.

4. ***What are the diagnosis and prognosis, and which organisms are commonly associated with this condition?***
   - Diagnosis: necrotizing fasciitis.
   - High mortality rate: 15–40% quoted for treated cases, and much higher if untreated.
   - Common organisms include clostridia, group A streptococci and anaerobes; but increasingly combinations of aerobes and anaerobes are possible, including MRSA.

OSCE SCENARIO ANSWER 21.2

A 68-year-old male patient develops acute retention of urine after repair of a right inguinal hernia. An indwelling urethral catheter was inserted and he has now developed a urinary tract infection. He was started on appropriate broad-spectrum antibiotics and is now systemically much better. He has asked to speak to one of the surgical team as he is upset about developing a hospital-acquired infection (HAI).

1. ***Answer the patient's questions about HAI.***

The tone of this conversation should be considerate to this man's feelings and to provide him with information about the condition in language he can understand. Important things to mention would include:

- The need for a catheter when a patient develops postoperative retention, to avoid renal failure.
- The risk of developing an infection at the time of catheter insertion (despite this risk being reduced by the use of aseptic technique) or from organisms that can travel up the catheter whilst it is indwelling.
- That you have sent off a sample of his urine to try to identify the particular bug causing the infection, so that the antibiotics can be tailored to this.
- Explain that you understand he is feeling upset, and that you regret he suffered a complication of the treatment.

He is satisfied with your explanation and feels much happier now; however, he is worried about the possibility of getting an MRSA infection whilst he is in hospital, as he has read so much about it in the newspapers.

2. ***Explain what MRSA is, the different sources of infection and methods of spread.***
   - MRSA is a type of bacteria that normally lives on people's skin, particularly around the nose, armpits and groin.
   - The reason that MRSA is different from the normal type of this bug is that it has developed resistance to the more common types of antibiotics used to treat it.
   - It can be a very serious infection, and MRSA infection risk is increased in the elderly, those who have been in hospital for a long time, or have been in and out of hospital a lot, and those who have been on lots of antibiotics and have wounds.
   - It is most commonly spread by touch.
3. ***Explain the methods employed in hospitals for prevention and control of HAI.***

The methods employed by hospitals to reduce HAI include:

- Staff and patient/visitor education and awareness, e.g. handwashing teaching, posters.
- Good sterile techniques before examinations or procedures.
- Sterilization and disinfection of equipment.
- Protective clothing and barrier nursing when treating those infected.
- Careful tracking of hospital/ward infection rates.

OSCE SCENARIO ANSWER 21.3

A 31-year-old male patient who admits to regular intravenous drug use is admitted with cellulitis of his right groin, which began 48 h after repeated attempts to inject his femoral vessels. He saw his GP and was started on oral antibiotics but tells you the redness is increasing, though he is systemically well. On examination, the area is warm, pink and swollen but there is no evidence of abscess.

1. ***Which two bacterial species are the most likely to be the cause of this patient's infection?***

Staphylococcus and Streptococcus.

Microbiology culture results of a wound swab taken by the patient's GP report that a resistant organism has been isolated.

2. ***Explain how organisms develop and spread resistance to antimicrobials.***

Resistance can be:

- Intrinsic (innate) – e.g. when the organism lacks the target site for the agent or is impermeable to the antibiotic.
- Acquired – resistance develops in organisms that were previously susceptible to the antibiotic by:
  - altering the target site of the antibiotic
  - altering antibiotic uptake (by changing cell permeability or actively pumping drug out of the cell)
  - antibiotic-inactivating enzymes, e.g. β-lactamase.

Resistance is spread by:

- Chromosomal mutations causing altered protein expression.
- Genes on transmissible plasmids.
- Transposons.

The antibiotics are changed, but as the erythema settles, the patient develops a fluctuant area in the skin, consistent with an abscess. The patient is prepped for theatre.

3. ***What considerations and precautions should be taken when operating on this patient?***

Special precautions should be taken when operating on a patient who is high risk for a blood-borne virus. These measures include:

- Informing personnel involved in patient care of the potential/actual risk.
- Arrangements for disposal of contaminated material.
- Minimizing theatre staff present to essential personnel only.
- Removal of all but essential equipment.
- Disposable drapes and gowns.
- Double-gloving and indicator gloves.
- Visors to prevent splash injuries.
- Blunt suture needles or staples.
- Use of kidney dishes to pass all instruments.

- Thorough post-operative cleansing of theatre.

In addition, an ultrasound scan of this man's groin would help to reassure the surgeon that the abscess did not communicate with a false aneurysm.

OSCE SCENARIO ANSWER 21.4

A 67-year-old male patient was admitted with perforated duodenal ulcer that necessitated laparotomy and repair. Postoperatively, he recovered on the high-dependency unit and was stepped down to the ward and deemed medically fit for discharge. He was commenced on H. pylori eradication therapy and was awaiting a social package. However, he developed severe diarrhoea a few days later along with abdominal pain and distension. He had T of 39.5°C, PR of 140/min, RR of 25/min and his blood tests showed WBC count of 35,000 × 10^6/dL. Abdominal X-ray showed very dilated colon.

1. ***What is the most likely diagnosis and responsible microorganism?***

The diagnosis is consistent with colitis due to *Clostridium difficile*, which is a gram-positive spore-forming anaerobic bacillus. It is present in the gut of 3% of healthy adults and remains the most common cause of hospital-acquired infectious diarrhoea. It can cause a spectrum of illnesses ranging from mild diarrhoea to life-threatening pseudomembranous colitis, paralytic ileus, peritonitis and death.

2. ***What are the predisposing risk factors for acquiring this infection in this context?***

Risk factors for *C. difficile* colonization/ infection include:

- Antibiotic use, especially broad-spectrum antibiotics.
- Acid-suppressing medication (especially proton pump inhibitors).
- Significant co-morbidity e.g. chronic renal failure, pre-existing bowel pathology, malignancy.
- Naso-gastric feeding.
- Alteration in gut motility, e.g. by laxatives.
- Age over 65.
- Recent healthcare intervention/stay in care facility.

The above patient had recent surgery and hospitalization, was commenced on broad-spectrum antibiotics and PPI and likely had postoperative NG feeding. Although the biggest risk factor for *C. difficile* is prior exposure to antibiotics, cases have been associated with no obvious antibiotic exposure. Almost all antibiotics have been implicated as they all cause disruption of commensal microbiota including paradoxically metronidazole and vancomycin, which are antibiotics used for treatment of *C. difficile*. However, the highest-risk antibiotics are broad-spectrum antibiotics such as penicillins, cephalosporins and clindamycin. Quinolones are high risk for the 027 strain of *C. difficile*, which is hyper virulent and hyper transmissible.

3. ***How do you confirm the diagnosis?***

This requires sending a stool sample immediately to test for *C. difficile*. If *C. difficile* toxin is detected; this means the patient has *C. difficile* and should be treated in the context of symptoms. The case would be also subject to mandatory reporting to the Department of Health.

Occasionally *C. difficile* toxin is not detected, but *C. difficile* toxin gene is detected. This indicates that the patient is likely colonized with *C. difficile*. They should be reviewed and assessed for treatment, but it does not trigger mandatory reporting to the Department of Health.

4. ***How do you manage this condition?***

Suspected infectious diarrhoea must be managed by applying the SIGHT mnemonic.

S Suspect that a case may be infective where there is no clear alternative cause for diarrhoea.

I Isolate the patient and consult with the infection prevention and control team while determining the cause of diarrhoea.

G Gloves and aprons must be used for all contacts with the patient and their environment.

H Hand washing with soap and water should be carried out before and after each contact with the patient and the patient's environment.

T Test the stool for *C. difficile* by sending a specimen immediately.

5. ***What are the precautions required to prevent this infection from occurring and spreading in hospitals?***

Ward staff must isolate symptomatic patients on first suspicion of *C. difficile* at the onset of symptoms in a single room, preferably with en suite toilet facilities. Isolation can be discontinued when the patient has been symptom-free for at least 72 h and has passed formed stool or stool is normal for the patient within that time. There is no requirement to submit further faeces samples for toxin detection, as toxin may be present in the gut for some time after the patient has become asymptomatic. All staff and visitors on entering an isolation room should put on disposable gloves and aprons. PPE must be removed, and hands washed with soap and water before leaving the isolation room. Alcohol-based hand sanitizers are not effective against *C. difficile*. Stool chart should be commenced and hospital's antibiotic policy for treating *C. difficile* should be consulted. Generally, this is based on the severity of symptoms and includes oral or i.v. metronidazole and oral vancomycin.

OSCE SCENARIO ANSWER 21.5

You attend the minor operation room to perform excision of skin lesions under local anaesthesia. Your consultant reminds you of using the pink disinfectant for skin preparation and performing the procedures under strict sterile measures using sterile instruments, gloves and gowns.

1. ***What disinfection agents are used on skin?***

There are several available skin disinfectants. The commonest are alcohol, chlorhexidine and povidine–iodine.

- Alcohol: effective against Gram-positive and Gram-negative organisms and has some antiviral activity; however, it is relatively inactive against spores and fungi. Avoid pooling as it is inflammable. It can also irritate sensitive areas.
- Chlorhexidine: non-toxic to skin and mucous membranes in aqueous solution (0.5%), while 4% solution is used as surgical scrub. It is more effective against Gram-positive, but has moderate activity against Gram-negative; hence, 0.5% concentration is frequently mixed with 70% alcohol for local antisepsis as it is more effective than aqueous preparations, but caution should be taken with diathermy to avoid fire.
- Povidine–iodine: broad spectrum against bacteria, spores, fungi, viruses (hepatitis B and HIV). In addition to skin disinfection, it is used for wound antisepsis, but can get inactivated by organic material such as pus, blood and faeces.

2. ***What is the difference between cleaning, disinfection, and sterilization?***
   - Cleaning is the process of physically removing contamination, but it does not inactivate microorganisms.
   - Disinfection is the process of reducing the number of viable microorganisms; however, bacterial spores and viruses may survive.
   - Sterilization is the process of complete eradication of all microorganisms including spores and viruses.
3. ***What are the four main methods of sterilization?***
   - Heat:
     - moist heat (autoclave): most used in hospitals: 121°C for 15 min or 134°C for 3 min
     - dry heat: higher heat; hence, not suitable for plastics and other material that cannot withstand such heat: 160°C for 2 h
   - Irradiation: for heat labile articles, such as lines, catheters, syringes.
   - Filtration: used to sterilize drugs for injection.
   - Chemicals:
     - ethylene oxide: used for electrical equipment, sutures
     - glutaraldehyde: used for endoscopes, needs 3 h to kill all microbes
     - formaldehyde: for heat labile instruments.

OSCE SCENARIO ANSWER 22.1

A 28-year-old right-handed female attends A&E with a wound on the radial and volar border of her right index finger, just proximal to the PIPJ. She explains that she cut it last night with a knife whilst washing dishes, and complains of radial numbness distal to the wound.

1. ***Outline how you would examine the patient's finger to establish what structures have been injured other than the digital nerve.***
   - Need to elicit numbness distal to the wound with loss of light touch sensation.
   - Establish that the finger is well vascularized by testing capillary refill.
   - Examine the tendons of the finger to ensure that extensor digitorum communis (EDC), flexor digitorum superficialis (FDS), and flexor digitorum profundus (FDP) are intact.
2. ***Explain to the examiners what would happen pathologically and clinically if the nerve injury was left untreated.***

Histopathologically

- Wallerian degeneration would occur: degeneration of the axons and myelin distal to the wound.
- Regeneration would start to occur 3–4 days post-injury and the axons would grow at 1–2 mm/day.
- Schwann cells would perform remyelination.
- However, if the perineurium has been disrupted, then the regeneration may not be successful.

Clinically

- Permanent loss of sensation is likely if the nerve has been transected.
- A painful neuroma may form.

3. ***Explain your management plan to the patient and answer any questions she may have.***
   - It is likely that the nerve has been cut, and to ensure that no neuroma occurs and to have the best chance of sensation returning, surgical repair is advised.
   - If we repair it, there is a chance that the sensation will return, but this is not always the case and is often not exactly the same as before the injury.
   - Nerves grow very slowly, so there will be a long wait to see how much recovery the nerve will get.
   - The most important reason for repairing the nerve is to try to avoid a neuroma, which is uncontrolled re-growth of the nerve endings that can be painful and irritating.
   - The side of the index finger you have injured is one that you use to grasp objects (e.g. pens) against your

thumb, so we consider this even more important to try to keep your hand functioning well.

OSCE SCENARIO ANSWER 22.2

A 19-year-old male attends your outpatient clinic with a 3-month history of right knee pain and swelling. The pain and swelling are worsening, waking him at night, and he now walks with a limp. He denies any traumatic injury, is otherwise fit and well, and on no medications. An X-ray arranged by his GP whilst waiting for his referral is shown below (Fig. 22.2Q).

1. ***Describe the pathological signs on the X-ray** (Fig. 22.2A).*
    - Bone destruction.
    - Soft tissue invasion.
    - Growth of bone outside of the cortex and elevating periosteum.
    - Deposition of periosteal bone (Codman's triangle) – single arrow.
    - Spicules of radiating bone ('sunray' spicules) –double arrow.
2. ***What is the likely diagnosis, given the history and the X-ray?***

Osteosarcoma (osteogenic sarcoma) of the lower femur.

3. ***What other investigations could you arrange?***
    - Alkaline phosphatase.
    - ESR.
    - CT.

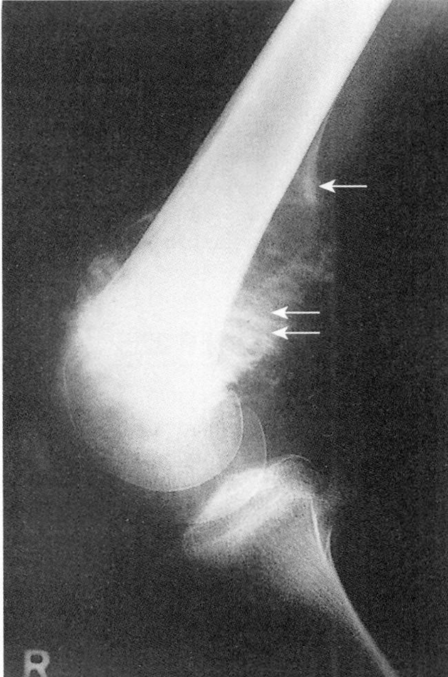

Fig. 22.2A X-ray of the patient's right knee.

    - MRI.
    - CXR/CT chest.
    - Bone biopsy.
4. ***What are the management options?***

Medical

- Neo-adjuvant chemotherapy to shrink the tumour and/or lung metastases.
- Post-operative chemotherapy.

Surgical

- Wide local excision with chemotherapy.
- Amputation.
- Resection of pulmonary metastases if appropriate.

OSCE SCENARIO ANSWER 22.3

A 45-year-old female has presented in A&E after falling down some steps. She is alert and her pulse and blood pressure are normal, though her oxygen saturations are only 80% on high-flow oxygen. She is complaining bitterly of pain down her right chest wall, though only grazes are present.

1. ***How will you approach the assessment of this patient?***

Using ATLS principles:

- Airway with C-spine control
- Breathing
- Circulation.

2. ***Her chest X-ray is shown below** (Fig. 22.3Q). **What is the condition shown? What is the likely cause?***
    - A right-sided closed pneumothorax (Fig. 22.3A).
    - Though rib fractures cannot be seen, it is possible that this is the cause, given the history.
3. ***How would you treat this condition?***
    - If oxygenation is severely compromised, needle decompression of the pneumothorax in the 2nd intercostal space in the midclavicular line is appropriate.
    - Definitive treatment is with insertion of a chest drain connected to an underwater seal.
4. ***Explain to the examiners the classification of causes and types of this condition, and how you would have treated the patient if she had presented with tracheal deviation and haemodynamic instability.***

Types of pneumothorax

- Open.
- Closed.
- Tension.

Causes

- Spontaneous (primary and secondary).
- Traumatic (open and closed).
- Iatrogenic.

Treatment

- If the patient had presented with tracheal deviation and haemodynamic instability with clinical signs of a pneumothorax, you would suspect a tension pneumothorax.

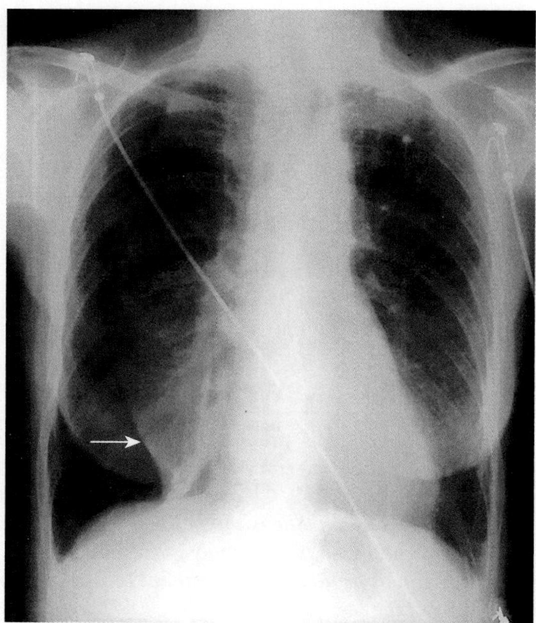

Fig. 22.3A The patient's chest X-ray. A pneumothorax is visible on the right side. The lung edge is visible (arrow).

- As this is a life-threatening condition which can rapidly cause death, a swift needle decompression WITHOUT waiting for a chest X-ray would be the appropriate management.

OSCE SCENARIO ANSWER 22.4

A 14-year-old boy attends your clinic with his mother, who is concerned that her son seems to be developing breasts. The boy is overweight, with a BMI of 29, but both he and his mother state that he has lost weight recently and his breasts are still enlarging. His examination reveals enlarged nipples with small firm breast bud development.

1. ***What is the likely diagnosis? What questions would you like to ask to confirm this?***
   - Pubertal physiological gynaecomastia.

   Relevant points to elicit would include:
   - A full drug history to exclude drug-induced gynaecomastia; note that the patient's mother is in the room and therefore answers regarding cannabis and anabolic steroid use may have to be asked at a confidential time, e.g. during examination.
   - Anything to suggest hypogonadism, i.e. undescended testes, lack of body hair, bilateral torsion, Kleinfelter's syndrome.
   - Any testicular swellings (testicular tumour).
   - Any visual disturbance/lactation (pituitary cause).
   - Anything to suggest male breast carcinoma (nipple discharge or retraction, hard lump, lymphadenopathy).
   - Family history of gynaecomastia or hypogonadism.
2. ***Explain the diagnosis and its causes in layman's terms, and outline the options for investigation and management.***

Important to perform this very sensitively as the patient is likely to be embarrassed and confused. Points to raise would include:

- All men have some breast tissue, and in some men this tissue can grow – we call this gynaecomastia and it can happen to babies, teenagers or older men and it's actually not that rare.
- This is different to just being 'overweight' as it is breast tissue and not just fat causing the swelling, though weight loss may help.
- This can happen at puberty because of hormonal imbalances, but often we don't really know why it happens.
- Sometimes there are specific causes such as certain drugs, which can reduce your male hormones or increase female hormones, or medical conditions.
- If we aren't sure of the cause then certain blood tests, X-rays and even taking a tissue sample can help, though often we don't need to do this if we think the cause is puberty.
- General options for treatment include:
  - removing the cause (i.e. stop any medications causing it)
  - nothing – 90% of physiological gynaecomastia goes away by itself, though it can take a few weeks or a couple of years
  - medication to reduce oestrogen or increase testosterone
  - surgery to remove the breast tissue – but this will leave scarring.

OSCE SCENARIO ANSWER 22.5

A 62-year-old male attends A&E with acute onset of severe abdominal pain radiating to the back. He is pale and sweaty with a tense, distended, tender abdomen. A CT of his abdomen is shown below (Fig. 22.5Q).

1. ***What pathology is shown?***

A leaking abdominal aortic aneurysm (Fig. 22.5A).

The patient is still in the radiology department and his blood pressure is stable at 90 mmHg systolic.

2. ***Outline the immediate management of this patient.***
   - Immediate surgery is needed to try to save this man's life.

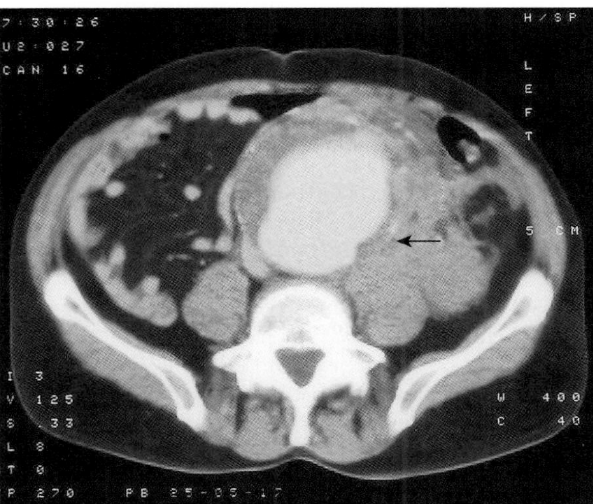

Fig. 22.5A CT scan of the patient's abdomen. There is a large leaking abdominal aortic aneurysm (arrow).

- Explain the diagnosis to the patient and the urgent need for surgery.
- Arrange for immediate transfer to theatre.
- Alert the senior anaesthetist on call, the on-call theatre team and the senior surgeon.
- Ensure that the patient has had FBC/U&Es/LFT/clotting screen taken and is cross-matched for 10 units of blood.
- Ensure the patient's family is kept informed.

3. ***What risk factors exist for this condition?***
    - Smoking.
    - Hypertension.
    - Male sex.
    - Family history.
4. ***What is the operative mortality risk for this condition?***

30–50%.

5. ***Explain to the examiners the different types of this condition, their classification and their aetiology.***
    - Can be classified in the following ways:
        - true: where the wall of the aneurysm contains all three elements of intima, media and adventitia (can be subdivided by shape into fusiform and saccular)
        - false: pulsating haematoma with a cavity in continuity with the lumen.
    - Or as:
        - congenital: 'berry' aneurysms around the circle of Willis
        - acquired: aneurysms which develop in life for various reasons (listed below).
    - Or by cause:
        - atheromatous
        - mycotic
        - syphilitic
        - dissecting
        - arteriovenous aneurysms (aneurysmal varices associated with A/V fistulae).

OSCE SCENARIO ANSWER 22.6

A 37-year-old female attends your clinic having been referred by her GP with excessive sweating, diarrhoea and neck swelling.

1. ***Ask this patient about her symptoms and give the examiners your differential diagnosis.***
    - Elicit goitre features:
        - How long present for? Is it enlarging?
        - Painful?
        - Problems swallowing?
        - Problems breathing in?
        - Change in voice?
        - Enlarging?
    - Elicit features of hyperthyroidism:
        - excessive sweating/heat intolerance
        - weight loss; check not intentional, i.e. not dieting
        - anxiety/irritability
        - palpitations/tremor
        - insomnia
        - diarrhoea
        - menorrhagia.
    - Differential diagnosis is thyrotoxicosis, secondary to:
        - a toxic goitre (single/multinodular)
        - Graves' disease
        - functioning adenoma.
2. ***What physical signs may you expect to see on examination?***
    - Clubbing.
    - Wet palms/excessive sweating.
    - Tachycardia/irregular heart rate/AF.
    - Eye signs (exophthalmos/lid lag).
    - Tremor.
    - Pretibial myxoedema/hyper-reflexia.
    - Proximal myopathy.
3. ***What investigations might you arrange?***
    - FBC/ESR/TFTs.
    - USS (ultrasound scan) of goitre.
    - Radioisotope scan of goitre.
    - FNA of goitre.

The results of your investigations suggest a benign toxic goitre with a dominant nodule.

4. ***What treatment options are available?***
   - Medical treatment for symptoms (e.g. beta-blockers).
   - Medical treatment to block thyroid hormone production (e.g. carbimazole).
   - Radioactive iodine treatment.
   - Surgical removal (e.g. total/subtotal thyroidectomy – will need thyroxine treatment afterwards).
5. ***If the patient opts for surgery, which nerves are at risk of intra-operative damage?***
   - Recurrent laryngeal nerve (related to the inferior thyroid artery).
   - External branch of the superior laryngeal nerve (related to the superior thyroid artery).

OSCE SCENARIO ANSWER 22.7

The blood results displayed below are those taken from a 49-year-old male ex-alcoholic, feeling generally unwell with vague abdominal pain, whose GP has referred him to your clinic.

Bilirubin 57 µmol/L
Albumin 22 g/L
Total protein 64 g/L
Alkaline phosphatase (ALP) 152 IU/L
Alanine aminotransferase (ALT) 188 IU/L
Aspartate aminotransferase (AST) 220 IU/L
Gamma glutamyltransferase (GGT) 129 IU/L

1. ***What biochemical abnormalities are shown?***
   - Raised levels of bilirubin, AST/ALT/GGT, and to a lesser extent ALP.
   - Reduced levels of albumin.
2. ***Explain to the examiners the different types of jaundice and give examples of the causes of each type.***

Pre-hepatic jaundice

This is due to intravascular haemolysis and some causes include:

- Congenital defects, e.g. Gilbert's disease.
- Congenital red cell defects, e.g. sickle cell, hereditary spherocytosis.
- Acquired red cell defects, e.g. malaria, autoimmune disease, hypersplenism.

Hepatic jaundice

This is due to intrinsic liver pathology and some causes include:

- Acute hepatocellular disease due to:
  - infections, e.g. hepatitis, CMV, leptospirosis
  - drugs, e.g. paracetamol, anaesthetics
  - autoimmune disease.
- Chronic hepatocellular disease due to:
  - infections, e.g. chronic viral hepatitis
  - chronic autoimmune disease
  - end-stage liver disease, e.g. alcohol, cirrhosis, Wilson's disease.

Post-hepatic/cholestatic jaundice

This is due to either intrahepatic cholestasis or post-hepatic biliary obstruction and some causes include:

- Intrahepatic causes due to:
  - pregnancy
  - drugs/nutrition, e.g. chlorpromazine; TPN
  - primary biliary cirrhosis.
- Extrahepatic causes due to obstruction in:
  - lumen, e.g. gallstones or parasite infestation (schistosomiasis)
  - wall, e.g. strictures, cholangitis, cholangiocarcinoma
  - outside of wall, e.g. tumour in head of pancreas, nodes in porta hepatis, chronic pancreatitis.

3. ***Which type is this patient's likely to be from the blood results?***

Blood results suggest a chronic hepatocellular form of jaundice, possibly due to alcoholic cirrhosis. Chronic element is suggested due to low levels of albumin.

4. ***Closer questioning reveals that the patient has developed abnormal stools which are pale, float, and are difficult to flush away. What other condition is the patient likely to have developed?***

Chronic pancreatitis due to chronic alcoholism.

OSCE SCENARIO ANSWER 22.8

An 82-year-old male is brought into the emergency department with an acutely painful right leg. The symptoms include the leg feeling cold, looking very pale and pins and needles. The patient's ECG is shown below (Fig. 22.8Q).

GET AN AF ECG

1. ***What is the likely diagnosis?***

The likely diagnosis given the symptoms and ECG findings are an acute arterial embolism leading to acute ischaemia of the right leg. The ECG shows the classic signs of Atrial Fibrillation (AF) - irregularly irregular pulse and lack of P waves.

2. ***What are the causes?***

Causes of acute ischaemia can be divided broadly into luminal and extra-luminal causes.

- Luminal causes include embolism, thrombosis (including clotting disorders), arterial dissection.
- Extra-luminal causes include trauma, external compression, popliteal entrapment, and cystic adventitial disease (the last two rarely present acutely).

3. ***What other symptoms can occur and which are the most clinically important?***

The classic symptoms of an acutely ischaemic limb are the 6 P's: Pain, Pulseless, Perishingly cold, Paralysis, Paraesthesia, and Pallor. The most clinically important of these are the degree of paraesthesia and paralysis; nerves are very sensitive to ischaemia. It is very common to have mild pins and needles or a mild difference in sensation; paralysis is often absent in the early stages. However, as ischaemia persists, a limb which is paralysed and insensate may not be salvageable. The 6 P's does not draw attention to the importance of pain on muscle squeezing; a patient with pain on compression of the gastrocnemius or anterior compartment has severe limb ischaemia and is at high risk of compartment syndrome.

4. ***What investigations would you perform?***

Bit of a trick question this one – it may be none. In a patient in AF with no previous vascular surgery/interventions and normal pulses on the opposite side and severe symptoms, the patient may be taken to theatre for an urgent embolectomy. If, however, the diagnosis is not so clear cut then a CT angiogram or duplex ultrasound will give the required information.

5. ***Are you aware of any classification systems for this condition?***

The most widely used classification system is by Rutherford; it divides the severity into viable, threatened and irreversible on the grounds of capillary return, degree of paralysis and sensory loss and whether there are audible arterial and venous Doppler signals.

6. ***If the patient had a paralysed and insensate leg with a purple discolouration which did not blanch under pressure, what would be the likely management plan?***

This sadly sounds like a Rutherford stage 3 ischaemia; the leg is irreversibly ischaemic; the classic sign is the deep purple discolouration of the leg does not blanch after digital pressure. The only treatment is primary amputation or in patients where this would be inappropriate then palliation.

OSCE SCENARIO ANSWER 22.9

A 56-year-old male is admitted with severe dehydration and vomiting, his urea and creatinine are raised at 15 mmol/L and 215 μmol/L. A blood gas shows the following abnormalities: pH 7.55, PO_2 10.9 kPa, CO_2 6.9 kPa and HCO_3 is 21.

1. ***What type of metabolic abnormality is this patient displaying?***

The patient has a metabolic alkalosis – this is indicated by the pH showing alkalosis. The fact that is it metabolic in nature is indicated by the raised CO_2 (compensatory hypoventilation) and the low HCO_3 (compensatory loss by the kidneys). The fact that the HCO_3 is low would suggest the cause of the alkalosis is loss of H ions rather than excess HCO_3.

2. ***How has it occurred?***

Vomiting results in a loss of H ions and thus a metabolic alkalosis.

3. ***The patient has a 'succussion splash' on examination – what is the diagnosis?***

A 'succussion splash' is a characteristic finding in gastric outlet obstruction which leads to severe vomiting. It is an examination finding where you literally shake the patient's abdomen from side to side and can hear the fluid in the stomach moving.

4. ***How would you manage this condition?***

The management of this condition would fall into –

- Resuscitation and correction of electrolyte abnormalities.
- Investigation as to the cause – OGD and or CT scan.
- Management of the cause – the commonest causes are peptic ulcer disease or malignancy. If due to malignancy then surgical resection of the tumour or palliative gastro-jejunostomy would be appropriate. If due to peptic ulcer disease then initial medical management with i.v. PPI is appropriate for 48–72 h. If there is no improvement then surgical resection may be deemed appropriate.

OSCE SCENARIO ANSWER 22.11

A 62-year-old male is in the A&E department and is complaining of epigastric pain. This feels like his normal heartburn but has not been relieved by antacids. In addition he is sweating and has a bradycardia. An ECG is performed and shows raised ST segments.

1. ***From the history, what type of myocardial infarction is the patient having and in what leads would you expect to see the ST segment rises?***

The symptoms are suggestive of an inferior MI – this is an often overlooked differential diagnosis for acute epigastric pain and explains why an ECG is essential in patients presenting with upper abdominal pain. Classically the leads showing raised ST segment changes are leads II, III and aVF.

2. ***Which coronary artery is involved?***

The right coronary artery supplies the territory involved in an inferior MI. Occlusion of the left anterior descending artery (LAD) leads to an anterior and or septal MI. Occlusion of the circumflex branch of the left coronary artery leads to a lateral MI. Occlusion of the right coronary artery leads to an inferior MI (as mentioned) and also may lead to a right ventricle and atrial infarction. Occlusion of the circumflex branch of the right coronary artery can occasionally cause an inferior MI but more usually a posterior MI.

3. ***Why is it common to see a bradycardia?***

In approximately 60% of the population the SA node is supplied by the right coronary artery and thus infarctions involving this territory may present with bradycardia and conduction problems.

INDEX

Page numbers followed by "*f*" indicate figures, "*t*"indicate tables, and "*b*" indicate boxes.

A

B

C

F

G

H

M

P

T

W

X

Y

Z